Yearbook of Intensive Care and Emergency Medicine 1998

Edited by J.-L. Vincent

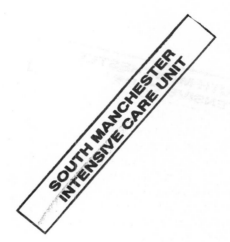

Springer

Berlin
Heidelberg
New York
Barcelona
Budapest
Hong Kong
London
Milan
Paris
Santa Clara
Singapore
Tokyo

Yearbook of Intensive Care and Emergency Medicine 1998

Edited by J.-L. Vincent

With 156 Figures and 92 Tables

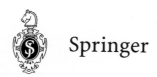

Springer

Prof. Jean-Louis Vincent
Clinical Director, Department of Intensive Care
Erasme Hospital, Free University of Brussels
Route de Lennik 808, B-1070 Brussels, Belgium

ISBN 3-540-63798-2 Springer-Verlag Berlin Heidelberg New York

ISSN 0942-5381

Production: PRO EDIT, Heidelberg
Typesetting and printing: Zechnersche Buchdruckerei, Speyer
Bookbinding: J. Schäffer, Grünstadt

SPIN: 10629822   19/3133-5 4 3 2 1 0 – Printed on acid-free paper

Contents

Host Responses in Sepsis and ARDS

Cardiocirculatory Alterations

Oxygen Carriers

Epidemiology and Markers of Sepsis – Clinical Trials

Severe Infections

Measuring Lung Mechanics

Modes of Mechanical Ventilation

Lung Stretching and Barotrauma

Weaning from Mechanical Ventilation

Non-Invasive Mechanical Ventilation

The Gut

Head Trauma

Surgery and Obstetrics

ICU Performance – Evaluation

List of Contributors

Adrie C
Dept of Intensive Care,
Cochin Hospital,
27 rue du Faubourg Saint Jacques,
75014 Paris, France

Alia I
Dept of Intensive Care,
University Hospital,
Carretera de Toledo Km 12,500,
28905 Getafe, Madrid, Spain

Aliverti A
Dept of Anesthesiology and Intensive
Care, Ospedale Maggiore di Milano,
35 Via Francesco Sforza,
20122 Milan, Italy

Allen SJ
Dept of Anesthesiology,
The University of Texas,
Houston TX 77030, USA

Angus DC
Dept of Critical Care Medicine,
Room 606B Scaife Hall,
University of Pittsburgh,
200 Lothrop Street,
Pittsburgh PA 15213, USA

Anning PB
Dept of Critical Care, Imperial College
of Science, Technology and Medicine
at the National Heart and Lung
Institute, Dovehouse Street,
London SW3 6LY, United Kingdom

Appendini L
Dept of Pulmonary Diseases,
"Clinica del Lavoro",
Foundation IRCCS,
Medical Center of Rehabilitation,
13, Via per Revislate,
28010 Veruno NO, Italy

Arnaud S
Dept of Anesthesiology,
Critical Care and Trauma Center,
North Hospital,
Chemin des Bourrellys,
13915 Marseille Cedex 20, France

Aslanian P
Dept of Intensive Care,
University Hospital, Pavillon St Luc,
1058 St Denis, Montreal,
Quebec H2X 3J4, Canada

Balligand JL
Dept of Medicine, Pharmacology Unit,
FATH 53.49, University of Louvain
Medical School,
Tour Pasteur +2, 53 Avenue E.
Mounier, 1200 Brussels, Belgium

Bennett ED
Dept of Intensive Care,
St George's Hospital,
Blackshaw Road, Tooting,
London SW17 0QT, United Kingdom

Bihari D
Dept of Intensive Care,
The St George Hospital,
Gray Street, Kogarah NSW 2217,
Australia

Böhm SH
Dept of Anesthesiology,
Erasmus University,
PO Box 1738, 3000 RD Rotterdam,
The Netherlands

Boldt J
Dept of Anesthesiology
and Intensive Care Medicine,
Klinikum der Stadt Ludwigshafen,
Bremserstrasse 79,
67063 Ludwigshafen, Germany

Braga M
Dept of Surgery,
IRCCS San Raffaele Hospital,
60 Via Olgettina, 20132, Milan, Italy

Burchardi H
Dept of Anesthesiology,
University Hospital,
PO Box 3742,
37070 Göttingen, Germany

Carroll SF
Preclinical Research,
Xoma Corporation,
2910 Seventh Street, Berkeley CA
94710, USA

Cassiere HA
Dept of Thoracic
and Cardiovascular Surgery,
Winthrop University Hospital,
259 First Street, Mineola, NY 11501,
USA

Chee HL
Dept of Intensive Care,
The St George Hospital,
Gray Street, Kogarah NSW 2217,
Australia

Chiche J-D
Dept of Anesthesiology
and Critical Care Medicine,
Massachusetts General Hospital,
32 Fruit Street,
Boston MA 02114, USA

Clark RSB
Dept of Anesthesiology and Critical
Care Medicine, Safar Center
for Resuscitation Research,
University of Pittsburgh,
3434 Fifth Avenue,
Pittsburgh PA 15260, USA

Coakley J
Dept of Intensive Care,
Homerton Hospital,
Homerton Row, London E9 6SR,
United Kingdom

Cohen J
Dept of Infectious Diseases, Royal
Postgraduate Medical School,
Hammersmith Hospital,
Du Cane Road, London W12 0NN,
United Kingdom

Cook DJ
Dept of Epidemiology and Medicine,
St Joseph's Hospital,
50 Charlton Avenue East,
Hamilton ON L8N 4A6, Canada

Darouiche RO
Dept of Infectious Diseases
(Rm 4B-370), Veterans Affairs
Medical Center,
2002 Holcombe Boulevard,
Houston TX 77030, USA

De Backer D
Dept of Intensive Care,
Erasme University Hospital,
808 Route de Lennik,
1070 Brussels, Belgium

Deby C
Center for the Biochemistry
of Oxygen, Institut de Chimie,
Domaine Universitaire
du Sart Tilman, B6a,
4000 Liège, Belgium

Deby-Dupont G
Dept of Anesthesiology and
Intensive Care, University Hospital,
Domaine Universitaire
du Sart Tilman, B35,
4000 Liège, Belgium

Delclaux C
Dept of Intensive Care,
Henri Mondor Hospital,
51 Avenue du Maréchal de Lattre de
Tassigny, 94010 Créteil, France

Dellaca R
Dept of Anesthesiology and
Intensive Care, Ospedale Maggiore
di Milano, 35 Via Francesco Sforza,
20122 Milan, Italy

Dinh-Xuan AT
Laboratory of Respiratory Physiology,
Cochin Hospital,
27 rue du Faubourg Saint Jacques,
75014 Paris, France

Donner CF
Dept of Pulmonary Diseases,
"Clinica del Lavoro",
Foundation IRCCS, Medical Center
of Rehabilitation, 13 Via per Revislate,
28010 Veruno NO, Italy

d'Ortho MP
Dept of Physiology,
Henri Mondor Hospital,
51 Avenue du Maréchal de Lattre de
Tassigny, 94010 Créteil, France

Eddleston J
Dept of Anesthesiology
and Intensive Care,
Manchester Royal Infirmary,
Oxford Road, Manchester M13 9WL,
United Kingdom

Eichelbroenner O
London Health Sciences Center,
University of Western Ontario,
Victoria Hospital, Room 16A,
Health Services Building,
375 South Street,
London ON N6A 4G5, Canada

Eggimann P
Dept of Internal Medicine,
University Hospital,
24 rue Micheli-du-Crest,
1211 Geneva 14, Switzerland

Ellis CG
London Health Sciences Center,
University of Western Ontario,
Victoria Hospital, Room 16A,
Health Services Building,
375 South Street,
London ON N6A 4G5, Canada

Esteban A
Dept of Intensive Care,
University Hospital,
Carretera de Toledo Km 12,500,
28905 Getafe, Madrid, Spain

Evans DC
Dept of Surgery, McGill University,
Montreal General Hospital,
Montreal, Canada

Evans TW
Dept of Critical Care,
Royal Brompton Hospital,
Sydney Street, London SW3 6NP,
United Kingdom

Feihl F
Institute of Pathophysiology,
University Hospital,
BH-19, 1011 Lausanne,
Switzerland

Frass M
Dept of Internal Medicine and
Intensive Care, University Hospital,
18-20 Währinger Gürtel,
1090 Vienna, Austria

Georgopoulos D
Dept of Intensive Care, University of
Crete, School of Medicine,
PO Box 1352, Heraklion 71110 Crete,
Greece

Gianotti L
Dept of Surgery, IRCCS San Raffaele
Hospital, 60 Via Olgettina,
20132 Milan, Italy

Girbes ARJ
Dept of Surgery, University Hospital,
PO Box 30.001, 9700 RB Groningen,
The Netherlands

Giroir BP
Dept of Pediatric Critical Care
Medicine, UT Southwestern
Medical Center,
5323 Harry Hines Boulevard,
Dallas TX 75235-9063, USA

Gordo F
Dept of Intensive Care,
University Hospital,
Carretera de Toledo Km 12,500,
28905 Getafe, Madrid, Spain

Görlach A
Institute for Physiology,
University of Zurich-Irchel,
190 Winterthurstrasse,
8057 Zurich, Switzerland

Groeneveld ABJ
Dept of Intensive Care,
Free University Hospital,
1117 De Boelelaan,
1081 HV Amsterdam,
The Netherlands

Groth M
Dept of Critical Care, Winthrop
University Hospital, 259 First Street,
Mineola, NY 11501, USA

Hébert PC
Dept of Medicine, Ottawa General
Hospital, 501 Smyth Road,
LM11, Ottawa ON K1H 8L6, Canada

Hillman K
Dept of Critical Care,
Liverpool Hospital,
Liverpool NSW 2170, Australia

Hoogenberg K
Dept of Internal Medicine,
University Hospital,
PO Box 30.001, 9700 RB Groningen,
The Netherlands

Ilkka L
Dept of Intensive Care,
Kuopio University Hospital,
70210 Kuopio, Finland

Ince C
Dept of Anesthesiology,
Academic Medical Center,
University of Amsterdam,
9 Meibergdreef, 1105 AZ Amsterdam,
The Netherlands

Kacmarek RM
Dept of Anesthesiology,
Massachusetts General Hospital,
55 Fruit Street, Ellison 401,
Boston Ma 02114-2696, USA

Karzai W
Dept of Anesthesiology,
Friedrich Schiller University,
Bachstrasse 18, 07740 Jena,
Germany

Keays R
Dept of Anesthesiology
and Intensive Care, Chelsea
and Westminster Hospital,
369 Fulham Road, London SW10 9NH,
United Kingdom

Kellum JA
Dept of Critical Care Medicine,
University of Pittsburgh Medical
Center, 200 Lothrop Street,
Pittsburgh PA 15213-28582, USA

Kleen M
Institute for Surgical Research
and Institute of Anesthesiology,
Ludwig Maximilian University,
Klinikum Grosshadern,
Marchioninistrasse 15,
81366 Munich, Germany

Kochanek PM
Dept of Anesthesiology
and Critical Care Medicine,
Safar Center for Resuscitation
Research, University of Pittsburgh,
3434 Fifth Avenue,
Pittsburgh PA 15260, USA

Kofler J
Dept of Internal Medicine and
Intensive Care, University Hospital,
18–20 Währinger Gürtel,
1090 Vienna, Austria

Kollef MH
Dept of Pulmonary and Critical Care,
Washington University School
of Medicine,
Box 8052, 660 South Euclid Avenue,
St Louis MO 63110, USA

Kumle B
Dept of Anesthesiology
and Intensive Care Medicine,
Klinikum der Stadt Ludwigshafen,
Bremserstrasse 79,
67063 Ludwigshafen, Germany

Lachmann B
Dept of Anesthesiology,
Erasmus University,
PO Box 1738, 3000 RD Rotterdam,
The Netherlands

Lamy M
Dept of Anesthesiology and
Intensive Care, University Hospital,
Domaine Universitaire
du Sart Tilman, B35, 4000 Liège,
Belgium

Leclerc J
Dept of Anesthesiology and Intensive
Care, University Hospital of Lille,
Place de Verdun, 59037 Lille Cedex,
France

Leverve XM
Laboratoire de Bioénergétique
Fondamentale et Appliquée,
Université J Fourier,
38041 Grenoble, France

Liaudet L
Dept of Internal Medicine (Service B),
University Hospital,
BH-19, 1011 Lausanne, Switzerland

Mancebo J
Dept of Intensive Care,
Hospital de Sant Pau,
167 Avenida S.A.M. Claret,
08025 Barcelona, Spain

Marshall JC
Dept of Surgery and Critical Care
Medicine Programme,
Eaton North 9-234, Toronto General
Hospital, 200 Elizabeth Street,
Toronto ON M5G 2C4, Canada

Martin C
Dept of Anesthesiology
and Critical Care and Trauma Center,
North Hospital,
Chemin des Bourrellys,
13915 Marseille Cedex 20, France

Meduri GU
Dept of Pulmonary
and Critical Care Medicine,
The University of Tennessee,
956 Court Avenue, Room H314,
Memphis TN 38163, USA

Meier-Hellmann A
Dept of Anesthesiology,
Friedrich Schiller University,
Bachstrasse 18, 07740 Jena, Germany

Mentges D
Dept of Anesthesiology
and Intensive Care Medicine,
Klinikum der Stadt Ludwigshafen,
Bremserstrasse 79,
67063 Ludwigshafen, Germany

Messmer K
Institute for Surgical Research,
Ludwig Maximilians University,
Klinikum Grosshadern,
Marchioninistrasse 15, 81366 Munich,
Germany

Moreno R
Dept of Intensive Care,
Hospital de St Antonio dos Capuchos,
Alameda de St Antonio dos Capuchos,
1150 Lisboa, Portugal

Morley P
Dept of Intensive Care,
Royal Melbourne Hospital,
Grattan Street, 3430 Parkville,
Victoria, Australia

Mustafa I
Dept of Surgical Intensive Care,
Cardiac Medical Center,
Jakarta, Indonesia

Nevière RR
Dept of Intensive Care,
Calmette University Hospital of Lille,
Boulevard Pr. Leclercq,
59037 Lille Cedex, France

Newman PJ
Dept of Intensive Care,
St George's Hospital,
Blackshaw Road, Tooting,
London SW17 0QT,
United Kingdom

Niederman MS
Dept of Pulmonary
and Critical Care Medicine,
Winthrop University Hospital,
222 Station Plaza North,
Mineola, NY 11501, USA

Parviainen I
Dept of Intensive Care,
Kuopio University Hospital,
70210 Kuopio, Finland

Pelosi P
Dept of Anesthesiology
and Intensive Care,
Ospedale Maggiore di Milano,
35 Via Francesco Sforza,
20122 Milan, Italy

Peronnet F
Laboratoire de Bioénergétique
Fondamentale et Appliquée,
Université J Fourier,
38041 Grenoble, France

Piek J
Klinik für Neurochirurgie,
Ernst Moritz Arndt University,
Ferdinand-Sauerbruch Strasse 8,
17487 Greifswald, Germany

Piek M
Institut für Epidemiologie
und Sozialmedizin,
Ernst Moritz Arndt University,
Ferdinand-Sauerbruch Strasse 8,
17487 Greifswald, Germany

Pinsky MR
Dept of Anesthesiology and Critical
Care, University of Pittsburgh,
3550 Terrace Street,
Pittsburgh PA 15208, USA

Puybasset L
Dept of Anesthesiology,
La Pitié-Salpêtrière Hospital,
47-89 Boulevard de l'Hôpital,
75013 Paris, France

Raad II
Dept of Medical Specialties,
Section of Infectious Diseases,
The University of Texas Anderson
Cancer Center, Houston TX 77030,
USA

Reinhart K
Dept of Anesthesiology,
Friedrich Schiller University,
Bachstrasse 18, 07740 Jena, Germany

Rhodes A
Dept of Intensive Care,
St George's Hospital,
Blackshaw Road, Tooting,
London SW17 0QT, United Kingdom

Rouby J-J
Dept of Anesthesiology,
La Pitié-Salpêtrière Hospital,
47-89 Boulevard de l'Hôpital,
75013 Paris, France

Roussos CT
Dept of Critical Care and Pulmonary,
Evangelismos Hospital,
45-47 Ipsilandou Street,
106 75 Athens, Greece

Rossi S
Dept of Intensive Care,
Ospedale Policlinico,
35 Via F Sforza, 20122 Milan, Italy

Rotelli S
Dept of Intensive Care,
Ospedale Policlinico,
35 Via F Sforza, 20122 Milan, Italy

Sair M
Dept of Critical Care,
Royal Brompton Hospital,
Sydney Street, London SW3 6NP,
United Kingdom

Scannon PJ
Preclinical Research,
Xoma Corporation,
2910 Seventh Street,
Berkeley CA 94710, USA

Schaller MD
Dept of Internal Medicine (Service B),
University Hospital,
BH-19, 1011 Lausanne, Switzerland

Schröder CH
Dept of Nephrology
and Renal Transplantation,
Wilhelmina Children's Hospital,
PO Box 18009, 3501 CA Utrecht,
The Netherlands

Schultz MJ
Dept of Infectious Diseases,
Tropical Medicine and AIDS,
Academic Medical Center,
F4-222, 9 Meibergdreef,
1105 AZ Amsterdam, The Netherlands

Sibbald WJ
London Health Sciences Center,
University of Western Ontario,
Victoria Hospital, Room 16A,
Health Services Building,
375 South Street,
London ON N6A 4G5, Canada

Siegemund M
Laboratory of Experimental
Anesthesiology, Academic Medical
Center, University of Amsterdam,
9 Meibergdreef, 1105 AZ Amsterdam,
The Netherlands

Silva E
Dept of Intensive Care,
Erasme University Hospital,
808 Route de Lennik, 1070 Brussels,
Belgium

Sinuff T
Dept of Medicine,
St Joseph's Hospital,
50 Charlton Avenue East,
Hamilton ON L8N 4A6, Canada

Slutsky AS
Dept of Surgery,
Mount Sinai Hospital,
600 University Avenue, Suite 656A,
Toronto, ONT M5G 1X5, Canada

Spahn DR
Institute of Anesthesiology,
University Hospital,
Rämistrasse 100, 8091 Zurich,
Switzerland

Sreeram N
Pediatric Heart Center,
Wilhelmina Children's Hospital,
PO Box 18009, 3501 CA Utrecht,
The Netherlands

Stocchetti N
Dept of Intensive Care,
Ospedale Policlinico,
35 Via F Sforza, 20122 Milan, Italy

Stoiser B
Dept of Internal Medicine and
Intensive Care, University Hospital,
Währinger Gürtel 18-20,
1090 Vienna, Austria

Studer W
Dept of Anesthesiology and Research,
University of Basel, Kantonsspital,
4031 Basel, Switzerland

Sugrue M
Dept of Critical Care,
Liverpool Hospital,
Liverpool NSW 2170, Australia

Sydow M
Dept of Anesthesiology,
University Hospital,
PO Box 3742, 37070 Göttingen,
Germany

Takala J
Dept of Intensive Care,
Kuopio University Hospital,
70210 Kuopio, Finland

Thiemermann C
The William Harvey Research
Institute, St Bartholomew's
and the Royal London School
of Medicine and Dentistry,
Charterhouse Square,
London EC1M 6BQ, United Kingdom

Tremblay LN
Dept of Surgery,
Mount Sinai Hospital,
600 University Avenue, Suite 656A,
Toronto, ONT M5G 1X5, Canada

Vallet B
Dept of Anesthesiology
and Intensive Care,
University Hospital of Lille,
Place de Verdun, 59037 Lille Cedex,
France

van der Poll T
Laboratory of Experimental
Internal Medicine,
Academic Medical Center,
9 Meibergdreef, 1105 AZ Amsterdam,
The Netherlands

van Deventer SJH
Laboratory of Experimental
Internal Medicine,
Academic Medical Center,
9 Meibergdreef, 1105 AZ Amsterdam,
The Netherlands

van Vught AJ
Dept of Pediatric Intensive Care,
Wilhelmina Children's Hospital,
PO Box 18009, 3501 CA Utrecht,
The Netherlands

Vassilakopoulos T
Dept of Critical Care and Pulmonary,
Evangelismos Hospital,
45-47 Ipsilandou Street,
106 75 Athens, Greece

Vazquez de Anda GF
Dept of Anesthesiology,
Erasmus University,
PO Box 1738, 3000 RD Rotterdam,
The Netherlands

Vignali A
Dept of Surgery,
IRCCS San Raffaele Hospital,
60 Via Olgettina, 20132 Milan, Italy

Vincent J-L
Dept of Intensive Care,
Erasme University Hospital,
808 Route de Lennik, 1070 Brussels,
Belgium

Viviand X
Dept of Anesthesiology and
Critical Care and Trauma Center,
North Hospital,
Chemin des Bourrellys,
13915 Marseille Cedex 20, France

Watson D
Dept of Intensive Care,
Homerton Hospital,
Homerton Row,
London E9 6SR, United Kingdom

Werner C
Dept of Anesthesiology,
University Hospital,
Ismaninger Strasse 22,
81675 Munich, Germany

Wray G
The William Harvey Research
Institute, St Bartholomew's and the
Royal London School of Medicine
and Dentistry, Charterhouse Square,
London EC1M 6BQ, United Kingdom

Wrigge H
Dept of Anesthesiology,
University Hospital,
PO Box 3742, 37070 Göttingen,
Germany

Wysocki M
Dept of Intensive Care,
Institut Mutualiste Montsouris,
42 Boulevard Jourdan, 75674 Paris,
France

Zakynthinos S
Dept of Critical Care
and Pulmonary Medicine,
Evangelismos Hospital,
45-47 Ipsilandou Street,
106 75 Athens, Greece

Zinserling J
Dept of Anesthesiology and
Intensive Care, University Hospital,
Bonn, Germany

Zwissler B
Institute of Anesthesiology,
Ludwig-Maximilians-University,
Klinikum Grosshadern,
Marchioninistrasse 15, 81366 Munich,
Germany

Common Abbreviations

ACE	Angiotensin-converting enzyme
ADP	Adenosine diphosphate
ALI	Acute lung injury
AMI	Acute myocardial infarction
APACHE	Acute physiology, age, chronic health evaluation
ARDS	Acute respiratory distress syndrome
ARF	Acute renal failure or Acute respiratory failure
ATLS	Advanced trauma life support
ATP	Adenosine triphosphate
BAL	Broncho-alveolar lavage
BIPAP	Biphasic positive airway pressure
BPI	Bactericidal permeability-increasing protein
CABG	Coronary artery bypass graft
cAMP	Cyclic adenosine monophosphate
CBF	Cerebral blood flow
cGMP	Cyclic guanosine monophosphate
cNOS	Constitutive nitric oxide synthase
CNS	Central nervous system
COP	Colloid osmotic pressure
COPD	Chronic obstructive pulmonary disease
CPAP	Continuous positive airway pressure
CPB	Cardiopulmonary bypass
CPP	Cerebral perfusion pressure
CPR	Cardiopulmonary resuscitation
CRP	C-reactive protein
CSF	Cerebro-spinal fluid
CT	Computerized tomography
DIC	Disseminated intravascular coagulation
DNA	Desoxyribonucleic acid
DO_2	Oxygen delivery
EBM	Evidence-based medicine

ECMO	Extracorporeal membrane oxygenation
EKG	Electrocardiogram
ELISA	Enzyme-linked immunosorbent assay
EMG	Electromyograph
EN	Enteral nutrition
eNOS	Endothelial nitric oxide synthase
FFA	Free fatty acids
FRC	Functional residual capacity
GCS	Glasgow coma score
G-CSF	Granulocyte-colony stimulating factor
GFR	Glomerular filtration rate
GI	Gastrointestinal
GM-CSF	Granulocyte macrophage-colony stimulating factor
GSH	Gluthatione
I/R	Ischemia/reperfusion
IABP	Intraaortic balloon counterpulsation
IAP	Intraabdominal pressure
ICAM	Intercellular adhesion molecule
ICP	Intracranial pressure
ICU	Intensive care unit
IFN-γ	Interferon gamma
IL	Interleukin
IL-1ra	IL-1 receptor antagonist
iNOS	Inducible nitric oxide synthase
IPPV	Intermittent positive pressure ventilation
IRV	Inverse ratio ventilation
IV	Intravenous
LBP	LPS binding protein
L-NAA	N^w-amino-L-arginine
L-NAME	N^G-nitro-L-arginine methyl ester
L-NMA	N^G-methyl-L-arginine
L-NMMA	N^G-nitro-monomethyl-L-arginine
L-NNA	N^w-nitro-L-arginine
LOS	Length of stay
LPS	Lipopolysaccharide
LTA	Lipoteichoic acid
MAb	Monoclonal antibodies
MAP	Mean arterial pressure
MCT	Medium chain triglycerids
MEGX	Monoethylglycinexylidide

MODS	Multiple organ dysfunction syndrome
MOF	Multiple organ failure
MPO	Myeloperoxidase
mRNA	Monoclonal ribonucleid acid
NAC	N-acetylcysteine
NAD	Nicotinamide adenine dinucleotide
NF-κB	Nuclear factor-kappa B
NIV	Non invasive ventilation
NMDA	N-methyl-D-aspartate
NO	Nitric oxide
NOS	Nitric oxide synthase
O_2	Oxygen
PAF	Platelet activating factor
PAV	Proportional assist ventilation
PBS	Protected brush specimen
PDH	Pyruvate dehydrogenase
PDT	Percutaneous dilational tracheostomy
PEEP	Positive end-expiratory pressure
pHi	Gastric intramucosal pH
PMN	Polymorphonuclear leukocyte
PSV	Pressure support ventilation
PTCA	Percutaneous transluminal coronary angioplasty
REE	Resting energy expenditure
ROC	Receiver operating characteristic (curve)
ROS	Reactive oxygen species
rt-PA	Recombinant tissue plasminogen activator
SAH	Subarachnoid hemorrhage
SAPS	Simplified acute physiologic scoring system
SIRS	Systemic inflammatory response syndrome
SOD	Superoxide dismutase
SVR	Systemic vascular resistance
TGF	Transforming growth factor
TISS	Therapeutic intervention scoring system
TNF	Tumor necrosis factor
TPN	Total parenteral nutrition
VAP	Ventilator-associated pneumonia
VO_2	Oxygen consumption/uptake
WOB	Work of breathing
XO	Xantine oxidase
ZEEP	Zero end-expiratory pressure

Host Responses
in Sepsis and ARDS

Balancing the Inflammatory Response in Sepsis

M. R. Pinsky

Introduction

Human sepsis is associated with the activation and systemic expression of host in-flammatory pathways via stimulation of the host immune effector cells to synthesize and release potent mediators of cell inflammation [1]. Accordingly, some have sug-gested that it be referred to as the systemic inflammatory response syndrome (SIRS) [2]. Altbough some of the initial mediators of this process are cytokines, a vast array of protein and lipid mediator species is expressed subsequently in a complex net-work [3, 4]. We [5] and others [6, 7] have documented that sustained elevations of the pro-inflammatory cytokine tumor necrosis factor (TNF)-α and the immuno-modulating cytokine interleukin (IL)-6, rather than their peak serum levels, identify those patients who will subsequently develop multiple organ dysfunction and death. However, in patients with established sepsis pro-inflammatory cytokines, such as TNF-α, IL-1, IL-6, and IL-8, and anti-inflammatory species, such as IL-1 receptor antagonist (IL-1ra), IL-10, and the soluble TNF-α receptors I and II (sTNFrI and sTNFrII), co-exist in the circulation and presumably within the tissues [8–10]. Thus, sepsis may be more accurately described as a dysregulation of the systemic inflammatory response to external stress, rather than merely the over expression of either pro- or anti-inflammatory substances. Accordingly, we proposed over 10 years ago to use the term "malignant intravascular inflammation" to describe this process. This paradoxical expression in the blood of pro-inflammatory mediators and anti-inflammatory molecular species creates an internal milieu that in sustained sepsis induces impaired host adaptability.

Associated with these interacting humoral effects is a process known as "inflam-matory-stimuli-induced-anergy" [11]. This phenomenon describes the universal process commonly referred to as "endotoxin tolerance." Apparently, this process is induced by anti-inflammatory cytokines, such as transforming growth factor (TGF)-β, IL-10, IL-4 and somewhat by IL-1, but not by TNF-α, IL-6 or IL-8. Further-more, it is associated with altered intracellular metabolism of the important pro-in-flammatory regulatory protein, nuclear factor-kappa B (NF-κB). NF-κB is the intra-cellular species that once cleaved into its active portion binds to promoter sites on the genome stimulating messenger ribonucleic acid (mRNA) synthesis of genes cod-ing for pro-inflammatory cytokines, like TNF-α. During an endotoxin tolerant state, induced by prior exposure to small amounts of endotoxin, subsequent endotoxin exposure can induce the initial steps of signal transduction up to NF-κB, but NF-κB appears to be dysfunctional. Once released NF-κB dimerizes into either an active form made up of one p50 and one p65 monomer, or an inactive form of two p50 monomers. This NF-κB dysfunction reflects both an excess p50 homodimer production, which lacks transcription activity [12], and excess synthesis of the inhibitor of NF-κB, IκB-α [13]. The balance of NF-κB species is very sensitive to transcription rates, with ratios of NF-κB p50–p65 heterodimer to p50 homodimer of 1.8 ± 0.6 conferring activation of the inflammatory pathways, while a ratio of 0.8 ± 0.1 confers lack of stimulation in response to LPS, or endotoxin tolerance. However, these NF-κB-related processes can only explain the down-regulation of the overall inflammatory process. They cannot explain why both pro- and anti-inflammatory activation seem to be sustained throughout the course of severe stress, such as may occur during sepsis, following trauma and burns, or in pancreatitis.

Cytokine-mediated cell signaling can alter intracellular function of the same cell (autocrine), adjacent cells (paracrine) or remote cells (endocrine) [3]. Using this framework, sepsis can be thought of as the endocrine expression of cytokine effects because it requires a systemic response from signals that normally function on an autocrine or paracrine level [5]. Some degree of systemic activation of the host's inflammatory response is probably protective in combating infection and trauma. Fever, for example, decreases bacterial growth rate, and malaise tends to inhibit additional stressful activities by the host allowing the host to conserve energy. However, if this systemic inflammatory response is sustained it can lead to remote tissue injury and death. Thus, severe sepsis may be considered as an uncontrolled form of intravascular inflammation [14]. Serum cytokine levels can change within minutes [15] and may be very different in adjacent tissue compartments [16, 17]. Thus, the measure of their blood levels may not characterize well the overall balance of the systemic inflammatory process. Furthermore, the down-regulation of monocyte activation appears to reflect autocrine and potentially paracrine functions, suggesting that the overall picture of SIRS is one of a multi-layered immunological process in which compartmentalization of the responses may be occurring between the blood stream and the tissues.

Circulating Immune Effector Cells in Sepsis

Clearly humoral factors play an important role in initiating a systemic inflammatory response and in modulating the ultimate outcome from sepsis. Furthermore, local autocrine and paracrine factors alter local responsiveness despite common circulating levels of systemic inflammatory mediators. Still, the primary effector organ for cell injury in SIRS is the activated immunocyte, including polymorphonuclear leukocytes (PMN), monocyte-macrophages, and lymphocytes. These immune effector cells are those which may induce organ system dysfunction across different vascular beds and at sites remote from the initiating stimulus. Furthermore, activation of immune effector cells occurs rapidly, within minutes, does not require new protein synthesis, and thus reflects an alternative arm of the normal activation pathways, in parallel with NF-κB-induced gene transcription.

One method of assessing the activation state of circulating immunocytes is to measure the intensity of display of cell surface proteins essential for effector functions. In that regard, we previously demonstrated in septic patients with liver failure

[18] that both circulating PMNs and monocytes are activated. This is characterized by loss of L-selectin, a constitutively expressed cell surface protein necessary for weak cell adhesion, and increasing display of both CD11b, a β2 integrin essential for firm adhesion of circulating PMNs to endothelial cells, and CD35, a complement receptor. Furthermore, these changes in circulating immunocyte display correlated with mean serum IL-6 levels and with the degree of organ dysfunction but not with the level of shock severity.

Since circulating PMNs are potentially an important contributor to both host defense against infection and organ injury, they are a logical indicator of the overall immune state of the patient with SIRS. In fact, studies have reported that PMNs are both overactive [19, 20] and dysfunctional [21–24] in SIRS. Similarly, CD11b display on circulating PMNs has been reported to be either decreased [25, 26] or increased [27–30] in critically ill and septic patients. Thus, we hypothesized that the *de novo* display of L-selectin and CD11b on circulating PMNs and their subsequent expression of both CD11b and its avid form in response to *in vitro* stimulation by TNF-α would characterize the state of activation and responsiveness of these cells. If the PMNS were stimulated then their *de novo* display of CD11b would be increased with an associated loss of L-selectin. If, on the other hand, their immune responsiveness was suppressed then they may or may not display CD11b in increased levels *de novo*, but would demonstrate an attenuated up-regulation of both CD11b and its avid form in response to an *in vitro* TNF-α challenge. Thus, functional assessment of circulating immune effector cells may represent an accurate method of assessing functional immune tolerance, activation or anergy during sepsis and other stress states. For example, if circulating PMNs displayed increased CD11b but did not respond to *in vitro* TNF-α challenge, then this would characterize a dysfunctional state of increased pro-inflammatory presence (increased CD11b) but impaired responsiveness (decreased response to TNF-α challenge).

Furthermore, if therapies were to improve the normal immune balance one would expect this profile to change accordingly. Thus, therapies that minimized the presence of non-specific inflammatory stimuli should restore normal responsiveness to TNF-α stimulation. Potentially, such therapies may include pressure-limited ventilation and continuous veno-venous hemofiltration at high flow rates. Therapies which pushed the immune balance more toward a pro-inflammatory state may increase CD11b expression, but, based on this hypothesis, would only change functional status if they restored the *in vitro* TNF-α responsiveness.

In support of these hypotheses, we recently showed in a preliminary report [31] that circulating PMNs from septic humans have a constantly activated phenotype with high CD11b and low L-selectin expression. Paradoxically, they are impaired in their ability to up-regulate CD11b further or to change surface CD11b to the avid state. The up-regulation of total CD11b density was less impaired than was the transition to the avid form. Interestingly, cell surface TNF-α receptor density was not reduced in the cells of these septic patients. These data agree with reports of others showing that TNF-α tolerance does not reflect receptor down-regulation, but rather decreased intracellular responsiveness through expression of stress proteins [32]. The hypo-reponsiveness we observed [31], as manifest by a blunted increased display of CD11b and its avid form in response to exposure to TNF-α *in vitro*, was extended to virtually all circulating PMN and monocytes and correlated to the severity of ill-

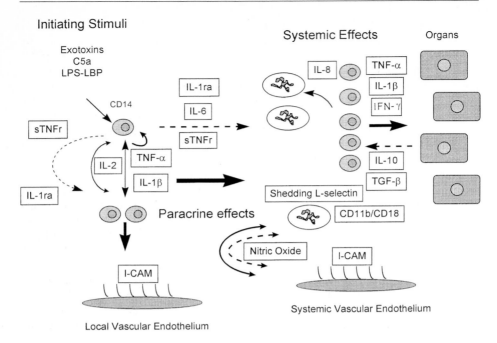

Fig. 1. A schematic representation of the network of pro- (solid lines) and anti- (dashed lines) inflammatory processes that occur in sepsis as they influence immune effector cells, endothelium and parenchymal cells. TNF-α and IL-1β are the initiating cytokines that stimulate IL-2 and interferon (IFN)-γ, while the chemokine IL-8 activates polymorphonuclear leukocytes. IL-6 induces an antioxidant acute phase protein synthesis by the liver and along with IL-2 promotes the febrile response. High levels of nitric oxide induce profound oxidative stress damaging numerous aspects of the cell. Low levels of nitric oxide are anti-inflammatory, as are IL-6, IL-10, TGF-β. Release of soluble TNF receptors (sTNFr) and IL-1ra minimize inflammation by competitive inhibition of the biological activity of circulating TNF-α and IL-1β, respectively

ness. This hypo-responsiveness may be a consequence of multiple mechanisms. The decreased responsiveness of the CD11b adhesion mechanism may protect tissues from the influx of large numbers of activated leukocytes. On the other hand, it may significantly impair anti-microbial defenses during SIRS. Prior studies have shown that cultured monocytes from septic patients have reduced intracellular storage of IL-1β and blunted synthesis of IL-1β in response to lipopolysaccharide (LPS) challenge [33]. These as of yet poorly described interactions that tend to balance the inflammatory processes are summarized in Figure 1. This schematic is, by necessity, an over simplification of the actual interactions as we presently understand them, but it aids in grouping primary systemic processes with their effects.

Mechanisms for Hypo-responsiveness of Immunocytes in Sepsis

Peripheral PMNs in patients with severe sepsis have a general up-regulation of β2-integrin (CD11b) with an accompanying loss of L-selectin, compatible with an activated phenotype. However, they also exhibit a significantly decreased CD11b. Patients with SIRS have shown impaired phagocytosis [21], oxygen burst capacity [23, 34] and adhesiveness [35]. Furthermore, circulating monocytes also exhibit CD11b hypo-responsiveness in SIRS. These data support the work of other investigators showing a profound impairment of cytokine production and antigen presenting capacity of circulating monocytes from patients with SIRS [36]. Thus, the phagocytes in the intravascular space during SIRS are very impaired in regard to several mechanisms that are important for host defense from infection. Conversely, they are also down-regulated in inflammatory capacity, which may limit host tissue injury.

Thus, an abnormal immunologic state is created in sepsis and SIRS by which sustained basal activation (increased *de novo* CD11b expression), impaired subsequent responsiveness (decreased response to endotoxin, TNF-α), and impaired phagocytosis of circulating immune effector cells leads to an increased likelihood of subsequent infection. Since these processes require no new RNA transcription, these aspects of sepsis may not be under the same influences as those that regulate NF-κB activity. However, this seems unlikely for several reasons. First, increased oxidant activity precedes activation of NF-κB; second, such oxidant stress can alter mitrochondrial function; and third, non-enzymatic production of isoprostanes occurs during this same interval. Thus, the combined shedding of L-selectin and up-regulation of CD11b and its avid form, reflect a series of non-transcriptional activities early on in inflammation.

The cell surface alterations of the non-adherent intravascular immune effector cells in sepsis may be an artefact of selection, in that more adherent cells produced by the bone marrow would be quickly removed from the circulation and not be measured by blood testing. If this were so, the tissue supply of monocytes and PMNs may be fully functional, with non-adherent poorly functional cells left behind in the circulation. This scenario is unlikely based on the fact that flow cytometry allows examination of cell populations at the single cell level. The hypo-responsiveness that we observed affected every monocyte and PMN in the blood. It is unlikely that significant numbers of normally reacting leukocytes are transiting the circulation without comprising even one percent of the cells there at any given time. Thus, the vast majority of monocytes and PMNs available to tissue appear to be very hypo-responsive to inflammatory stimuli.

Leukocyte responsiveness to mediators is crucial for host defense from infection in both the circulation and the tissues. On the other hand, cellular inflammatory mechanisms account for tissue injury in many models of SIRS. Since organ dysfunction and recurrent infection frequently complicate SIRS, understanding the mechanisms and the consequences of altered cellular responsiveness in SIRS may provide a logical therapeutic target. There are currently multiple agents available that can stimulate or suppress immunocyte function.

The mechanism of hypo-responsiveness to TNF-α in severe sepsis is probably complex. The modulation of CD11b by TNF-α is a multi-step process and a diminished response in cells from septic patients relative to naive cells could be induced by alterations at any one of many steps. As an initial mechanism, this hypo-responsiveness could reflect inhibitory effects of circulating anti-inflammatory stimuli. Since most patients with severe SIRS, including all those in our preliminary study, had high levels of soluble TNF-α receptors in the plasma, some blockade of exoge-nous TNF-α effect in our assay on that basis is inevitable.

Second, many pro-inflammatory mediators decrease PMN responsiveness to TNF-α via a down-regulation of the cell surface TNF-α receptor density. TNF-α it-self, IL-8, N-formyl-methionyl-leucyl-phenylalanine (MLP), platelet activating fac-tor (PAF), leukotriene B4, complement fragment C5a, and endotoxin have also been shown to down-regulate TNF-α receptors on the PMN *in vitro* [37, 38]. Potentially, the PMNs in the circulation of our patients with SIRS had down-regulated their TNF-α receptors and were insensitive to TNF-α stimulation on that basis. Schleif-fenbaum and Fehr [37] demonstrated that PMNs in culture lost TNF-α receptors in response to pertussis toxin stimulation, suggesting that receptor loss may be a pro-cess explaining PMN desensitization.

Third, exposure of circulating cells to inflammatory mediators can down-regulate their responsiveness to TNF-α by mechanisms other than TNF-α receptor loss. Upon PMN activation by cytokines, a coordinated chain of events is activated which allows the PMN to move along the endothelial surface by a combination of gripping, releasing and cell shape change. This is accomplished by a rapidly reversible avidity of CD11b for counter-receptors and intracellular association with the cytoskeleton. This sequence is believed to be driven by a concentration gradient of activator(s) bound to the endothelial surface. Continuous exposure to soluble IL-8, however, disrupts this chain of events and causes cell rounding, and loss of avidity of CD11b after about one hour [39, 40]. PMN-endothelium adhesion is inhibited and adherent cells detach. Re-stimulation with fresh IL-8 does not cause a return of CD11b avidity, i.e., the cells remain desensitized to IL-8.

Fourth, the developmental stage of circulating immune cells is another factor that can influence TNF-α responsiveness. The vigorous stimulation of bone marrow in SIRS produces many immature PMNs in the circulation, i.e. the "left shift." These immature cells may not be capable of normal adhesion responses. If this were the cause of hypo-responsiveness, then there should be a correlation between the degree of PMN desensitization to TNF-α to the immature PMN (band) count. Babcock and Rodeberg [41] did not find a correlation between these two factors in their study. At the opposite extreme, circulating PMNs could be senescent in SIRS. Many of the me-diators of inflammation, including TNF-α, extend the lifetime of PMNs by inhibiting apoptosis [42, 43]. Moreover, preliminary studies on the PMNs of patients with SIRS indicated a delay in apoptotic cell death [44]. The circulating cells may be relatively older and dysfunctional due to any number of intracellular defects.

Finally, failure of CD11b response could also be due to exhaustion of the CD11b supply within the cells. CD11b is stored in intracellular granules, which are rapidly released to the surface upon cell activation [45]. The intracellular pool of CD11b could be depleted by continuous activation. It is likely that a combination of intra-cellular depletion of stored CD11b, altered intracellular signaling and perhaps depletion of key regulatory moieties in the transduction pathway from cell surface receptor to NF-κB activation all play a role in developing a decreased responsiveness of CD11b in SIRS patients.

The site for the altered immune response in sepsis and SIRS appears to be localiz-ed to an impaired signal transduction following LPS or TNF-α binding to cell sur-face receptors but before transcription via NF-κB activation. Although either dysfunctional NK-κB or excess IκB-α may reduce autocrine release of TNF-α and IL-1, it should have a minimal effect on the expression of pre-formed adhesion molecules whose expression does not require transcription. To the extent that exhaustion of specific heat shock proteins (HSP), which function as intracellular chaperones, occurs, then multiple intracellular signaling processes may be affected. This hypothesis is attractive because it would explain both non-specific depression of transcription and impaired expression of appropriate cell surface adhesion molecules.

Mitochondrial Oxidative Stress and Heat Shock Protein Protection in Sepsis

Recent work has shown that an initial step in the intracellular activation of the inflammatory pathway is the production of reactive oxygen species and an associated oxidative stress on the mitochondria [32]. If mitochondrial oxidation does not occur then NF-κB does not become activated. Using sensitive bioassays of "redox" state, Polla et al. [32] have shown that a specific HSP, HSP-70, prevents this oxidative stress and blunts the inflammatory response. Numerous other studies have shown that HSP are a basic cellular defense mechanism against numerous stresses, such as fever, trauma, and inflammation [46]. They constitute a significant proportion of the intracellular protein pool, representing 2% of the resting cellular protein component and up to 20% of the stressed cellular protein component. They also minimize nitric oxide (NO), oxygen free radical and stretozotocin cytotoxicity [47]. HSP-70 has been shown to be an inducible protective agent in the myocardium against ischemia, reperfusion injury and NO toxicity [48], but requires some initial NO synthesis for its activation. Such NO-induced HSP synthesis blunts the inflammatory response to endotoxin and TNF-α *in vitro*. These data suggest that HSP, in general, and HSP-70, in particular, may be important in modulating the intracellular inflammatory signal acting at the level of NK-κB. The interaction between the HSP system and the pro-inflammatory pathway represents an exciting and potentially very important aspect of the molecular control of immunomodulation of the inflammatory response.

Thus, the initiation and inhibition of the intracellular inflammatory responses in sepsis should reflect a balance between these normal processes. As such, they should also be present in any cell line capable of mounting an inflammatory response. Several intracellular events must occur prior to the activation of NK-κB. Most of these events, surprisingly require intracellular oxidative stress. It is not clear if any specific oxidative stress is capable of stimulating these responses. Several processes, such as NO synthesis and hydrogen peroxide can markedly stimulate NF-κB activation. These stimulate a counter-regulatory process via stimulation of HSP, as well as other anti-oxidants, such as manganese superoxide dismutase. Thus, NF-κB activation may be prevented by blunting the synthesis of TNF-α in response to a new stress [32]. Importantly, these intracellular responses need not be associated with changes in TNF-α cell receptor density or affinity [46]. Furthermore, continued inflammatory stimulation must deplete intracellular pools of NF-κB, as the NF-κB is released from I-κB, and then migrates into the nucleus. Thus, the subsequent inflammatory state will depend on synthesis of new NF-κB.

The Clinical Paradox

Multiple immune cell types are dysfunctional in septic patients. The impairment of monocyte antigen presentation and inflammatory cytokine production has been correlated to the development of organ failure and mortality [36]. The dysfunction of PMN phagocytosis and oxygen burst has been linked to an unfavorable outcome from sepsis in some studies but not others [49–51]. Nonetheless, circumstantial evidence suggests that PMN function is important in sepsis:

1) Neutropenic hosts are extremely susceptible to infection and the development of a severe septic state;
2) pre-treatment with anti-CD11b antibodies exacerbates infection [52, 53];
3) finally, congenital deficiency of CD11b display predisposes to recurrent infection in humans [54].

Similarly, in situations where continued infection determines outcome, PMN activation is beneficial [55]. On the opposite side of the spectrum, clear evidence exists that PMN activation can be very destructive in acute lung injury and sepsis. In balance, these data suggest that PMNs are beneficial in some settings and harmful in others.

Based on these data, it is important to define which patient populations benefit from augmenting monocyte and PMN function by assessing cellular functional markers in addition to the customary parameters during trials of new therapies. Only in this fashion can the impact of therapy on immunocyte function be discerned and related to outcome. The alternative, treatment without immune monitoring, risks exacerbating inflammatory injury or impairing host defense against infection.

Conclusion

The clinical expression of sepsis has classically suggested a common process of inflammation and tissue injury induced by the combined assault of the outside environment and the host's pro-inflammatory response. As with most of clinical medicine, when a deeper understanding of the molecular and cellular mechanisms involved in the expression and evolution of a major biological process is developed, such simplistic models and therapeutic paradigms disappear. Likewise, sepsis reflects the complex interaction of both pro- and anti-inflammatory processes often simultaneously expressed, that together create the clinical picture. Conceptually, sepsis involves networks of reciprocating, complimentary and differentially active biological processes that may be antagonistic as often as they are synergistic. Accordingly, therapeutic measures that inhibit only one arm of this process or block only one step in either pro-inflammatory or anti-inflammatory limbs will be universally ineffective for large heterogeneous groups of critically ill patients. Using this logic, several lines of diagnostic and therapeutic approach appear promising. First, bioassays of the state of pro- versus anti-inflammatory balance in specific patients may allow for titration of less aggressive immunomodulation to allow the system to return to a state of balance. Second, therapies that reduce blood levels of grossly elevated immunomodulating agents should reduce the overall cacophony of the stimuli assaulting the immune competent cells of the body. Finally, conventional therapies that further limit direct or remote organ injury will, in themselves, reduce the inflammatory load on the patient. As new understanding of the molecular mechanisms of sepsis develops, both our diagnostic and therapeutic options expand. Maintaining a balanced perspective on how we evolved genetically, and how we create our natural equilibrium and adapt to stress, will aid greatly in our effective application of these new data for the overall benefit of the critically ill patient and society.

References

1. Schlag G, Redl H (1996) Mediators of injury and inflammation. World J Surg 20:406–410
2. Bone RC (1996) Toward a theory regarding the pathogenesis of the systemic inflammatory response syndrome: what we do and do not know about cytokine regulation. Crit Care Med 24:163–172
3. Marsh CB, Wewers MD (1996) The pathogenesis of sepsis. Factors that modulate the response to gram-negative bacterial infection. Clin Chest Med 17:183–197
4. Crowley SR (1996) The pathogenesis of septic shock. Heart & Lung 25:124–134
5. Pinsky MR, Vincent JL, Deviere J, Alegre M, Kahn RJ, Dupont E (1993) Serum cytokine levels in human septic shock. Relation to multiple-system organ failure and mortality. Chest 103:565–575
6. Thijs LG, Hack CE (1995) Time course of cytokine levels in sepsis. Intensive Care Med 21 (Suppl 2):S258–S263
7. Blackwell TS, Christman JW (1996) Sepsis and cytokines: current status. Br J Anaesth 77:110–117
8. Goldie AS, Fearon KC, Ross JA, et al (1995) Natural cytokine antagonists and endogenous anti-endotoxin core antibodies in sepsis syndrome. The Sepsis Intervention Group. JAMA 274:172–177
9. Vanderpoll T, Malefyt RD, Coyle SM, Lowry SF (1997) Anti-inflammatory cytokine responses during clinical sepsis and experimental endotoxemia – sequential measurements of plasma soluble interleukin (IL)-1 receptor type Ii, IL-10, and IL-13. J Infect Dis 175:118–122
10. Ertel W, Scholl FA, Trentz O (1996) The role of anti-inflammatory mediators for the control of systemic inflammation following severe injury. In: Faist E, Baue AE, Schildberg FW (eds) The immune consequences of trauma, shock, and sepsis – mechanisms and therapeutic approaches. Pabst Science Publishers, Lengerich, pp 453–470
11. Cavaillon JM (1995) The nonspecific nature of endotoxin tolerance. Trends in Microbiol 3:320–324
12. Ziegler-Heitbrock HWL, Wedel A, Schraut W, et al (1994) Tolerance to lipopolysaccharide involves mobilization of nuclear factor κB with predominance of p50 homodimers. J Biol Chem 269:17001–17004
13. Larue KEA, McCall CE (1994) A liable transcriptional repressor modulates endotoxin tolerance. J Exp Med 180:2269–2275
14. Pinsky MR (1994) Clinical studies on cytokines in sepsis: role of serum cytokines in the development of multiple-systems organ failure. Nephrol Dial Transplant 9 (Suppl 4):94–98
15. Martich GD, Boujoukos AJ, Suffredini AF (1993) Response of man to endotoxin. Immunobiol 187:403–416
16. Boutten A, Dehoux MS, Seta N, et al (1996) Compartmentalized IL-8 and elastase release within the human lung in unilateral pneumonia. Am J Respir Crit Care Med 153:336–342
17. Hauser CJ (1996) Regional macrophage activation after injury and the compartmentalization of inflammation in trauma. New Horizons 4:235–251
18. Rosenbloom AJ, Pinsky MR, Bryant JL, Shin A, Tran T, Whiteside T (1995) Leukocyte activation in the peripheral blood of patients with cirrhosis of the liver and SIRS. Correlation with serum interleukin-6 levels and organ dysfunction. JAMA 274:58–65

19. Tschaikowsky K, Sittl R, Braun GG, Hering W, Rugheimer E (1993) Increased fMet-Leu-Phe receptor expression and altered superoxide production of neutrophil granulocytes in septic and posttraumatic patients. J Clin Invest 72:18–25

20. Trautinger F, Hammerle AF, Poschl G, Micksche M (1991) Respiratory burst capability of poly-morphonuclear neutrophils and TNF-alpha serum levels in relationship to the development of septic syndrome in critically ill patients. J Leukocyte Biol 49:449–454

21. Wenisch C, Parschalk P, Hasenhundl M, Griesmacher A, Graninger W (1995) Polymorpho-nuclear leukocyte dysregulation in patients with gram-negative septicemia assessed by flow cytometry. Eur J Clin Invest 25:418–424

22. McCall CE, Grosso-Wilmoth LM, LaRue K, Guzman RN, Cousart SL (1993) Tolerance to endo-toxin-induced expression of the interleukin-1 beta gene in blood neutrophils of humans with the sepsis syndrome. J Clin Invest 91:853–861

23. Vespasiano MC, Lewandoski JR, Zimmerman JJ (1993) Longitudinal analysis of neutrophil superoxide anion generation in patients with septic shock. Crit Care Med 21:666–672

24. Sorrell TC, Sztelma K, May GL (1994) Circulating polymorphonuclear leukocytes from patients with gram-negative bacteremia are not primed for enhanced production of leukotriene B4 or 5-hydroxyeicosatetraenoic acid. J Infect Dis 169:1151–1154

25. Nakae H, Endo S, Inada K, Takakuwa T, Kasai T (1996) Changes in adhesion molecule levels in sepsis. Res Comm Mol Pathol Pharmacol 91:329–338

26. Fasano MB, Cousart S, Neal S, McCall CE (1991) Increased expression of the interleukin 1 re-ceptor on blood neutrophils of humans with the sepsis syndrome. J Clin Invest 88:1452–1459

27. Brom J, Koller M, Schluter B, Muller-Lange P, Ulrich Steinau H, Konig W (1995) Expression of the adhesion molecule CD11b and polymerization of actin by polymorphonuclear granulocytes of patients endangered by sepsis. Burns 21:427–431

28. Ljunghusen O, Berg S, Hed J, et al (1995) Transient endotoxemia during burn wound revision causes leukocyte beta 2 integrin up-regulation and cytokine release. Inflammation 19:457–468

29. Lin RY, Astiz ME, Saxon JC, Saha DC, Rackow EC (1994) Relationships between plasma cytokine concentrations and leukocyte functional antigen expression in patients with sepsis. Crit Care Med 22:1595–1602

30. Lin RY, Astiz ME, Saxon JC, Rackow EC (1993) Altered leukocyte immunophenotypes in septic shock. Studies of HLA-DR, CD11b, CD14, and IL-2R expression. Chest 104:847–853

31. Rosenbloom AJ, Levann D, Ray B, Nguyen S, Pinsky MR (1996) Density and avidity changes of Cd11b on circulating polymorphonuclear leukocytes (PMN) in systemic inflammatory re-sponse syndrome (SIRS). Am J Respir Crit Care Med 153(4):A123 (Abst)

32. Polla BS, Jacquier-Sarlin MR, Kantengwa S, et al (1996) TNFα alters mitochondrial membrane potential in L929 but not in TNFα-resistance L929.12 cells: relationship with the expression of stress proteins, annexin 1 and superoxide dismutase activity. Free Rad Res 25:125–131

33. Munoz C, Carlet J, Fitting C, Misset B, Bieriot J-P, Cavaillon J-M (1991) Dysregulation of in vitro cytokine production by monocytes during sepsis. J Clin Invest 88:1747–1754

34. Babcock GF, Rodeberg DA, White-Owen CL (1996) Changes in neutrophil function following major trauma or thermal injury. In: Faist E, Baue AE, Schildberg FW (eds) The immune conse-quences of trauma, shock and sepsis – mechanisms and therapeutic approaches. Pabst Science Publishers, Lengerich, pp 194–201

35. Terregino CA, Lubkin C, Thom SR (1997) Impaired neutrophil adherence as an early marker of systemic inflammatory response syndrome and severe sepsis. Ann Emerg Med 29:400–403

36. Docke WD, Syrbe U, Meinecke A, et al (1994) Improvement of monocyte function – A new therapeutic approach? In: Reinhart K, Eyrich K, Sprung C (eds) Sepsis: current perspectives in pathophysiology and therapy. Springer-Verlag, Berlin, Heidelberg, New York, pp 473–500

37. Schleiffenbaum B, Fehr J (1990) The tumor necrosis factor receptor and human neutrophil func-tion. Deactivation and cross-deactivation of tumor necrosis factor-induced neutrophil respon-ses by receptor down-regulation. J Clin Invest 86:184–195

38. van der Poll T, Calvano SE, Kumar A, Braxton CC, Coyle SM, Barbosa K, Moldawer LL, Lowry SF (1995) Endotoxin induces downregulation of tumor necrosis factor receptors on circulating monocytes and granulocytes in humans. Blood 86:2754–2759

39. Detmers PA, Powell DE, Walz A, Clark-Lewis I, Baggiolini M, Cohn ZA (1991) Differential effects of neutrophil-activating peptide 1/IL-8 and its homologues on leukocyte adhesion and phago-cytosis. J Immunol 147:4211–4217

40. Luscinskas FW, Kiely JM, Ding H, et al (1992) In vitro inhibitory effect of IL-8 and other chemo-attractants on neutrophil-endothelial adhesive interactions. J Immunol 149:2163–2171
41. Babcock GF, Rodeberg DA (1996) The effect of thermal injury and lipopolysaccharide exposure on neutrophil b2 integrin and CD14 expression. In: Faist E, Baue AE, Schildberg FW (eds) The immune consequences of trauma, shock and sepsis – mechanisms and therapeutic approaches. Pabst Science Publishers, Lengerich, pp 202–210
42. Biffl WL, Moore EE, Moore FA (1996) Interleukin-6 delays neutrophil apoptosis. Arch Surg 131:24–30
43. Colotta F, Re F, Polentarutti N, Sozzani S, Mantovani A (1992) Modulation of granulocyte survival and programmed cell death by cytokines and bacterial products. Blood 80:2012–2020
44. Marshall JC, Watson RWG (1997) Apoptosis in the resolution of systemic inflammation. In: Vincent JL (ed) Yearbook of intensive care and emergency medicine. Springer-Verlag, Berlin, Heidelberg, New York, pp 100–108
45. Singer II, Scott S, Kawka DW, Kazazis DM (1989) Adhesomes: specific granules containing receptors for laminin, C3bi/fibrinogen, fibronectin, and vitronectin in human polymorpho-nuclear leukocytes and monocytes. J Cell Biol 109:3169–3182
46. Jaaettla M, Wising D (1993) Heat shock proteins protect cells from monocyte cytotoxicity: possible mechanism of self protection. J Exp Med 177:231–236
47. Bellmann K, Wenz A, Radons J, Burkart V, Kleemann R, Kolb H (1995) Heat shock induces resistance in rat pancreatic islet cells against nitric oxide, oxygen radicals and streptozototocin toxicity in vitro. J Clin Invest 95:2840–2845
48. Malyshev IY, Malugin AV, Golubeva LY, et al (1996) Nitric oxide donor induces HSP70 accumulation in the heart and in cultured cells. FEBS Lett 391:21–23
49. Alexander JW, Ogle C, Stinnett J, MacMillan BG (1978) A sequential prospective analysis of immunological abnormalities and infection following severe thermal injury. Ann Surg 188:809–816
50. Deitch E, McDonald J (1982) Influence of serum on impaired neutrophil chemotaxis after thermal injury. J Surg Res 33:251–257
51. Christou NV, Tellado JM (1989) In vitro polymorphonuclear neutrophil function in surgical patients does not correlate with anergy but with "Activating" processes such as sepsis or trauma. Surgery 106:718–724
52. Rosen H, Gordon S (1990) The role of the type 3 complement receptor in the induced recruitment of myelomonocytic cells to inflammatory sites in the mouse. Am J Respir Cell Mol Biol 3:3–10
53. Conlan JW, North RJ (1992) Monoclonal antibody NIMP-R10 directed against the CD11b chain of the type 3 complement receptor can substitute for monoclonal antibody 5C6 to exacerbate listeriosis by preventing the focusing of myelomonocytic cells at infectious foci in the liver. J Leukocyte Biol 52:130–132
54. Lipnick RN, Iliopoulos A, Salata K, Hershey J, Melnick D, Tsokos GC (1996) Leukocyte adhesion deficiency: report of a case and review of the literature. Clin Exper Rheumatol 14:95–98
55. Karzai W, Reinhart K (1997) Is it beneficial to augment or to inhibit neutrophil function in severe infections and sepsis? In: Vincent JL (ed) Yearbook of intensive care and emergency medicine. Springer-Verlag, Berlin, Heidelberg, New York, pp 122–132

Bactericidal/Permeability-Increasing Protein (BPI): Structure, Function, and Clinical Applications

B. P. Giroir, S. F. Carroll, and P. J. Scannon

Introduction

Bactericidal/permeability-increasing protein (BPI) is a basic protein found in the azurophilic granules of neutrophils, which has multiple anti-infective properties. BPI was first described by Weiss and Elsbach in the mid-1970s as a cationic protein fraction from rabbit polymorphonuclear leukocytes which had potent bactericidal activity against Gram-negative bacteria and which bound bacterial lipopolysaccharides (LPS or endotoxin) [1, 2]. Since then, BPI has been cloned and characterized, and genetically engineered fragments of the native molecule have been generated. Additional bioactivities of BPI and proteins derived from its N-terminal domain have been discovered. After 20 years of research and development, bioactive BPI N-terminal protein is now undergoing clinical trials for multiple indications. The purpose of this review is to summarize information relating to the structure of BPI, its activity *in vitro*, in animal models and in humans, as well as its current clinical development.

Native BPI

BPI is a 55kD protein which is 45% identical in its amino acid sequence to lipopolysaccharide binding protein (LBP). The genes for both BPI and LBP have been localized to chromosome 20 in humans [3]. The BPI protein is organized into two domains, the N-terminal domain and the C-terminal domain. The N-terminal domain is rich in basic amino acids and is overall amphipathic, with alternating hydrophobic and hydrophilic segments. The C-terminal domain is essentially neutral, with hydrophobic regions that are postulated to serve a membrane-anchoring function. Placed between the termini is a hydrophilic, proline-rich linker sequence.

The novel boomerang-shaped three dimensional structure of BPI has recently been described (Fig. 1) [4]. Although the N- and C-terminal domains share less than 20% amino acid sequence homology, they share striking structural similarity such that each domain is barrel-shaped and is connected together by a central β-sheet structure. After the amino acid sequence had been placed in the electron density maps, a phosphatidylcholine molecule was found bound in each apolar pocket on the concave surface of each domain, primarily through interactions with the acyl chains of phosphatidylcholine. These data suggest that the apolar pockets represent sites of BPI binding to lipids and, possibly, to the lipid A portion of LPS.

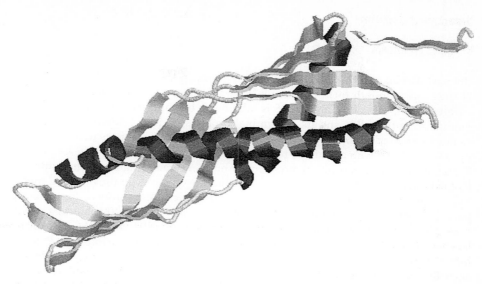

Fig. 1. Structural model of recombinant bactericidal/permeability-increasing protein (rBPI$_{21}$). Cartoon diagram illustrating the secondary and tertiary structure of rBPI$_{21}$, based upon the X-ray crystal structure of human BPI [4]. Alpha-helical segments of the protein are shown as coils, and beta-strands are shown as arrows. The image was prepared using the program RasMol

N-Terminal Constructs

In 1987 Ooi and coworkers [5] purified a 25kD N-terminal fragment of the native holo-protein following long-term storage. This 25kD fragment was as bactericidal (on a molar basis) as the holo-protein against rough strains of *E. coli* (J5), but the 25kD fragment was five-fold more potent in killing smooth strains of *E. coli*, i.e., strains with longer polysaccharide chains. In contrast, the C-terminal fragment had no bactericidal properties. These data immediately suggested that holo-BPI could be functionally divided, and that the anti-infective properties which might have clinical utility were uniquely present in the N-terminal fragment of the molecule.

Following cloning of the human gene in 1989, multiple recombinant N-terminal BPI (rBPI) proteins were produced and characterized, and two have been extensively investigated: rBPI$_{23}$, a 199 amino acid N-terminal fragment of the holo-protein, and rBPI$_{21}$, a modified 193 amino acid N-terminal fragment of the holo-protein in which the cysteine at position 132 is replaced by an alanine in order to improve homogeneity and stability. Both rBPI$_{23}$ and rBPI$_{21}$ retain the anti-infective properties of the holo-protein, and in some circumstances, have improved bioactivity.

Bioactive Properties

BPI Binds Endotoxin

BPI and its bioactive N-terminal proteins have been shown to bind a broad range of rough and smooth form LPS in a fashion that is specific, saturable, and of high affinity. The specific binding to LPS is inhibitable by competition with lipid A. The binding affinity of BPI and its N-terminal proteins is similar when tested against isolated LPS *in vitro* [6]. Importantly, however, there are differences in the ability of the 55kD holo-protein and the N-terminal proteins to bind smooth-type LPS on the bacterial membrane surface or presumably on membrane fragments shed into the circulation. Both $rBPI_{23}$ and $rBPI_{21}$ bind to smooth-type LPS on the bacterial membrane significantly better than holo-BPI, possibly due to the ability of long, tightly packed polysaccharide chains on the bacterial membrane to inhibit binding of the holo-protein compared to N-terminal fragments [7]. Binding of $rBPI_{23}$ and $rBPI_{21}$ has been demonstrated to LPS from *Esherichia coli*, *Klebsiella pneumoniae*, *Pseudomonas aeruginosa* (including clinical isolates), to a multitude of clinically relevant smooth strain serotypes, and to mutant LPS. Data confirm that the binding of BPI and the N-terminal proteins to LPS is via lipid A, and that this binding involves both electrostatic and hydrophobic interactions.

BPI Kills Bacteria

Despite recent crystallographic data indicating that both the N- and C-terminal domains bind phoshphatidylcholine (and possibly LPS), only the holo-protein and its bioactive N-terminal proteins are bactericidal, whereas the C-terminal fragment is not [5, 8]. It is currently thought that BPI binds to endotoxin in the bacterial outer membrane, leading rapidly to increased permeability of the bacterial cytoplasmic membrane, activation of enzymes which degrade membrane phospholipids and peptidoglycans, and ultimate death of the bacteria [9]. The molecule has been shown to be bactericidal against numerous Gram-negative organisms, including *Escherichia coli*, *Klebsiella pneumoniae*, *Pseudomonas aeruginosa*, *Neisseria meningitidis*, and others. Killing occurs following brief incubations of N-terminal proteins with the bacteria, and occurs at concentrations of $rBPI_{21}$ that are clinically achievable in humans (see below). Both smooth and rough strains are sensitive to killing by the holo-protein, but killing with the N-terminal proteins is consistently more effective than killing by the holoprotein.

Although BPI and its N-terminal proteins are bactericidal by themselves, their antibacterial effects are enhanced by the presence of complement, antibiotics, phospholipase, and p15s [10]. Of interest, although LBP alone has no bactericidal effect, the presence of even small quantities of LBP has been shown to decrease by 10 000 fold the concentration of BPI necessary to kill rough Gram-negative organisms *in vitro*. The mechanism of enhancement by LBP is not yet understood.

BPI Neutralizes Endotoxin

In 1990, Marra and colleagues [11] determined that purified holo-BPI was able to prevent up-regulation of complement receptors CR1 and CR3 on the surface of human neutrophils stimulated with both rough and smooth LPS chemotypes, but did not prevent neutrophil stimulation by tumor necrosis factor (TNF) and the peptide N-formylmethionyl-leucyl-phenylalanine (FMLP). Since that time, extensive data have been generated on the normal processes of LPS signaling, and as a result, the mechanisms by which BPI and its N-terminal proteins interrupt that signaling.

The mechanisms by which LPS activates macrophages, endothelial cells, and other effector cells have been elucidated [12]. LPS is first bound to LBP, a 60kD acute phase protein synthesized in the liver. LBP is thought to serve a LPS-transfer function, such that LPS is efficiently transferred to the CD14 receptor on macrophages, or to soluble CD14 for activation of CD14-negative cells such as endothelial cells. CD14 is a glycophosphatidylinosilol (GPI)-linked protein which is postulated to be associated with at least one additional protein and is responsible for intracellular signal transduction, which occurs via protein kinase cascades.

BPI and its bioactive N-terminal proteins compete with LBP for binding to LPS [13]. $rBPI_{21}$ and $rBPI_{23}$ were shown to have an affinity for LPS in the range of 30–100 fold greater than LBP. The ability of the N-terminal proteins to neutralize free endotoxin from rough or smooth strains is at least equivalent to that of the holoprotein. The C-terminal domain also has endotoxin binding and neutralizing properties, but is 5–10 fold less potent on a molar basis than holo-BPI or the N-terminal proteins. Of major importance is that BPI and N-terminal proteins are able to bind to, and thus neutralize, not only free endotoxin in the circulation, but also endotoxin on the outer membrane of intact bacteria, and from bacterial membrane fragments shed from bacteria following antibiotic treatment [14]. Included among the endotoxin-induced activities inhibited by BPI, $rBPI_{23}$ and $rBPI_{21}$ are [15–18]:

1) TNF release by human whole blood and peripheral blood mononuclear cells;
2) interleukin (IL)-1, IL-6, and IL-8 release by mononuclear cells;
3) generation of free radicals by whole human blood;
4) release of nitric oxide;
5) expression of tissue factor by human peripheral blood mononuclear cells and human endothelial cells;
6) LPS-induced adhesion of human neutrophils to human endothelial cells;
7) complement activation induced by lipid A.

Of importance to endotoxin neutralization are issues of endotoxin kinetics, i.e., whether there is any rationale for neutralization once endotoxin is already present. Current data indicate that ongoing expression of cytokines and adhesion molecules requires the constant presence of LPS. *In vitro* data demonstrating only transient expression of inflammatory mediators reflects clearance of endotoxin by normal plasma components [19]. Conversely, continued addition of endotoxin, as might be expected to occur during a clinical infection, leads to more prolonged expression of inflammatory mediators. Consequently, inhibition of endotoxin even after the initial induction of pro-inflammatory genes is associated with a rapid down-regula-

tion of these factors. In clinical conditions such as abdominal sepsis or meningococcal disease, during which plasma endotoxin may be elevated for many hours or
even days, clearance and neutralization of endotoxin would, based on *in vitro* data,
result in a more rapid down-regulation of the host response. In the specific case of
rBPI$_{21}$, inflammation might also be mitigated by direct bactericidal effects or anti-
biotic-enhancing effects against both Gram-negative and Gram-positive organisms.

Animal Models

Endotoxin Infusion

BPI and its bioactive N-terminal proteins have been shown to be effective in numerous animal models. BPI protects against mortality following endotoxin challenge in
mice, rats, and rabbits. BPI administration reduced serum levels of TNF-α, IL-1, and
IL-6 compared to controls, and was effective in reducing mortality as long as one
hour after endotoxin infusion [20]. In other studies, rBPI$_{23}$ mitigated endotoxin-induced alterations in serum glucose, lactate, and TNF-α in rats [21]. In both rats and
rabbits, administration of rBPI was associated with maintenance of baseline heart
rate, blood pressure, and normal sympathetic tone following LPS challenge, and also
with maintenance of tissue microperfusion to the left ventricle, kidneys, liver, and
skeletal muscle [22]. In pigs, rBPI$_{23}$ was shown to reduce neutrophil transmigration
into alveoli and significantly ameliorated LPS-induced hypoxemia [23]. BPI was
shown to be superior compared to HA-1A and E5 both in its ability to clear and neutralize endotoxin *in vitro*, and also in improving survival in CD-1 mice challenged
with lethal doses of endotoxin [24].

Bacteremia

In a murine peritonitis model [25] utilizing either *E. coli* or *P. aeruginosa*, rBPI$_{21}$
significantly increased survival, reduced serum cytokine levels, and enhanced clearance of bacteria from the blood and peritoneal cavity. Although when administered
alone rBPI$_{21}$ was found to be ineffective against *E. coli* O111:B4 in this model rBPI$_{21}$
was shown to improve survival and enhance bacterial clearance when given with
antibiotics, compared to a group which received antibiotics alone. Similarly, a chi-
meric BPI molecule improved mortality and reduced serum endotoxin levels in
neutropenic rats challenged with *P. aeruginosa* [26]; and rBPI$_{23}$ improved survival,
enhanced bacterial clearance, ameliorated hemodynamic alterations, and reduced
pulmonary edema, microvascular congestion and hepatic steatosis in a neutropenic
rat model challenged with an intravenous infusion of *E. coli* [27].

In a conscious rabbit model of *E. coli* bacteremia, rBPI$_{21}$ alone and rBPI$_{21}$ together
with cefamandole inhibited the rise in endotoxin levels, accelerated clearance of
bacteria, and minimized sepsis-induced derangements in hemodynamics and pulmonary function [28]. Finally, both BPI and its bioactive N-terminal proteins were
shown to improve survival in two independent models of severe Gram-negative bacteremia in baboons [29, 30].

Healthy Human Volunteer Studies

There have been seven randomized, double-blind, placebo-controlled phase I pharmacokinetic and safety trials of rBPI$_{23}$ in healthy human volunteers, and nine such trials using rBPI$_{21}$. All of these studies indicate that bioactive N-terminal BPI proteins are safe and devoid of immunogenicity in healthy humans at the doses tested. Pharmacokinetic analysis indicates that rBPI$_{21}$ has a short half life in the circulation, with systemic mean residence times following 30 min infusions varying between 8 and 35 minutes (in a dose related fashion) [31].

Although data suggest that rBPI$_{21}$ is not immunogenic in normal humans, there have been questions raised concerning the use of rBPI$_{21}$ in patients with anti-BPI anti-neutrophil cytoplasmic autoantibodies (ANCA). These ANCA antibodies, which have been detected in patients with vasculitis, inflammatory bowel disease, and cystic fibrosis, recognize native holo-BPI. However, studies conducted to date indicate that these anti-BPI ANCA antibodies are directed against the C-terminal region of BPI and do not react with rBPI$_{21}$.

In addition to these studies, 8 male volunteers were challenged with endotoxin and concurrently with rBPI$_{23}$ or placebo in a randomized, double blind, placebo-controlled, crossover study. Compared to placebo, rBPI$_{23}$ significantly reduced the concentration of circulating endotoxin, TNF, TNF soluble receptors, IL-6, IL-8, IL-10, and neutrophil activation and degranulation [32]. In addition, rBPI$_{23}$ blunted LPS-induced procoagulant activation and activation of the fibrinolytic response.

BPI in Human Disease

Several reports have described the levels of BPI in humans during the course of disease. Wong and colleagues [33] prospectively examined the plasma BPI concentrations in critically ill children with or without sepsis. They documented that patients with sepsis had a significantly higher level of BPI than non-septic patients, and that BPI levels were positively associated with the pediatric risk of mortality (PRISM) score. Similarly, Calvano et al. [34] reported elevations in BPI and LBP following endotoxin challenge in humans, and further showed that BPI expression on neutrophils was up-regulated in surgical ICU patients with Gram-negative sepsis. In other studies, BPI has been detected not only in plasma, but also in bronchoalveolar lavage fluid, in pleural fluid, in wound fluid, in peritoneal fluid, and in the gut mucosa.

Clinical Trials

Bioactive N-terminal BPI proteins possess multiple anti-infective properties which together are associated with improved biochemical values, clinical physiology, and survival in numerous models of infection in rodents, rabbits, and pigs, and in non-human and human primates under a variety of experimental conditions. Coupled with a favorable safety profile, clinical trials in ill patients using rBPI$_{21}$ were begun in mid-1995.

Meningococcemia

Rationale

Severe invasive infection with the Gram-negative diplococci *Neisseria meningitidis* is associated with high mortality and morbidity including gangrene of extremities. These infections are associated with markedly elevated plasma levels of bacterial endotoxin (both on intact bacteria and on bacterial membranes shed into the circulation), and subsequent induction of inflammatory responses including cytokines, nitric oxide, and coagulation. $rBPI_{21}$ has multiple anti-infective properties to this disease, including direct bactericidal activity against *Neisseria meningitidis*, as well as binding to bacterial endotoxin and bacterial membranes resulting in clearance and neutralization.

Clinical Study

This was an open label, dose escalation, multicenter trial in pediatric patients (1–18 years) conducted in the United States [35]. Patients had a clinical diagnosis of meningococcemia and were required to have severe disease according to the Glasgow meningococcal septicemia prognostic score. Twenty-six patients were enrolled and received a short 30 minute infusion of $rBPI_{21}$ (to quickly achieve high levels in the blood) followed by a continuous infusion over 24 hours. All patients received standard care in the ICU including parenteral antibiotics. Plasma levels of $rBPI_{21}$ were consistent with those predicted from data in healthy adults, and were in the range required for bacterial killing. One of the twenty-six patients died (mortality 4%), compared to an expected mortality of at least 20% based on a matched historical series or independent prognostic indices. All adverse events were considered "probably not related" to $rBPI_{21}$, but were consistent with common complications of meningococcemia [35].

Ongoing Studies

A phase III, randomized, placebo-controlled multicenter trial in pediatric patients (12 weeks – 18 years) with severe meningococcemia is currently underway in the United States, Canada, and the United Kingdom.

Major Liver Resection

Rationale

Major hepatic resection, including hemihepatectomy, is associated with high postoperative morbidity including hepatic failure, disseminated intravascular coagulation, and infection. It has been shown that liver damage after surgery results from an inflammatory activation, believed to be induced by translocation of intestinally derived bacteria and their components. Animal studies indicate that the multiple anti-infective properties of $rBPI_{21}$ reduce hepatic damage following major liver resection in rodents.

Clinical Study

This was a randomized, double-blind, placebo-controlled, multicenter dose escalation study in patients undergoing major liver resection. The first twelve patients were enrolled in the low dose phase, and there was one death in the placebo group of six patients occurring during the 28-day study period. In this low dose group, the pharmacokinetics of $rBPI_{21}$ were consistent with data from healthy adults. There were no safety concerns noted for $rBPI_{21}$. When compared to the controls, the $rBPI_{21}$ treated group showed trends toward fewer days in the hospital, fewer days in the ICU, and decreased time on ventilators.

Ongoing Study

A higher dose phase of the study has begun, in which additional patients will be enrolled and followed for a 28-day study period.

Hemorrhage Due to Trauma

Rationale

Acute trauma with hemorrhage results in substantial mortality, morbidity, and cost. Among patients who survive the initial insult, a significant proportion develop infections and infectious complications such as multiple organ failure. There are compelling data in rodents, primates, and humans, that the hemorrhagic trauma is associated with translocation of bacteria and bacterial products from the gut. Such translocation may be critical in the development of late mortality and morbidity. For example, in a rat hemorrhage and reperfusion model [36], treatment with $rBPI_{21}$ reduced mortality from 62% to 31%, decreased levels of circulating bacterial endotoxin, and reduced the incidence of multiorgan damage. The multiple anti-infective properties of $rBPI_{21}$, including direct bacterial killing and clearance/neutralization of endotoxin on bacterial membranes raises the possibility that $rBPI_{21}$ might be useful in preventing infections and infectious complications following hemorrhagic trauma.

Clinical Trial

A multicenter, randomized, double-blind, placebo-controlled phase II study has completed accrual. In this study, 401 adult patients with traumatic injuries requiring at least two units of blood replacement were treated with $rBPI_{21}$ or placebo, in addition to standard care. Additionally, a multicenter, randomized, single-blind, placebo controlled phase II trial comparing placebo treatment and $rBPI_{21}$ treatment given as 3 treatment regimens has also completed accrual.

Ongoing Study

A phase III trial in hemorrhagic trauma is expected to begin during the fall of 1997.

Cystic Fibrosis

Rationale

Cystic fibrosis (CF) is an autosomal recessive disease which results from a defective chloride transporter. Clinically, patients suffer chronic pulmonary infections and develop bronchiectasis and chronic lung disease. Pathogens typically isolated from CF patients' lungs include *Staphylococcus aureus*, *Haemophilus influenza*, and *Pseudomonas aeruginosa*. Early aggressive treatment of pulmonary infectious exacerbations, combined with aggressive nutritional support, has resulted in improved duration and quality of life for CF patients. However, pulmonary flora rapidly become resistant to conventional antibiotics, limiting the effectiveness of traditional therapeutics and leading to progressive disease. Recently, *in vitro* studies using clinical bacterial isolates from CF patients and $rBPI_{21}$ alone or in combination with a panel of antibiotics, have demonstrated that isolates representing several genera were either killed by $rBPI_{21}$ alone, or were made more sensitive to conventional antibiotics when tested in the presence of clinically achievable concentrations of $rBPI_{21}$.

Ongoing Study

An open label, pharmacokinetic study of $rBPI_{21}$ in patients with CF (6 years and older) has recently begun. After initial safety and pharmacokinetics have been assessed, a dose escalation phase is planned.

Conclusion

$rBPI_{21}$ is a novel human protein which has multiple anti-infective properties, including direct killing of bacteria and enhancement of the anti-bacterial effects of conventional antibiotics, as well as binding to bacterial endotoxin (whether present on intact bacteria, on shed bacterial membrane fragments, or freely dispersed in the circulation), resulting in clearance and neutralization. These properties make $rBPI_{21}$ distinct from previous monoclonal antibodies used in phase III trials for sepsis. Additional biological properties of the molecule that may have clinical application are currently under investigation.

References

1. Weiss J, Elsbach P, Olsson I, Odeberg H (1978) Purification and characterization of a potent bactericidal and membrane active protein from the granules of human polymorphonuclear leukocytes. J Biol Chem 253.8:2664–2672
2. Weiss J, Olsson I (1987) Cellular and subcellular localization of the bactericidal/permeability-increasing protein of neutrophils. Blood 69:652–659
3. Gray PW, Corcorran AE, Eddy RL, Byers MG, Shows TB (1993) The genes for the lipopolysaccharide binding protein (LPB) and the bactericidal/permeability-increasing protein (BPI) are encoded in the same region of human chromosome 20. Genomics 15:188–190
4. Beamer LJ, Carroll SF, Eisenberg D (1997) Crystal structure of human BPI and two bound phospholipids at 2.4 Angstrom resolution. Science 276:1861–1864
5. Ooi CE, Weiss J, Elsbach P, Frangione B, Mannion B (1987) A25-kDa NH2-terminal fragment carries all the antibacterial activities of the human neutrophil 60-kDa bactericidal/permeability-increasing protein. J Biol Chem 262:14891–14894
6. Appelmelk BJ, An Y-Q, Thijs BG, MacLaren DM, De Graaff J (1994) Recombinant human bactericidal/permeability-increasing protein (rBPI$_{21}$) is a universal lipopolysaccharide-binding ligand. Infect Immun 62:3564–3567
7. Capodici C, Chen S, Sidorczyk Z, Elsbach P, Weiss J (1994) Effect of lipopolysaccharide (LPS) chain length on interactions of bactericidal/permeability-increasing protein and its bioactive 23-Kilodalton NH2-Terminal fragment with isolated LPS and intact proteus mirabilis and Escherichia coli. Infect Immun 62:259–265
8. Weiss J, Elsbach P, Shu C, et al (1992) Human bactericidal/permeability-increasing protein and a recombinant NH2-Terminal fragment cause killing of serum-resistant gram-negative bacteria in whole blood and inhibit tumor necrosis factor release induced by the bacteria. J Clin Invest 90:1122–1130
9. Veld Gl, Mannion B, Weiss J, Elsbach P (1988) Effects of the bactericidal/permeability-increasing protein of polymorphonuclear leukocytes on isolated bacterial cytoplasmic membrane vesicles. Infect Immun 56:1203–1208
10. Levy O, Ooi CE, Weiss J, Lehrer RI, Elsbach P (1994) Individual and synergistic effects of rabbit granulocyte proteins on Escherichia coli. J Clin Invest 94:672–682
11. Marra MN, Wilde CG, Griffithe JE (1990) Bactericidal/permeability-increasing protein has endotoxin-neutralizing activity. J Immunol 144:662–666
12. Ulevitch RJ, Tobias PS (1995) Receptor-dependent mechanisms of cell stimulation by bacterial endotoxin. Annu Rev Immunol 13:437–457
13. Gazzano-Santoro H, Meszaros K, Birr C, et al (1994) Competition between rBPI$_{23}$, a recombinant fragment of bactericidal/permeability-increasing protein, and lipopolysaccharide (LPS)-binding protein for binding to LPS and gram-negative bacteria. Infect Immun 62:1185–1191
14. Katz SS, Chen K, Doerfler ME, Elsbach P, Weiss J (1996) Potent CD14-mediated signalling of human leukocytes by Escherichia coli can be mediated by interaction of whole bacteria and host cells without extensive prior release of endotoxin. Infect Immun 64:3592–3600
15. Huang K, Fishwild DM, Wu H-M, Dedrick R (1995) Lipopolysaccharide-induced E-selectin expression requires continuous presence of LPS and is inhibited by bactericidal/permeability-increasing protein. Inflammation 19:389–404
16. Corradin SB, Heumann D, Gallay P, Smith J, Mauel J, Glauser MP (1994) Bactericidal/permeability-increasing protein inhibits induction of macrophage nitric oxide production by lipopolysaccharide. J Infect Dis 169:105–111
17. Meszaros K, Parent JB, Gazzano-Santoro H, et al (1993) A recombinant amino terminal fragment of bactericidal/permeability-increasing protein inhibits the induction of leukocyte responses by LPS. J Leukocyte Biol 54:558–563
18. Arditi M, Zhou J, Huang SH, Luckett PM, Marra MN, Kim KS (1994) Bactericidal/permeability-increasing protein protects vascular endothelial cells from lipopolysaccharide-induced activation and injury. Infect Immun 62:3930–3936
19. Dedrick R, Conlon PJ (1995) Prolonged expression of lipopolysaccharide (LPS)-induced inflammatory genes in whole blood requires continual exposure to LPS. Infect Immun 63:1362–1368

20. Fisher CJ, Marra MN, Palardy JE, Marchbanks CR, Scott RW, Opal SM (1994) Human neutrophil bactericidal/permeability-increasing protein reduces mortality from endotoxin challenge: a placebo-controlled study. Crit Care Med 22:553–558

21. Lin Y, Kohn FR, Kung AHC, Ammons WS (1994) Protective effect of a recombinant fragment of bactericidal/permeability increasing protein against carbohydrate dyshomeostasis and tumor necrosis factor-a elevation in rat endotoxemia. Biochem Pharmacol 47:1553–1559

22. Ammons WS, Kung AHC (1993) Recombinant amino terminal fragment of bactericidal/permeability-increasing protein prevents hemodynamic responses to endotoxin. Circ Shock 41: 176–184

23. Vandermeer TJ, Menconi MJ, O'Sullivan BP, et al (1994) Bactericidal/permeability-increasing protein ameliorates acute lung injury in porcine endotoxema. J Appl Physiol 76:2006–2014

24. Marra MN, Thornton MB, Snable JL, Wilde CG, Scott RW (1994) Endotoxin-binding and -neutralizing properties of recombinant bactericidal/permeability-increasing protein and monoclonal antibodies HA-1A and E5. Crit Care Med 22:559–565

25. Ammons WS, Kohn FR, Kung AHC (1994) Protective effects of an N-terminal fragment of bactericidal/permeability-increasing protein in rodent models of gram-negative sepsis: Role of bactericidal properties. J Infect Dis 170:1473–1482

26. Opal SM, Palardy JE, Jhung JW, et al (1995) Activity of lipopolysaccharide-binding protein-bactericidal/permeability-increasing protein fusion peptide in an experimental model of pseudomonas sepsis. Antimicrob Agents Chemother 39:2813–2815

27. Lechner AJ, Lamprech KE, Johanns CA, Matuschak GM (1995) The recombinant 23-kDa N-terminal fragment of bactericidal/permeability-increasing protein (rBPI-23) decreases Escherichia coli-induced mortality and organ injury during immunosuppression-related neutropenia. Shock 4:298–306

28. Lin Y, Leach WJ, Ammons WS (1996) Synergistic effect of a recombinant N-terminal fragment of bactericidal/permeability-increasing protein and cefamandole in treatment of rabbit gram-negative sepsis. Antimicrob Agents Chemother 40:65–69

29. Rogy MA, Oldenburg HSA, Calvano SE, et al (1994) The Role of bactericidal/permeability-increasing protein in the treatment of primate bacteremia and septic shock. J Clin Immunol 14:120–133

30. Rogy MA, Moldawer LL, Oldenburg HSA, et al (1994) Anti-endotoxin therapy in primate bacteremia with HA-1A and BPI. Ann Surg 220:77–85

31. Bauer RJ, White ML, Nelson BJ, et al (1996) A phase I safety and pharmacokinetic study of a recombinant amino terminal fragment of bactericidal/permeability-increasing protein in healthy male volunteers. Shock 5:91–96

32. von der Mohlen MAM, Kimmings AK, Wedel NI, et al (1995) Inhibition of endotoxin-induced cytokine release and neutrophil activation in humans by use of recombinant bactericidal/permeability-increasing protein. J Infect Dis 172:144–151

33. Wong HR, Doughty LA, Wedel N, et al (1995) Plasma bactericidal/permeability-increasing protein concentrations in critically ill children with the sepsis syndrome. Pediatr Infect Dis J 14:1087–1091

34. Calvano SE, Thompson WA, Marra MN, et al (1994) Changes in polymorphonuclear leukocyte surface and plasma bactericidal/permeability-increasing protein and plasma lipopolysaccharide binding protein during endotoxemia or sepsis. Arch Surg 129:220–226

35. Giroir BP, Quint PA, Barton P, et al (1997) Preliminary evaluation of recombinant amino-terminal fragment of human bactericidal/permeability-increasing protein in children with severe meningococcal disease. Lancet 350:1439–1443

36. Yao YM, Bahrami S, Leichtfried G, Redl H, Schlag G (1995) Pathogenesis of hemorrhage-induced bacteria/endotoxin translocation in rats. Ann Surg 221:398–405

Inhibition of the Activation of Nuclear Factor-κB as a Novel Therapeutic Approach for SIRS and Septic Shock

G. Wray and C. Thiemermann

Introduction

It is now widely accepted that the release of pro-inflammatory cytokines [e.g., tumor necrosis factor-α (TNF-α), interleukin-1 (IL-1), IL-6], the expression on endothelium and neutrophils of adhesion molecules, and the overproduction of vasoactive mediators (e.g., nitric oxide, eicosanoids) play important roles in the pathophysiology of sepsis and septic shock. The expression of inducible genes leading to the formation of these proteins and autacoids relies on transcription factors which are either controlled by (other) inducible genes and, hence, require *de novo* protein synthesis or alternatively by so-called "primary transcription factors". Among the latter, nuclear factor-kappa B (NF-κB) has received a considerable amount of attention because of its unique mechanism of activation, its active role in cytoplasmic/nuclear signaling, and its rapid response to pathogenic stimulation of cells [1, 2]. NF-κB was first identified some 10 years ago as a regulator of the expression of the kappa-light chain gene in murine B lymphocytes, but has subsequently been identified in most, if not all cell types studied [3–5]. In the last few years, it has become apparent that NF-κB plays a central role in the regulation of many genes responsible for the generation of proteins and mediators which play a role in local and systemic inflammation as well as circulatory shock. This article reviews the mechanisms involved in the regulation of the activation of NF-κB, highlights the consequences of the activation of this transcription factor and points to novel therapeutic approaches aimed at preventing the activation of NF-κB in animal models of endotoxin shock. We propose that interventions which interfere with the activation of NK-κB may be useful in the therapy of circulatory shock or other disorders associated with local or systemic inflammation.

Regulation of the Activation of NF-κB

NF-κB is the prototype of a family of dimeric transcription factors made from monomers that have approximately 300 amino acid Rel regions which bind to deoxyribonucleic acid (DNA), interact with each other, and bind the IκB inhibitors. The most frequent form of human NF-κB is a dimer composed of two DNA-binding proteins, namely NF-κB1 (or p50) and RelA (or p65), although other dimeric combinations (which may include RelA and p50, Rel B, c-Rel and p52) also exist [6]. Under physiological conditions, NF-κB is held (in an inactive or "dormant" form) in

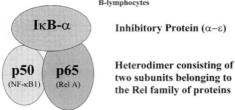

Nuclear factor-κ B (NF-κB)

identified as a factor that regulates κ-light-chain expression in murine
B-lymphocytes

IκB-α   **Inhibitory Protein (α–ε)**

p50   **p65**   **Heterodimer consisting of**
(NF-κB1) (Rel A)   **two subunits belonging to**
                        the Rel family of proteins

Fig. 1. Schematic representation of the
structure of human NF-κB

the cytoplasm by the inhibitory protein IκB-α, which avidly binds to most hetero-
dimers including the NF-κB1/Rel A heterodimer. This inhibitory subunit can be
considered as a cytoplasmatic anchor, as it prevents the nuclear uptake of NF-κB
(Fig. 1).

Activation of NF-κB involves the release of the inhibitory subunit IκB-α from a
cytoplasmic complex, which IκB forms together with the DNA-binding subunit
Rel A and NF-κB1 [4, 5]. Activation of NF-κB allows the p50/p65 subunits to translocate to the nucleus and to induce the expression of specific genes. There is some
evidence that p50 and p65 can be independently transported into the nucleus due to
a conserved cluster of positively charged amino acid residues in the C-terminal end
of their NRD domains serving as nuclear location signals [9].

The cascade of events leading to the activation of NF-κB involves the signal-induced phosphorylation of IκB-α (Fig. 2a) resulting in its ubiquitination and proteolytic degradation in proteosomes (Fig. 2b) and ultimately in the release of NF-κB
from its cytoplasmatic anchor (Fig. 2c). NF-κB then translocates into the nucleus,

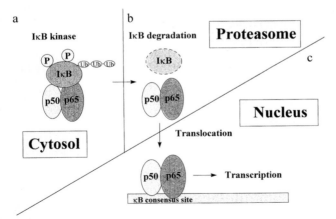

Fig. 2. Cascade of events leading to the activation of NF-κB including (**a**) activation of IκB kinase in
the cytosol leading to the phosphorylation of IκB and ubiquitination (Ub) of this inhibitor, (**b**) pro-
tealytic degradation of IκB in the proteasome leading to the release of p50/p65 which (**c**) is now
able to translocate into the nucleus where it binds to a κB consensus site

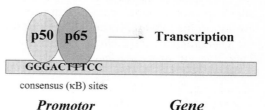

Proteolysis of IκB uncovers nuclear localization signals on the Rel proteins, which results in rapid translocation of NF-κB to the nucleus

Fig. 3. Binding of p50/p65 to the κB consensus motif in the 5'region of the promotor of specific target genes results in their expression

consensus (κB) sites

Promotor   *Gene*

where it binds to consensus (or κB) sites located in the upstream (5′) promotor region of a variety of genes (Fig. 3) [10].

Activation of NF-κB

NF-κB is itself activated by the exposure of cells to endotoxin (lipopolysaccharide, LPS), pro-inflammatory cytokines e.g. TNF-α and IL-1, or oxidants to name but a few. Table 1 provides an (incomplete) list of the many factors which have been reported to result in the activation of NF-κB [3, 7–11]. The signaling pathway which ultimately leads to the expression of certain genes by NF-κB comprises phosphorylation, ubiquitination (in proteasomes) and finally degradation of IκB. The

Table 1. Factors activating NF-κB

Cytokines	Tumor necrosis factor-α (TNF-α)
	Lymphtoxin (TNF-β)
	Interleukin-1β
	Interleukin-2
	Leukotriene B4
	Lymphocyte inhibitory factor
Bacterial products	Lipopolysaccharide
	Exotoxin B
	Toxic shock syndrome toxin 1
	Muramyl peptides
Viruses	Human immunodeficiency virus 1 (HIV-1)
	Human T-cell leukemia virus type 1 (HTLV-1)
	Herpes simplex virus type 1
	Epstein-Barr virus (EBV)
	Adenovirus
	Influenzavirus
	Rhinovirus
Oxidants	Hydrogen peroxide
	Ozone
Physical stress	Ultraviolet radiation
	γ radiation

first step in the activation of NF-κB is the activation of IκB kinase(s) in the cytosol which results in the phosphorylation of IκB on serine 32 and 36 of the protein (Fig. 2a). This event leads to the subsequent conjugation with ubiquitin which allows the degradation of the IκB in proteasomes (see below). Although the exact events leading to the activation of IκB kinase are unclear, there is good evidence that the generation of intracellular oxygen-derived free radicals plays a pivotal role. Thus, it is not surprising that

- the intracellular "redox status" of the cell is of the utmost importance,
- many oxidants facilitate the activation of NF-κB, while,
- many anti-oxidants may function as inhibitors of this transcription factor.

As the gene for IκBα also contains a κB recognition site in its promotor region, NF-κB itself induces the synthesis of IκB, which, when encountering activated NF-κB, binds to this activated transcription factor resulting in the (re)generation of a "dormant" cytosolic form.

Role of the Proteasome in the Activation of NF-κB

The multicatalytic proteinase or the "proteasome" is a highly conserved cellular structure which is responsible for the adenosine triphosphate (ATP)-dependent rapid degradation (proteolysis) of many rate-limiting enzymes (e.g., ornithine decarboxylase), critical regulatory proteins (e.g., cyclins in cell growth) and transcription factors, such as NF-κB [12]. Despite the abundance, characteristic appearance, and unique properties of the proteasome, progress in the understanding of its function has, until recently, been slow. The 20S proteasome (700-kDa) is a complex containing multiple subunits (20–35-Kda each) which contains a large internal cavity or "proteolytic pore". The 20S proteasome (in eukaryotes) contains at least 5 identifiable proteolytic activities. Although the 20S proteasome does contain a proteolytic pore, it cannot degrade proteins *in vivo* unless it is complexed with a 19S cap, at either end of its structure, which itself contains multiple ATPase activities. This larger structure, termed 26S proteasome, will rapidly degrade proteins that have been targeted for degradation by the addition of multiple molecules of the 8.5-Kda polypeptide, ubiquitin (reviewed in [12]). Hence, this ubiquitination step in the activation of the proteasome serves as a regulatory mechanism and allows for the degradation of specific proteins, such as NF-κB.

Proteins Regulated by NF-κB

Activation of NF-κB results in the expression of the genes of the following pro-inflammatory cytokines, many of which play an important role in the pathophysiology of systemic inflammatory response syndrome (SIRS) and septic shock: TNF-α, Il-1, IL-2, Il-6, IL-8, granulocyte-colony stimulating factor (G-CSF) and macrophage-colony stimulating factor (M-CSF). In addition, activation of NF-κB results in the expression of the genes of several chemokines (Table 2, Fig. 4), adhesion molecules, such as intercellular adhesion molecule-1 (ICAM-1) and vascular adhesion mole-

Table 2. Proteins regulated by NF-κB

Cytokines/chemokines	Tumor necrosis factor-α (TNF-α)
	Interleukin-1β
	Interleukin-2
	Interleukin-6
	Interleukin-8
	Granulocyte colony stimulating factor (G-CSF)
	Macrophage colony stimulating factor (M-CSF)
Inflammatory enzymes	Inducible nitric oxide synthase (iNOS)
	Inducible cyclooxygenase-2 (COX II)
	5-lipoxygenase
	Phospholipase A_2
Acute phase proteins	Angiotensinogen
	Serum amyloid A precursor
	Complement factor B
	Complement factor C4
Adhesion molecules	Intercellular adhesion molecule 1 (ICAM 1)
	Vascular adhesion molecule 1 (VCAM 1)
	E-selectin
Receptors	T-cell receptor (β chain)
	Interleukin-2 receptor (α chain)

cule-1 (VCAM-1), as well as certain pro-inflammatory enzymes. The latter include the inducible isoform of nitric oxide synthase (iNOS or NOS II) [13, 14], the expression of which results in an overproduction of nitric oxide (NO) which contributes to the circulatory failure (hypotension and vascular hyporeactivity of the vasculature to vasoconstrictor agents) in animals and man with endotoxin or septic shock [15].

Interestingly, lipoteichoic acid (LTA), a fragment of the cell wall of Gram-positive bacteria, which synergizes with peptidoglycan to cause the induction of iNOS, shock and multiple organ failure (in the rat) also causes the activation of NF-κB in macrophages, as the induction of iNOS caused by LTA is prevented by several agents which interfere with the activation of NF-κB [16] (Fig. 4). In addition to iNOS, activation of NF-κB is essential for the expression of the inducible isoform of cyclooxygenase (or COX-2) and phospholipase A_2, both of which importantly contribute to the well documented overproduction of prostaglandins in shock. Last, but not least, activation of NF-κB results in the expression of the gene for 5-lipoxygenase and, hence, may contribute to an enhanced formation of chemotactic and vasoactive 5-lipoxygenase metabolites. It should also be noted that NF-κB regulates the expression of the genes of the receptors for IL-2 as well as the T-cell receptor (α chain). Some (but not all) of the proteins regulated by NF-κB are depicted in Table 2.

Inhibition of the Activation of NF-κB

Some naturally occuring inhibitors of NF-κB have been identified including gliotoxin derived from *aspergillus* [17]. The activation of IκB kinase can be prevented by various agents known to be radical scavengers. These include rotenone, butylated

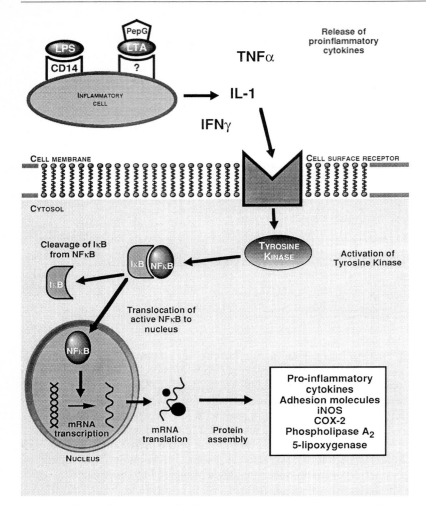

Fig. 4. Signal transduction events leading to the expression of genes regulated by NF-κB in cells activated, e.g., with pro-inflammatory cytokines. Binding of endotoxin (LPS) or lipoteichoic acid (LTA), together with peptidoglycan (PepG) to their receptors, e.g., on macrophages, leads to the release of TNF-α, IL-1 and interferon-γ (IFN-γ). These cytokines bind to specific receptors on target cells, which leads to the tyrosine kinase-dependent activation of NF-κB resulting in the expression of specific target genes

hydroxyanisole (BHA) and pyrrolidine dithiocarbamate (PDTC). Moreover, aspirin, sodium salicylate and N-acetylcysteine (at very high concentrations) attenuate the activation of NF-κB by a mechanism which may involve anti-oxidant effects of these agents. Interestingly, IL-10 (which has been reported to improve survival in animal models of endotoxin shock) also prevents the activation of NF-κB [11].

In addition to preventing the activation of IκB-kinase, the activation of NF-κB can be attenuated or prevented by inhibiting the proteolytic degradation of IκB in the proteasome. In recent years, several serine protease inhibitors have been reported to inhibit the proteolytic cleavage of proteins in the proteasome. These include the peptide aldehydes N-acetyl-l-leucinyl-l-leucinyl-l-norleucinyl (ALLN), a compound which is better known as "calpain I inhibitor" or "calpain inhibitor I". In addition to calpain inhibitor I, other peptide aldehydes including N-acetyl-L-leucinyl-l-leucinyl-methional (LLM) and N-carboxybenzoxyl-l-leucinyl-l-leucinyl-norvalinal (MG115) are also potent inhibitors of the 20S proteasome [18]. A series of α-ketocarbonyl and boronic ester derived dipeptides [19] and epoxyketones [20] have also been described that are new inhibitors of the proteasome. Most notably, Lum and colleagues [21] have recently described a series of potent and specific inhibitors of the 20S proteasome, termed CVT-634. The following paragraphs review the effects of some of these agents on the activation of NF-κB, the release of pro-inflammatory cytokines, shock and multiple organ failure.

The molecular evidence of the effects of glucocorticoids in inflammation is not well understood, but there is recent evidence that glucocorticoids inhibit the action of the transcription factors AP-1 and NF-κB [11]. It is now well established that glucocorticoids bind to cytosolic receptors which then translocate into the nucleus and bind (as a homodimer) to glucocorticoid-response elements located on the promotor of target genes. This results in an increase in transcription of many proteins including lipocortin 1 [22]. There is some evidence that there is a direct protein-protein interaction between the activated glucocorticoid receptor and NF-κB, resulting in prevention of its binding to the κB consensus motif on the promotor of its target genes. In addition, glucocorticoids enhance the formation of IκBα, which results in an excess of this inhibitory factor in the nucleus and cytosol. Thus, activated NF-κB (following the degradation of IκB in the proteasome) when "travelling" to the nucleus meets with and binds to IκBα to form its "dormant" (inactive) cytosolic form. For a detailed review of the mechanisms by which glucocorticoids interfere with the activation of NFκB, the interested reader is referred to a recent, excellent review of this topic [11].

Inhibition of the Activation of NF-κB in Cells Challenged with Endotoxin

In RAW macrophages activated with endotoxin, calpain inhibitor I attenuates the degradation of IκB in the proteasome as well as the processing of the p65/p50 complex to p50. This results in the accumulation of IκB in the cytosol of LPS-activated macrophages, whereas this cannot be detected in macrophages which have not been pre-treated with calpain inhibitor I. Thus, calpain inhibitor I specifically interferes with the proteolytic cleavage of IκB and hence prevents the activation of NF-κB [23]. In addition to preventing the activation of cells challenged with endotoxin, calpain inhibitor I also attenuates the activation of murine macrophages challenged with wall fragments of Gram-positive bacteria. The mechanism(s) by which Gram-positive bacteria cause circulatory failure and multiple organ dysfunction was, until recently, largely unknown. We have reviewed the synergism of two wall fragments from the Gram-positive bacterium *Staphylococcus aureus*, namely LTA and peptidoglycan (PepG) to cause shock and multiple organ dysfunction syndrome (MODS) [24] (Fig. 4). Interestingly, the circulatory failure caused by coadministration of LTA and PepG [25] was attenuated by inhibitors of NOS activity as well as prevented by dexamethasone. In cultured macrophages, LTA causes the expression and activation of iNOS protein. The expression afforded by LTA in these cells is attenuated by inhibitors of protein tyrosine kinase (such as genistein or tyrphostins) (Fig. 4) as well as by various interventions known to intefere with the activation of NF-κB. These include the radical scavengers rotenone and BHA as well as PDTC and L-1-tosylamido-2-phenylethyl chloromethyl ketone (TPCK) [26]. These studies indicate that the induction of iNOS caused by LTA *in vitro* requires the activation of NF-κB. In addition, we have compared the effects of

- agents known to attenuate the activation of NF-κB [e.g., calpain inhibitor I, TPCK, N-carbobenzoxy-L-phenylalanine chloromethyl ketone (ZPCK)],
- proteases which do not attenuate the activation of NF-κB [e.g., chymostatin, leupeptins, (negative control)] and
- dexamethasone (positive control) on the accumulation of nitrite in the supernatant of murine macrophages (cell line J774.2) activated with endotoxin.

Activation of J774.2 macrophages resulted, within 24 h, in a significant increase in nitrite in the cell supernatant (from 0.9 ± 0.2 μM to 36 ± 1 μM). Calpain inhibitor I, TPCK, ZPCK (IC_{50}: ~ 10 μM) and dexamethasone (IC_{50}: ~ 0.1 μM) all caused concentration-dependent inhibition of the formation of nitrite elicited by LPS. In contrast, neither chymostatin nor leupeptin, which are inhibitors of cysteine and serine protease activity, respectively, and which do not prevent the activation of NF-κB [27], did not attenuate the increase in nitrite formation in the supernatant of macrophages activated with LPS [28]. Thus, the induction of iNOS activity afforded by either LTA or LPS in cultured macrophages also requires the activation of NF-κB (Fig. 4).

Inhibition of the Activation of NF-κB in Animal Models of Endotoxemia

Knowing that NO plays a pivotal role in the pathophysiology of shock of various etiologies [15, 29] and based on the above *in vitro* findings, we proposed in 1996 that the prevention of NF-κB activation may be useful in the therapy of circulatory shock. To test this hypothesis, we have investigated the effects of calpain inhibitor I, chymostatin and dexamethasone on the circulatory failure, the multiple organ dysfunction, and the induction and activity of iNOS and COX-2 protein in rats with endotoxic shock [28].

Beneficial Hemodynamic Effects of Calpain Inhibitor I in Shock

In anesthetized rats, administrazion of LPS (10 mg·kg^{-1}) caused a rapid (within 15 min), but transient fall in mean arterial pressure (MAP) which had partly recovered by 180 min. After 180 min, there was a second, further fall in MAP from 102 ± 4 mmHg to 73 ± 5 mmHg at 360 min. This delayed fall in MAP, was abolished by both dexamethasone (1 mg·kg^{-1}) and calpain inhibitor I (3 or 10 mg·kg^{-1}). Injection of LPS resulted, within 360 min, in a more than 50% reduction in the pressor response elicited by norepinephrine (vascular hyporeactivity). This vascular hyporeactivity to norepinephrine was attenuated by both dexamethasone and calpain inhibitor I. The circulatory failure was, however, not affected by administration of calpain inhibitor I ($10 \text{ mg} \cdot \text{kg}^{-1}$) given 2 h after LPS (late administration), suggesting that agents which prevent the activation of NF-κB have to be given early on in endotoxemia to achieve a maximal therapeutic benefit. Similarly, the serine protease inhibitor chymostatin did not affect the circulatory failure caused by LPS, suggesting that the observed beneficial hemodynamic effects of calpain inhibitor I were indeed due to prevention of the activation of NF-κB, and not due to its ability to inhibit the activity of (other) serine proteases.

Calpain Inhibitor I Attenuates the Multiple Organ Dysfunction Syndrome Caused by Endotoxin in the Rat

Endotoxemia for 6 h was associated with a significant rise in the plasma levels of urea and creatinine (indicators of renal failure); bilirubin, alanine amino transferase

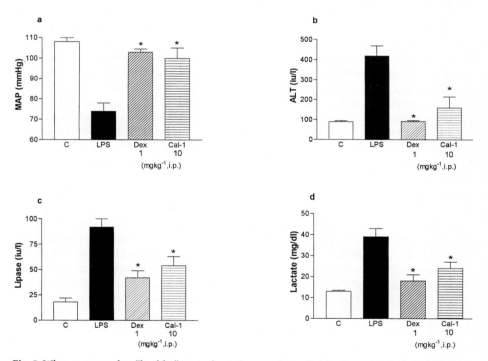

Fig. 5. When compared to "healthy" control rats (open columns), injection of endotoxin (black columns) leads within 6 h to (a) a substantial fall in mean arterial blood pressure (MAP), (b) a significant rise in the serum levels of alanine aminotransferase (ALT) indicating the development of hepatocellular injury, (c) a significant rise in the serum levels of lipase, indicating the development of pancreatic injury, and (d) a rise in serum lactate. Pre-treatment of rats with either dexamethasone (Dex, diagonal striped columns) or calpain inhibitor I (Cal-1, horizontally striped columns) prevents the hypotension as well as the multiple organ injury caused by endotoxin. *$p<0.05$ when compared to LPS control, ANOVA followed by Dunnett's *post hoc* test

(ALT) and aspartate amino transferase (AST), and γ-glutamyl transpeptidase (γGT) [all indicators of liver injury or failure]; lipase (an indicator of pancreatic injury); and lactate (Fig. 5). Dexamethasone, but not calpain inhibitor I, reduced the rise in the plasma levels of urea and creatinine caused by endotoxin. In contrast, pre-treatment with calpain inhibitor I prior to injection of rats with LPS attenuated the rises in the plasma levels of bilirubin, ALT (Fig. 5), AST and γGT, while the late administration of calpain inhibitor I (2 h after LPS) or chymostatin had no effect. Calpain inhibitor I also reduced the increase in the plasma levels of lipase and lactate caused by endotoxin (Fig. 5).

Injection of LPS also resulted in an increase in the serum level of TNF-α, which was attenuated by dexamethasone, but not by calpain inhibitor I. This study [28] provided the first evidence that calpain inhibitor I attenuates the circulatory failure as well as the liver injury/dysfunction and the pancreatic injury caused by endotoxin in the rat. There are several explanations for the effects of calpain inhibitor I in modifying the circulatory failure and MODS associated with endotoxemia. One could argue that some of the effects of calpain inhibitor I are due to the ability of this agent to inhibit the activity of serine or cysteine proteases. This is, however, unlikely as chymostatin, a potent inhibitor of such proteases [27], did not affect the circulatory failure nor the MODS caused by LPS. Thus, inhibition of protease activity is unlikely to account for the beneficial effects of calpain inhibitor I observed. We therefore proposed [28] that the effects of calpain inhibitor I are due to the inhibition of the activation of the transcription factor NF-κB. Clearly, activation of NF-κB plays an important role in the expression of iNOS [13, 14, 30]. An enhanced formation of NO by iNOS contributes to the circulatory failure caused by LPS in the anesthetized rat, as the selective inhibition of iNOS activity with 1400-W or L-NIL attenuates the delayed hypotension caused by LPS in this species (unpublished observation). Pretreatment of rats with calpain inhibitor I attenuates the increase in iNOS protein and activity in lungs and livers of rats with endotoxic shock [28]. Thus, the reduction in the expression of iNOS by calpain inhibitor I, this inhibitor of NF-κB, may contribute to (or account for) the attenuation of the circulatory failure caused by LPS in the rat.

TNF-α causes the activation of NF-κB [31] which, in certain cells, may result in the induction of iNOS (see above). Endogenous TNF-α also mediates the induction of iNOS [32] and, hence, the circulatory collapse [32, 33] as well as the liver injury [34, 35] caused by endotoxin. Interestingly, calpain inhibitor I does not attenuate the rise in the serum levels of TNF-α caused by endotoxin in the rat [28]. Thus, a reduction in the formation of TNF-α does not explain the inhibition by calpain inhibitor I of the expression of iNOS (and COX-2; see below) protein.

The promotor region of the murine and human COX-2 genes contains binding sites for NF-κB [36, 37]. The expression of the COX-2 gene is activated by oxidant stress [38], and reactive oxygen intermediates cause the activation of NF-κB [39] suggesting that NF-κB is one of the transcription factors involved. The increase in prostaglandin formation (COX activity) by murine osteoblasts (cell line MC3T3-E1) involves the activation of NF-κB [40]. In rats with endotoxemia, calpain inhibitor I attenuates the expression of COX-2 protein (in lung and liver) as well as the increase in the plasma levels of 6-keto-prostaglandin $F_{1\alpha}$ [28]. The reduction of the expression of COX-2 protein and activity by calpain inhibitor I is associated with beneficial hemodynamic effects (see above), but it is unclear whether the formation of arachidonic metabolites (by COX-2) contributes importantly to the pathophysiology of septic shock. Although there is some evidence that prostaglandins contribute to the hemodynamic alterations and the liver injury associated with endotoxic shock [41], the effects of selective inhibitors of COX-2 activity [42] on circulatory failure or MODS have not been investigated. Moreover, there are (to our knowledge) no studies evaluating the effects of anti-sense oligonucleotides against COX-2 mRNA in animal models of shock. Therefore, we cannot exclude that an enhanced formation of arachidonic acid metabolites by COX-2 contributes to the observed pathophysiology. It is impossible to predict if, and to what degree, reduction of the expression of COX-2 protein and activity contributes to the beneficial effects of calpain inhibitor I in rats with endotoxic shock. There is, however, evidence that the formation of arachidonic acid metabolites by COX-2 contributes to the inflammatory response caused by injection of carageenan into a subcutaneous air pouch of the rat, as this response is blocked by NS-393 as well as dexamethasone [43]. Thus, we propose that the reduction by calpain inhibitor I of the expression of COX-2 (caused, e.g., by cytokines) results in a potent anti-inflammatory effect of this inhibitor of IκBα proteolysis.

Like calpain inhibitor I, dexamethasone reduced the expression of iNOS and COX-2 and attenuated the circulatory failure, the hepatocellular injury and the pancreatic injury caused by LPS [28]. Indeed, the effects of dexamethasone and calpain inhibitor I were, with two exception, prevention of renal failure by dexamethasone, but not calpain inhibitor I, and reduction of the rise in serum levels of TNF-α by dexamethasone, but not calpain inhibitor I. These similar effects suggest a similar mechanism of action. Indeed, dexamethasone induces the transcription of the IκBα gene resulting in an increase in the synthesis of IκBα protein. Stimulation by TNF-α causes the release of NF-κB from IκBα (i.e. the activation of NF-κB). In cells pretreated with dexamethasone, the NF-κB released by TNF-α rapidly reassociates with (the newly synthesized) IκBα [31]. Thus, both dexamethasone (see above) and calpain inhibitor I significantly reduce the amounts of NF-κB which are able to translocate to the nucleus to initiate transcription of genes including those for COX-2 and iNOS.

Conclusion

There is increasing evidence, derived primarily from in vitro studies, that the activation of the transcription factor NF-κB plays a pivotal role in local or systemic inflammation. In 1997, we demonstrated that an agent which prevents the activation of NF-κB also attenuates the circulatory failure and the multiple organ dysfunction caused by endotoxin in the rat. The mechanism of the beneficial effect of this agent, calpain inhibitor I, is not entirely clear, but may include prevention of the expression of inducible enzymes (e.g., iNOS, COX-2, phospholipase A_2), adhesion molecules and cytokines. Thus, prevention of the activation of NF-κB may represent a novel approach for the therapy of circulatory shock (and other diseases associated with local or systemic inflammation) and deserves further investigation.

References

1. Nabel G, Baltimore D (1987) An inducible transcription factor activates expression of human immunodeficiency virus in T cells. Nature 326:711–713
2. Grimm S, Bauerle PA (1993) The inducible transcription factor NF-kappa B: structure function relationship of its protein subunit. Biochem J 290:297–308
3. Sen R, Baltimore D (1986) Inducibility of kappa immunoglobulin enhancer binding protein NF-kappa B by a posttranslation mechanism. Cell 47:921–928
4. Baeuerle PA, Baltimore D (1988) Activation of DNA-binding activity in an apparently cytoplasmic precursor of the NF-kappa B transcription factor. Cell 53:211–217
5. Baeuerle PA, Baltimore D (1988) I kappa B: a specific inhibitor of the NF-kappa B transcription factor. Science 242:540–546
6. Siebenlist U, Franzoso G, Brown K (1994) Structure, regulation and function of NF-kappa B. Ann Rev Cell Biol 10:405–455
7. Lowenthal JW, Ballard DW, Boehnlein E, Greene WC (1989) Tumor necrosis factor alpha induces proteins that bind specifically to kappa B-like enhancer elements and regulate interleukin 2 receptor alpha-chain gene expression in primary human T lymphocytes. Proc Natl Acad Sci USA 86:2331–2335
8. Arima N, Kuziel WA, Gardine TA, Greene WC (1992) IL-2-induced signal transduction involves the activation of nuclear NF-kappa B expression. J Immunol 149:83–91
9. Bauerle PA, Henkel T (1994) Function and activation of NF-κB in the immune system. Annu Rev Immunol 12:141–179
10. Henkel T, Machleidt T, Alkalay I, Kroenke M, Ben-neriah Y, Bauerle PA (1993) Rapid proteolysis of IKB-α is necessary for activation of transcription factor NF-κB. Nature 365:182–185
11. Barnes PJ, Karin M (1997) Nuclear factor-κB – A pivotal transcription factor in chronic inflammatory disease. N Eng J Med 336:1066–1071
12. Coux O, Tanaka K, Goldberg AL (1996) Structure and functions of the 20S and 26S proteasomes. Annu Rev Biochem 65:801–847
13. Griscavage JM, Wilk S, Ignarro LJ (1995) Serine and cysteine proteinase inhibitors prevent nitric oxide production by activated macrophages by interfering with transcription of the inducible NO synthase gene. Biochem Biophys Res Commun 215:721–729
14. Griscavage JM, Wilk S, Ignarro LJ (1996) Inhibitors of proteosome pathway interfere with induction of nitric oxide synthase in macrophages by blocking activation of transcription factor NF-kappa B. Proc Natl Acad Sci USA 93:3308–3312
15. Thiemermann C (1997) The use of selective inhibitors of inducible nitric oxide synthase in septic shock. Sepsis (in press)
16. Kengatharan M, De Kimpe SJ, Thiemermann C (1996) Analysis of the signal transduction in the induction of nitric oxide synthase by lipotechoic acid in macrophages. Br J Pharmacol 117:1163–1170
17. Pahl HL, Krauss B, Schulze-Osthoff K (1996) The immunosuppressive fungal metabolite gliotoxin specifically inhibits the transcription factor NF-κB. J Exp Med 183:89–96
18. Iqbal M, Chatterjee S, Kauer JC, et al (1996) Potent inhibitors of proteasome. J Med Chem 38:2276–2277
19. Iqbal M, Chatterjee S, Kauer JC, et al (1996) Potent a-ketocarbonyl and boronic ester derived inhibitors of proteasome. Biorg Med Chem Lett 6:287–290
20. Spaltenstein A, Leban JJ, Huang JJ, et al (1996) Design and synthesis of novel protease inhibitors tripeptide α',β'-epoxyketones as nanomolar inactivators of the proteasome. Tet Lett 37:1334–1346
21. Lum RT, Kerwar SS, Meyer SM, et al (1998) A new structural class of proteasome inhibitors that prevent NF-κB activation. Biochem Pharmacol (in press)
22. Wu CC, Croxtall JD, Perretti M, et al (1995) Lipopcortin-1 mediates the inhibition by dexamethasone of the induction by endotoxin of nitric oxide synthase in the rat. Proc Natl Acad Sci USA 92:3473–3477
23. Schow SR, Joly A (1997) N-acetyl-leucinyl-leucinyl-norleucinal inhibits lipopolysaccharide-induced NF-κB activation and prevents TNF and IL-6 synthesis in vivo. Cell Immunol 175:199–202

24. Kengatharan M, Thiemermann C (1997) Importance of cell wall components of gram-positive bacteria in gram-positive septic shock. In: Vincent JL (ed) 1997 Yearbook of intensive care and emergency medicine. Springer-Verlag, Berlin, Heidelberg, New York, pp 3–13

25. De Kimpe SJ, Hunter ML, Bryant CE, Thiemermann C, Vane JR (1995) Delayed circulatory failure due to the induction of nitric oxide synthase by lipoteichoic acid from Staphylococcus aureus in anaesthetized rats. Br J Pharmacol 114:1317–1323

26. Kengatheran M, De Kimpe SJ, Thiemermann C (1996) Analysis of the signal transduction in the induction of nictric oxide synthase by lipoteichoic acid in macrophages. Br J Pharmacol 117:1163–1170

27. Lin YC, Brown K, Siebenlist U (1995) Activation of NFκB requires proteolysis of the inhibitor IκB-α: Signal-induced phosphorylation of IκB-α alone does not release active NFκB. Proc Natl Acad Sci USA 92:552–556

28. Ruetten H, Thiemermann C (1997) Effect of calpain inhibitor I, an inhibitor of the proteolysis of IκB, on the circulatory failure and multiple organ dysfunction caused by endotoxin in the rat. Br J Pharmacol 121:695–704

29. Thiemermann C (1994) The role of arginine: nitric oxide pathway in circulatory shock. Adv Pharmacol 28:45–79

30. Xie Q, Kashiwabara Y, Nathan C (1994) Role of transcription factor NF-κB/Rel in induction of nitric oxide. J Biol Chem 269:4705–4708

31. Scheinman RI, Cogswell PC, Lofquist AK, Baldwin AS (1995) Role of transcriptional activation of I kappa B alpha in mediation of the immunosuppression by glucocorticostroids. Science 270:283–286

32. Thiemermann C, Wu CC, Szabo C, Perretti M, Vane JR (1993) Role of tumour necrosis factor in the induction of nitric oxide synthase in a rat model of endotoxic shock. Br J Pharmacol 110:177–182

33. Mozes T, Ben-efraim S, Tak CJ, Heiligers JP, Saxene PR, Bonta IL (1991) Serum levels of tumor necrosis factor determine the fatal or non-fatal course of endotoxic shock. Immunol Lett 27:157–162

34. De La-Mata M, Meager A, Rolando N, et al (1990) Tumour necrosis factor production in fulminant hepatic failure: relation to aetiology and superimposed microbial infection. Clin Exp Immunol 82:479–484

35. Hewett JA, Jean PA, Kunkel SL, Roth RA (1993) Relationship between tumor necrosis factor-alpha and neutrophils in endotoxin-induced liver injury. Am J Physiol 265:G1011–G1015

36. Sirois J, Levy LO, Simmons DL, Richards JS (1993) Characterization and hormonal regulation of the promoter of the rat prostaglandin endoperoxide synthase-2 gene in granulosa cells. Identification of functional and protein-binding regions. J Biol Chem 268:12199–12206

37. Appleby SB, Ristimaki A, Neilson K, Narko K, Hla T (1994) Structure of the human cyclo-oxygenase-2 gene. Biochem J 302:723–727

38. Feng L, Xia Y, Garcia GE, Hwang D, Wilson CB (1995) Involvement of reactive oxygen intermediates in cyclooxygenase-2 expression induced by interleukin-1, tumor necrosis factor-α, and lipopolysaccharide. J Clin Invest 95:1669–1675

39. Schreck R, Rieber P, Baeuerle PA (1991) Reactive oxygen intermediates as apparently widely used messengers in the activation of the NF-kappa B transcription factor and HIV-1. EMBO J 10:2247–2258

40. Yamamoto K, Arakawa T, Ueda N, Yamamoto S (1995) Transcriptional roles of nuclear factor κB and nuclear factor interleukin-6 in the tumor necrosis factor α-dependent induction of cyclo-oxygenase-2 in MC3T3-E1 cells. J Biol Chem 270:31315–31320

41. Feuerstein G, Hallenbeck JM (1987) Prostaglandins, leukotrienes, and platelet-activating factor in shock. Annu Rev Pharmacol Toxicol 27:301–313

42. Griswold DE, Adams JL (1996) Constitutive cyclooxygenase (COX-1) and inducible cyclooxygenase (COX-2): rationale for selective inhibition and progress to date. Med Res Rev 16:181–206

43. Masferrer JL, Zweifel BS, Manning PT, et al (1994) Selective inhibition of inducible cyclooxygenase 2 in vivo is antiinflammatory and nonulcerogenic. Proc Natl Acad Sci USA 91:3228–3232

The Role of the Host Defense Response in the Progression and Outcome of ARDS

G. U. Meduri

Introduction

Acute respiratory distress syndrome (ARDS) describes the clinical syndrome associated with the morphologic lesion termed diffuse alveolar damage (DAD). At presentation, (early) ARDS manifests with acute and diffuse injury to the endothelial and epithelial lining of the terminal respiratory units and causes increased vascular permeability with protein-rich exudative edema. In non-survivors of ARDS, DAD rapidly advances through three histological phases (exudative, fibroproliferative, and fibrotic) with different clinico-physiologic features. The objective of this review is to describe systematically the pathophysiology of unresolving ARDS relating to mechanisms of its development, structural alterations induced in the lung, and functional consequences of these morphologic changes.

Most ARDS patients (85–95%) survive the initial, direct or indirect, insult that precipitated acute respiratory failure and progress into the reparative stage, where outcome varies (Table 1) from complete recovery (group 3) to rapid death due to accelerated pulmonary fibrosis (group 5) [1]. In patients who recover, the per-

Table 1. Clinical classification of ARDS

Clinical group	1	2	3	4	5
Source of injury controlled	no	yes	yes	yes	yes
Percentage of patients	5–15 %	10%	20–40%	40–60%	5–10%
Average duration of ARF	≤3 days	≤7 days	7–28	7–28	≤7 days
Evolution	rapidly fatal	rapid recovery	slow improvement	slow deterioration	rapidly fatal
Survival	no	yes	yes	no	no
Causes of death	MODS	–	–	10–40% pulmonary 60–90% MODS	pulmonary
Histological findings	exudative phase of ALI	– –	fibroproliferation	55% extensive fibrosis 69% pneumonia	severe fibrosis

ARF = acute respiratory failure; MODS = multiple organ dysfunction syndrome; ALI = acute lung injury. Reproduced from [2] with permission

meability defect and gas exchange abnormalities improve (adaptive response) [1]. Conversely, ineffective repair is manifest by progression of fibroproliferation, inability to improve lung function (groups 4 and 5), and unfavorable outcome (maladaptive response) [2]. Most non-survivors die after a prolonged period of ventilatory support (group 4), and invariably develop fever, systemic inflammatory response syndrome (SIRS), clinical manifestations of sepsis [3], and multiple organ dysfunction syndrome (MODS) antemortem [1].

Tissue Homeostasis and the Host Defense Response

Tissue consists of organized groups of cells attached to an extracellular matrix (ECM) and is surrounded by a network of blood vessels. The ECM occupies a significant proportion of the volume of any tissue and is indispensable for its structural integrity [1]. Steady state, or homeostasis, is maintained by coordinating cell growth and proliferation with the production and turnover of ECM [1]. Cells achieve a remarkable coordination by constant signaling to themselves (autocrine activity) and each other (paracrine activity) by means of polypeptides called cytokines (also known as growth factors). Cell-cell and cell-matrix interactions, through cytokine networking, is essential not only for maintaining homeostasis but also for providing a rapid defense (stress) response against intrinsic or extrinsic disturbing (infectious and non-infectious) forces.

The host defense response (HDR) to insults is similar regardless of the tissue involved and consists of an interactive network of simultaneously activated pathways that work in synergy to increase the host's chance of survival. Among this complex cascade of integrated pathways, five aspects of the HDR (Table 2) are important for understanding the clinical development and evolution of ARDS: Inflammation; coagulation (intravascular clotting and extravascular fibrin deposition); modulation of the immune response; tissue repair; and activation of the hypothalamic-pituitary-adrenal (HPA) axis with production of glucocorticoids. Sympathetic system release of catecholamines and hepatic production of acute-phase reactants are an integral part of the HDR and are under the influence of glucocorticoids. The HDR is essentially a protective response which serves to destroy, dilute, or wall off injurious agents and to repair any consequent tissue damage. Repair consists of replacing injured tissue by regenerating native parenchymal cells and filling defects with fibroblastic tissue. Three aspects of the HDR, inflammation, coagulation, and tissue repair, can be analyzed separately to explain the histologic and physiologic changes occurring at tissue level in unresolving ARDS.

Cellular responses in HDR are regulated by a complex interaction of cytokines with final local and systemic effects not directly induced by the initiating insult. In this regard, cytokines have concentration-dependent biologic effects [4]. At low concentration, they regulate homeostasis, and at progressively higher concentrations, they mediate proportionally stronger local and then systemic responses. From a broad spectrum of proximal mediators, cytokines interleukin-1 (IL-1) and tumor necrosis factor (TNF) appear uniquely important in initiating all key aspects of the HDR (for a review see reference [5]). TNF-α and IL-1β stimulate their own and each other's production, and both promote the release of IL-6 (NF-IL6 is the transcription

Table 2. Components of the host defense response

Inflammation
- Vasodilation and stasis
- Increased expression of adhesion molecules
- Increased permeability of the microvasculature with exudative edema
- Leukocyte extravasation [a]
- Release of leukocyte products potentially causing tissue damage

Coagulation
- Activation of coagulation
- Inhibition of fibrinolysis
- Intravascular clotting
- Extravascular fibrin deposition

Modulation of the immune response
- Fever
- Induction of heat-shock proteins
- Release of neutrophils from the bone marrow
- Priming of phagocytic cells
- T-cells proliferation
- Antibody production

Tissue repair
- Angiogenesis
- Epithelial growth
- Fibroblast migration and proliferation
- Deposition of extracellular matrix and remodeling

Activation of the hypothalamic-pituitary-adrenal axis
- Release of ACTH with cortisol production
- ACTH and cortisol modulation of the sympathetic nervous system
- Cortisol modulation of acute phase proteins production by the liver [b]

[a] Initially polymorphonuclear cells and later monocytes
[b] Elevated levels of circulating glucocorticoids synergize with IL-6 in inducing hepatic synthesis and secretion of "acute phase" reactants such as fibrinogen, protease inhibitors, complement C3, ceruloplasmin, haptoglobin, and C-reactive protein

factor responsible for IL-6 gene activation after IL-1 stimulation). The term "inflammatory cytokines" (as they are commonly known) is restrictive, because their action extends well beyond this essential pathway of the HDR to include (among others) activation of coagulation, fibroproliferation, and stimulation of the HPA axis [1]. The cell most commonly associated with initiating the HDR cascade is the tissue macrophage or the blood monocyte [5]. Once released, TNF-α and IL-1β act on epithelial cells, stromal cells (fibroblasts and endothelial), the ECM, and recruited circulating cells (neutrophils, platelets, lymphocytes) to cause secondary waves of cytokine release, with amplification of the HDR [5]. Generation of inflammatory cytokines is normally controlled by a number of homeostatic regulatory mechanisms including shedding of specific cytokine receptors on host cells, synthesis of endogenously generated cytokine antagonists, synthesis of anti-inflammatory cytokines, down-regulation, and activation of the HPA axis with production of glucocorticoids [1].

The Host Defense Response in ARDS

ARDS is characterized by acute onset of diffuse and severe HDR of the lung parenchyma to a direct or indirect insult that disrupts the alveolocapillary membrane
with loss of compartmentalization [1]. The magnitude of the initial HDR appears to
be a major determinant of progression and outcome in ARDS. Our group recently
reported that non-survivors of ARDS had on day 1 of mechanical ventilation significantly (P<0.0001) higher plasma (Fig. 1) and bronchoalveolar lavage (BAL)
TNF-α, IL-1β, IL-2, IL-4, IL-6, and IL-8 levels than survivors [6, 7]. Although cytokine levels may not reflect activity, these findings are similar to those reported by
others and agree with studies indicating that the evolution of ARDS is determined
by the extent of initial pulmonary HDR in the form of alveolar denudation, basement membrane destruction, vascular permeability, and quantity of intraalveolar
exudate [1].

Of significant importance, during the progression of ARDS, we have found non-
survivors to have persistent and marked elevation of plasma (Fig. 1) and BAL inflammatory cytokine levels over time, while survivors had a rapid reduction in

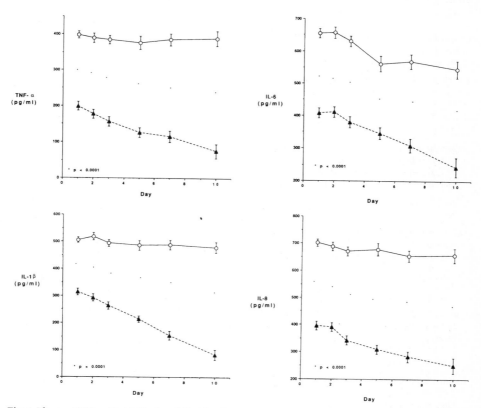

Fig. 1. Plasma TNF-α, IL-1β, IL-6, and IL-8 levels over time in survivors and non-survivors of ARDS.
Open circles represent non-survivors. Closed triangles represent survivors. (Reproduced from [6]
with permission)

inflammatory cytokine levels [6, 7]. Other groups have also reported non-survivors of ARDS or sepsis to have persistent elevation of inflammatory cytokines (Table 3) or other components of the HDR (i.e., phospholipase A_2, leukotrienes, and complement) over time [8–10]. This finding is important in understanding why treatment modalities of limited duration may be ineffective in ARDS. It is well accepted that during ARDS the HDR is not limited to the lung [1]. In patients with unresolving ARDS, disruption of the alveolo-capillary membrane [11] causes release of cytokines into the systemic circulation and contributes to the development and/or maintenance of SIRS and MODS [1]. Strong correlation among TNF-α, IL-1β, IL-6, and IL-8 levels at the onset of ARDS and over time is consistent with a broad and integrated HDR [6].

Overall, evidence strongly supports the view that an overaggressive and protracted HDR, rather than the etiologic condition precipitating respiratory failure, is the major factor influencing outcome in ARDS [3]. In agreement with this statement

Table 3. Host defense response and progression of ARDS

Variables at day 3–7 of ARDS	Survivors	Non-survivors	Ref
Clinical manifestations of inflammation			
Body temperature	↓	↑	[60]
Mean arterial blood pressure	↑	–↓	[49, 60]
Laboratory manifestations of inflammation			
Blood inflammatory cytokine levels	↓	↑	[6, 9, 61]
BAL inflammatory cytokine levels	↓	↑	[7, 62]
Blood phospholipase A_2 levels	↓	↑	[8, 9]
Complement activation	↓	NA	[10, 61]
Laboratory manifestations of pulmonary endothelial permeability			
BAL neutrophil percentage	↓	–↑	[10, 37, 38, 40, 41, 62]
BAL albumin and protein concentration	↓	–↑	[7, 37, 38]
Increased gallium-67 pulmonary uptake	↓	–	[43]
Clinical Manifestations of systemic endothelial permeability			
Positive fluid balance	↓	↑	[49, 60]
Laboratory manifestations of coagulation			
Platelet count	↓	↑	[16 ,61]
BAL antifibrinolytic activity	↓	–↑	[14, 63]
Physiologic and radiographic manifestations of fibroproliferation			
$PaO_2 : FiO_2$	↑	–↓	[7, 14, 34, 35, 37, 49, 60, 61]
PEEP requirements	↓	–↑	[49, 61]
Static compliance	↑	↓	[34]
Dead space ratio	↓	↑	[34, 51]
Pulmonary artery pressure	↓	–↑	[34, 49]
Alveolar infiltration	↓	↑	[11, 35, 61]
Laboratory manifestations of fibroproliferation			
BAL procollagen-III	↓	↑	[64]
Serum procollagen-III	↓	↑	[30–32, 64]

Variables on day 3–7 of ARDS in comparison to day 1: – = no change; ↑ = increased; ↓ = decreased; NA = not available

are the findings that ARDS patients may not improve despite appropriate treatment of the precipitating disease, while mortality is decreased when the HDR is adequately suppressed by sustained glucocorticoid administration (discussed later) [12]. In the absence of inhibitory signals, the continued exaggerated production of HDR mediators prevents effective restoration of lung anatomy and function (maladaptive response) by sustaining ongoing injury, coagulation, and fibroproliferation (the three act in synergy). Histology of lung tissue obtained by open lung biopsy in patients with unresolving ARDS (8 to 22 days into ARDS) showed new injury to previously spared endothelial and epithelial surfaces occurring concurrently with an amplified reparative (coagulation and fibroproliferation with deposition of extracellular matrix) process of previously injured areas (airspaces, interstitium, respiratory bronchioles, and walls of the intraacinar microvessels) [11]. Persistent endothelial and epithelial injury protracts vascular permeability in the lung and systemically. Intravascular coagulation decreases the available pulmonary vascular bed, while intraalveolar fibrin deposition promotes cell-matrix organization by fibroproliferation [1]. Most clinical and physiological derangements observed in unresolving ARDS are attributable to unrestrained coagulation and fibroproliferation and are discussed below.

Coagulation

During ARDS, normal intraalveolar fibrinolytic activity (urokinase-like plasminogen activators produced by alveolar macrophages) and endothelium anti-clotting activity (heparin-like molecules, thrombomodulin) are severely compromised and lead to accelerated vascular and extravascular fibrin deposition [13]. In patients with ARDS, BAL has increased procoagulant activity due to tissue factor associated with factor VII (1, 14] and concomitant depression of fibrinolytic activity attributable to increased levels of both plasminogen activator inhibitor-1 (PAI-1) and antiplasmin [1, 14]. In humans [14, 15], derangements of intraalveolar fibrin turnover occur early (1–3 days) and persist for ≥ 14 days. Depressed BAL fibrinolytic activity at day 7 of ARDS correlated with poor outcome [14]. Despite a depression in fibrinolytic activity, BAL fibrinogen degradation products (FDP) are markedly increased and remain elevated over time, and correlate significantly with BAL total protein concentration and number of neutrophils [15]. Patients with ARDS also have marked and prolonged systemic procoagulant activity and rapid exhaustion of the fibrinolytic system [1]. Virtually all ARDS patients have increased circulating FDP levels [16]. Disseminated intravascular coagulation (DIC) is a frequent finding in ARDS and carries a higher mortality rate [1]. Even in patients without DIC, a reduction in circulating platelets of at least 50% of the initial values is frequently observed during the course of ARDS, and non-survivors have a greater degree of thrombocytopenia than survivors [1]. Thrombocytopenia is not due to decreased platelet production, but to decreased platelet survival (one third of normal), due to increased pulmonary sequestration [17].

Patients with early ARDS as well as patients with late unresolving ARDS show diffuse pulmonary sequestration of intravenously administered radiolabeled fibrinogen [18].

Pathways for increased fibrinogen uptake include:
1) increased microvascular permeability with exudation of fibrinogen into pulmonary interstitial and intraalveolar edema;
2) intravascular and extravascular fibrin formation;
3) fibrinogen binding to injured endothelial cells [18].

Recovery from lung injury is associated with normalization of radiolabeled fibrinogen uptake [18]. Cytokines TNF-α, IL-1β, and IL-6 alter the surface of the endothelium from an anticoagulant into a procoagulant moiety, due to down-regulation of thrombomodulin and the expression of tissue factor, and are able to enhance the synthesis of PAI-1 [19].

Pulmonary thromboemboli are a frequent histological finding in patients with unresolving ARDS subjected to open-lung biopsy [11] and are found on postmortem examination in 95% of ARDS non-survivors [20, 21]. Macrothrombi (in arteries greater than 1 mm diameter) are found by postmortem angiography in 86% of patients and are more prevalent in patients who died in the early phase of ARDS [21]. Microthrombi are as prevalent as macrothombi but tend to be distributed throughout all phases of ARDS. In one study, filling defects at angiography correlated with the severity of ARDS, the degree of pulmonary hypertension, and the presence of DIC [20]. Unfortunately, anticoagulant treatment, in common with other treatments directed at one single facet of the complex host response does not improve outcome in ARDS [20]. Ischemic or avascular necrosis, particularly in the subpleural regions, is a common feature of unresolving ARDS (see section on barotrauma) [11, 20].

Fibrin deposition also influences the course of tissue injury and repair. Thrombin, fibrin and its degradation products play an important role in amplifying inflammation by promoting neutrophil chemotaxis and adhesiveness, and by directly causing increased endothelial permeability [22]. Thrombin is also a potent inducer of platelet degranulation with additional release of HDR mediators. Coagulation and fibrinolysis are also interactive with the kallikrein/kinin system with release of bradykinin. Bradykinin increases vascular permeability and stimulates collagen production by fibroblasts [1].

Animal studies have demonstrated that intraalveolar fibrin deposition is typical of DAD, even when injury resolves without fibrosis, indicating that fibrin deposition of limited duration is essential for effective lung repair [23]. In the presence of a protracted HDR, however, persistent intraalveolar fibrin deposition contributes to air-space organization and fibrosis [13, 23, 24]. *In vitro* data demonstrate that fibrin forms a matrix on which fibroblasts may aggregate and secrete collagen [1]. In addition, thrombin binds to thrombin receptors on fibroblasts and promotes their proliferation [1].

Fibroproliferation

Fibroproliferation is a stereotypical reparative response to injury. In ARDS, pulmonary fibroproliferation is manifest by the accumulation of myofibroblasts and their connective tissue products in the airspaces, interstitium, respiratory bronchioles, and walls of the intraacinar microvessels [11, 25]. Pulmonary fibroproliferation is a diffuse process, as indicated by the findings of chest computed tomography [11] gross inspection at surgery, microscopic analysis of biopsies from different lobes [26], and bilateral BAL findings [7]. At microscopy, however, regional heterogeneity exists, and focal areas of normal parenchyma are occasionally found [27]. Continuing fibroproliferation results in extensive fibrotic remodeling of the lung parenchyma. Macroscopically, the lung shows irregular zones of diffuse scarring with formation of numerous microcystic reorganized airspaces measuring between 1 and 2 mm, most prominent in the subpleural zones [11].

Pulmonary fibroproliferation in ARDS shares a common pathogenetic mechanism with other fibroproliferative diseases, where degree and duration of the HDR dictate the ultimate reparative outcome [28]. In this "linear" concept of tissue response to injury, mediators of the HDR sustain the fibrotic process [1]. Fibrosis ensues when the HDR is intense and prolonged, leading to released pro-fibrotic moieties and trophic factors for mesenchymal cells. Experimental work indicates that the severity of acute lung injury determines the intensity of chronic inflammation and fibrosis [1]. In agreement, we have found that patients with higher plasma IL-6 on days 1–3 of ARDS are more likely to develop accelerated fibroproliferation unresponsive to glucocorticoid rescue treatment [12].

Morphometric analysis of lung tissue in late ARDS has shown that intraalveolar fibroproliferation predominates over interstitial fibroproliferation [25]. The histological sequence leading to intraalveolar fibroproliferation had been clearly characterized [25]. Epithelial injury provides focal discontinuities (gaps) in the alveolar basement membrane resulting in direct communication of interstitial cells and matrix elements with the alveolar airspaces [11, 24]. Activated myofibroblasts from the interstitium migrate into the alveoli in response to chemotactic signals and attach to the luminal surface of the damaged basement membrane [24, 25]. Once they have migrated into the alveoli, the myofibroblasts proliferate and produce collagen [24], transforming the initially fibrinous intraalveolar exudate into myxoid connective tissue matrix and eventually into dense acellular fibrous tissue. TNF-α and IL-1β, among other HDR mediators, stimulate chemotaxis and are important modulators of fibroblast proliferation and collagen deposition [1].

Morphometric studies in non-survivors of ARDS have shown intraalveolar (and, to a lesser degree, interstitial) fibroproliferation occurring within 7 days of the onset of ARDS and rapidly increasing in the second and third week of respiratory failure [25]. The rate of progression varies [1, 29]. Newly produced matrix stains intensely for cell-associated fibronectin and type III procollagen [24]. Type III collagen (newly formed, flexible, and more susceptible to digestion by collagenase) predominates in the intermediate proliferative phase, while type I collagen (composed of thick fibrils, more resistant to digestion) is the major collagen present in the late fibrotic phase. In non-survivors, the collagen content of the lung is increased 2- to 3-fold after 2 weeks of ARDS, and it parallels the development of fibrosis [11]. Patients with ARDS dying after 7 days of respiratory failure have, in contrast to survivors, persistent elevation of extracellular matrix components (procollagen III) in the BAL and serum indicating ongoing fibrogenesis (Table 3) [30–33]. Patients with BAL procollagen III level greater than 1.75 U/ml on day 7 had a 72% mortality rate compared with a 20% mortality rate in patients with a procollagen III level less than 1.75 U/ml [33]. BAL procollagen III levels correlate with histological evidence of intraalveolar fibrosis [1]. Fibrosis present on open-lung or transbronchial biopsy is a poor prognostic factor [1].

The patterns of fibrous reorganization of the lung in ARDS have been described [11]. Intraalveolar fibroblastic aggregation is continuous with a similar process in the terminal bronchioles, respiratory bronchioles, alveolar ducts, and the interstitium [11]. The bronchiolar intraluminal (bud-like) fibrosis found in patients with fibroproliferation is similar to the one described in interstitial lung disorders [11]. The coexistence of unaffected bronchioles surrounded by parenchymal interstitial and alveolar space fibrosis indicates that lung injury induced patchy bronchial epithelial and basement membrane damage. In our experience, intraluminal fibrosis at open-lung biopsy in patients with unresolving ARDS predicts reversibility of fibroproliferation with glucocorticoid rescue treatment [29], similar to the response observed in patients with bronchiolitis obliterans organizing pneumonia.

Of significance, we, and others, have described microscopic and ultrastructural evidence of ongoing epithelial and endothelial injury in patients with advanced fibroproliferation [11, 21, 27, 29]. Despite the high turnover rate and ability of endothelial cells to repair themselves, acute endothelial injury is more pronounced in the proliferative phase than in the exudative phase of ARDS [21, 27], consistent with a continuous injury process. Fibrocellular intimal proliferation, the sequel of endothelial injury, involves predominantly the small arteries, but also the veins and lymphatics. Absence of arteriolar subintimal fibroproliferation at open-lung biopsy in patients with unresolving ARDS predicts the reversibility of fibroproliferation with glucocorticoid rescue treatment [29].

Clinical and Physiological Manifestations of the Host Defense Response in Unresolving ARDS

Morphological changes at epithelial and endothelial levels, caused by recurrent injury, ongoing coagulation, and amplified fibroproliferation can explain the physiologic and laboratory findings seen in patients with unresolving ARDS.

Gas Exchange and Lung Mechanics

As shown in Figure 2, gaps in the alveolar basement membrane in unresolving ARDS [11] allow communication between the alveoli and the interstitium for entrance of vascular and interstitial components into the airspaces. Myofibroblasts migrate, proliferate, and produce collagen. Progressive fibroproliferation leads to obliteration of the respiratory units, changing their mechanical properties (loss of inflection point in the pressure-volume [P-V] curve and lack of recruitability by positive end-expiratory pressure [PEEP]), increasing dead space ventilation (V_D/V_T), and further compromising gas exchange [34]. A concomitant reduction in capillary volume and thickening of the alveolar septa additionally contributes to reducing gas transfer and increasing V_D/V_T [27]. In several studies (Table 3), the $PaO_2:FiO_2$ ratio, although similar at the onset of ARDS, clearly separated survivors (increased) from non-sur-

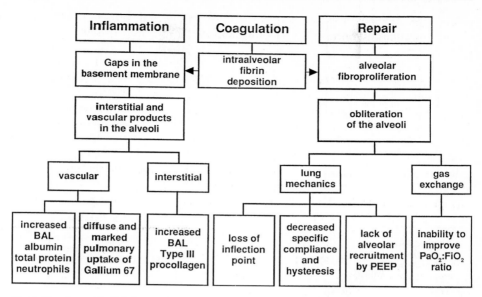

Fig. 2. Alveolar epithelial changes in unresolving ARDS. (Modified from [11] with permission)

vivors (decreased or no change) by day 3–7. In one report, the mortality rates in patients with and without improvement in lung function by day 7 of ARDS were 43% and 97% respectively [35].

Pulmonary Vascular Permeability

As shown in Figure 3, endothelial injury in unresolving ARDS favors the passage of vascular products in the alveoli [11]. Among the many cells and substances that exude in the airspaces, the following have been the subject of clinical investigations: Albumin; proteins, neutrophils, and gallium 67 (^{67}Ga).

BAL albumin and total protein are markers of pulmonary endothelial permeability in ARDS [36]. At the onset of ARDS, we have found BAL albumin and total protein levels to be similar in survivors and non-survivors. In agreement with others [37, 38], we have found in survivors, in contrast to non-survivors, a progressive decline in BAL albumin and total protein levels over time, suggesting effective repair of the alveolar-endothelial surface. We have also identified a consistent correlation between BAL albumin and total protein levels and BAL TNF-α, IL-1β, IL-6, and IL-8 levels [7].

BAL neutrophilia ($\geq 70\%$) is invariably found in early ARDS [38]. The percentage of BAL neutrophils parallels BAL protein [37] and albumin [7] concentration and correlates with the severity in gas exchange [38]. We and others have identified a positive correlation between total neutrophil count and BAL TNF-α, IL-1β, and IL-8 levels [7, 39]. Persistent elevation of neutrophils in the BAL by days 7 and 14 of ARDS is associated with poor outcome [40, 41]. Resolution of ARDS, on the contrary, is

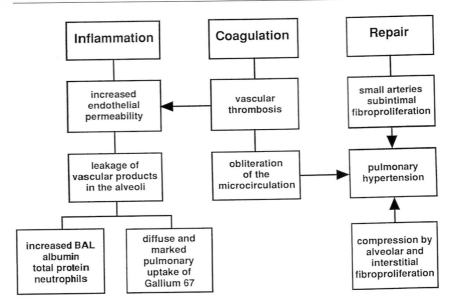

Fig. 3. Pulmonary endothelial changes in unresolving ARDS. (Modified from [11] with permission)

associated with a dramatic fall in neutrophils and increased number of macrophages [40].

The origin of neutrophils recovered by BAL in unresolving ARDS requires clarifi-
cation. In patients with unresolving ARDS subjected to both bronchoscopy and
open-lung biopsy after an average of 14 days respiratory failure, we have found a
significant discrepancy between marked BAL neutrophilia (60% of recovered cells)
and an almost complete absence of neutrophils in the airways, alveoli, and interstitium at histology [29]. It has been recognized that the alveolo-capillary membrane is permeable to fluids and that in normal patients 39% of the aspirated BAL
fluid originates from the circulation [42]. In conditions associated with disruption of vascular and epithelial integrity, such as unresolving ARDS, the circulatory
component of BAL effluent becomes more significant, and cells such as neutrophils
and erythrocytes are aspirated into the alveoli when negative pressure is applied
during suction [42]. Therefore, BAL neutrophilia in unresolving ARDS is a marker
of endothelial permeability [29, 37], not a reflection of "neutrophilic alveolitis," and
it is unlikely that neutrophils play a major role in the progression of unresolving
ARDS.

^{67}Ga uptake in the lung is an additional marker of endothelial permeability [1].
The mechanism of ^{67}Ga uptake was recently reviewed [43]. In the lung, ^{67}Ga concentration is normally low. Diffuse ^{67}Ga uptake has been used as a sensitive but non-
specific test to identify patients with active pulmonary inflammation who may
respond to glucocorticoid treatment. Five reports (total of 44 patients) have described marked and diffuse uptake of ^{67}Ga in the lungs of patients with unresolving
ARDS and who subsequently responded to glucocorticoid rescue treatment [29,
44–46]. Diffuse and marked pulmonary uptake of ^{67}Ga in unresolving ARDS corre-

lates with BAL neutrophilia [43]. Decreased pulmonary ^{67}Ga uptake correlates with improvement in gas exchange [43]. The diagnostic role of ^{67}Ga scintigraphy in ARDS has been reported [43].

Pulmonary Hypertension

While in early ARDS the pulmonary vasculature is available for dilation and/or recruitment, vascular changes in unresolving ARDS are less responsive to vasodilator treatment [47]. In these patients, vascular obstruction from thrombosis, subintimal fibroproliferation of the small arteries, and compression from alveolar and interstitial expansion significantly reduces the capacity of the pulmonary microcirculation (Fig. 3) [27], and subjects the patent vascular bed to abnormally high flow, stimulating medial hypertrophy of the muscular and partially muscular arteries [48]. These changes are similar to those seen in pulmonary hypertension of thromboembolic origin [48] and they worsen with progression of fibroproliferation [34, 49]. In early ARDS, there is a marked elevation in circulating levels of endothelin-1, a mediator of vascular remodeling and pulmonary hypertension [50]. With the progression of ARDS, endothelin-1 levels drop to normal values in patients with improving lung function, but remain elevated in patients who worsen [50]. Persistent elevation or worsening of pulmonary artery pressure is a poor prognostic sign. In the final stages of ARDS, the mean pulmonary artery pressure can exceed 40 mmHg due to a 4-fold elevation of vascular resistance [47].

Barotrauma

In unresolving ARDS, vascular obstruction with subpleural tissue necrosis and endoluminal fibrosis with intraparenchymal pseudocyst formation contribute to alveolar rupture. Barotrauma may manifest as intraparenchymal and subpleural pneumatoceles, large compliant air collections or bullae, pulmonary interstitial emphysema, pneumomediastinum, pneumothorax, subcutaneous emphysema, and rarely pneumoperitoneum. Barotrauma in ARDS is related to the severity of lung dysfunction and is associated with a higher mortality [51, 52]. An increase in the alveolar-arterial pressure gradient, from either hyperinflation and/or reduced blood flow, causes disruption at the common border between the alveolar base and the vascular sheath [48]. Partial obliteration (endoluminal fibrosis) of terminal airways leads to cyst formation by a valvular mechanism and by compensatory dilatation of neighboring bronchioles [52]. Tissue necrosis distal to pulmonary artery thrombi [20] is prominent in the subpleural regions where insufficient collateral blood flow makes lung tissue particularly susceptible to ischemia [53]. At angiography, a "picket-fence" appearance is seen, caused by dilated subpleural arteries bridging regions of oligemia and necrosis distal to the thrombotic arterial occlusion [53]. With progressive fibroproliferation, preferential ventilation of these hypoperfused peripheral areas may occur, contributing to the development of barotrauma [53].

Fever of Infectious and Non-Infectious Origin

Fever is caused by the systemic release of endogenous pyrogens: TNF-α, IL-1β, and IL-6. On reaching the hypothalamic thermoregulatory center, these cytokines induce an abrupt release of prostaglandins that increase the thermostatic set point and produce heat. Fever induces production of heat shock proteins, that have an important role in cell survival under stress (cytoprotection). Fever and SIRS invariably develop during the course of unresolving ARDS, even in the absence of infection [3, 44]. Clinical studies have attributed the frequent occurrence of fever and SIRS in late ARDS to ventilator-associated pneumonia (VAP), and the assumption was made that in these patients, nosocomial infections (mainly VAP) amplify SIRS and lead to MODS and death [1].

Correlation Between Nosocomial Infections and Cytokine Response

In a study involving serial measurements of plasma and BAL inflammatory cytokines and careful search for and diagnosis of infections, we found that nosocomial infections (either definitive or presumed) developing in 34 patients with ARDS on mechanical ventilation for > 72 h caused neither a transient nor a sustained increase in plasma and BAL inflammatory cytokine levels (TNF-α, IL-1β, IL-6, and IL-8) or in the SIRS score [3]. These findings are similar to those reported by others [54] and question the prior hypothesis, based on clinical criteria, that in unresolving ARDS, nosocomial infections amplify SIRS leading to MODS and death [1]. Down-regulation in the presence of nosocomial infection most likely represents cytoprotection from overwhelming cytokinemia and not a detrimental form of immunosuppression.

Systemic Effects of the Host Defense Response

Figure 4 displays the local and systemic effects of a protracted HDR in ARDS. Systemic release of HDR mediators causes; (1) SIRS; (2) development and progression of MODS (by a mechanism similar to the one causing progression of ARDS); and (3) increased systemic endothelial permeability.

Fever is a common clinical denominator to noninfectious SIRS and nosocomial infections. The diagnostic evaluation of fever in patients with ARDS has been reviewed [55].

Response to Glucocorticoid Therapy in Unresolving ARDS

Although, large randomized clinical trials have clearly shown no benefit when a short course (≤ 48 h) of high-dose intravenous glucocorticoids is administered in early sepsis and ARDS [56], we [29, 44] and others [45, 46, 57] have reported a significant improvement in lung function during prolonged glucocorticoid administration in patients with unresolving ARDS (rescue treatment).

We recently completed a prospective, randomized, double-blind, placebo-controlled trial [58]. Twenty-four patients with severe ARDS who had failed to improve

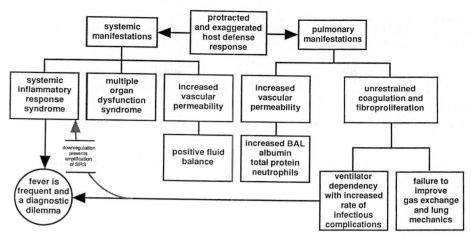

Fig. 4. Pathopohysiology of unresolving ARDS.

their lung injury score (LIS) by the 7th day of respiratory failure entered the study. The decision to stop the study was made when the statistical power for difference in intensive care unit (ICU) mortality reached 0.79. Sixteen patients received methylprednisolone and 8 received placebo. The methylprednisolone dose was initially 2 mg/kg/day and the duration of treatment was 32 days. Surveillance bronchoscopy to identify occult pneumonia was performed on study day 5 and weekly while intubated. Patients failing to improve their LIS by at least 1 point after 10 days of treatment were blindly crossed over to the alternative treatment. The primary outcome measures were improvement in lung function and mortality. The secondary outcome measures were improvement in MODS and development of nosocomial infections. Physiologic characteristics at the onset of ARDS were similar in both groups. At study entry (day 9 ± 1 of ARDS), the two groups had similar LIS, $PaO_2 : FiO_2$, and MODS score. ICU mortality for the treatment group versus the placebo group was 0% versus 62% ($P = 0.002$); hospital-associated mortality for the two groups was 12% versus 62% ($P = 0.03$). Changes observed by study day 10 are reported for methylprednisolone versus placebo: LIS (1.7 ± 0.1 vs 3.0 ± 0.2; $P < 0.0001$), $PaO_2 : FiO_2$ (262 ± 19 vs 148 ± 35; $P = 0.0003$), MODS score (0.7 ± 0.2 vs 1.8 ± 0.3; $P = 0.0008$), and successful extubation (7 vs 0; $P = 0.051$). The rate of infections per day of treatment was similar in both groups, and pneumonia was frequently detected in the absence of fever. These findings indicate that prolonged administration of methylprednisolone in patients with unresolving ARDS is associated with rapid improvement in lung injury and MODS scores and a significant reduction in mortality. Methylprednisolone treatment was associated with a rapid and sustained reduction in plasma and BAL procollagen type I and III aminoterminal propetide levels, while no change was observed in the control patients [59]. These findings provide additional confirmation of the association between biological efficacy and physiologic response during prolonged methylprednisolone treatment of unresolving ARDS.

In the randomized study [58], improvement in LIS and survival were correlated. The degree of improvement in LIS was similar to the response we previously observed in 20 (rapid responders) of 34 ARDS patients receiving methylprednisolone rescue treatment [12, 29]. In rapid responders, this treatment was associated with: (1) decrease in plasma and BAL TNF-α, IL-1β, IL-6, and IL-8 levels that paralleled reductions in LIS and BAL albumin; (2) normalization of ^{67}Ga pulmonary uptake; (3) restoration of normal alveolar architecture (follow-up histology); and (4) a lower mortality rate [12, 29]. The striking parallel between improvement in lung function and reduction in cytokine levels during glucocorticoid treatment conclusively supports the link between HDR and progression of ARDS. Of importance, when effective, glucocorticoid treatment suppressed production of all measured inflammatory cytokines. A similar degree of anti-inflammatory action may not be achieved by specific anti-mediator therapy (i.e., monoclonal antibody directed at TNF or antagonist directed at IL-1 receptors).

Conclusion

The HDR to insults is similar regardless of the tissue involved and results from an interactive network of specialized and interconnected pathways. An exaggerated and protracted HDR plays a key role in ARDS outcome and is accountable for the histologic, laboratory, clinical, and physiologic findings seen during the course of unresolving ARDS. Continued elevated production of HDR mediators, such as TNF-α, IL-1β, and IL-6, prevents effective restoration of lung anatomy and function by sustaining inflammation, coagulation, and fibroproliferation. Predictors of poor outcome in ARDS as reported in the literature are in actuality manifestations of a persistent and exaggerated HDR. During ARDS, down-regulation of the HDR, is responsible for the lack of laboratory and clinical amplification of SIRS with nosocomial infections. These findings dispute the hypothesis, based on clinical criteria, that in unresolving ARDS, nosocomial infections amplify SIRS and lead to MODS and death. Spontaneous or treatment-induced suppression of the exaggerated and autonomous pulmonary HDR is associated with improvement in lung function and outcome.

References

1. Meduri GU (1996) The role of the host defense response in the progression and outcome of ARDS: pathophysiological correlations and response to glucocorticoid treatment. Eur Respir J 9:2650–2670
2. Meduri GU (1993) Late ARDS. New Horizons 1:563–577
3. Headley AS, Tolley E, Meduri GU (1997) Infections and the inflammatory response in acute respiratory distress syndrome. Chest 111:1306–1321
4. Cerami A (1992) Inflammatory cytokines. Clin Immunol Immunopathol 62:S3–S10
5. Baumann H, Gauldie J (1994) The acute phase response. Immunol Today 15:74–80
6. Meduri GU, Headley S, Kohler G, et al (1995) Persistent elevation of inflammatory cytokines predicts a poor outcome in ARDS. Plasma IL-1β and IL-6 are consistent and efficient predictors of outcome over time. Chest 107:1062–1073
7. Meduri GU, Kohler G, Headley S, Tolley E, Stentz F, Postlethwaite A (1995) Inflammatory cytokines in the BAL of patients with ARDS. Persistent elevation over time predicts poor outcome. Chest 108:1303–1314

8. Vadas P, Pruzanski W, Stefanski E, et al (1988) Concordance of endogenous cortisol and phospholipase A_2 levels in gram-negative septic shock: a prospective study. J Lab Clin Med 111: 584–590

9. Romaschin AD, DeMajo WC, Winton T, et al (1992) Systemic phospholipase A_2 and cachectin levels in adult respiratory distress syndrome and multiple-organ failure. Clin Biochem 25: 55–60

10. Robbins RA, Russ WD, Rasmussen JK, Clayton MM (1987) Activation of the complement system in the adult respiratory distress syndrome. Am Rev Respir Dis 135:651–658

11. Meduri GU, ElTorky M, Winer-Muram HT (1995) The fibroproliferative phase of late adult respiratory distress syndrome. Semin Respir Infect 10:154–175

12. Meduri GU, Headley S, Tolley E, Shelby M, Stentz F, Postlethwaite A (1995) Plasma and BAL cytokine response to corticosteroid rescue treatment in late ARDS. Chest 108:1315–1325

13. Idell S (1994) Extravascular coagulation and fibrin deposition in acute lung injury. New Horizons 2:566–574

14. Idell S, Koenig KB, Fair DS, Martin TR, McLarty J, Maunder RJ (1991) Serial abnormalities of fibrin turnover in evolving adult respiratory distress syndrome. Am J Physiol 261: L240–L248

15. Fuchs-Buder T, de Moerloose P, Ricou B, et al (1996) Time course of procoagulant activity and D dimer in bronchoalveolar fluid of patients at risk for or with acute respiratory distress syndrome. Am J Respir Crit Care Med 153:163–167

16. Carvalho AC (1985) Blood alterations during ARDS. In: Zapol WM, Falke KJ (eds) Acute respiratory failure. Marcel Dekker, New York, pp 303–346

17. Schneider RC, Zapol WM, Carvalho AC (1980) Platelet consumption and sequestration in severe acute respiratory failure. Am Rev Respir Dis 122:445–451

18. Quinn DA, Carvalho AC, Geller E, et al (1987) ^{99m}Tc-fibrinogen scanning in adult respiratory distress syndrome. Am Rev Respir Dis 135:100–106

19. Taylor FB (1994) The inflammatory-coagulant axis in the host response to gram-negative sepsis:regulatory roles of proteins and inhibitors of tissue factor. New Horizons 2:555–565

20. Greene R, Zapol WM, Snider MT, et al (1981) Early bedside detection of pulmonary vascular occlusion during acute respiratory failure. Am Rev Respir Dis 124:593–601

21. Tomaseski JF, Davies P, Boggis C, Greene R, Zapol WM, Reid LM (1983) The pulmonary vascular lesions of the adult respiratory distress syndrome. Am J Pathol 112:112–126

22. Leavell KJ, Peterson MW, Gross TJ (1996) The role of fibrin degradation products in neutrophil recruitment to the lung. Am J Respir Cell Mol Biol 14:53–60

23. McDonald JA (1990) The yin and yang of fibrin in the airways. N Engl J Med 322:929–931

24. Kuhn C III, Boldt J, King TE, Crouch E, Vartio T, McDonald JA (1989) An immuno histochemical study of architectural remodeling and connective tissue synthesis in pulmonary fibrosis. Am Rev Respir Dis 140:1693–1703

25. Fukuda Y, Ishizaki M, Masuda Y, Kimura G, Kawanami O, Masugi Y (1987) The role of intraalveolar fibrosis in the process of pulmonary structural remodeling in patients with diffuse alveolar damage. Am J Pathol 126:171–182

26. Lamy M, Fallat RL, Koeniger E, et al (1976) Pathologic features and mechanisms of hypoxemia in adult respiratory distress syndrome. Am Rev Respir Dis 114:267–284

27. Bachofen M, Weibel ER (1977) Alterations of the gas exchange apparatus in adult respiratory insufficiency associated with septicemia. Am Rev Respir Dis 116:589–615

28. Kovacs EJ, Dipietro LA (1994) Fibrogenic cytokines and connective tissue production. FASEB J 8:854–861

29. Meduri GU, Chinn AJ, Leeper KV, et al (1994) Corticosteroid rescue treatment of progressive fibroproliferation in late ARDS. Patterns of response and predictors of outcome. Chest 105: 1516–1527

30. Entzian P, Huckstadt A, Kreipe H, Barth J (1990) Determination of serum concentrations of type III procollagen peptide in mechanically ventilated patients. Pronounced augmented concentrations in the adult respiratory distress syndrome. Am Rev Respir Dis 142:1079–1082

31. Kropf J, Grobe E, Knoch M, Lammers M, Gressner AM, Lennartz H (1991) The prognostic value of extracellular matrix component concentrations in serum during treatment of adult respiratory distress syndrome with extracorporeal CO_2 removal. Eur J Clin Chem Clin Biochem 29:805–812

32. Waydhas C, Nast-Kolb D, Trupka A, et al (1993) Increased serum concentrations of procollagen type III peptide in severely injured patients: An indicator of fibrosing activity? Crit Care Med 21:240–247
33. Clark JG, Milberg JA, Steinberg KP, Hudson LD (1995) Type III procollagen peptide in the adult respiratory distress syndrome. Association of increased peptide levels in bronchoalveolar lavage fluid with increased risk for death. Ann Intern Med 122:17–23
34. Shimada Y, Yoshiya I, Tanaka K, Sone S, Sakurai M (1979) Evaluation of the progress and prognosis of adult respiratory distress syndrome: simple respiratory physiologic measurement. Chest 76:180–186
35. Bernard GR, Luce JM, Sprung CL, et al (1987) High-dose corticosteroids in patients with the adult respiratory distress syndrome. N Engl J Med 317:1565–1570
36. Holter JF, Weiland JE, Pacht ER, Gadek JE, Davis WB (1986) Protein permeability in the adult respiratory distress syndrome. Loss of size selectivity of the alveolar epithelium. J Clin Invest 78:1513–1522
37. Sinclair DG, Braude S, Haslam PL, Evans TW (1994) Pulmonary endothelial permeability in patients with severe lung injury. Chest 106:535–539
38. Weiland JE, Davis WB, Holter JF, Mohammed JR, Dorinsky PM, Gadek JE (1986) Lung neutrophils in the adult respiratory distress syndrome. Clinical and pathophysiologic significance. Am Rev Respir Dis 133:218–225
39. Miller EJ, Cohen AB, Magao S, et al (1992) Elevated levels of NAP-1/interleukin-8 are present in the airspaces of patients with the adult respiratory distress syndrome and are associated with increased mortality. Am Rev Respir Dis 146:427–432
40. Steimberg KP, Milberg JA, Martin TR, Maunder RJ, Cockrill BA, Hudson LD (1994) Evolution of bronchoalveolar lavage cell population in the adult respiratory distress syndrome. Am J Respir Crit Care Med 150:113–122
41. Gunther K, Baughman RP, Rashkin M, Pattishall E (1993) Bronchoalveolar lavage results in patients with sepsis-induced adult respiratory distress syndrome: evaluation of mortality and inflammatory response. Am Rev Respir Dis 147:A346 (Abst)
42. Kelly CA, Fenwick JD, Corris PA, Fleetwood A, Hendrick DJ, Walters EH (1988) Fluid dynamics during bronchoalveolar lavage. Am Rev Respir Dis 138:81–84
43. Meduri GU, Belenchia JM, Massey JD, ElTorky M (1996) ^{67}Ga scintigraphy in diagnosing sources of fever in ventilated patients. Intensive Care Med 22:395–403
44. Meduri GU, Belenchia JM, Estes RJ, Wunderink RG, ElTorky M, Leeper KV Jr (1991) Fibroproliferative phase of ARDS. Clinical findings and effects of corticosteroids. Chest 100:943–952
45. Hooper RG, Kearl RA (1990) Established ARDS treated with a sustained course of adrenocortical steroids. Chest 97:138–143
46. Hooper RG, Kearl RA (1996) Established adult respiratory distress syndrome successfully treated with corticosteroids. South Med J 89:359–364
47. Zapol WM, Snider MT (1977) Pulmonary hypertension in severe acute respiratory failure. N Engl J Med 296:476–480
48. Snow RL, Davies P, Pontoppidan W, Zapol WM, Reid L (1982) Pulmonary vascular remodeling in adult respiratory distress syndrome. Am Rev Respir Dis 126:887–892
49. Sloane PJ, Gee MH, Gottlieb JE, et al (1992) A multicenter registry of patients with acute respiratory distress syndrome. Am Rev Respir Dis 146:419–426
50. Langleben D, Demarchie M, Laporta D, et al (1993) Endothelin-1 in acute lung injury and the adult respiratory distress syndrome. Am Rev Respir Dis 148:1646–1650
51. Gattinoni L, Bombino M, Pelosi P, et al (1994) Lung structure and function in different stages of severe adult respiratory distress syndrome. JAMA 271:1772–1779
52. Rouby JJ, Lherm T, de Lassale EM, et al (1993) Histologic aspects of pulmonary barotrauma in critically ill patients with acute respiratory failure. Intensive Care Med 19:383–389
53. Tomasheski JR Jr (1990) Pulmonary pathology of the adult respiratory distress syndrome. Clin Chest Med 11:593–619
54. Kristiansson M, Soop M, Saraste L, Sundqvist KS (1993) Post-operative circulating cytokine patterns – the influence of infection. Intensive Care Med 19:395–400
55. Meduri GU (1994) Fever in late adult respiratory distress syndrome: Etiology, pathophysiology, and diagnostic evaluation. Semin Respir Med 15:308–324

56. Lefering R, Neugebauer EAM (1995) Steroid controversy in sepsis and septic shock: A meta-analysis. Crit Care Med 23:1294–1303

57. Ashbaugh DG, Maier RV (1985) Idiopathic pulmonary fibrosis in adult respiratory distress syndrome. Diagnosis and treatment. Arch Surg 120:530–535

58. Meduri GU, Headley AS, Golden E, et al (1998) Prolonged methylprednisolone treatment improves lung function and outcome in patients with unresolving acute respiratory distress syndrome. Results of a randomized, double-blind, placebo-controlled trial. Am J Respir Crit Care Med (In press)

59. Meduri GU, Headley EA, Tolley A, Chin A, Stentz F, Postlethwaite A (1998) Plasma and BAL procollagen type I & III levels during ARDS and in response to prolonged methylprednisolone treatment. Am J Resp Crit Care Med (In Press)

60. Simmons RS, Berdine GG, Seidenfeld JJ, et al (1994) Fluid balance and the adult respiratory distress syndrome. Am Rev Respir Dis 135:924–929

61. Groeneveld ABJ, Raijmakers PGHM, Hack CE, Thijs LG (1995) Interleukin 8-related neutrophil elastase and the severity of the adult respiratory distress syndrome. Cytokine 7:746–752

62. Baughman RP, Gunther KL, Rashkin MC, Keeton DA, Pattishall EN (1996) Changes in the inflammatory response of the lung during acute respiratory distress syndrome: Prognostic indicators. Am J Resp Crit Care Med 154:76–81

63. Gando S, Nakanishi Y, Tedo I (1995) Cytokines and plasminogen activator inhibitor-1 in post-trauma disseminated intravascular coagulation: Relationship to multiple organ dysfunction syndrome. Crit Care Med 23:1835–1842

64. Lotz M, Guerne PA (1991) Interleukin-6 induces the synthesis of tissue inhibitor of metallo-proteinases-1/erythroid potentiating activity (TIMP-1/EPA). J Biol Chem 266:2017–2020

The Role of Cytokines in the Pathogenesis of Pneumonia

M. J. Schultz, S. J. H. van Deventer, and T. van der Poll

Introduction

Bacterial pneumonia is a major cause of morbidity and mortality worldwide, despite the armamentarium of antibacterial agents, advanced diagnostic technologies and sophisticated, sometimes aggressive treatments used in intensive care facilities. In developing countries community-acquired pneumonia causes ten times as many deaths as all infectious diseases together [1]. Pneumonia is the second most frequent cause of hospital-acquired infection in the United States [2].

Adult patients on the intensive care unit receiving mechanical ventilation suffer the highest occurrence rate and mortality is particulary high in these critically ill patients. Treatment of bacterial pneumonia is hampered by the increased antibiotic-resistance of pathogens [3]. Immune host defense continues to play an important role in the outcome of bacterial pneumonia, and modulation of the inflammatory response has been considered as an adjunctive treatment strategy.

Normally, bacteria are prevented from reaching the alveoli by several defense mechanisms located along the upper airway. Bacteria reaching the alveoli are usually phagocytosed and killed by alveolar macrophages. When these normal protective mechanisms are overwhelmed, several complex defense systems are triggered. The invasion of pathogens produces a vigorous inflammatory response, including the recruitment of neutrophils. Neutrophils exert microbicidal effects involving several oxidative and enzymatic processes [4, 5]. In addition, complement products can promote the killing of bacteria by neutrophils and macrophages [6, 7].

Multiple lines of scientific evidence have demonstrated the crucial role of a complex network of cytokines in the initiation and maintenance of inflammation during bacterial infection. Much of our understanding of the role of cytokines is based on results from studies on overwhelming immune activation in the absence of a localized source, such as is induced by intravenous administration of bacterial products. Although excessive pro-inflammatory cytokine production during severe infection may have deleterious effects, more recent studies support the beneficial role of pro-inflammatory cytokines in local host defense.

Cytokines in Systemic Infections and Experimental Endotoxemia

Cytokines are small glycoproteins (6–30 kD) that can be produced by, and have effects on a large variety of cell types. The affinity of cytokines for their receptors is very high, enabling effects at picomolar concentrations. Mononuclear activation by bacteria or bacterial products, like lipopolysaccharide (LPS), leads to the production of the pro-inflammatory cytokines tumor necrosis factor-alpha (TNF-α), interleukin (IL)-1, IL-6 and IL-8 [8, 9], as well as the anti-inflammatory cytokine IL-10 [8]. TNF, IL-10 and interferon-γ (IFN-γ) are also produced by T cells and B cells after anti-genic stimulation. The pro- and anti-inflammatory cytokines interact in a complex network, in which they can influence each other's production and/or activity.

Much of our knowledge about the function of the cytokine network is derived from studies on systemic infections. Severe bacterial infection can result in profound physiologic changes including hypotension, fever, tissue necrosis, multiple organ dysfunction and finally death. In Gram-negative infections, these changes are due, at least in part, to endotoxin, the LPS component of the bacterial cell wall. Injection of LPS into animals produces changes that are typical of the sepsis syndrome. During such overwhelming immune activation, TNF and IL-1 are considered to be important mediators of systemic inflammatory responses [9, 10]. TNF and IL-1β have pleiotropic effects, including activation of neutrophils and the extrinsic pathway of coagulation, and stimulation of neutrophilic adherence to endothelial cells. It is clear that these cytokines play an orchestrating role in the generation of inflammation after an intravenous bolus of LPS in healthy humans. TNF is the first cytokine to appear [8] with peak plasma levels reached within 90 minutes following LPS administration. After the release of TNF, serum concentrations of other cytokines such as IL-6 and IL-8 increase. TNF is responsible for the release of these cytokines, since neutralization of TNF activity prevents the appearance of these secondary cytokines during endotoxemia [11]. Elimination of IL-6 activity does not affect the induction of other cytokines [12], indicating that IL-6 is a more distal cytokine in the LPS-induced cytokine cascade.

IL-10 is produced under different conditions of immune activation by different cell types, including T-cells, B-cells and monocytes [13]. In sepsis and after LPS administration, circulating levels of IL-10 are elevated. IL-10 production is also enhanced in various models of infection, like experimental endotoxemia, staphylococcal enterotoxin B-induced lethal shock, and septic peritonitis. IL-10 can inhibit the LPS-stimulated production of pro-inflammatory cytokines *in vitro* and *in vivo*. IL-10 plays a protective role in models of overzealous inflammation, since administration of IL-10 reduces LPS-mortality in animals, and neutralization of IL-10 results in increased lethality in LPS-challenged mice [13].

An important problem in interpreting models of Gram-negative sepsis and experimental endotoxemia is that they do not provide insight into the local production and interactions of cytokines at the site of an infection, e.g., within the lung during pneumonia. In recent years, several studies have provided information about local cytokine production during pneumonia, in human as well as in animal models.

The Cytokine Cascade in Pulmonary Infection

In local infection, like pneumonia, the initiation, maintenance and resolution of inflammation are considered to be dependent upon the expression of the complex network of pro-inflammatory and anti-inflammatory cytokines. In the last decade numerous studies have been performed to determine systemic and local levels of pro-inflammatory and anti-inflammatory cytokines in patients with pneumonia. In a study comprising 64 patients with community-acquired pneumonia with a well-defined etiology, Kragsbjerg et al. [14] found high concentrations of TNF, IL-6, IL-8 and IFN-γ in sera taken on admission to the hospital. Serum TNF was elevated in most patients, irrespective of the etiology, while serum IL-6 was highest in patients with pneumococcal pneumonia, and patients with pneumonia due to *Legionella* species. None of the patients with pneumonia due to pathogens like *Haemophilus influenzae, Moraxella catarrhalis* and *Chlamydia pneumoniae*, had a serum IL-6 level above 500 pg/ml. On the other hand, serum IFN-γ concentrations were elevated in most of the patients with viral or intracellular bacterial disease, the highest values being detected in patients with pneumonia due to *Legionella* species and *Chlamydia pneumoniae*. Elevated IFN-γ levels were seen in a minority of patients with pneumococcal pneumonia. In the second study by Kragsbjerg et al. [15], involving 63 patients with acute respiratory tract infection, serum IL-8 levels on admission were significantly higher among patients with bacteremic pneumococcal pneumonia, than in patients with *Chlamydia* pneumonia, *Legionella* pneumonia or influenza A virus infection. Other studies have confirmed the presence of elevated serum concentrations of TNF, IL-1β and IL-6 in patients with community-acquired pneumonia [16, 17].

Investigations examining cytokine concentrations in pleural and bronchoalveolar lavage (BAL) fluid have suggested that during pneumonia, cytokines are produced locally at the site of the infection. In a study of 102 patients with pleural effusion of different etiologies, Silva-Mejias et al. [18] found that IL-1 levels were elevated in pleural fluids of all 14 patients with empyema. In pleural effusions of other etiologies (transudates, parapneumonic, tuberculous, neoplastic and miscellanous), only 3 patients, 2 with parapneumonic pleural effusion and 1 with tuberculous pleural effusion, had elevated IL-1β levels in the pleural fluid [18]. Broaddus et al. [19] found higher IL-8 levels in pleural empyema fluids, compared with other types of effusion. IL-8 levels correlated with neutrophil counts in pleural fluid, and pleural fluid neutrophil chemotactic activity [19]. Interestingly an anti-IL-8 antibody decreased the neutrophil chemotactic activity of pleural fluid, suggesting that IL-8 plays an important role in the recruitment of neutrophils in empyema.

Dehoux et al. [20] and Boutten et al. [21] studied local cytokine production by measuring cytokine levels in BAL fluid from 15 patients admitted for unilateral community-acquired pneumonia. Cytokine concentrations in BAL fluid from the infected lung were compared with those in BAL fluid from the contralateral, non-involved lung and in BAL fluid from healthy individuals. In addition, cytokine levels were determined in sera, to enable comparison between local and systemic cytokine concentrations. It was found that TNF, IL-1β, IL-6 and IL-8 concentrations were significantly higher in the infected lung than in the non-involved lung or serum, indicating that the cytokine response during unilateral pneumonia is compartmentalized and limited to the site of infection (Fig. 1). Schutte et al. [22] compared cytokine concentrations in BAL fluid and serum of patients with acute respiratory failure due to cardiogenic pulmonary edema (6 patients), adult respiratory distress syndrome (ARDS, 12 patients), primary severe pneumonia (38 patients) or a combination (pneumonia and ARDS, 18 patients). In all patients with ARDS and/or pneu-

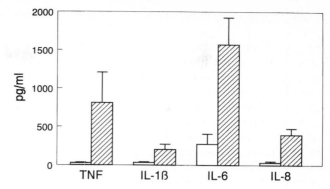

Fig. 1. Compartmentalized cytokine production during pneumonia. Mean (±SE) cytokine concentrations in bronchoalveolar lavage (BAL) fluid obtained from patients with unilateral community acquired pneumonia. Open bars represent cytokine levels in BAL fluid from the non-involved lung, hatched bars represent cytokine levels in BAL fluid from the infected lung. (Adapted from [20] and [21] with permission)

monia elevated BAL fluid levels of IL-6 and IL-8 were detected. Serum IL-6 levels were also elevated in these patients, whereas IL-8 levels were increased inconsistently.

In addition to cytokine measurements in BAL fluid and serum, Dehoux et al. [20] also examined cytokine production by alveolar and peripheral macrophages *ex vivo*. Alveolar macrophages recovered from the infected lung spontaneously released more TNF, IL-1β and IL-6 into cell culture supernatants than macrophages evacuated from the non-involved lung. The spontaneous release of these cytokines by macrophages from the non-involved lung was comparable to those from lungs of healthy controls. After stimulation with LPS *ex vivo*, cytokine concentrations reached in cell culture supernatants were similar when cells from the involved lung and non-involved lung of the patients were compared, but much lower than those measured in control subjects. This hypo-responsiveness to *in vitro* LPS stimulation was not observed in the cultures of peripheral monocytes. These data are in line with reports on LPS hyporesponsiveness of mononuclear cells from peripheral blood of patients with severe systemic infections [23], and support the existence of a compartmentalized inflammatory response during pneumonia. Huang et al. [24] measured cytokine release from alveolar macrophages obtained from patients with acquired immunodeficiency syndrome (AIDS) and *Pneumocystis carinii* pneumonia who received or did not receive corticosteroids. LPS stimulation resulted in significantly less TNF and IL-1β release from alveolar macrophages of patients receiving corticosteroids, indicating that local cytokine production can be downregulated by this steroid hormone.

At present no studies have been published concerning the local production of anti-inflammatory cytokines in pneumonia in humans.

Studies on Cytokine Production in Animal Models of Pneumonia

Recently, several studies in animals with experimental respiratory tract infections have confirmed the suggestion that in pneumonia, like in systemic infections, inflammation is orchestrated by pro-inflammatory and anti-inflammatory cytokines (Table 1). In murine pneumococcal pneumonia, induced by intranasal instillation of 10^6 colony forming units (CFU) of *Streptococcus pneumoniae*, increased levels of TNF were found from day 1 in serum and from day 3 in lungs, concomitant with an increase in bacterial counts in lungs [25]. The experimental infection was worsened by intravenous administration of an anti-TNF antibody, since this treatment enhanced bacterial proliferation in the blood, compared with mice treated with normal rabbit serum. These results suggest that TNF prevents the onset of bacteremia, and plays a protective role in experimental pneumococcal pneumonia. Indeed mortality was significantly higher in anti-TNF-treated mice. Similar results were obtained in another murine pneumococcal pneumonia investigation [26]. Intranasal inoculation of 10^6 CFU of *Streptococcus pneumoniae* resulted in a sustained release of TNF in lung homogenates reaching a plateau between 12 and 72 hours. Intraperitoneal treatment with a neutralizing anti-TNF antibody two hours before inoculation strongly reduced TNF levels in lungs, while IL-1β levels were only modestly affected and IL-6, IL-10 and IFN-γ concentrations were unchanged. Mice treated with anti-TNF had four fold more *Streptococcus pneumoniae* CFU isolated from lungs than control mice 40 hours after inoculation, and died significantly earlier from pneumococcal pneumonia (Fig. 2). Compelling evidence in support of TNF as an important mediator in bacterial pneumonia with other than Gram-positive pathogens is derived from models of Gram-negative bacterial respiratory tract infections. In murine pneumonia induced by an intratracheal challenge with 10^2 CFU of *Klebsiella pneumoniae*, anti-TNF treatment was associated with a markedly decreased survival, increased bacterial growth in lung homogenates and blood, and a significant reduction in BAL neutrophils at 48 hours after inoculation [27]. Anti-TNF had the same effect on growth of *Legionella pneumophila* in lungs in a pneumonia model induced by intratracheal inoculation of 10^6 CFU of this microorganism [28]. In mice with pneumonia caused by *Pneumocystis carinii* anti-TNF almost completely prevented the clearance of *Pneumocystis* from the lungs [29]. In addition, treatment of granulocytopenic mice with low doses of TNF and/or IL-1β significantly diminished mortality and enhanced pulmonary clearance of *Pseudomonas*

Table 1. Role of endogenous cytokines, produced within the pulmonary compartment, during pneumonia in mice

Protective	Detrimental
TNF	IL-10
IL-6	
IFN-γ	
IL-12	
MIP-2	

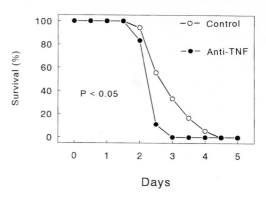

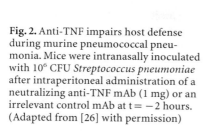

Fig. 2. Anti-TNF impairs host defense during murine pneumococcal pneumonia. Mice were intranasally inoculated with 10^6 CFU *Streptococcus pneumoniae* after intraperitoneal administration of a neutralizing anti-TNF mAb (1 mg) or an irrelevant control mAb at t = −2 hours. (Adapted from [26] with permission)

aeruginosa during severe pneumonia [30]. Hence, endogenously produced TNF is important for host defense during experimental pneumonia induced by different microorganisms.

Macrophage inflammatory protein-2 (MIP-2) is an important mediator of inflammation, inducing potent chemotaxis of neutrophils. Greenberger et al. [31] found time-dependent expression of MIP-2 mRNA and protein within the lung during murine *Klebsiella* pneumonia. Treatment of mice with an anti-MIP-2 antibody caused a 60% decrease in lung neutrophil influx, a significant increase of *Klebsiella pneumoniae* CFU in lungs and liver homogenates, and a decrease in early survival. These results indicate the important role of MIP-2 in neutrophil influx and bacterial clearance during pneumonia.

Evidence for the importance of IL-6 in host defense is obtained from a study on pneumococcal pneumonia in IL-6 deficient mice [32]. Intranasal inoculation of 10^6 CFU of *Streptococcus pneumoniae*, resulted in sustained expression of IL-6 mRNA and protein in lungs. Higher levels of the pro-inflammatory cytokines TNF, IL-1β and IFN-γ and the anti-inflammatory cytokine IL-10 were found in the lungs of IL-6 deficient mice with pneumonia. IL-6 deficient mice had more CFU of *Streptococcus pneumoniae* in their lungs, and died significantly earlier than normal mice. Hence, IL-6 down-regulates the activation of the cytokine network within the lung during pneumonia and contributes to host defense.

IFN-γ is another pro-inflammatory cytokine that seems to be important for resistance against Gram-positive respiratory tract infections. IFN-γ production is enhanced during murine pneumococcal pneumonia [26, 33], and IFN-γ deficient mice show a markedly increased susceptibility to infection with *Streptococcus pneumoniae* [33]. However, anti-IFN-γ treatment had no detectable effect on the clearance of *Pneumocystis carinii* from lungs [29].

The importance of another pro-inflammatory cytokine, IL-12, was recently demonstrated in mice suffering from pneumonia with *Klebsiella pneumoniae* [34]. Intratracheal challenge with 10^2 CFU *Klebsiella pneumoniae* resulted in a time dependent expression of IL-12 mRNA and protein in the lung. Passive immunization with a polyclonal anti-IL-12 antibody at the time of infection with *Klebsiella pneumoniae* resulted in a marked increase in bacterial counts in lung homogenates 48 hours after inoculation, as compared with mice receiving control serum. Moreover, treatment with anti-IL-12 decreased survival. Overexpression of IL-12 within the lung by intratracheal administration of an adenoviral vector containing the human cytomegalovirus promoter and cDNA coding for IL-12, resulted in 45% long term survival in *Klebsiella* pneumonia, while none of the mice receiving control adenovirus survived. In the same experiment [34], passive immunization against TNF or IFN-γ led to a failure of IL-12 overexpression to protect mice, indicating that IL-12 does not act alone in the defense against invading microorganisms.

Considerable evidence exists that the anti-inflammatory cytokine IL-10 plays a detrimental role in the clearance of bacteria during pulmonary infections [35, 36]. Intratracheal installation of 10^3 CFU *Klebsiella pneumoniae* was associated with increased IL-10 mRNA and protein levels in lung homogenates [35]. Passive immunization of mice with a polyclonal anti-IL-10 antibody resulted in significantly higher levels of TNF in lung homogenates, than in mice that received pre-immune serum. Importantly, *Klebsiella pneumoniae* CFU in lungs of mice treated with anti-IL-10 were approximately eight fold less, than in mice treated with pre-immune serum, while *Klebsiella pneumoniae* CFU in plasma were over a hundred fold less. Although intratracheal instillation of *Klebsiella pneumoniae* resulted in 100% lethality in all mice, survival was significantly longer in anti-IL-10 treated mice. Similar results were obtained in studies with experimental pneumonia with Gram-positive bacteria [36]. Intranasal administration of *Streptococcus pneumoniae* resulted in a marked increase in IL-10 in lung homogenates, the highest lung IL-10 levels being measured at 72 hours after inoculation with pneumococci. Treatment of mice with recombinant IL-10 resulted in a decrease in lung TNF levels, while administration of an anti-IL-10 antibody resulted in a three and a half fold rise in lung TNF and IFN-γ levels. In animals treated with anti-IL-10, bacterial counts from lung and blood were lower and survival was significantly increased (Fig. 3). Together with the results from the study of Greenberger et al. [35], these results indicate that during pneumonia, IL-10 attenuates the pro-inflammatory cytokine response within the lungs, hampers effective clearance of infection and shortens survival.

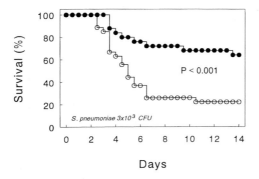

Fig. 3. Anti-IL-10 protects mice against lethality during pneumococcal pneumonia. Mice were intranasally inoculated with 3×10^3 CFU *Streptococcus pneumoniae* after intraperitoneal administration of a neutralizing anti-IL-10 mAb (2 mg; closed circles) or an irrelevant control mAb (open circles) at $t = -2$ hours. (Adapted from [36] with permission)

Conclusion

As in systemic infection, inflammation during pneumonia is orchestrated by locally produced pro-inflammatory and anti-inflammatory cytokines. There are however some important differences between the role of cytokines during localized infection and during fulminant systemic infection. Whereas excessive production of pro-inflammatory cytokines at the systemic level causes organ failure and death in animal models of fulminant sepsis, the local production of these cytokines importantly contributes to host defense against pneumonia. Conversely, while the anti-inflammatory cytokine IL-10 is protective in models of overzealous immune activation, it impairs host defense during pneumonia. These findings emphasize the importance of clinically relevant animal models to fully understand the role of cytokines in the pathogenesis of bacterial infection. Local modulation of the cytokine network may serve as an important addition to antibiotic therapy, especially when faced with multi-drug resistant organisms and/or immunocompromised hosts.

References

1. British Thoracic Society Research Committee (1987) Community-acquired pneumonia in adults in British hospitals in 1982–1983: A survey of aetiology, mortality, prognostic factors and outcome. Q J Med 62:195–220
2. Horan T, Culver D, Jarvis W (1988) Pathogens causing nosocomial infections. Antimicrob Newsletter 5:65–67
3. Davies J (1994) Inactivation of antibiotics and the dissemination of resistance genes. Science 264:375–382
4. Weiss SJ (1989) Tissue destruction by neutrophils. N Engl J Med 320:365–375
5. Tsai WC, Strieter RM, Zisman DA, et al (1997) Nitric Oxide is required for effective innate immunity against Klebsiella pneumoniae. Infect Immun 65:1870–1875
6. Hopken UE, Lu B, Gerard NP, Gerard C (1996) The C5a chemoattractant receptor mediates mucosal defense to infection. Nature 383:86–89
7. Winkelstein JA (1981) The role of complement in the host's defense against Streptococcus pneumoniae. Rev Infect Dis 3:289–297
8. Pajkrt D, van der Poll T, van Deventer SJH (1997) Inflammatory responses during human endotoxemia. In: Vincent JL (ed) 1997 Yearbook of intensive care and emergency medicine. Springer-Verlag, Berlin, Heidelberg, pp 14–30
9. Van der Poll T, Lowry SF (1995) Tumor necrosis factor in sepsis: Mediator of multiple organ failure or essential part of host defense? Shock 3:1–12
10. Dinarello CA (1996) Biological basis for interleukin 1 in disease. Blood 87:2095–2147
11. Suffredini AF, Reda D, Banks SM, Tropea M, Agosti JM, Miller R (1995) Effects of recombinant dimeric TNF receptor on human inflammatory responses following intravenous endotoxin administration. J Immunol 155:5038–5045
12. Van der Poll T, Levi M, Hack CE, et al (1994) Elimination of interleukin 6 attenuates coagulation activation in experimental endotoxemia in chimpanzees. J Exp Med 179:1253–1259
13. Moore KW, O'Garra A, de Waal Malefyt R, Vierra P, Mosmann TR (1993) Interleukin-10. Annu Rev Immunol 11:165–190
14. Kragsbjerg P, Vekerfors T, Holmberg H (1993) Serum levels of interleukin 6, tumor necrosis factor alpha, interferon gamma and C-reactive protein in adults with community-acquired pneumonia. Serodiagn Immunoth Infect Disease 5:156–160
15. Kragsbjerg P, Jones I, Vikerfors T, Holmberg H (1995) Diagnostic value of blood cytokine concentrations in acute pneumonia. Thorax 50:1253–1257
16. Puren AJ, Feldman C, Savage N, Becker PJ, Smith C (1995) Patterns of cytokine expression in community-acquired pneumonia. Chest 107:1342–1349

17. Moussa K, Michie HJ, Cree IA, et al (1994) Phagocyte function and cytokine production in community-acquired pneumonia. Thorax 49:107–111
18. Silva-Mejias C, Gamboa-Antinolo F, Lopez-Cortez LF, Cruz-Ruiz M, Pachon J (1995) Interleukin 1 beta in pleural fluids of different etiologies. Its role as inflammatory mediator in empyema. Chest 108:942–945
19. Broaddus VC, Hebert CA, Vitangcol RV, Hoeffel JM, Bernstein MS, Bylan AM (1992) Interleukin-8 is a major neutrophil chemotactic factor in pleural liquid of patients with empyema. Am Rev Respir Dis 146:825–830
20. Dehoux MS, Boutten A, Ostinelli J, et al (1994) Compartmentalized cytokine production within human lung in unilateral pneumonia. Am J Resp Crit Care Med 150:710–716
21. Boutten A, Dehoux MS, Seta N, et al (1996) Compartmentalized IL-8 and elastase release within the human lung in unilateral pneumonia. Am J Respir Crit Care Med 153:336–342
22. Schutte H, Lohmeyer J, Rosseau S, et al (1996) Bronchoalveolar and systemic cytokine profiles in patients with ARDS, severe pneumonia and cardiogenic pulmonary oedema. Eur Respir J 9:1858–1867
23. Munoz C, Carlet J, Fitting C, Misset B, Bleriot JP, Cavaillon JM (1991) Dysregulation of in vitro cytokine production by monocytes during sepsis. 88:1747–1754
24. Huang ZB, Eden E (1993) Effect of corticosteroids on IL-1β and TNF alpha release by alveolar macrophages from patients with AIDS and Pneumocystis carinii pneumonia. Chest 104:751–755
25. Takashima K, Tateda K, Matsumoto T, Iizawa Y, Nakao M, Yamaguchi K (1997) Role of tumor necrosis factor alpha in the pathogenesis of pneumococcal pneumonia in mice. Infect Immun 65:257–260
26. Van der Poll T, Keogh CV, Buurman WA, Lowry SF (1997) Passive immunization against tumor necrosis factor alpha impairs host defense during pneumococcal pneumonia. Am J Resp Crit Care Med 155:603–608
27. Laichalk LL, Kunkel SL, Strieter RM, Danforth JM, Bailie MB, Standiford TJ (1996) Tumor necrosis factor mediates lung antibacterial host defense in murine Klebsiella pneumonia. Infect Immun 64:5211–5218
28. Brieland JK, Remick DG, Freeman PJ, Hurley MC, Fontane JC, Engleberg NC (1995) In vivo regulation of replicative Legionella pneumophila lung infection by endogenous tumor necrosis factor alpha and nitric oxide. Infect Immun 63:3253–3258
29. Chen W, Havell EA, Harmsen AG (1992) Importance of endogenous tumor necrosis factor alpha and interferon gamma in host resistence against Pneumocystis carinii infection. Infect Immun 60:1279–1284
30. Amura C, Fontan PA, Sanjuan N, Sordelli DO (1994) The effect of treatment with interleukin-1 and tumor necrosis factor on Pseudomonas aeruginosa lung infection in a granulocytopenic mouse model. Clin Immunol Immunopath 2:261–266
31. Greenberger MJ, Strieter RM, Kunkel SL, et al (1996) Neutralization of macrophage inflammatory protein-2 attenuates neutrophil recruitment and bacterial clearance in murine Klebsiella pneumonia. J Infect Dis 173:159–165
32. Van der Poll T, Keogh CV, Guirao X, Buurman WA, Kopf M, Lowry SF (1997) Interleukin-6 gene deficient mice show impaired defense against Streptococcal pneumonia. J Infect Dis 176:439–444
33. Rubins JB, Pomeroy C (1997) Role of gamma interferon in the pathogenesis of bacteremic pneumococcal pneumonia. Infect Immun 65:2975–2977
34. Greenberger MJ, Kunkel SL, Strieter RM, et al (1996) IL-12 gene therapy protects mice in lethal Klebsiella pneumonia. J Immunol 157:3006–3012
35. Greenberger MJ, Strieter RM, Kunkel SL, Danforth JM, Goodman RE, Standiford TJ (1995) Neutralizing of IL-10 increases survival in a murine model of Klebsiella pneumonia. J Immunol 155:722–729
36. Van der Poll T, Marchant A, Keogh CV, Goldman M, Lowry SF (1996) Interleukin-10 impairs host defense in murine pneumococcal pneumonia. J Infect Dis 174:994–1000

A Central Role of Interleukin-8 in the Pathogenesis of ARDS

A. B. J. Groeneveld

Introduction

The pathogenesis of the acute respiratory distress syndrome (ARDS) remains incompletely understood. It is generally believed that extrapulmonary factors, such as sepsis and trauma, or intrapulmonary factors, such as aspiration of gastric contents or pneumonia, lead to microvascular neutrophil entrapping in the lungs and migration into the interstitium and alveolar air space, resulting in structural damage, increased permeability and altered lung mechanics and gas exchange. The factor(s) primarily responsible for this neutrophil response remains unclear, and even the primary role of the neutrophil itself can be questioned.

The goal of this chapter is to present the arguments for a central role of interleukin (IL)-8 in the development and course of ARDS. In fact, IL-8 is believed to be a central and powerful neutrophil chemoattracting and activating agent [1, 2].

Properties and Actions of IL-8

Origin and Stimuli for Release

A variety of cell types are able to produce the small molecular (8 kD) cytokine (chemokine) IL-8, in response to a variety of stimuli [1, 2] (Table 1). Table 2 describes the classic conditions in which IL-8 has been reported or suggested to play a role in man. *In vitro*, endotoxin, tumor necrosis factor (TNF)-α and IL-1β are major IL-8 inducers [1, 3–7]. Hypoxia/re-oxygenation is also a potent stimulus for IL-8 production by endothelium and macrophages/monocytes *in vitro*, even in the absence of release of other cytokines, and oxyradicals released during reperfusion may play an intermediary role [8, 9]. This seemingly selective IL-8 production is enhanced by endotoxin [8]. In endotoxin-stimulated blood, inhibition of oxyradicals may ame-

Table 1. Origin and stimuli for release of IL-8

Stimuli
Endotoxin, IL-1β, IL-2, TNF-α, activated complement C5a
Cell types
Monocytes and neutrophils, endothelium, synovial cells, (alveolar) macrophages, hepatocytes, (alveolar and tubular) epithelial cells, mesangial cells, fibroblasts

Table 2. Conditions associated with IL-8 production and increased risk of ARDS in man

- Endotoxemia
- TNF-α infusion
- Sepsis
- Cardiopulmonary bypass
- Respiration
- Pneumonia
- Hemodialysis
- Major vascular surgery

liorate IL-8 release but not that of other cytokines [8]. These phenomena may also apply to ischemia/reperfusion *in vivo*. After coronary occlusion and reperfusion in dogs, IL-8 is expressed in the infarcted area and this is believed to contribute to neutrophil-mediated myocardial injury [7, 10]. Hypoxic mice demonstrate IL-8 dependent pulmonary leukostasis [9]. Some evidence exists that these mechanisms also operate in man. During aortic surgery in man, resulting in ischemia/reperfusion of the lower body and occasionally in pulmonary complications, a rapid rise in IL-8 plasma levels occurs peaking within hours after the start of reperfusion [11–13]. This, in turn, is accompanied by a rise in pulmonary microvascular permeability [11, 13] and, in another study, by some discrete radiographic, lung mechanical and gas exchange abnormalities [12]. The 77-amino acid endothelial form of IL-8 has less potent neutrophil activating capacity than the 72-amino acid form from monocytes [14], but the former may be cleaved, at least *in vitro*, to the more potent 72-amino acid form by thrombin, among others [14]. By this mechanism coagulation and inflammation may interact. Intravascular coagulation is thus a stimulus for IL-8 release by endothelial and mononuclear cells [14, 15].

Actions

IL-8 is considered as a potent neutrophil (and T-lymphocyte) chemoattractant and activator [1]. It may induce neutrophil conformational (cytoskeleton) changes, increase adhesive properties, promote degranulation, and enhance the respiratory burst [1, 10]. However, the role of IL-8 as a potent neutrophil activating agent has been modified somewhat, since in some studies IL-8 appears to activate neutrophils to release oxyradicals *in vitro* only if primed, for instance by other cytokines or activated complement products [16, 17]. Conversely, IL-8 is able to prime neutrophils and to enhance their response to other agonists [16]. Intratrachealy administered IL-8 is able to recruit neutrophils into the lungs in rats, but is unable to induce degranulation on its own [18].

IL-8 secreted by the endothelium is a central chemoattractant for circulating neutrophils [3, 6, 7, 19]. It enhances adhesion and neutrophil transmigration through endothelium, thereby increasing permeability [3, 6, 7]. IL-8 is also able to increase endothelial permeability independently of (activated) neutrophils [20]. These are clearly pro-inflammatory effects [1]. However, IL-8 may play a dual role,

since circulating IL-8, for instance released into the circulation by endothelium activated by endotoxin or cytokines, may decrease the adhesive capacity of neutrophils
to endothelium [4, 6, 7, 14, 21]. This may explain why locally injected IL-8 may induce an inflammatory response, that can be inhibited by intravascularly administered IL-8 [19]. Part of the anti-inflammatory effect is related to shedding, IL-8 desensitization and to a change in the cytoskeleton of the neutrophils [4, 6, 21, 22].

A change in the neutrophil cytoskeleton would inhibit their ability to adhere to
vascular endothelium but on the other hand would promote, as a result of stiffening,
their ability to sequestrate in the pulmonary microvasculature [22] This would explain the rapid but transient leukopenia attributed to lung microvascular sequestration of neutrophils after intravenous injection of IL-8 in healthy animals [5, 19]. The
neutropenia reverses into neutrocytosis following bone marrow recruitment until
the IL-8 infusion is stopped [5, 19]. The injected animals, however, do not release
other cytokines nor have adverse sequelae, i.e., gas exchange or pulmonary radiographic abnormalities, after the IL-8 dose, raising doubt about the toxicity of circulating IL-8 [5].

The neutrophil pulmonary entrapping effect of IL-8 could only partly explain the
occurrence of remote organ, i.e., pulmonary damage, after an extrapulmonary insult
such as lower body ischemia/reperfusion associated with aortic surgery and a local
release of IL-8 into the circulation [11–13]. To explain the suggested harmful role of
circulating IL-8 in ARDS predisposing conditions in man [11–13, 23, 24], one therefore has to surmise the involvement of other initiating, priming or synergistic factors affecting neutrophils, which may include oxyradicals and activated complement
products [11–13].

Interaction with Other Inflammatory Mediators

The release of IL-8 is, under certain circumstances, partly dependent on TNF-α and
IL-1β, and the neutrophil chemoattractant and activating properties of TNF-α and
IL-1β are partly accomplished through IL-8 [1]. Anti-TNF-α may, in some models,
thus reduce IL-8 responses in sepsis. The effect of IL-1β and TNF-α on neutrophil
transendothelial migration is also partly dependent on endothelial production of
IL-8 [6]. When considering the time course, the rise in IL-8 in blood usually lags
behind the rise in TNF-α and IL-1β after stimulation *in vivo* or *in vitro* [21]. This
reinforces the idea that some of the effects of the primary cytokines are mediated
through IL-8 *in vivo*. Finally, complement activation products may increase the
monocyte production of IL-8. As far as plasma levels are concerned, circulating IL-8
levels generally correlate with those of IL-6 during sepsis and allied conditions,
suggesting a similar origin, stimulus and kinetics of release, and making it difficult
to attribute biological effects to one cytokine or the other [11–15, 23–28].

Modulators

Table 3 shows some modulators of IL-8. IL-8 can be complexed to erythrocytes, α_2-
macroglobulin and endogenous anti-IL-8 antibodies [29, 30]. Binding to anti-IL-8

Table 3. Some modulators of IL-8

Release inhibitors	IL-8 binding
Anti-TNF-α	α_2-macroglobulin
IL-1-receptor antagonist	Erythrocytes
IL-10	Anti-IL-8 (auto)antibodies
Gamma-interferon	
Prostaglandin E_2	
Steroids	
Oxyradical scavengers	
Anti-C5a	
Platelet activating factor antagonist	
Pentoxifylline	
Nitric oxide inhibitors	

antibodies or erythrocytes limits the activity of the free form, while binding to α_2-macroglobulin prevents IL-8 from proteolytic breakdown and enhances its active form [30]. In fact, some of these mechanisms may play a role in the alveolar space during ARDS [29, 30].

Potential Pathogenetic Role of IL-8 in ARDS

Various extrapulmonary conditions are risk factors for ARDS, such as sepsis, multiple trauma, shock, major vascular surgery and cardiopulmonary bypass. Severe inhalation injury, aspiration or pneumonia may also result in ARDS. The syndrome is characterized by diffuse alveolar consolidations on the chest radiograph, a non-compliant lung and severe gas exchange abnormalities, supposedly caused by alveolar inflammation and protein-rich exudate, in response to a critical illness.

During ARDS, neutrophils are believed to play a central role, even though ARDS may also occur in patients with neutropenia. Recruitment into the alveolar space and activation of neutrophils is thought to be accomplished by a chemoattractant substance produced in the alveolar space. A likely candidate for this role is IL-8, whether or not it is induced by other cytokines like IL-1β [27, 28, 31–39]. In fact, the severity of radiographic, lung mechanical, and gas exchange abnormalities, expressed as the lung injury score (LIS), may be directly related to the degree of neutrophil activation during ARDS [25, 35]. Alveolar macrophages, epithelial cells and pulmonary fibroblasts can produce IL-8 [34, 40] in response to certain stimuli such as IL-1β and TNF-α but the main stimuli for induction of ARDS-associated inflammation are still conjectural.

After an intrapulmonary injury such as pneumonia or aspiration, it can be presumed that the local inflammatory reactions involve IL-8-associated neutrophil recruitment. In ARDS associated with extrapulmonary disease, a similar mechanism may be operative, and indeed authors have suggested higher IL-8 levels in bronchoalveolar lavage (BAL) fluid than in blood in extrapulmonary ARDS, i.e., gradients that would favor neutrophil attraction into the lungs [27, 33], but the reason for this greater pulmonary than systemic production of IL-8 is unclear. In fact, IL-8 may be produced outside the lungs, with elevated circulating levels found in sepsis, cardio-pulmonary bypass, hemodialysis, lower body ischemia/reperfusion and other etio-logic risk factors for ARDS (see below) [11–13, 23, 24, 41–45]. Circulating IL-8 may on the one hand impair extrapulmonary extravasation at inflammatory sites by leukocyte adhesion inhibition, but may on the other hand, stiffen neutrophils for entrapment in the lungs and promote, if primed by some prior stimulus, the release of harmful products (see above). This may indeed explain the relation between cir-culating IL-8 levels and pulmonary changes in patients with extrapulmonary risk factors for ARDS (Fig. 1) [15], and the relation between circulating IL-8 levels and the severity and course of established ARDS from mainly extrapulmonary sources, as described before [25]. During ischemia/reperfusion-associated aortic surgery in man, it has also been suggested that circulating IL-8 is the primary cytokine in-volved in the post-operative pulmonary changes of neutrophil-mediated acute lung injury, since blood levels shortly after completing surgery are elevated, and unlike activated complement products, correlate with neutropenia, elevated pulmonary vascular protein permeability and the LIS [11–13]. Nevertheless, complement acti-vation may have primed neutrophils in these conditions [12]. These mechanisms may explain why conditions eliciting high circulating IL-8 levels constitute risk fac-tors for ARDS development.

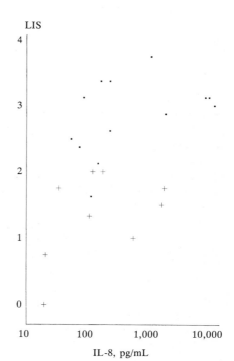

Fig. 1. Correlation betweeen plasma IL-8 levels and the lung injury score (LIS), expressing the clinical severity of pulmonary injury, in pa-tients at risk for ARDS (+) and in those with established ARDS (●): $r_s = 0.46$, $p < 0.05$. Nor-mal IL-8 levels are < 20 pg/mL. (Data from [15])

IL-8 Levels During ARDS

Blood

Elevated blood levels of IL-8 in man have been found during sepsis, multiple organ failure, endotoxemia, trauma, and hemodialysis, all known risk factors for ARDS [21, 23, 24, 28, 33, 38, 41, 44, 45]. During cardiopulmonary bypass, (leukocyte associated) IL-8 levels may also increase [42, 43]. Elevated blood levels have been found in human ARDS, particularly if caused by sepsis, but not all authors agree on this [9, 15, 23–26, 28, 33–35, 38, 41, 44]. Blood cytokine levels may even be higher during intra-pulmonary (pneumonia complicated by sepsis) than extrapulmonary ARDS [26, 28, 33, 35]. Moreover, IL-8 levels in blood have been found to correlate with neutrophil activation and degranulation products such as elastase during sepsis and ARDS, supporting a role for the cytokine in neutrophil activation *in vivo* and thereby, perhaps, in the pathogenesis of ARDS [24, 25, 35]. Shortly after ischemia/reper-fusion-involving aortic surgery, a risk factor for ARDS in man, however, elevated elastase levels correlated with activated complement products rather than with elevated IL-8 levels [12]. It was suggested that priming of neutrophils by activated complement was necessary for circulating IL-8 to induce neutrophil-mediated pulmonary microvascular changes in this condition.

Bronchoalveolar Lavage

Many authors reported elevated BAL/edema fluid IL-8 levels in pneumonia, ARDS and other inflammatory lung diseases, compared with levels in edema fluid from hydrostatic pulmonary edema patients, while some studies found no difference in BAL IL-8 levels during pneumonia and ARDS [27–32, 35–39, 40]. However, other studies found a higher BAL IL-8 level in pneumonia (and sepsis)-associated ARDS than in extrapulmonary ARDS, but the gradient to blood levels may be similar [27, 33, 38]. It has been reported that BAL IL-8 levels are more elevated than those in blood, and that this increased gradient could be responsible for attracting neu-trophils into the lungs, with subsequent activation and tissue damage [27, 32–34, 37, 38, 42, 46]. IL-8, of all the inflammatory mediators, appeared to correlate best with BAL (activated) neutrophil numbers [27, 28, 31–33, 35, 37–39, 42, 46], thus suggesting that this cytokine was primarily responsible for neutrophil recruit-ment into alveolar spaces. When serially obtained, BAL neutrophil counts seem to parallel changes in IL-8 concentration [46]. Furthermore, BAL IL-8 levels may correlate with and parallel changes in albumin/protein levels, suggesting that IL-8 is, directly or indirectly, involved in the increased permeability in these conditions, but this correlation may be less clear than the correlation with neutrophil numbers [27, 28, 31, 32, 39, 46]. Taken together, these data suggest a direct role of IL-8 in alveolar exudation.

Association with ARDS Development

In some studies blood and BAL IL-8 levels were elevated, in patients at risk of ARDS but not yet fulfilling the criteria for the syndrome [7, 31, 34, 42, 43]. These recognized risk factors included sepsis, trauma, major vascular surgery, and cardiopulmonary bypass. For instance, cardiopulmonary bypass, a known risk factor for ARDS may result in increased blood and particularly BAL IL-8 levels [31, 42, 43]. Some authors have noted higher circulating levels in patients developing ARDS in the course of sepsis, trauma or other risk factors, than in those with risk factors but without subsequent ARDS development (Fig. 1) [15, 41], supporting a pathogenetic role for circulating IL-8 in ARDS. This has not, however, been confirmed in other studies, so that the predictive value of circulating IL-8 in this respect, even if serially measured in at risk patients, is still unclear [7, 15, 24, 34, 44]. For instance, patients developing ARDS after trauma may have higher circulating IL-8 levels at, and after, a diagnosis of ARDS than patients without ARDS [44], disfavoring a cause-effect relation although a late ARDS diagnosis cannot be ruled out. In other studies, however, trauma patients with the highest plasma IL-8 levels post-injury were more likely to develop ARDS [41]. This predictive value of circulating IL-8 seemed higher than that of circulating IL-6 and activated complement products. During aortic surgery-associated ischemia/reperfusion, IL-8 levels in the blood may transiently increase, and this may be accompanied by a transient increase in directly measured pulmonary microvascular permeability and slight radiographic, ventilatory, lung mechanical and gas exchange abnormalities [11–13]. Since no patient with this mild form of acute lung injury developed full blown ARDS, the predictive value of these changes, including an elevated IL-8 level, for the development of ARDS remained uncertain [11–13, 24]. In other studies, at risk patients ultimately developing ARDS had more elevated BAL IL-8 levels than at risk patients without ARDS development, in the presence of similar blood levels, so that BAL IL-8 levels predicted ARDS occurrence [31, 34]. Taken together, these data suggest a major role of IL-8 in the pathogenesis of ARDS in patients at risk.

Correlation with ARDS Severity and Course

A relation between IL-8 levels and the clinical severity and course of ARDS would also favor a pathogenetic role for IL-8 in the syndrome. In fact, several investigators have shown that the course of blood IL-8 levels, but also the level of other cytokines, during ARDS of extrapulmonary origin parallels the clinical course with a fall during ARDS recovery, a rise during worsening of the syndrome, and a direct relation with the LIS [25, 26, 35]. For BAL IL-8 levels a similar phenomenon has been described: Persistence of elevated levels in patients not recovering from ARDS, a fall towards normal levels in recovering patients, and a direct relation with the LIS [27, 35, 37]. Jorens et al. [31] described a direct correlation of BAL IL-8 levels with oxygenation impairment during (pre-) ARDS.

Correlation with ARDS Outcome

Like IL-6 levels, blood IL-8 levels also appear to be of prognostic significance during sepsis [24–26], a leading cause of ARDS. Serial blood and BAL values may separate survivors from non-survivors in patients with ARDS or at risk of ARDS [25, 26, 46]. In fact many, but not all, authors found that (persistently) elevated BAL IL-8 levels (and their ratio to plasma values) were associated with a poor outcome, i.e., increased mortality, during ARDS [25, 27–30, 32, 33, 36, 37, 46].

Interventions Aimed at Suppressing IL-8 in Experimental Models

Although a variety of agents are known to inhibit IL-8 release, as demonstrated mainly in *in vitro* experiments (Table 3), administration of anti-IL-8 antibodies has been tried in experimental models of lung ischemia/reperfusion [47], immune complex vasculitis of the lungs [48], aspiration [49] and endotoxemia/sepsis [50]. In these models, intravenously administered anti-IL-8 almost completely blocked the inflammatory response in the lungs, even if given after the challenge rather than before [47–50]. The efficacy of circulating anti-IL-8 is also remarkable in models where intrapulmonary challenges mainly leads to local IL-8 production. Anti-IL-8 antibodies may block the chemoattractant activity in human BAL fluid *in vitro* [32, 37]. A word of caution is necessary, however, since circulating IL-8 may have an anti-inflammatory effect as alluded to above so that an anti-IL-8 antibody may enhance rather than inhibit neutrophil-endothelial interactions [7]. Monoclonal antibodies against human IL-8 have been developed [47, 48].

Conclusion

The available evidence suggesting that the cytokine IL-8 may play a fundamental role in the pathogenesis, severity and course of ARDS has been collected. This may prompt exploratory pilot studies in man on the prophylactic and therapeutic value of anti-IL-8 antibodies or other more, or less, specific IL-8 neutralizing or blocking agents.

References

1. Matsushima K, Baldwin ET, Mukaida N (1992) Interleukin-8 and MCAF: novel leukocyte recruitment and activating cytokines. In: Kishimoto T (ed) Interleukins: molecular biology and immunology. Karger, Basel, pp 236–265
2. Hack CE, Aarden L, Thijs LG (1997) Role of cytokines in sepsis. Adv Immunol 66:101–195
3. Kuijpers TW, Hakkert BC, Roos D (1992) Neutrophil migration across monolayers of cytokine-prestimulated endothelial cells: a role for platelet-activating factor and IL-8. J Cell Biol 117:565–572
4. Luscinskas F, Kiely J-M, Ding H, et al (1992) In vitro inhibitory effect of IL-8 and other chemo-attractants on neutrophil-endothelial adhesive interactions. J Immunol 149:2163–2171
5. Van Zee KJ, Fisher E, Hawes AS, et al (1992) Effects of intravenous IL-8 administration in non-human primates. J Immunol 148:1746–1752
6. Smith WB, Gamble JR, Clark-Lewis I, Vadas MA (1993) Chemotactic desensitization of neutrophils demonstrates interleukin-8 (IL-8) dependent and IL-8-independent mechanisms of transmigration through cytokine-activated endothelium. Immunology 78:491–497

7. Takahashi M, Masuyama J-I, Ikeda U, et al (1995) Effects of endogenous endothelial interleukin-8 on neutrophil migration across an endothelial monolayer. Cardiovasc Res 29:670–675
8. DeForge LE, Preston AM, Takeuchi E, Kenney J, Boxer LA, Remick DG (1993) Regulation of interleukin-8 gene expression by oxidant stress. J Biol Chem 268:25568–25576
9. Karakurum M, Shreeniwas R, Chen J, et al (1994) Hypoxic induction of interleukin-8 gene expression in human endothelial cells. J Clin Invest 93:1564–1570
10. Kukielka GL, Smith CW, LaRosa GJ, et al (1995) Interleukin-8 gene induction in the myocardium after ischemia and reperfusion in vivo. J Clin Invest 95:89–103
11. Raijmakers PGHM, Groeneveld ABJ, Rauwerda JA, et al (1995) Transient increase in interleukin-8 and pulmonary microvascular permeability following aortic surgery. Am J Respir Crit Care Med 151:698–705
12. Groeneveld ABJ, Raijmakers PGHM, Rauwerda JA, Hack CE (1998) The inflammatory response to vascular surgery-associated ischemia and reperfusion in man: effect on postoperative pulmonary function. Eur J Vasc Endovasc Surg (In press)
13. Raijmakers PGHM, Groeneveld ABJ, Rauwerda JA, Teule GJJ, Hack CE (1997) Acute lung injury after aortic surgery: the relation between lung and leg microvascular permeability to [111]Indium-transferrin and circulating mediators. Thorax 52:866–871
14. Hébert CA, Luscinskas FW, Kiely J-M, et al (1990) Endothelial and leukocyte forms of IL-8. Conversion by thrombin and interactions with neutrophils. J Immunol 145:3033–3040
15. Groeneveld ABJ, Kindt I, Raijmakers PGHM, Hack CE, Thijs LG (1997) Systemic coagulation and fibrinolysis in patients with or at risk for the adult respiratory distress syndrome. Thromb Haemost 78:1444–1449
16. Yuo A, Kitagawa S, Kasahara T, Matsushima K, Takaku F (1991) Stimulation and priming of human neutrophils by interleukin-8: cooperation with tumor necrosis factor and colony-stimulating factors. Blood 78:2708–2714
17. Wozniak A, Betts WH, Murphy GA, Rokicinski M (1993) Interleukin-8 primes human neutrophils for enhanced superoxide anion production. Immunology 79:608–615
18. Jorens PG, Richman-Eisenstat JBY, Housset BP, et al (1992) Interleukin-8 induces neutrophil accumulation but not protease secretion in the canine trachea. Am J Physiol 263:L708–L713
19. Hechtman DH, Cybulsky MI, Fuchs HJ, Baker JB, Gimbrone GA (1991) Intravascular IL-8. Inhibitor of polymorphonuclear leukocyte accumulation at sites of acute inflammation. J Immunol 147:883–892
20. Biffl WL, Moore EE, Moore FA, Carl VS, Franciose RJ, Banerjee A (1995) Interleukin-8 increases endothelial permeability independent of neutrophils. J Trauma 39:98–103
21. Solomkin JS, Bass RC, Bjornson HS, Tindal CJ, Babcock GF (1994) Alterations of neutrophil responses to tumor necrosis factor alpha and interleukin-8 following human endotoxemia. Infect Immun 62:943–947
22. Sham RL, Phatak PD, Ihne TP, Abboud CN, Packman CH (1993) Signal pathway regulation of interleukin-8-induced actin polymerization in neutrophils. Blood 82:2546–2551
23. Hack CE, Hart N, Strack van Schijndel RJM, et al (1992) Interleukin-8 in sepsis: relation to shock and inflammatory mediators. Infect Immun 60:2835–2842
24. Marty C, Misset B, Tamion F, Fitting C, Carlet J, Cavaillon J-M (1994) Circulating interleukin-8 concentrations in patients with multiple organ failure of septic and nonseptic origin. Crit Care Med 22:673–679
25. Groeneveld ABJ, Raijmakers PGHM, Hack CE, Thijs LG (1995) Interleukin-8 related neutrophil elastase and the severity of the adult respiratory distress syndrome. Cytokine 7:745–752
26. Meduri GU, Headley S, Kohler G, et al (1995) Persistent elevation of inflammatory cytokines predicts a poor outcome in ARDS. Plasma IL-1β and IL-6 levels are consistent and efficient predictors of outcome over time. Chest 107:1062–1073
27. Meduri GU, Kohler G, Headley S, Tolley E, Stentz F, Postlewaite A (1995) Inflammatory cytokines in the BAL of patients with ARDS. Persistent elevation over time predicts poor outcome. Chest 108:1303–1314
28. Schütte H, Lohmeyer J, Rosseau S (1996) Bronchoalveolar and systemic cytokine profiles in patients with ARDS, severe pneumonia and cardiogenic pulmonary oedema. Eur Respir J 9:1858–1867
29. Kurdowska A, Miller EJ, Noble JM, et al (1996) Anti-IL 8 autoantibodies in alveolar fluid from patients with the adult respiratory distress syndrome. J Immunol 157:2699–2706

30. Kurdowska A, Carr FFK, Stevens MD, Baughman RP, Martin TR (1997) Studies on the interaction of IL-8 with human plasma α_2-macroglobulin. Evidence of the presence of IL-8 complexed to α_2-macroglobulin in lung fluids with patients with adult respiratory distress syndrome. J Immunol 158:1930–1940

31. Jorens PG, Van Damme J, De Backer W, et al (1992) Interleukin-8 (IL-8) in the bronchoalveolar lavage fluid from patients with the adult respiratory distress syndrome (ARDS) and patients at risk for ARDS. Cytokine 4:492–497

32. Miller EJ, Cohen AB, Nagao S, et al (1992) Elevated levels of NAP/Interleukin-8 are present in the airspaces of patients with the adult respiratory distress syndrome and are associated with increased mortality. Am Rev Respir Dis 148:427–432

33. Chollet-Martin S, Montravers P, Gibert C, et al (1993) High levels of interleukin-8 in the blood and alveolar spaces of patients with pneumonia and adult respiratory distress syndrome. Infect Immun 61:4553–4559

34. Donnelly SC, Strieter RM, Kunkel SL, et al (1993) Interleukin-8 and development of adult respiratory distress syndrome in at-risk patient groups. Lancet 341:643–647

35. Chollet-Martin S, Jourdain B, Gibert C, Elbim C, Chastre J, Gougerot-Pocidalo MA (1996) Interactions between neutrophils and cytokines in blood and alveolar spaces during ARDS. Am J Respir Crit Care Med 153:594–601

36. Donnelly SC, Strieter RM, Reid PT, et al (1996) The association between mortality rates and decreased concentrations of interleukin-10 and interleukin-1 receptor antagonist in the lung fluids of patients with the adult respiratory distress syndrome. Ann Int Med 125:191–196

37. Goodman RB, Strieter RM, Martin DP, et al (1996) Inflammatory cytokines in patients with persistence of the acute respiratory distress syndrome. Am J Respir Crit Care Med 154:602–611

38. Miller EJ, Cohen AB, Matthay MA (1996) Increased interleukin-8 concentrations in the pulmonary edema fluid of patients with acute respiratory distress syndrome from sepsis. Crit Care Med 24:1448–1454

39. Martin TR, Rubefeld GD, Ruzinski JT, et al (1997) Relationship between soluble CD14, lipopolysaccharide binding protein, and the alveolar inflammatory response in patients with acute respiratory distress syndrome. Am J Respir Crit Care Med 155:937–944

40. Standiford TJ, Kunkel SL, Basha MA, et al (1990) Interleukin-8 gene expression by a pulmonary epithelial cell line. A model for cytokine networks in the lung. J Clin Invest 86:1945–1953

41. Donnelly TJ, Meade P, Jagels M, et al (1994) Cytokine, complement, and endotoxin profiles associated with the development of the adult respiratory distress syndrome after surgery. Crit Care Med 22:768–776

42. Jorens PG, De Jongh R, De Backer W, et al (1993) Interleukin-8 production in patients undergoing cardiopulmonary bypass. The influence of pretreatment with methylprednisolone. Am Rev Respir Dis 1148:890–895

43. Kalfin RE, Engelman RM, Rousou JA, et al (1993) Induction of interleukin-8 expression during cardiopulmonary bypass. Circulation 88:401–406

44. Meade P, Shoemaker WC, Donnelly TJ, et al (1994) Temporal patterns of hemodynamics, oxygen transport, cytokine activity, and complement activity in the development of adult respiratory distress syndrome after severe injury. J Trauma 36:651–657

45. Nakanishi I, Moutabariik A, Kitamura E (1994) Interleukin-8 in chronic renal failure and dialysis patients. Nephrol Dial Transplant 9:1435–1442

46. Baughman RP, Gubther KL, Rashkin MC, Keeton DA, Pattishall H (1996) Changes in the inflammatory response of the lung during acute respiratory distress syndrome: prognostic indicators. Am J Respir Crit Care Med 154:76–81

47. Sekido N, Mukalda N, Harada A, Nakanishi I, Watanabe Y, Matsushima K (1993) Prevention of lung reperfusion injury in rabbits by a monoclonal antibody against interleukin-8. Nature 365:654–657

48. Mulligan MS, Jones ML, Bolanowski MA, et al (1993) Inhibition of lung inflammatory reactions in rats by an anti-human IL-8 antibody. J Immunol 150:5585–5595

49. Folkesson HG, Matthay MA, Hebert CA, Broaddus VC (1995) Acid aspiration-induced lung injury in rabbits is mediated by interleukin-8-dependent mechanisms. J Clin Invest 96:107–116

50. Yokoi K, Makaida N, Harada A, Watanabe Y, Matsushima K (1997) Prevention of endotoxemia-induced acute respiratory distress syndrome-like lung injury in rabbits by a monoclonal antibody to IL-8. Lab Invest 76:375–384

Neutrophil Myeloperoxidase:
Effector of Host Defense and Host Damage

G. Deby-Dupont, C. Deby, and M. Lamy

Introduction

Myeloperoxidase (MPO) is a heme peroxidase present in azurophilic (primary) granules of neutrophils and in monocytes. It gradually disappears from these cells as they differentiate into macrophages [1, 2]. Eosinophils contain eosinophil peroxidase (EPO), a peroxidase which shares similar functions with MPO, but is immunologically distinct, since antisera obtained against MPO do not cross react with EPO. MPO is synthesized as a precursor glycosylated polypeptide (MW $\pm$ 90,000 Da) in promyelocytes [3]. This precursor is trimmed to $\pm$ 60,000 and 15,000 Da polypeptides, the heavy and light chains respectively, which by association form the protomer. Two protomers, joined by a disulphide bond, then constitute the mature enzyme, which thus carries 2 identical prosthetic groups [4]. MPO is a heme enzyme and contains ferric ion (Fe^{3+}): The incorporation of the heme group precedes the maturation process [5], so that the precursor is enzymatically active [6]. Human neutrophil MPO was purified over 20 years ago and its amino acid sequence has been completely elucidated [7, 8]. The cDNA coding for MPO has been cloned and characterized [9]. Human recombinant MPO can now be produced from genetically engineered Chinese hamster ovary cell lines as a glycosylated monomeric, heme-containing, single-chain precursor of 84,000 Da, with enzymatic activity and strong similarity to the native human enzyme [10, 11].

Oxidant Species: Products of the Enzymatic Activity of MPO (Fig. 1)

The reactive oxidant species generated by phagocytes are of central importance in host defense, in tumor surveillance, and in inflammation. During the respiratory burst, phagocytes generate superoxide anion, which in turn dismutates into hydrogen peroxide (H_2O_2) [12]. Peroxidases are heme enzymes that use H_2O_2 as an electron acceptor to catalyze several oxidative reactions. In neutrophils, MPO catalyzes the conversion of H_2O_2, using chloride anion (Cl^-) as the electron donor, to produce cytotoxic chlorinating or oxidizing species with similar reactivities to hypochlorite [13]. The hypochlorous acid (HOCl) thus formed is a potent oxidant species which further reacts with amines to form chloramines, some of which are also considered to be potent oxidants. When chloramines approach tyrosyl residues in a protein structure, they are capable of chlorinating the tyrosines. However, it now appears

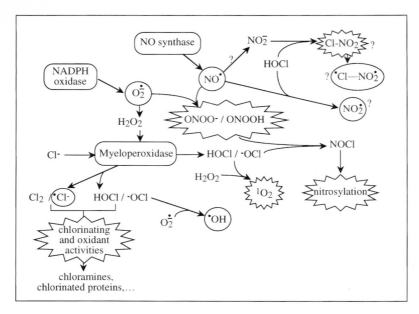

Fig. 1. Active oxidant species produced by the activity of myeloperoxidase. NO$^{\bullet}$: nitrogen monoxide (= nitric oxide); ONOO^{-}: peroxynitrite; NO$_2^{-}$: nitrite; NO$_2^{\bullet}$: nitrogen dioxide; NOCl nitrosyl chloride; Cl-NO$_2$: nitryl chloride; HOCl: hypochlorous acid; $^{\bullet}$OH: hydroxyl radical; O$_2^{-}$: superoxide anion; H$_2$O$_2$: hydrogen peroxide; ^{1}O$_2$: singlet oxygen; $^{\bullet}$Cl: nascent chlorine

that chlorine (Cl$_2$) and even monoatomic chlorine (nascent chlorine, Cl$^{\bullet}$) is produced in equilibrium with HOCl; these species could carry out the oxidation/halogenation reactions that have previously been attributed to HOCl/ClO^{-} [14]. The production of chlorine is favored by the acidic pH found in the phagolysosome (Fig. 2), and would seem to imply the possibility of free radical mechanisms, as suggested by the synthesis of dityrosine by human neutrophils [15]. This production of radicals would occur when MPO uses compounds other than Cl^{-} as electron donors for the

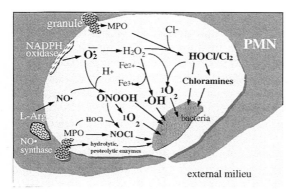

Fig. 2. Neutrophil function of phagocytosis: Active products within the phagolysosome (see legend of figure 1 for symbol identification)

reduction of H_2O_2. Such compounds, of which tyrosine is an example, would be converted into radical species that could subsequently initiate lipoperoxidation or crosslinking of proteins. Whatever the mechanism of MPO activity (production of $Cl^•$, Cl_2, ClO^- or chloramines), chlorinated low density lipoproteins [16], chlorinated sterols [17] and chlorinated tyrosyl residues [18, 19] are formed by MPO activity. These chlorinated tyrosines have been considered to be specific markers of MPO activity in inflammatory tissue damage [18]. MPO can use other halogens to produce hypohalogenous acids and the corresponding gases, and its reactivity with iodide anion (I^-) may be higher than with Cl^- [20, 21], but the relative rarity of I^- in vivo limits the iodination activity of MPO.

Other active oxygen species appear to be produced by MPO. One is singlet oxygen, an excited form of oxygen ($^1O_2$), whose marked energetic instability makes it able to react with most organic compounds. Singlet oxygen is easily produced by the reaction of H_2O_2 with HOCl; both of these compounds can be simultaneously produced by activated neutrophils. However, while the synthesis of singlet oxygen is theoretically possible during MPO activity, and has been demonstrated under in vitro conditions, the reality of its production in vivo is far from being firmly demonstrated, so that the production of singlet oxygen by stimulated neutrophils remains a matter of discussion [22, 23]. MPO activity has also been implicated in the production of hydroxyl radical ($^•OH$) by stimulated neutrophils. Here, HOCl would react with superoxide anion to produce $^•OH$, using a mechanism different from the Fenton reaction, and independent of the presence of metal ions [24, 25].

Neutrophils produce superoxide anion and nitrogen monoxide (NO), two radical species that react at a rate controlled by diffusion to produce peroxynitrite ($ONOO^-$), a strongly oxidizing agent [26]. MPO activity interferes with both NO and $ONOO^-$ production. The reaction of NO with HOCl, yielding nitrogen dioxide ($NO_2^•$) can occur, but cannot efficiently compete with the reaction of superoxide anion with H_2O_2 yielding peroxynitrite. Interestingly however, HOCl can react with peroxynitrite to form nitrosyl chloride, a strong oxidant and nitrosylating agent for organic compounds [27]. It has also been reported that HOCl can react with NO_2^-, the autoxidation product of NO, to form reactive intermediate species capable of nitrating phenolic substrates such as tyrosine, at physiological pH. These reactions would occur via radical compounds and transient species similar to nitryl-chloride ($Cl-NO_2$) [28].

The activity of MPO is thus responsible for the synthesis of many oxidant species (Fig. 1) which participate in normal host defense, and in the complex chemiluminescence that is observed when isolated neutrophils are stimulated in vitro. The use of a specific technique for detection of free radicals (electron spin resonance with spin trapping) proves that free radicals are produced during in vitro neutrophil activation, and that MPO activity is involved in this synthesis.

A Beneficial Role of MPO: Microbicidal Activity

The MPO-H_2O_2-Cl^- system is of primary importance in microbial killing by neutrophils, but also in cytotoxicity against tumor cells, in tissue damage at sites of inflammation, and in the modulation of the inflammatory response.

Monocytes and neutrophils kill pathogenic microorganisms by sequestration within phagocytic vacuoles (phagolysosomes), where toxic oxygen species are delivered together with granulocytic enzymes (Fig. 2) [12]. MPO has been proven to be active against many microorganisms, presumably by initiating oxidant attack at various sites, and by a variety of mechanisms, most of which remain uncharacterized. It acts on *Escherichia coli* by oxidation of iron centers (perhaps at the cytoplasmic membrane electron transport chain) leading to the loss of microbial iron, loss of aerobic respiration, and decreased viability [29, 30]. It is active against *Candida albicans* and would appear to bind to the target yeast walls via the mannan component [31].

Monocytes were found to lose their granule MPO during culture *in vitro*; this loss was correlated with decreased killing activity towards protozoa. Killing activity could be restored by coating the microorganisms with EPO [1]. Similar results were obtained for *Pseudomonas aeruginosa* killing by human macrophages. We [2] demonstrated that cultured human macrophages were rapidly overwhelmed by these microorganisms which, despite being incorporated into the phagocytes remained alive and capable of multiplying. Indeed, their polysaccharide capsules protected them against the proteolytic and hydrolytic machinery of macrophages. But when these cultured macrophages were pre-incubated with human neutrophil MPO, in order to restore their MPO-H_2O_2-Cl^- system, the enzyme was internalized, remained active, and enhanced the killing capacity of these cells against *Pseudomonas aeruginosa* [2]. With murine peritoneal macrophages, it was also demonstrated that the addition of exogenous recombinant MPO at physiological concentrations enhances phagocytosis and killing of *Escherichia coli*, together with increased production of reactive oxygen species, as measured by luminol-dependent chemiluminescence [32]. A macrophage mannose receptor, which is very sensitive to oxidant stress, would appear to be a regulator of exogenous MPO uptake (which occurs without loss of MPO activity) and its delivery to the lysosomal compartment of macrophages [33]. MPO is also taken up by endothelial cells and fibroblasts, which affords these cells a self-protective capacity that they normally lack [34].

MPO: Modulator of Cellular Functions

MPO is transported to the site of infection via diapedesis of chemotactically attracted neutrophils, and is then released by degranulating or dying neutrophils at the site of inflammation. MPO will thus catalyze locally the production of potent oxidant species, capable of diffusing into neighboring biological structures and can thus directly or indirectly affect most living cells and tissues, modulating the functions of many cells when in close contact with them.

MPO triggers cytokine production [tumor necrosis factor (TNF)-α, interleukin (IL)-1 and interferon (IFN)-γ] by macrophages [35] in a dose-dependent manner, and induces the cytotoxicity of macrophages for target cells. While the exact mechanism of this induction remains unknown, it may proceed via internalization of the enzyme by mannose receptors present on macrophages. After this uptake, MPO could enhance the cytotoxicity of macrophages by increasing their production of active oxygen species. The increase in cytokine production may be due to a direct action of MPO, but could also be the result of an induction of signal transduction by the specific activity of MPO.

When MPO is added to normal neutrophils, it decreases phagocytosis (attachment and ingestion of particles). These data indicate that, in addition to being a potent antimicrobial effector, the oxidizing activity of the MPO-H_2O_2-halide system may modulate the inflammatory response by impairing certain receptor-mediated recognition mechanisms of phagocytic cells, which otherwise could elicit inflammatory reactions and tissue injury [36]. In vivo, the activity of natural killer cells in tumor tissue is decreased when they are placed in the presence of phagocytes. In vitro, the natural killer activity of lymphocytes showed a marked decrease when these cells were exposed to stimulated purified neutrophils and monocytes. The reactive oxygen species produced by the phagocytes were at least partially responsible for this immunosuppression, and more particularly the MPO-H_2O_2-Cl^- system since MPO deficient neutrophils or the absence of chloride anion limit this inhibition of natural killer cell functions [37]. This functional impairment of adjacent immunocompetent cells is most often sublethal, influenced in situ by the number, the state of activation, and the proximity of the neutrophils, as well as by the antioxidant potential of the microenvironment.

When neutrophils are marginated in capillaries, and bound to adhesion receptors of endothelial cells, they can be activated locally, with resulting degranulation and release of MPO in close contact with endothelial cells. These cells can then take up active enzyme into the endothelium where it can interfere with endothelial function [34]. These effects of trapped MPO on endothelial cell function under physiological conditions remain, however, largely unexplored. Trapping of MPO by alveolar macrophages can also occur, when neutrophils are attracted into the alveoli and degranulate, or are phagocytosed by the stimulated macrophages. This uptake of MPO can reinforce the microbicidal activity of macrophages, as described above [2].

MPO: Responsible for Oxidant Stress

When phagocytes are activated in excess, they degranulate, releasing MPO into the extracellular milieu in close contact with cells and tissues, potentially leading to local oxidant stress. The oxidant species produced by neutrophils have been implicated in the pathogensis of diseases ranging from atherosclerosis to ischemia/reperfusion injury and cancer. The MPO-H_2O_2-Cl^- system reacts with a wide variety of biological compounds, including heme proteins and porphyrins (oxidative bleaching), unsaturated lipids, iron sulfur centers, thiols, reduced pyridine nucleotides, DNA, amines and amino acids. This lack of target specificity makes it potentially dangerous [13, 38–41]. The reaction products are often active compounds such as unsaturated aldehydes formed from hydroxy amino acids, and chlorohydrins formed from unsaturated fatty acids, which are responsible for membrane disruption and cytotoxicity [42, 43]. Extracellularly, at physiological pH, the MPO system can inactivate thiol functions, suppressing the anti-protease activities of essential antiproteases such as α_1 proteinase inhibitor and α_2-macroglobulin [44, 45]. Fortunately, in plasma many other compounds bearing thiol functions (such as albumin) are present, so that a large excess of oxidant would be required to destroy the anti-proteases.

However, local damage by MPO activity cannot be excluded in cases of excessive inflammatory reaction. MPO is taken up and internalized by macrophages, fibroblasts and endothelial cells, so that it exerts its activity within the cells themselves, sometimes leading to undesirable oxidant effects. We [46] have demonstrated that human endothelial cells incorporate exogenous human MPO, which retains its enzymatic activity. After this uptake, the cells can undergo oxidative stress if H_2O_2 is produced intracellularly, as occurs during ischemia/reperfusion phenomena. Under these conditions, the cells undergo an oxidant stress, leading to variable degrees of cytotoxicity. When neutrophils are recruited and activated in an uncontrolled manner, they degranulate close to the endothelium or in the target organs or tissues. The $MPO-H_2O_2-Cl^-$ system, released by the degranulating cells, could then become the source of oxidative damage [47, 48]. This oxidant stress can be encountered in diseases characterized by excessive inflammation and neutrophil activation, such as severe sepsis, acute lung injury (ALI), and acute respiratory distress syndrome (ARDS). Using a specific radioimmunological technique, we demonstrated that plasma concentrations of MPO increased in many intensive care patients in whom leukocyte activation could conceivably occur. Increased plasma concentrations of MPO were observed in critically ill patients (trauma, shock, sepsis, acute pancreatitis) and in cardiac surgery patients (Fig. 3). The highest plasma MPO values (up to 100 times the mean normal value) were measured in sepsis, and persisted for several days. In trauma, the release of MPO occurred early (within the first hours after injury) and was concomitant with the release of elastase, another neutrophil enzyme, indicating degranulation of these cells into the extracellular milieu [49]. In cardiac surgery, MPO release paralleled the increase in neutrophil number, and appeared to be a consequence of neutrophil stimulation by the complement cascade, activated by contact with the foreign surfaces of the extracorporeal circulation device [50]. MPO was also found in the bronchoalveolar lavage (BAL) fluid of intensive care patients with bronchopneumonia and ARDS, together with other products of neutrophil activation (elastase, lactoferrin) and with oxidant activity of BAL [51–53]. The enzyme was found to be active, and its levels in BAL fluid were demonstrated to correlate with cytotoxicity for alveolar cells in culture [54]. This

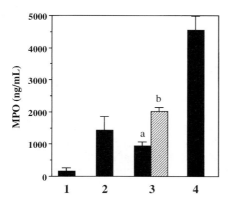

Fig. 3. MPO levels in critically ill patients.
1. Control levels in plasma of healthy volunteers (n = 152). 2. Plasma levels in trauma (first 24 h after injury) (n = 15). 3. Plasma levels in cardiac surgery patients; a: immediateiy after heparin administration; b: on declamping (cardiac reperfusion) (n = 30). 4. Plasma levels in severe sepsis (n = 22)

activity would appear to be a marker of the presence of activated neutrophils in the alveoli.

Compounds able to inhibit MPO activity could be useful, but known inhibitors are either not specific for MPO (such as the thiol compounds), or not specific for neutrophil MPO such as methimazole, a competitive inhibitor which however, also blocks thyroid peroxidase.

MPO in Cell Signaling

Reactive oxygen species are responsible for the activation of nuclear transcription factors such as nuclear factor-kappa B (NF-κB), and are now considered to be second messengers in the induction of gene transcription [55]. They are involved in cellular mutagenesis via the nitrosylating activity of compounds derived from ONOO$^-$ [56]. Hydrogen peroxide has been demonstrated to be active in the phosphorylation of protein kinase C and in the NF-κB transcription [57, 58]. This activating role has also been noted with HOCl. The activity of MPO is thus responsible for modulating the cellular signaling process, via production of oxidant species such as HOCl, but also without doubt by its chlorinating activity of tyrosine residues. Tyrosine is an essential residue in many proteins active in cellular signaling, such as the cytoplasmic protein kinases (PKs). The phosphorylation of tyrosyl residues is a key step in the transmission of signals leading to the activation of the cellular machinery [57]. In the activation of NF-κB, tyrosyl phosphorylation results in the activation of PKs, which starts a sequence of reactions leading to the cleavage of the NF-κB inhibitor by a proteasome (a multicatalytic protease complex). This allows the nuclear factor to enter the nucleus where it triggers mRNA synthesis and protein transcription (Fig. 4). The activity of PKs is controlled by the phosphotyrosine phosphatases (PTP) which dephosphorylate the PKs and so regulate the level of signal transduction [57]. The PTP are themselves tyrosine proteins. The nitrosylation of the tyrosyl residues of PKs and PTP by peroxynitrite destroys the normal functions of these proteins and alters membrane structure when this protein is located in the cell membrane [56, 57]. It is highly probable that the chlorination of tyrosyl residues by HOCl or chloramines would lead to similar loss of protein function. In this perspective, MPO activity would impair cell signaling, leading to alterations of cellular func-

Fig. 4. Schematic view of the role of reactive oxygen species (ROS) in transcriptional nuclear factor activation (NF-κB is taken as an example). ROS are produced outside or in the cell. p50 p60 I: NF-κB complex; p50 p65 = NF-κB; I: Inhibitor of NF-κB; P: phosphate group; PK: protein kinase; PTP: phosphotyrosine phosphatase; MPC: multicatalytic protease complex (proteasome)

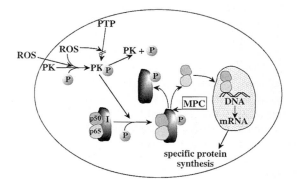

tion and secretion, including inhibition of active mediator production and deregulation of the control of specific protein synthesis. HOCl and MPO have recently been shown to act on signaling in T-lymphocyte cell lines [59]. This activation of nuclear transcription factors has different effects, which could be beneficial for the host, but also deleterious, particularly when this transcription leads to the synthesis of inflammatory mediators, such as TNF-α and IL-8, occurring in patients with severe sepsis, acute inflammation, ARDS or systemic inflammatory response syndrome [60].

Myeloperoxidase in Disease States

MPO in Atherosclerosis

Elevated levels of low density lipoproteins (LDL) are considered to be a major risk for the development of atherosclerosis. However, it has been suggested that LDL must be oxidized to trigger the development of this disease. The MPO system plays an important role in atherosclerosis because hypoxic conditions are likely to render the arterial wall acidic, favoring chlorination and oxidation. Indeed, MPO can be provided by monocytes and neutrophils which infiltrate the intima during the early stage of atherosclerosis [61] and is present in active form in human atherosclerotic lesions [62]. This enzyme is capable of modifying LDL into a high uptake-form for macrophages [63]. Oxidation of LDL may contribute to the early stages of atherosclerosis, and oxidized LDL have been recognized in diseased human aortas and in plasma of humans with established cardiovascular disease. Recently the *in vivo* oxidants responsible for generation of oxidized LDL have been identified as hypochlorite and molecular chlorine, products of MPO activity. Indeed, activated phagocytes generate chlorinated LDL cholesterol and amino acid-derived aldehydes [17, 64], and hypochlorite-modified LDL and elevated levels of 3-chlorotyrosine are present in human atherosclerotic lesions [16, 65].

MPO Deficiency

MPO deficiency is the most common neutrophilic lysosomal enzyme deficiency. Humans have been found to present an hereditary MPO deficiency, and case studies indicate that individuals with this MPO deficiency are susceptible to serious infection in the presence of co-existing conditions such as diabetes mellitus. In these diabetic patients with MPO deficiency, granulocyte microbicidal activity is partially diminished with regard to *Staphylococcus aureus* and is almost nil with regard to *Candida albicans*. Moreover, MPO deficiency seems to be associated with chronic granulomatous disease, and anti-MPO-ANCA (autoantibodies to neutrophil cytoplasmic antigens) have been detected in the plasma of patients with idiopathic forms of necrotizing glomerulonephritis and necrotizing alveolar capillaritis (idiopathic pulmonary hemorrhage) [66, 67].

MPO deficiency can be partial or complete with total lack of HOCl production. Humans lacking MPO do not usually show altered inflammatory responses, in contrast to several other biochemical defects in polymorphonuclear neutrophils. But, MPO deficient neutrophils present strikingly decreased luminol-enhanced chemiluminescence, while lucigenin-enhanced chemiluminescence (a marker of superoxide anion production) is significantly increased compared to normal granulocytes. These neutrophils also have increased phagocytic activity [36]. In patients with MPO deficiency, the activity of peroxidase in eosinophils is not affected, despite a 70% homology in the DNA sequences of EPO and MPO [68].

The lack of MPO therefore appears to be compensated by increased phagocytic activity, increased production of superoxide anion, and an alternative route of H_2O_2 metabolism, explaining the absence of severe infections in these patients [69]. The microbicidal activity of neutrophils thus seems to be the result of overlapping antimicrobial systems. Indeed, MPO-deficient neutrophils remain capable of killing *Escherichia coli*, indicating that non-oxidative microbicidal systems are sufficient for full microbicidal effect, and that the contribution of MPO may even be somewhat redundant. However, normal neutrophils rapidly suppress *E. coli* DNA synthesis [70], an effect that is not observed with MPO-deficient neutrophils. Furthermore, some pathogens coated with polysaccharide capsules, which are resistant to proteolytic enzymes, and require a full oxidative system to be inactivated, would likely remain unkilled by MPO-deficient neutrophils.

Conclusion

MPO plays a primary adaptive role in host defense by its ability to produce aggressive oxygen and chlorine species which are deleterious to microorganisms, and by acting in concert with hydrolytic and proteolytic enzymes within the phagolysosome. When removed from this phagocytic vacuole, however, MPO is far from being an innocuous enzyme. When MPO is taken up by macrophages, it conserves a beneficial role, helping these cells in the killing of pathogens. However, when released in excess onto endothelium or into alveolar spaces, MPO exerts oxidizing activities leading to essential protein inactivation and cytotoxicity. Until now the control of this deleterious activity remains impossible, as we have no safe specific inhibitors of MPO, and since it could be dangerous to inhibit MPO activity by repressing neutrophil activation, especially in critically ill patients.

References

1. Locksey RM, Nelson C, Fankhauser JE, Klebanoff SJ (1987) Loss of granule myeloperoxidase during in vitro culture of human monocytes correlates with decay in antiprotozoa activity. Am J Trop Med Hyg 36:541–548
2. Mathy-Hartert M, Deby-Dupont G, Melin P, Lamy M, Deby C (1996) Cultured macrophages acquire a bactericidal activity against Pseudomonas aeruginosa after incorporation of myeloperoxidase. Experientia 52:1–8
3. Olsson I, Persson AM, Strömberg K (1984) Biosynthesis, transport and processing of myeloperoxidase in the human leukaemic promyelocytic cell line HL-60 and normal marrow cells. Biochem J 223:911–920
4. Andrews PC, Krinsky NI (1981) The reductive cleavage of myeloperoxidase in half, producing enzymatically active hemi-myeloperoxidase. J Biol Chem 256:4211–4218

5. Arnljots K, Olsson I (1987) Myeloperoxidase precursors incorporate heme. J Biol Chem 262: 10430–10433
6. Taylor KL, Guzman GS, Burgess CA, Kinkade JM (1990) Assembly of dimeric myeloperoxidase during posttranslational maturation in human leukemic HL-60 cells. Biochemistry 29: 1533–1539
7. Bakkenist ARJ, Wever R, Vulsma T, Plat H, Van Gelder BF (1978) Isolation procedure and some properties of myeloperoxidase from human leukocytes. Biochim Biophys Acta 524:45–54
8. Miyasaki KT, Wilson ME, Cohen E, Jones PC, Genco RJ (1986) Evidence for and partial characterization of three major and three minor chromatographic forms of human neutrophil myeloperoxidase. Arch Biochem Biophys 246:751–764
9. Morishita K, Kubota N, Asano S, Kaziro Y, Nagata S (1987) Molecular cloning and characterization of cDNA for human myeloperoxidase. J Biol Chem 262: 3844–3851
10. Moguilevsky N, Garcia-Quintana L, Jacquet A, et al (1991) Structural and biological properties of human recombinant myeloperoxidase produced by Chinese hamster ovary cell lines. Eur J Biochem 197:605–614
11. Jacquet A, Deby C, Mathy M, et al (1991) Spectral and enzymatic properties of human recombinant myeloperoxidase: comparison with the mature enzyme. Arch Biochem Biophys 291:132–138
12. Klebanoff SJ, Waltersdorph AM, Rosen H (1984) Antimicrobial activity of myeloperoxidase. Meth Enzymol 105:399–403
13. Winterbourn CC (1985) Comparative reactivities of various biological compounds with myeloperoxidase-hydrogen peroxide-chloride, and similarity of the oxidant to hypochlorite. Biochim Biophys Acta 840:204–210
14. Hazen SL, Hsu FF, Mueller DM, Crowley JR, Heinecke JW (1996) Human neutrophils employ chlorine gas as an oxidant during phagocytosis. J Clin Invest 98:1283–1289
15. Heinecke JW, Li W, Daehnke HL, Goldstein JA (1993) Dityrosine, a specific marker of oxidation, is synthesized by the myeloperoxidase-hydrogen peroxide system of human neutrophils and macrophages. J Biol Chem 268:4069–4077
16. Hazen SL, Heinecke JW (1997) 3-Chlorotyrosine, a specific marker of myeloperoxidase-catalyzed chlorination is markedly elevated in low density lipoprotein isolated from human atherosclerotic intima. J Clin Invest 99:2075–2081
17. Hazen SL, Hsu FF, Duffin K, Heinecke JW (1996) Molecular chlorine generated by the myeloperoxidase-hydrogen peroxide-chloride system of phagocytes converts low density lipoprotein cholesterol into a family of chlorinated sterols. J Biol Chem 271:23080–23088
18. Domigan NM, Charlton TS, Duncan MW, Winterbourn CC, Kettle AJ (1995) Chlorination of tyrosyl residues in peptides by myeloperoxidase and human neutrophils. J Biol Chem 270: 16542–16548
19. Kettle AJ (1995) Neutrophils convert tyrosin residues in albumin to chlorotyrosine. FEBS Lett 379:103–106
20. Olsson, I, Olofsson T, Odeberg H (1972) Myeloperoxidase-mediated iodination in granulocytes. Scand J Haemat 9:483–491
21. Taurog A, Dorris ML (1992) Myeloperoxidase-catalyzed iodination and coupling. Arch Biochem Biophys 296:239–246
22. Kanofsky JR, Wright J, Miles-Richardson GE, Tauber A (1984) Biochemical requirements for singlet oxygen production by purified human myeloperoxidase. J Clin Invest 74:1489–1495
23. Cadenas E (1985) Biological chemiluminescence. In: Quintanilha A (ed) Reactive oxygen species in chemistry, biology and medicine. Plenum Press, New York, pp 117–141
24. Ramos CL, Pou S, Britigan BE, Cohen MS, Rosen GM (1992) Spin trapping evidence for myeloperoxidase-dependent hydroxyl radical formation by human neutrophils and monocytes. J Biol Chem 267:8307–8312
25. Kettle AJ, Winterbourn CC (1994) Superoxide-dependent hydroxylation by myeloperoxidase. J Biol Chem 269:17146–17151
26. Carreras MC, Pargament GA, Catz SD, Poderoso JJ, Boveris A (1994) Kinetics of nitric oxide and hydrogen peroxide production and formation of peroxynitrite during the respiratory burst of human neutrophils. FEBS Lett 341:65–68
27. Koppenol WH (1994) Thermodynamic considerations on the formation of reactive species from hypochlorite, superoxide and nitrogen monoxide. Could nitrosyl chloride be produced by neutrophils and macrophages? FEBS Lett 347:5–8

28. Eiserich JP, Cross CE, Jones AD, Halliwell B, van der Vliet A (1996) Formation of nitrating and chlorinating species by reaction of nitrite with hypochlorous acid. J Biol Chem 271:19199–19208
29. Rosen H, Klebanoff SJ (1982) Oxidation of *Escherichia coli* iron centers by the myeloperoxidase-mediated microbicidal system. J Biol Chem 257:13731–13735
30. Rakita RM, Michel BR, Rosen H (1990) Differential inactivation of *Escherichia coli* membrane dehydrogenases by a myeloperoxidase-mediated antimicrobial system. Biochemistry 29:1072–1080
31. Wright CD, Bowie JU, Gray GR, Nelson RD (1983) Candidacidal activity of myeloperoxidase: mechanisms of inhibitory influence of soluble cell wall mannan. Infect Immun 42:76–80
32. Lincoln JA, Lefkowitz DL, Cain T, et al (1995) Exogenous myeloperoxidase enhances bacterial phagocytosis and intracellular killing by macrophages. Infect Immun 63:3042–3047
33. Shepperd VL, Hoidal J (1990) Clearance of neutrophil-derived myeloperoxidase by the macrophage mannose receptor. Am J Respir Cell Mol Biol 2:335–340
34. Zabucchi G, Soranzo MR, Menegazzi R, Bertoncin P, Nardon E, Patriarca P (1989) Uptake of human eosinophil peroxidase and myeloperoxidase by cells involved in the inflammatory process. J Histochem Cytochem 37:499–508
35. Lefkowitz DL, Mills K, Morgan M, Lefkowitz S (1992) Macrophage activation and immunomodulation by myeloperoxidase. Proc Soc Exp Biol Med 199:204–210
36. Stendahl O, Coble BI, Dahlgren C, Hed J, Molin L (1984) Myeloperoxidase modulates the phagocytic activity of polymorphonuclear neutrophil leukocytes. Studies with cells from a myeloperoxidase-deficient patient. J Clin Invest 73:366–373
37. El-Hag A, Clark RA (1987) Immunosuppression by activated human neutrophils. J Immunol 139:2406–2413
38. Albrich JM, McCarthy, CA, Hurst JK (1981) Biological reactivity of hypochlorous acid: implications for microbicidal mechanisms of leukocyte myeloperoxidase. Proc Natl Acad Sci USA 78:210–214
39. Marquez LA, Dunford HB (1994) Chlorination of taurine by myeloperoxidase. J Biol Chem 269:7950-7956
40. Van den Berg J, Winterbourn CC (1994) Measurement of reaction products from hypochlorous acid and unsaturated lipids. Meth Enzymol 223:639–649
41. Prütz WA (1996) Hypochlorous acid interactions with thiols, nucleotides, DNA, and other biological substrates. Arch Biochem Biophys 332:110–120
42. Winterbourn CC, van den Berg JJM, Roitman E, Kuypers FA (1992) Chlorohydrin formation from unsaturated fatty acids reacting with hypochlorous acid. Arch Biochem Biophys 296: 547–555
43. Anderson MM, Hazen SL, Hsu FF, Heinecke JW (1997) Human neutrophils employ the myeloperoxidase-hydrogen peroxide-chloride system to convert hydroxy-amino acids into glycolaldehyde, 2-hydroxypropanal, and acrolein. A mechanism for the generation of highly reactive alpha-hydroxy and alpha, beta-unsaturated aldehydes by phagocytes at sites of inflammation. J Clin Invest 99:424–432
44. Clarke RA, Stone PJ, El-Hag AZ, Calore JD, Franzblau C (1981) Myeloperoxidase-catalyzed inactivation of α_1-proteinase inhibitor by human neutrophils. J Biol Chem 256:3348–3353
45. Deby-Dupont G, Croisier JL, Camus G, et al (1994) Inactivation of α_2 macroglobulin by activated human polymorponuclear leucocytes. Med Inflammation 3:117–123
46. Mathy-Hartert M, Deby-Dupont G, Deby C, Jadoul L, Vandenberghe A, Lamy M (1995) Cytotoxicity induced by neutrophil myeloperoxidase towards human endothelial cells: protection by ceftazidime. Med Inflammation 4:1–7
47. Weiss SJ (1989) Tissue destruction by neutrophils. N Engl J Med 320:365–376
48. Fujishima S, Aikawa N (1995) Neutrophil-mediated tissue injury and its modulation. Intensive Care Med 21:277–285
49. Deby-Dupont G, Faymonville ME, Adam A, Damas P, Lamy M (1997) Markers of early neutrophil activation in trauma patients. Med Inflammation 6:155 (Abst)
50. Faymonville ME, Pincemail J, Duchateau J, et al (1991) Myeloperoxidase and elastase as marker of leukocyte activation during cardiopulmonary bypass in human. J Thorac Cardiovasc Surg 102:309–317
51. Cochrane CG, Spragg RG, Revak SD, Cohen AB, McGuire WW (1983) The presence of neutrophil elastase and evidence of oxidation activity in bronchoalveolar lavage fluids of patients with adult respiratory distress syndrome. Am Rev Respir Dis 127:525–527

52. Weiland JE, Davis WB, Holter JF, Mohammed JR, Dorinsky PM, Gadek JE (1986) Lung neutrophils in the adult respiratory distress syndrome. Am Rev Respir Dis 133:218–225
53. Hällgren R, Samuelsson T, Venge P, Modig J (1987) Eosinophil activation in the lung is related to lung damage in adult respiratory distress syndrome. Am Rev Respir Dis 135:639–642
54. Damas P, Nys M, Mathy M, et al (1997) Cytotoxicity index and neutrophil products in BAL fluid from ventilator-associated penumonia and ARDS patients. Intensive Care Med 23:S106 (Abst)
55. Schulze-Osthoff K, Bauer M, Vogt M, Wesselborg S, Baeuerle PA (1997) Reactive oxygen intermediates as primary signals and second messengers in the activation of transcription factors. In: Forman HJ, Cadenas E (eds) Oxidative stress and signal transduction. Chapman and Hall, New York, pp 32–51
56. Spear N, Estevez AG, Radi F, Beckman JS (1997) Peroxynitrite and cell signaling. In: Forman HJ, Cadenas E (eds) Oxidative stress and signal transduction. Chapman and Hall, New York, pp 239–259
57. Schieven GL (1997) Tyrosine phosphorylation in oxidative stress. In: Forman HJ, Cadenas E (eds) Oxidative stress and signal transduction. Chapman and Hall, New York, pp 181–199
58. Konishi H, Tanaka M, Takemura Y, et al (1997) Activation of protein kinase by tyrosine phosphorylation in response to H_2O_2. Proc Natl Acad Sci USA 94:11233–11237
59. Schoonbroodt S, Legrand-Poels S, Best-Belpomme M, Piette J (1997) Activation of the NF-κB transcription factor in a T-lymphocytic cell line by hypochlorous acid. Biochemical J 321:777–785
60. Schwartz MD, Moore EE, Moore FA, et al (1996) Nuclear factor-κB is activated in alveolar macrophages from patients with acute respiratory distress syndrome. Crit Care Med 24:1285–1292
61. Gerrity RG (1981) The role of the monocyte in atherogenesis. I. Transition of blood-borne monocytes into foam cells in fatty lesions. Am J Pathol 103:181–190
62. Daugherty A, Dunn JL, Rateri DL, Heinecke JW (1994) Myeloperoxidase, a catalyst for lipoprotein oxidation, is expressed in human atherosclerotic lesions. J Clin Invest 94:437–444
63. Hazell LJ, Stocker R (1993) Oxidation of low-density lipoprotein with hypochlorite causes transformation of the lipoprotein into a high-uptake form for macrophages. Biochem J 290:165–172
64. Heinecke JW, Li W, Mueller DM, Bohrer A, Turk J (1994) Cholesterol chlorohydrin synthesis by the myeloperoxidase-hydrogen peroxide-chloride system: potential markers for lipoproteins oxidatively damaged by phagocytes. Biochemistry 33:10127–10136
65. Hazell LJ, Arbold L, Flowers D, Waeg G, Malle F, Stocker R (1996) Presence of hypochlorite-modified proteins in human atherosclerotic lesions. J Clin Invest 97:1535–1544
66. Bosch X, Mirapeix E, Font J, Ingelmo M, Revert L (1991) Anti-myeloperoxidase antibodies in crescentic glomerulonephritis. Nephron 59:504–505
67. Bosch X, Font J, Mirapeix E, Revert L, Ingelmo M, Urbano-Marquez A (1992) Antimyeloperoxidase autoantibody-associated necrotizing alveolar capillaritis. Am Rev Respir Dis 146:1326–1329
68. Rosen H, Michel BR (1997) Redundant contribution of myeloperoxidase- dependent systems to neutrophil-mediated killing of *Escherichia coli*. Infect Immun 65:4173–4178
69. Gerber CE, Kuci S, Zipfel M, Niethammer D, Bruchelt G (1996) Phagocytic activity and oxidative burst of granulocytes in persons with myeloperoxidase deficiency. Eur J Clin Chem Clin Biochem 34:901–908
70. Rosen H, Orman J, Ratika RM, Michel BR, Van-Devanter DR (1990) Loss of DNA interactions and cessation of DNA synthesis in myeloperoxidase treated *Escherichia coli*. Proc Natl Acad Sci USA 87:10048–10052

NAD(P)H Oxidase in Non-Phagocytic Cells

A. Görlach

Introduction

The importance of reactive oxygen intermediates (ROI) is evident from the vast literature describing the involvement of free radicals in the pathogenesis of various disorders including neurological (Alzheimer's disease, Parkinson's disease), viral human immunodeficiency virus (HIV) and acquired immunodeficiency syndrome (AIDS), and degenerative (atherosclerosis, cancer, cataract) diseases.

The generation of ROI is an activity normally associated with phagocytes. As part of the body's host defense system these cells are able, when stimulated by various agents including bacterial toxins, to generate large amounts of superoxide in the respiratory burst in order to kill invading microorganisms. Over the past ten years it has become increasingly apparent that non-phagocytic cells also share the capacity to generate oxygen radicals. Such activity has been detected in a wide variety of different cells including endothelial cells, vascular smooth muscle cells, mesangial cells, fibroblasts, oocytes, spermatozoa, Leydig cells, various tumor cells, thyroid cells, B-lymphocytes, adipocytes, platelets, chondrocytes and osteoblasts. Since the capacity to generate ROI is widespread, the risk-benefit relation for these potentially hazardous molecules becomes a matter of interest. Whereas the controlled generation of these highly reactive molecules may serve an important second messenger role in many different cell types, their uncontrolled production may contribute to the etiology of pathological conditions through the initiation and propagation of peroxidative damage. Therefore the identification of sources of ROI in non-phagocytic cells is of considerable interest.

Recently, evidence has accumulated that nicotinamide adenine dinucleotide (phosphate) [NAD(P)H] oxidases might also be present in non-phagocytic cells. However, the molecular identity and function of these systems are only beginning to be elucidated. This article will summarize current knowledge about the presence of NAD(P)H oxidases in non-phagocytic cells.

NADPH Oxidase in Phagocytes

NADPH oxidase is a highly regulated membrane-bound enzyme complex which was initially found in phagocytes. As the key enzyme for the respiratory burst, it catalyzes O_2^- production according to the following reaction [1]:

$$2\,O_2 + NADPH \rightarrow 2\,O_2^- + NADP^+ + H^+ \tag{1}$$

Although O_2^- is a free radical, it is unreactive towards many organic molecules and not an oxidant at neutral pH [2]. It is highly solute in water and is not expected to be transported through membranes or to penetrate into hydrophobic regions of cells and peroxide lipids. However, it readily, either spontaneously or catalyzed by superoxide dismutase (SOD), dismutes to hydrogen peroxide (H_2O_2) an oxidant, germicide and cytotoxic agent. This ROI is stable and carries no charge, allowing it to cross membranes and to travel freely to its targets. It readily participates in one-electron processes with metal ions such as the Fenton reaction, thereby generating highly reactive hydroxyl radicals. Other toxic weapons generated in phagocytes from O_2^- include oxidized halogens and singlet oxygen [3].

In resting cells NADPH oxidase is dormant and the protein components are segregated into cytoplasmic and plasma membrane compartments [1]. The enzyme can be activated by receptor-dependent stimuli such as complement fragment C5a, the chemotactic tripeptide N-formyl-methionyl-leucyl-phenylalanine (fMLP) and immune complexes, for example via the G-protein activated phospholipase C pathway, finally stimulating protein kinase C and phospholipase D. Receptor-independent stimuli include long-chain unsaturated fatty acids and phorbol-myristate-acetate (PMA) [4, 5].

On stimulation, the cytosolic proteins p47, p67 and p40 form a complex and translocate to the plasma membrane, where they associate with a membrane-bound flavocytochrome composed of two subunits, p22 and gp91 (Fig. 1) [4]. The low molecular weight guanosine tri-phosphate (GTP)-binding protein, rac, changes from an inactive guanosine diphosphate (GDP)-bound to an active GTP-bound form and translocates separately to the plasma membrane, where it probably modulates the function of one or more NADPH oxidase proteins [6]. The role of additional factors such as p40, which also translocates to the membrane, and the membrane bound rap1A, known as tumor suppressor gene, in the activation process are not

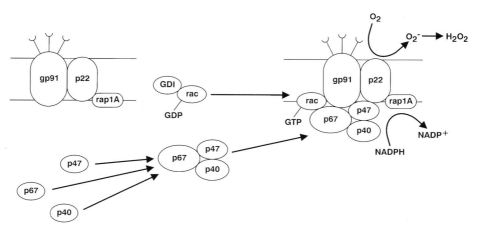

Fig.1. Assembly of the NADPH oxidase components in phagocytes. Under resting conditions membrane-bound components are separated from cytosolic factors. On activation, the cytosolic components assemble and translocate to the membrane where they associate with cytochrome b558. Independently, rac also translocates to the membrane

fully understood. Recently p40 has been suggested to down-modulate NADPH oxidase function [7].

The unusual low midpoint potentials of the two hemes in the cytochrome, -225 mV and -265 mV, facilitate the electron flow from NAD(P)H via flavin adenine dinucleotide (FAD) to the cytochrome and molecular oxygen [4]. Both, NADPH ($K_m \sim 30$ µM) and NADH ($K_m \sim 200$ µM), can be used as reducing agents. The K_m for oxygen, the other oxidase substrate, was determined around 10 µM (below 1% O_2 in water), suggesting that the enzyme can produce O_2^- even under hypoxic conditions such as in infected tissue. In contrast to other cytochromes, cytochrome b558 binds carbon monoxide (CO) with low affinity ($K_m \sim 1.4$ mM) and cannot be re-oxidized by respiratory chain inhibitors like cyanide or rotenone [3]. Protons arising from NADPH oxidation cross the membrane via a Cd^{2+}/Zn^{2+} sensitive proton channel probably located in the gp91 subunit of the cytochrome [8]. They act as compensating ions as they accompany the electrons that were moved electrogenically to reduce oxygen to superoxide. The dismutation of O_2^- then consumes H^+ to produce H_2O_2.

The importance of NADPH oxidase in host defense is made evident by a rare inherited disorder, chronic granulomatous disease (CGD), in which mutations in any of four components of this enzyme lead to a failure to generate O_2^-, rendering the patients highly susceptible to life threatening microbial infections [5]. The complementary deoxyribonucleic acids (cDNAs) for all components have been cloned and sequenced, and the genes encoding these proteins have been localized and characterized. Recently, at least one highly homologous pseudogene has been identified for the p47 gene [9]. The transcript for p22 is constitutively present in a variety of tissues, whereas gp91 as well as the cytosolic factors p40, p47 and p67 are considered to be predominantly expressed in the white cell line [5, 7]. Promoter elements in the gp91 and p47 genes have been identified as being responsible for this line confinement [10, 11].

NAD(P)H Oxidase in Non-Phagocytic Cells

The potential to generate low levels of superoxide has been described in several non-phagocytic cell types. Whereas some cell types spontaneously generate ROI, other cell types require, similar to phagocytes, activating stimuli such as cytokines, phorbol esters or calcium ionophores. The amount of ROI generated by non-phagocytic cells typically reaches around 1%–10% of the ROI levels produced in the respiratory burst by activated neutrophils [3]. Low levels of ROI are non-toxic and can lead to modulation of intracellular signaling, gene expression, cell proliferation and cell death [2]. The proliferation of several cell types, including fibroblasts and T-lymphocytes, can be stimulated by small amounts of superoxide [3]. Thus, the cellular functions of free radicals can be roughly summarized in five categories:
(1) cytokine, growth factor, and hormone action and secretion;
(2) ion transport;
(3) transcription;
(4) neuromodulation;
(5) apoptosis (for review see [12]).

Numerous signaling pathways are known to be affected by ROI including arachidonate metabolism, protein kinases and transcription factors such as nuclear factor-
kappa B (NF-κB) activator protein (AP-1), p53 and hypoxia inducible factor-1
(HIF-1). ROI are involved in the induction of immediate early response genes such
as *c-fos, c-jun, c-myc* and *egr-1*. Recently it has been suggested that they participate
in the activation of the ras pathway [13]. Given these multiple actions in various
tissues, the identification of potential sources of ROI in cellular systems is of major
importance.

Many oxygen radical producing systems are known to modulate the cellular redox
state including xanthine oxidase, lipoxygenases, cyclooxygenases, as well as the respiratory chain [12]. The identification of ROI generating systems relies mainly on
the use of more or less specific inhibitors of the various enzymes. Based on the
decrease of superoxide production by the application of diphenylene iodonium
(DPI), an inhibitor of NADPH oxidase, but not by inhibitors of other radical generating enzymes (see above), the presence of NAD(P)H oxidase was suggested in
various cell types including spermatozoa, pneumocytes, thyroid cells, and tumor
cells [3, 14]. However, DPI has been shown to be a rather non-specific inhibitor of
flavoprotein containing enzymes, among them nitric oxide synthase (NOS), and no
specific NADPH oxidase inhibitor is available at the moment [15]. The presence of
an NAD(P)H oxidase was also postulated when NADPH and/or NADH were required to generate superoxide. A number of cell types showed, in contrast to the
phagocyte NADPH oxidase, higher affinities for NADH than for NADPH. Therefore
it appears appropriate to suggest that in many non-phagocytic cell types NADPH/
NADH oxidases exist, and some of them might represent isoforms of the phagocyte
enzyme.

However, only a limited number of studies so far provide direct evidence for the
presence of non-phagocytic NAD(P)H oxidase. In a number of cells types a heme
protein exhibiting the characteristic features of cytochrome b558, such as an absorption maximum at 558 nm, a very low midpoint potential, and insensitivity to
cyanide, could be identified. However, non-phagocytic cells contained substantially
lower amounts of cytochrome b558 than phagocytes. Further proof for the presence
of NAD(P)H oxidase in non-phagocytic cells has been provided by the detection of
NADPH oxidase components at the mRNA and/or protein level in several cell types
(Table 1) which are described in more detail in the section below.

Oxygen Sensing Cells

Under hypoxic conditions specific adaptive responses are induced in order to sustain
and improve oxygen availability to the tissues. Specific chemoreceptive organs such
as the carotid body actively regulate ventilation and circulation. In the kidney, the
expression of the glycoprotein hormone erythropoietin is dramatically enhanced, to
stimulate erythropoiesis and thereby improve oxygen transport capacity to the
tissues. Moreover, many, if not all, other cell types are able to adapt their activity according to variations in oxygen availability, for example, by the modulation of channel activities and/or gene expression. Whereas oxygen dependent transcription factors such as HIF-1 have been identified in various cell types, the oxygen sensor

Table 1. NAD(P)H oxidase in non-phagocytic cells

Method of detection	Spectro-photo-metry	mRNA level (Northern, RT-PCR)	Protein level (Western, Immuno-fluorescence)	Cloning (cDNA)
Cell type				
Hepatoma HepG2	+	p22	p22, p47, p67, gp91	
Endothelial cells	+	p22, p47,p67, gp91	p47, p67	
Smooth muscle cells	+	p22	gp91	p22
Mesangial cells	+	p22, p47, p67	p22, gp91	
Fibroblasts	+	p22, p47, p67	p22, gp91	
Chondrocytes		p22, p40, P47	p67	
Carotid body, type I cells	+		p22, p47, p67, gp91	
Neuroepithelial bodies	+	p22, gp91	p22, p47, p67, gp91	
SIF cells[a]			p22	

[a] Small intensely fluorescent cells

This table summarizes NADPH oxidase components identified in non-phagocytic cells. By spectro-photometry, a low potential cytochrome b558 component was detected which could not be reoxidized by cyanide. No spectroscopic data were available from chondrocytes and SIF cells.

remains obscure. A heme protein has been suggested to act as an oxygen sensor by changing the conformational state according to the amount of oxygen available (for review see [16, 17]).

Based on spectrophotometric studies in erythropoietin-producing hepatoma cells a b-type heme protein similar to the cytochrome b558 was suggested to be involved in oxygen sensing [18]. This b-cytochrome was reducible by hypoxia but not by cyanide, and it had a low affinity to CO. The expression of all four NADPH oxidase components was demonstrated by either Western blot analysis or immuno-fluorescence [18]. These cells produced ROI depending on the oxygen availability. The addition of H_2O_2 resulted in a substantial decrease in hypoxic erythropoietin production whereas the presence of scavenging systems stimulated erythropoietin production already under normoxic conditions, suggesting that the decrease in ROI putatively generated by an NAD(P)H oxidase might allow the up-regulation of erythropoietin in hypoxia [19].

Similar studies were performed in chemoreceptive organs known to be crucially involved in oxygen sensing in the body. The addition of H_2O_2 inhibited the hypoxic nerve discharge in the carotid body [20]. The spectrophotometric detection of cyto-chrome b558 together with the identification of four NADPH oxidase components by immunofluorescence in hypoxia-responsive type I cells in the carotid body sug-gested again the involvement of NAD(P)H oxidase in oxygen sensing [21].

In pulmonary neuroepithelial bodies representing airway chemoreceptive organs in the lung, all NAD(P)H oxidase components were identified in close vicinity to oxygen sensitive K^+ channels in the membrane. Since the activity of these channels could be modulated by H_2O_2 it was suggested that an NAD(P)H oxidase might be involved in oxygen-dependent regulation of channel activity in neuroepithelial bodies [22, 23]. Moreover, p22 expression and H_2O_2 production have also been demonstrated in small intensely fluorescent cells (SIF), hypoxia-sensitive paragang-lionic structures found throughout the body [24], indicating that NAD(P)H oxidase might play a specific role in oxygen sensitive cells. However, the molecular identity of these components remains to be clarified. In CGD patients no defect in oxygen sensing has become apparent, indicating that either multiple overlapping oxygen sensing systems are present, or that NAD(P)H oxidase isoforms exist in oxygen sens-ing cells.

Vascular System

The potential to generate free radicals has long been recognized in the vascular system. In pig coronary arteries and rabbit aortas low basal values have been measured. Indirect evidence using DPI to inhibit ROI production suggests that an enzyme similar to NADPH oxidase is also present in vascular cells [3].

In calf small pulmonary arteries the presence of a low potential cytochrome b558 was demonstrated spectrophotometrically. The detection of gp91 expression by Western blot analysis suggested the presence of NAD(P)H oxidase. In contrast to other studies superoxide production increased from 1.4 to 73 nmol O_2^-/min/mg protein in these cells under hypoxic conditions. Since DPI could inhibit hypoxic superoxide production as well as hypoxic vasoconstriction, it was suggested that NAD(P)H oxidase might play a role in pulmonary hypoxic vasoconstriction [25].

Approximately 24% of ROI release has been accounted for as being derived from endothelial cells [26]. Cultured endothelial cells respond to a diverse range of stimu-li including cytokines, bradykinin, calcium ionophores, phorbol esters, and cyclic strain with the generation of low levels of ROI (for review see [26, 27]). Hypoxia/re-oxygenation stress is able to increase ROI production in endothelial cells whereas under hypoxic conditions superoxide production is strictly dependent on the PO_2 [28, 29]. Excess production of ROI has been related to the pathogenesis of athero-sclerosis. Under pathological conditions such as hypercholesterolemia, hyperten-sion and diabetes, ROI appear to participate in the deregulation of vascular tone [26]. Superoxide has also been suggested to be identical to the endothelial derived contracting factor in analogy to endothelial derived relaxing factor (EDRF) which has been identified as nitric oxide (NO) [3].

Human umbilical venous endothelial cells were able to generate seven times more superoxide when using NADH instead of NADPH. However, iodonium diphenyl (IDP), a flavoprotein inhibitor, impaired the response three times more efficiently when NADPH was used as substrate. The presence of NAD(P)H oxidase in human umbilical venous endothelial cells was supported by the identification of all four components (p22, gp91, p47, p67) of the NADPH oxidase by reverse transcriptase polymerase chain reaction (RT-PCR) using oligonucleotides derived from phago-cyte sequences [27]. Partial sequence analysis revealed a high homology to the neu-trophil sequences. Furthermore p47 and p67 expression could be detected by immu-nofluorescence and Western blot analysis. Although this study was the first to sug-gest gp91 transcripts in non-phagocytic cells, no evidence for a low-potential cyto-chrome b558 could be detected spectrophotometrically. It was speculated that a post-transcriptional block as has been observed in B-lymphocytes might also

impair the effective translation of gp91 in endothelial cells. Alternatively, heme availability might restrict the formation of a stable cytochrome b558. Additional studies
will have to analyze in more detail the structure and function of endothelial
NAD(P)H oxidase.

Whereas ROI have been shown to stimulate proliferation of vascular smooth
muscle cells (VSMC) [3], the generation of ROI by smooth muscle cells apparently
contributes significantly to the overall ROI production by different types of blood
vessels [26]. A variety of stimuli can activate the generation of ROI in smooth muscle
cells, such as growth factors, insulin and fatty acids. For example, the glycosphingolipid lactosylceramide stimulated the generation of superoxide in membrane fractions from human aortic smooth muscle cells in the presence of NADPH but not
NADH. Since DPI could inhibit the radical generation as well as the proliferation of
these cells, the presence of an NAD(P)H oxidase activated by this glycosphingolipid
was suggested as mediating the proliferative stimulus [30]. In rat VSMC, oxidase
activity could be measured using NADPH and NADH as substrates, leading to basal
levels of activity of 3.23 nmol O_2^-/min/mg protein and 16.76 nmol O_2^-/min/mg
protein respectively. DPI was more effective in inhibiting NADPH than NADH oxidase activity. The NAD(P)H oxidase activity was localized in the membrane fraction
and could be stimulated approximately four-fold by angiotensin II (ATII) [31]. Subsequent studies proved this finding *in vivo* and showed that ATII could up-regulate
p22 mRNA levels. Cloning of rat p22 from a rat VSMC library revealed a high
homology to the neutrophil component. Using an anti-sense approach, the ability to
generate O_2^- was found to be critically dependent on p22. Cytochrome b558 was
demonstrated spectrophotometrically in cells overexpressing p22, but could not be
detected in cells transfected with an anti-sense construct [33]. However, no evidence
for the presence of gp91 could be found in this study, suggesting that a structurally
distinct form of this protein is present in these cells. As ATII mediates hypertrophy
of smooth muscle cells which can lead to hypertension, NAD(P)H oxidase activity
has been related to ATII mediated hypertension [32]. These studies provide the first
evidence that NAD(P)H oxidase components are functional in non-phagocytic cells.

Kidney

Human kidney glomerular mesangial cells (HMC) produce ROI when stimulated
with tumor necrosis factor (TNF)-α, interleukin-1α (IL-1α), or IL-1β as well as with
calcium ionophores. ROI generation has been related to the pathogenesis of glomerular injury [34]. By RT-PCR, transcripts for p22 were detected in resting cells,
whereas p47 and p67 transcripts were only found in HMC treated with IL-1β.
Sequence analysis of the PCR fragments revealed approximately 98% homology
with the neutrophil sequence. Immunodetection studies showed the presence of
p22, p47, and p67. Although by spectroscopy a low potential cytochrome b558 in
HMC membranes could be demonstrated in a concentration of 60 pmol/mg membrane protein, gp91 could not be identified by RT-PCR or immunoblotting. In contrast, the presence of gp91 was demonstrated immunohistochemically in rat visceral
glomerular epithelial cells with passive Heymann nephritis [35] indicating that
NAD(P)H oxidase components or their homologs might be induced during inflam-

mation. Alternatively, isoforms of this enzyme may exist containing a differently composed cytochrome b558. Recently, in rabbit proximal tubular epithelial cells of the kidney, indirect evidence, provided by the inhibitory action of DPI on O_2^- production, indicated that arachidonic acid activates an NAD(P)H oxidase to release superoxide which stimulates *c-jun* N-terminal kinase [36].

Other Cell Types

In fibroblasts a low potential cytochrome b558 was detected spectrophotometrically in a concentration of about 10 pmol/mg protein [37]. ROI release could be observed in fibroblasts stimulated with various cytokines, calcium ionophores or PMA. However, a cell-cycle dependent, very low basal ROI production was also observed, consistent with the finding that ROI are involved in proliferation of fibroblasts [37]. Transcripts were found for p22, p47 and p67, using RT-PCR but not for gp91. The presence of p47 protein could also be demonstrated by Western blot analysis [38]. However, fibroblasts from healthy donors and gp91 deficient CGD patients did not differ in their ability to produce superoxide, indicating that the fibroblast cytochrome is genetically distinct from the neutrophil cytochrome b558 [37].

In porcine articular chondrocytes the calcium ionophore ionomycin stimulated superoxide production which could be inhibited by IDP [39]. The presence of transcripts for p22, p47 and p40 was shown by RT-PCR. Furthermore the expression of p67 could be demonstrated by Western blot analysis. The ability to generate ROI spontaneously or after stimulation with various cytokines has been noted previously [40]. The local production of ROI in chondrocytes may be important for the terminal differentiation of chondrocytes in the hypertrophic and calcified zones of the growth plates. The excess generation of ROI might play a role in the degradation of matrix in arthritis.

Evidence for an NAD(P)H oxidase expressing p22, gp91 and p47 as demonstrated by immunofluorescence has also been shown in osteoclasts [41]. As these cells derive from common myelo-monocytic precursors it can be speculated that they might contain a genetically identical NAD(P)H oxidase form. However, there are no reports to date demonstrating that osteoclasts derived from CGD patients contain non-functional NAD(P)H oxidase due to mutations in the enzyme subunits.

Conclusion

Many cell types have the potential to generate ROI. In contrast to the cytotoxic activity observed in phagocytes, non-phagocytic cells generate low rates of ROI which might serve as signaling molecules. NADPH oxidase plays an important role in the generation of ROI in phagocytes, but has also been identified in non-phagocytic cells. However, the substrate requirements for the phagocyte and non-phagocyte enzymes are different in that, in the latter, NADH is used more efficiently than NADPH. Although high sequence homologies appear to exist between the phagocyte and non-phagocytic enzyme components, the molecular and genetic identity of these proteins in non-phagocytic cells remains to be clarified. First reports in vascular smooth muscle cells have demonstrated that NAD(P)H oxidase components are functional and critically involved in the cell's potential to generate ROI. The identification of ROI generating systems in non-phagocytic cells will provide important insights into the role of oxygen generating systems in cellular signaling and might allow new therapeutic tools to be developed for various disease processes ranging from inflammatory disorders to ischemic diseases and cancer.

Acknowledgements. I thank C. Gasser for the art work, and Drs. C. Bauer and M. Gassmann for support.

References

1. Jones OTG (1994) The regulation of superoxide production by the NADPH oxidase of neutrophils and other mammalian cells. Bioessays 16:919–922
2. Khan AU, Wilson T (1995) Reactive oxygen species as cellular messengers. Chem Biol 2:437–445
3. Cross AR, Jones OTG (1991) Enzymatic mechanisms of superoxide production. Biochem Biophys Acta 1057:281–298
4. Leusen JHW, Verhoeven AJ, Roos D (1996) Interactions between the components of the human NADPH oxidase: Intrigues in the phox family. J Lab Clin Med 128:461–476
5. Curnutte JT (1993) Chronic granulomatous disease: the solving of a clinical riddle. Clin Immunol Immunopath 67:S2–S15
6. DeLeo FR, Quinn M (1996) Assembly of the phagocyte NADPH oxidase: molecular interaction of oxidase proteins. J Leukoc Biol 60:677–691
7. Saythyamoorthy M, deMendez I, Adams AG, Leto TL (1997) p40phox down-regulates NADPH oxidase activity through interactions with its SH3 domain. J Biol Chem 272:9141–9146
8. Henderson LM, Thomas S, Banting G, Chappell JB (1997) The arachidonate-activable, NADPH oxidase-associated H^+ channel is contained within the multi-membrane-spanning N-terminal region of gp91-phox. Biochem J 325:701–705
9. Görlach A, Lee PL, Roester J, et al (1997) A p47-*phox* Pseudogene carries the most common mutation causing p47-*phox*-deficient chronic granulomatous disease. J Clin Invest 100:1907–1918
10. Lien LL, Lee Y Orkin SH (1997) Regulation of the myeloid-cell-expressed human gp91phox gene as studied by transfer of yeast artificial chromosome clones into embryonic stem cells: suppression of a variegated cellular pattern of expression requires a full complement of distant cis elements. Mol Cell Biol 17:2279–2290
11. Li SL, Valente AJ, Zhao SJ, Clark RA (1997) Pu.1 is essential for p47(phox) promoter activity in myeloid cells. J Biol Chem 272:17802–17809
12. Lander HM (1997) An essential role for free radicals and derived species in signal transduction. FASEB J 11:118–124
13. Irani K, Xia Y, Zweier JL, et al (1997) Mitogenic signaling mediated by oxidants in Ras transformed fibroblasts. Science 275:1649–1652
14. van Klaveren RJ, Roelant C, Boogaerts M, Demedts M, Nemery B (1997) Involvement of an NAD(P)H oxidase-like enzyme in superoxide anion and hydrogen peroxide generation by rat type II cells. Thorax 52:465–471
15. O'Donnell VB, Tew DG, Jones OTG, England PJ (1993) Studies on the inhibitory mechanism of iodonium compounds with specific reference to neutrophil NADPH oxidase. Biochem J 290:41–49
16. Bunn HF, Poyton RO (1996) Oxygen sensing and molecular adaptation to hypoxia. Physiol Rev 76:839–885
17. Acker H (1994) Mechanisms and meaning of cellular oxygen sensing in the organism. Resp Physiol 95:1–10
18. Görlach A, Holtermann G, Jelkmann W, et al (1993) Photometric characteristics of haem proteins in erythropoietin-producing hepatoma cells (HepG2). Biochem J 290:771–776
19. Fandrey J, Frede S, Jelkmann W (1994) Role of hydrogen peroxide in hypoxia-induced erythropoietin production. Biochem J 303:507–510

20. Acker H, Bölling B, Delpiano MA, Dufau E, Görlach A, Holtermann G (1992) The meaning of H_2O_2 generation in carotid body cells for pO_2 chemoreception. J Auton Nerv Syst 41:41–52
21. Kummer W, Acker H (1995) Immunohistochemical detection of four subunits of neutrophil NAD(P)H oxidase in type I cells of carotid body. J Appl Physiol 78:1904–1909
22. Wang D, Youngson C, Wong V, et al (1996) NADPH-oxidase and a hydrogen peroxide-sensitive K^+ channel may function as an oxygen sensor complex in airway chemoreceptors and small lung cell carcinoma cell lines. Proc Natl Acad Sci USA 93:13182–13187
23. Youngson C, Nurse C, Yeger H, et al (1997) Immunocytochemical localization of O_2-sensing proteins (NADPH oxidase) in chemoreceptor cells. Microsc Res Tech 37:101–106
24. Kummer W, Acker H (1997) Cytochrome b558 and hydrogen peroxide production in small intensely fluorescent cells of sympathetic ganglia. Histochem Cell Biol 197:151–158
25. Marshall C, Mamary AJ, Verhoeven AJ, Marshall BE (1996) Pulmonary artery NADPH-oxidase is activated in hypoxic pulmonary vasoconstriction. Am J Resp Cell Mol Biol 15:633–644
26. Brandes RP, Barton M, Philippens KHM, Schweitzer G, Mügge A (1997) Endothelial-derived superoxide anions in pig coronary arteries: evidence from lucigene chemiluminescence and histochemical techniques. J Physiol 500:331–342
27. Jones SA, O'Donnell V, Wood JD, Broughton JP, Hughes EJ, Jones OTG (1996) Expression of phagocyte NADPH oxidase components in human endothelial cells. Am J Physiol 271: H1626–H1634
28. Zulueta JJ, Yu FS, Hertig IA, Thannickal VJ, Hassoun PM (1995) Release of hydrogen peroxide in response to hypoxia-reoxygenation: role of an NAD(P)H oxidase-like enzyme in endothelial cell plasma membrane. Am J Resp Cell Mol Biol 12:41–49
29. Kinnula VK, Mirza Z, Cerapo JD, Whorton AR (1993) Modulation of hydrogen peroxide release from vascular endothelial cells by oxygen. Am J Resp Cell Mol Biol 9:603–609
30. Bhunia AK, Han H, Snowden A, Chatterjee S (1997) Redox-regulated signaling by lactosylcera-mide in the proliferation of human aortic smooth muscle cells. J Biol Chem 272:15642–15649
31. Griendling KK, Minieri CA, Ollerenshaw JD, Alexander RW (1994) Angiotensin II stimulates NADH and NADPH oxidase activity in cultured vascular smooth muscle cells. Circ Res 74: 1141–1148
32. Rajagopalan S, Kurz S, Münzel T, et al (1996) Angiotensin II-mediated hypertension in the rat increases vascular superoxide production via membrane NADH/NADPH oxidase activation. J Clin Invest 97:1916–1923
33. Ushio-Fukai M, Mazia-Zafari A, Fukui T, Ishizaka N, Griendling KK (1996) p22phox is a critical component of the superoxide-generating NADH/NADPH oxidase system and regulates angiotensin II-induced hypertrophy in vascular smooth muscle cells. J Biol Chem 271:23317–23321
34. Jones SA, Hancock JT, Jones OTG, Neubauer A, Topley N (1995) The expression of NADPH oxidase components in human glomerular mesangial cells: detection of protein and mRNA for p47phox, p67phox, and p22phox. J Am Soc Nephrol 5:1483–1491
35. Neale TJ, Ullrich R, Ojha P, Poczewski H, Verhoeven AJ, Kerjaschki D (1993) Reactive oxygen species and neutrophil respiratory burst cytochrome b558 are produced by kidney glomerular cells in passive Heymann nephritis. Proc Natl Acad Sci USA 90:3645–3649
36. Cui XL, Douglas JG (1997) Arachidonic acid activates c-jun N-terminal kinase through NADPH oxidase in rabbit proximal tubular epithelial cells. Proc Natl Acad Sci USA 94:3771–3776
37. Meier B, Jesaitis AJ, Emmendoerfer A, Roesler J, Quinn MT (1993) The cytochrome b-558 molecules involved in the fibrobalst and polymorphonuclear leucocyte superoxide-generating NADPH oxidase systems are structurally and genetically distinct. Biochem J 289:481–486
38. Jones SA, Wood JD, Coffey MJ, Jones OTG (1994) The functional expression of p47-phox and p67-phox may contribute to the generation of superoxide by an NADPH oxidase-like system in human fibroblasts. FEBS Lett 355:178–182
39. Hiran TS, Moulton PJ, Hancock JT (1997) Detection of superoxide and NADPH oxidase in porcine articular chondrocytes. Free Rad Biol Med 23:736–743
40. Rathakrishanan C, Tiku K, Raghavan A, Tiku MT (1992) Release of oxygen radicals by articular chondrocytes: a study of luminol-dependent chemiluminescence and hydrogen peroxide secretion. J Bone Min Res 7:1139–1148
41. Steinbeck MJ, Appel WH, Verhoeven AJ, Karnovsky MJ (1994) NADPH-oxidase expression and in situ production of superoxide by osteoclasts actively resorbing bone. J Cell Biol 126: 765–772

Gelatinases and the Acute Respiratory Distress Syndrome

C. Delclaux and M. P. d'Ortho

Introduction

The acute respiratory distress syndrome (ARDS) is a clinical and pathophysiological entity characterized by acute, diffuse injury to the alveolar capillary barrier. In the area of gas exchange, this barrier is reduced to endothelial and epithelial cells separated by a thin extracellular matrix (ECM) resulting from fusion of the two basement membranes of the former lining cells. It has been demonstrated for many years that the epithelial barrier is the major component of the alveolar capillary wall defense against alveolar flooding, the characteristic of ARDS [1].

Passage of high-molecular mass proteins into the alveoli indicates the loss of size selectivity of the alveolar capillary barrier. Furthermore, basement membrane disruption has been documented, and degradation products of type IV collagen have been found in alveolar spaces during the course of ARDS [2]. This basement membrane injury is believed to result mainly from proteinase activity(ies), and oxygen metabolites do not seem to participate in this process. Among proteinases capable of degrading the basement membrane components, the serine protease leukocyte elastase has been the focus of several studies, which have yielded conflicting data [3]. Indeed, for a long time, polymorphonuclear neutrophils (PMN) were thought to be the major factor involved in the injury process but more recent experimental and clinical data support the hypothesis that the PMN is neither indispensable nor sufficient to create this injury [4, 5]. It is well-known that ARDS can occur in neutropenic patients and that neutrophil influx into airspaces does not imply a significant alveolar capillary wall degradation. Therefore, the participation of alveolar capillary wall cells, namely endothelial and alveolar epithelial cells, in the modulation of permeability became an exciting research field. The fact that non-inflammatory cells and proteinases other than leukocyte elastase are probably involved, led to recent interest in the possible involvement of the matrix metalloproteinase (MMP) family in ARDS pathophysiology [3].

Matrix Metalloproteinase Family

Although many proteases can cleave ECM molecules, the MMPs are believed to be the usual mediators of both normal ECM degradation in physiologic ECM turnover, and of the accelerated ECM destruction occurring in many diseases such as tumor metastasis, arthritis, aneurysm formation, atherosclerosis, and pulmonary emphysema. There are several reasons for this: the MMPs are secreted proteins, or some of them membrane anchored, placing them in the proper location for ECM degradation, and their enzymatic activities are most potent at pH values close to neutral. They are synthesized and secreted by connective tissue and some hematopoietic cells. Regulation of

MMP is stringent, occuring not only at gene expression but extracellularly after secretion, by the action of activators of pro-enzyme forms and specific inhibitors.

The MMPs are a family of zinc- and calcium-dependent proteases that are able to degrade the various components of ECM. Sixteen MMPs have been identified by cDNA cloning and sequencing. Comparison of these sequences, in conjuction with biochemical and immunological data, have indicated that these comprise two gelatinases, four collagenases, four stromelysins, four membrane-anchored MMP (membrane-type MMP, MT-MMPs), one metalloelastase and one recently identified MMP not yet classified in one of the above subfamilies, MMP-19 (Table 1).

Substrates

Among the MMPs, the two gelatinases are proposed to be important in basement membrane type IV collagen degradation in many situations. These gelatinases degrade type IV collagen, denatured collagens (gelatins), types V, VII, XI collagens, elastin and laminin. Gelatinase A (72 kD form) is produced by epithelial, endothelial and mesenchymal cells. Gelatinase B (92–95 kD form) is derived from macrophages and neutrophils, as well as some stimulated tissue cells and tumors.

The collagenases cleave the native helix of the fibrillar collagens at a single locus. Stromelysins 1 and 2 are able to degrade many ECM molecules including proteoglycans and laminin, and are potentiators of collagenase and gelatinase B activity.

Table 1. MMP family

Trivial name	MMP n°	Source	Substrates
Gelatinases			
Gelatinase A (72 kD)	MMP2	Most cell types	Collagen IV, V, VII, X and XI
Gelatinase B (95 kD)	MMP9	Inflammatory cells Connective tissue cells	Elastin, gelatin
Collagenases			
Fibroblast collagenase	MMP1	Connective tissue cells	Fibrillar collagens
Neutrophil collagenase	MMP8	Neutrophils, chondrocytes	
Collagenase-3	MMP13	Tumor cells	
Xenopus laevi collagenase	MMP18		
Stromelysins			
Stromelysin 1	MMP3	Connective tissue cells, macrophages	Proteoglycans, fibronectin, laminin gelatin, procollagenase, progelatinase B
Stromelysin 2	MMP10		
Stromelysin 3	MMP11	Macrophages Stromal cells of tumors	
Matrilysin (pump)	MMP7	Monocytes, tumor cells	
Metalloelastase	MMP12	Macrophage	Elastin, fibronectin
MT-MMP 1–4	MMP14–17	Stromal cells of tumors	Proteoglycans, fibronectin, laminin, progelatinase A
	MMP19	Liver tissue	unknown

The metalloelastase cleaves elastin as well as fibronectin. The MT1- and MT2-MMP have a broad spectrum of activity cleaving for example fibronectin or proteoglycans, but their role as membrane activators of progelatinase A and procollagenase 3 is the most defined [6].

MMPs cannot only cleave ECM molecules, but they play a role in-various diseases by directly cleaving pro-cytokines, growth factors, growth factor receptors, and cell surface receptors. Indeed, most MMPs cleave pro-tumor necrosis factor (proTNF) into mature TNF [7], as well as cleaving interleukin-1β (IL-1β). Stromelysins can cleave insulin-like growth factor (IGF) binding proteins; similarly, gelatinase A has been reported recently as being able to release the active soluble ectodomain of fibroblast growth factor (FGF) receptor-1. L-selectin levels on leukocytes can be regulated by MMPs.

The cDNA-predicted amino acid sequences of all MMPs can be aligned, demonstrating a high degree of conservation between each type of enzyme across several mammalian species. Domains with apparent specific functions can be delineated within these sequences, including a propetide lost during activation, a catalytic Zn^{2+}- and Ca^{2+}-binding domain, and a C-terminal vitronectin-like domain with sequence similarities to a number of ECM structural proteins. The C-terminal domain is found in all MMPs except matrilysin. The gelatinases also have a fibronectin-like gelatin-binding sequence inserted into the catalytic domain. Gelatinase B has a further collagen-like insertion C-terminal in the catalytic domain. The MT-MMPs have a stretch of hydrophobic amino acids in their C-terminal domain which anchors them at the cell surface.

Inhibitors

The major natural MMP inhibitors are α2-macroglobulin, and a family of inhibitors that are specific for MMP, the metalloproteinase tissue inhibitors (TIMPs). TIMPs are produced by many cell types and four have been identified to date [8]. Two TIMPs have been fully characterized in terms of their inhibitory activity against MMP, TIMP-1 is a 30 kD glycoprotein and TIMP-2 a 28 kD unglycosylated protein. Their cellular distribution appears to be very similar, although TIMP-1 is usually found in larger amounts. The TIMPs act specifically against the active forms of MMPs, but TIMP-1 can also bind to progelatinase B, and TIMP-2 to progelatinase A.

Regulation

The regulation of MMPs is complex and occurs at different levels, the first one being gene expression [9], regulated at the level of transcription and mRNA stability. The promotor regions of the genes of stromelysin-1 and -2, of the fibroblast collagenase, of collagenase 3 and of gelatinase B all contain TATA elements and have activator protein (AP)-1 and Pg enhancer activity (PEA)-3 sites. These sites regulate the basal MMP levels and the inducibility of these genes by a variety of agents, including cytokines and growth factors. Transcription factors that recognize and transactivate these elements are proto-oncogenes, including *c-fos* and *c-jun* which transactivate through the AP-1 element, and *c-ets*, which recognizes the PEA-3 element. This is an oversimplification, since there are several examples in which one of these genes is selectively activated without an effect on the other. More recent data indicate that basal transcription, as well as transactivation by phorbol-myristate-acetate (PMA), cytokines, and growth factors, requires the specific interaction of AP-1 with other cis-acting elements and particularly PEA-3. On the other hand, the AP-1 site plays a dominant role in repression of MMPs by transforming growth factor (TGF)-β, retinoids and glucocorticoids, although some AP-1 independent mechanisms may also contribute. While the AP-1 site is involved in tissue-specific expression of MMPs, the presence of one or more AP-2 elements appears critical. Thus, the AP-1 site, alone, does not regulate transcription of MMPs. Rather, there is an essential interaction with other cis-acting sequences in the promoters and with certain transcription factors that bind to these sequences. In contrast to collagenase, stromelysin and gelatinase B, the promoter regions of gelatinase A and of neutrophil collagenase lack the TATA box and the AP-1 site.

Regulation at the post-transcriptional but pre-translational level has been reported as well; for example fibroblast collagenase mRNA stability can be increased by IL-1, or bronchial epithelial cell gelatinase B mRNA by lipopolysaccharide (LPS) [10].

Post-translational regulation occurs extracellularly, ultimately controlling the level of enzyme activity in terms of matrix destruction, namely activation of secreted pro-enzyme forms and their subsequent inhibition by TIMPs.

The stepwise process of physiological pro-MMP activation by loss of the pro-peptide is initiated by exogenous proteolytic cleavage in the case of the collagenases, stromelysins and gelatinase B. Plasmin is thought to be one of the most important *in vivo* physiological activators. Pro-gelatinase A and pro-collagenase-3 are unlike the other MMPs in that they differ in their mechanism of extracellular activation, which is a membrane-mediated process sensitive to metalloproteinase inhibitors. The membrane activators of pro-gelatinase A and pro-collagenase-3 have been identified recently as MT-MMPs [6]. In disease states, alternate pathways of activation may be involved, such as activation of pro-gelatinase B and neutrophil pro-collagenase by free oxygen radicals and by leukocyte elastase [11]. It has been demonstrated recently that fibroblast and neutrophil pro-collagenase, as well as pro-gelatinase B, can be activated by various bacterial proteinases, especially by *Pseudomonas aeruginosa* elastase.

TIMPs are important regulators of MMP activity. In many cell model systems, the ability of TIMPs to prevent matrix degradation has been demonstrated. In some cell culture conditions such as LPS-stimulated bronchial epithelial cells, it has been shown that TIMP levels rise but do not compensate for the much larger increase in MMPs.

Methodologica Issues

Given the potential role of MMPs, and especially gelatinases, in ARDS, several studies have been published addressing this issue. In order to understand the sometimes conflicting results obtained, some methodological issues need to be explained. Methods of studying gelatinases at the protein level can be divided into two groups: Immunological methods; and assays for gelatinase activity.

Immunoassay Methods

Immunoassay methods using specific antibodies, such as enzyme-linked immunosorbent assay (ELISA), can determine the concentration of gelatinase and TIMPs, but do not evaluate biological activity which reflects total proteinase activity (gelatinase A plus B) versus total anti-proteinase activity (presence in biological samples of specific and non-specific inhibitors, namely TIMPs and α2-macroglobulin). Moreover, immunoassay methods cannot differentiate latent and active forms of gelatinases, nor the degradation products of proteinases.

Gelatinase Activity

Gelatinase assay on radiolabeled substrate measures non-complexed (free) gelatinase activity. Thus, activity found in a biological sample indicates an excess in active gelatinase(s) compared to antiproteinase(s). Aminophenylmercuric acid (APMA) is a mercurial compound that activates pro-gelatinase; therefore, radiolabeled assay in the presence of APMA evaluates the balance between total gelatinase activity (i.e., latent and active forms) and antiproteinase(s).

By contrast, zymography, because of the presence of sodium dodecyl sulfate (SDS-PAGE) during the electrophoresis, allows the determination and quantification of latent and free or complexed activated gelatinase(s) which are present in the biological sample. Samples are subjected to electrophoresis on polyacrylamide gels containing gelatin (which is degraded by gelatinases), in the presence of SDS-PAGE, under non-reducing conditions. Zones of enzymatic activity are indicated by negative staining; areas of proteolysis appear as clear bands against a blue background. Thus, different forms of gelatinases (gelatinase A and B, pro- and active forms) can be visualized, and molecular mass can be determined. Activities in the gel slabs can be quantified using image analysis to quantify both the surface area and the intensity of lysis bands, results are expressed as arbitrary units. It must be stressed that an activity demonstrated by zymography in a biological sample does not imply an imbalance in favour of gelatinase, because SDS artificially reveals activities even in the presence of pro-forms or in inhibitor excess.

Zymography *in situ*: the principle of this method is similar to the former, except that the gelatinase substrate, namely gelatin (photographic film) is covered by a frozen tissue section. Gelatinase activity (thus, free activity implying an excess of proteinase) appears as dark lysis spots.

Gelatinase and Permeability

Gelatinases are believed to be important for many of the normal processes requiring basement membrane turn over. In addition, it could be hypothesized that overexpression of these gelatinases could be involved in pathologic processes characterized by basement membrane injury. Indeed, gelatinase B has been implicated in blood-brain barrier injury, in changes in glomerular capillary permeability, and in TNF-α-induced increased microvascular endothelial permeability [12].

Gelatinases and Acute Lung Injury

Recent studies conducted in experimental settings and in humans suffering from ARDS suggest the involvement of these gelatinases in the alveolar capillary wall lesions observed during acute lung injury (ALI) (Table 2).

Results from our laboratory [13] first stressed this possible involvement as gelatinases A and B were found to be increased in bronchoalveolar lavage (BAL) fluid of guinea pigs challenged intratracheally by endotoxin. Pardo and colleagues [14], recently demonstrated increased expression of gelatinases in rat lung exposed to 100% oxygen, associated with gelatinolytic activity in frozen sections by *in situ* zymography of oxygen-exposed lungs but not in normal lungs. Interestingly, gelatinase A mRNA was diffusely distributed in the hyperoxic lungs whereas a more focal pattern was observed with the gelatinase B transcript, and expression of gelatinase A mRNA putatively involved type II alveolar epithelial cells [14].

Table 2. Gelatinases and ARDS

Authors	Study Design	Methodology	Main Results: injured-lung
Mulligan [17]	Rats: Immune complex Alveolar installation of TIMP-2	Index of lung injury (permeability, hemorrhage) Alveolar PMN influx (MPO content)	Decreased lung injury, modest decrease in PMN influx with TIMP-2
d'Ortho [13]	Guinea pigs: Endotoxin instillation Gelatinase evaluation	BAL fluid: Zymography, free activity	Increase in gelatinase A, presence of gelatinase B and increased free gelatinase activity
Pardo [14]	Rats: Hyperoxia Gelatinase evaluation	Lung tissue: Immuno-localization, mRNA hybridation, zymography *in situ* BAL fluid: Zymography, activity (with APMA)	Increased expression of gelatinase A and B and respective mRNA. Gelatinolytic activity *in situ*
Ricou [19]	Serial BAL in ARDS patients Balance gelatinase B/TIMP-1	Gelatinase B and TIMP-1: ELISA	Gelatinase B increased in BAL fluid, gelatinase B/TIMP ratio in BAL fluid remained elevated in late phases of prolonged ARDS: Involvement in fibrosis suspected
Torii [15]	BAL fluids of ARDS patients vs normal	Gelatinases A and B, TIMP-1 and TIMP-2: EIA (measurement of collagen 7S and laminin)	Increase in gelatinase A, B and TIMP-1 Correlation between gelatinases and markers of basement membrane disruption
Delclaux [4]	BAL fluids of ARDS patients vs ventilated patients	Gelatinases A and B: Zymography of BAL fluids and isolated-inflammatory cell supernatants Free gelatinolytic activity	Increase in gelatinase A, activated gelatinase A specific for ARDS patients, no free activity, correlation between sum of activated gelatinases and albumin
Foda [18]	Rats: Oxidant Synthetic MMP-inhibitor	Isolated perfused lung: wet/dry weight ratio Gelatinases A and B: BAL fluid zymography	Improvement of lung injury Prevention of activation of gelatinase A
Kossodo [20]	ARDS patients vs at risk patients	Gelatinases A and B: Zymography of BAL fluid	Increase in gelatinase A and B
Pugin [21]	ARDS patients vs hydrostatic edema patients	Gelatinases A and B: Zymography of BAL fluid	Increase in gelatinase B

BAL: bronchoalveolar lavage; PMN: polymorphonuclear neutrophil; MPO: myeloperoxidase

Two recent studies [4, 15] demonstrate the involvement of both gelatinase A and B in ARDS pathogenesis. These studies demonstrate the presence of gelatinases in air-spaces during ARDS, and suggest (statistical correlations) their involvement in base-ment membrane disruption [15] and permeability increase [4]. Interestingly, the in-volvement of the two gelatinases is stressed, thus inflammatory cells and non-inflam-matory cells seem to be involved in the injury process. Furthermore, we have recently demonstrated the production of gelatinases and TIMP-2 by alveolar epithelial cells *in vitro* [16].

Two experimental studies [17, 18] seem to demonstrate the causality of MMPs in this phenomenon, with alveolar instillation of TIMP-2 being beneficial during im-mune complex acute lung injury in rats [17], and a specific synthetic inhibitor of MMPs having a beneficial effect in a model of acute lung injury [18]. Nevertheless, in the former study, the beneficial effect seemed to be partially due to the inhibition of neutrophil influx in alveoli which is logical since gelatinase B is involved in neutro-phil migration across the basement membrane [11]. In the latter study (unpublished data), conducted in isolated ventilated perfused lungs, the inhibitor attenuated the increase in the wet/dry ratio (an index of pulmonary edema) and prevented the activation of gelatinase A (thus demonstrating the involvement of MMPs in gelati-nase A activation). However, MMPs are involved in pro-TNF-α activation which in turn increases gelatinase synthesis. Thus, the beneficial effect observed in this model could be due to either inhibition of gelatinase activity and/or inhibition of TNF-α pro-cessing [7].

In summary, evidence for a direct involvement of gelatinases in the increased permeability occurring during ALI is still lacking. Moreover, their are several theoret-ical arguments against a major involvement of gelatinases during ALI:

2) Alveolar capillary wall permeability is controlled by alveolar epithelial cells and hence their tight junctions; permeability of these junctions is highly regulated, and has been extensively investigated;

2) The kinetics of edema constitution seem to argue against a degradation phenom-enon. Indeed, in experimental models, lung edema appears early (within 3 hours) after the onset of injury, a fact that could more probably be related to paracellular permeability involvement.

Conclusion

The participation of alveolar epithelial cells in the regulation of alveolar capillary wall permeability is an exciting field of research. Extracellular matrix degradation products are found in the air spaces during the course of ARDS, related to the initial injury pro-cess and/or to the remodeling phenomenon occuring later. Due to the heavy alveolar neutrophil influx, leukocyte elastase was initially thought to be involved in this degra-dation process. However, studies conducted in the eighties yielded conflicting results. Moreover, there is some evidence in the literature arguing against a major role of the PMN in the injury process. Thus, the possible participation of MMPs secreted either by inflammatory (alveolar macrophages and PMNs and/or non-inflammatory (endothe-lial and epithelial cells, fibroblasts) cells, has been the subject of recent studies. From these investigations, it is apparent that gelatinases A and B, which are able to degrade all basement membrane components, are produced locally. Statistical correlations sup-port the hypothesis of the involvement of gelatinases in the degradation process lead-ing to increased permeability. Experimental studies utilizing natural or synthetic in-hibitors provide further arguments for a causal relationship.

References

1. Wangensteen OD, Wittmers LE, Johnson JA (1969) Permeability of the mammalian blood-gas barrier and its components. Am J Physiol 216:719–727
2. Kondoh Y, Taniguchi H, Taki F, Tagaki K, Satake T (1992) 7S collagen in bronchoalveolar lavage fluid of patients with adult respiratory distress syndrome. Chest 101:1091–1094
3. Pittet JF, Mackersie RC, Martin TR, Matthay MA (1997) Biological markers of acute lung injury: Prognostic and pathogenetic significance. Am J Respir Crit Care Med 155:1187–1205
4. Delclaux C, d'Ortho MP, Delacourt C, et al (1997) Gelatinases in epithelial lining fluid of patients with adult respiratory distress syndrome. Am J Physiol 272:L442–L451
5. Delclaux C, Rezaiguia-Delclaux S, Delacourt C, Brun-Buisson C, Lafuma C, Harf A (1997) Alveolar neutrophils in endotoxin-induced and bacteria-induced acute lung injury in rats. Am J Physiol 273:L104–L112
6. Sato H, Takino T, Okada Y, et al (1994) A matrix metalloproteinase expressed on the surface of invasive tumour cells. Nature 370:61–65
7. Gearing AJH, Beckett P, Christodoulou M, et al (1994) Processing of tumor necrosis factor-α precursor by metalloproteinases. Nature 370:555–557
8. Apte SS, Olsen BR, Murphy G (1995) The gene structure of tissue inhibitor of metalloproteinases (TIMP)-3 and its inhibitory activities define the distinct TIMP gene family. J Biol Chem 270:14313–14318
9. Benbow U, Brinckerhoff CE (1997) The AP-1 site and MMP gene regulation: what is all the fuss about? Matrix Biol 15:519–526
10. Yao PM, Buhler JM, d'Ortho MP, et al (1996) Expression of matrix metalloproteinase gelatinases A and B by cultured epithelial cells from human bronchial explants. J Biol Chem 271:15580–15589
11. Delclaux C, Delacourt C, d'Ortho MP, Boyer V, Lafuma C, Harf A (1996) Role of gelatinase B and elastase in human polymorphonuclear neutrophil migration across basement membrane. Am J Respir Cell Mol Biol 14:288–295
12. Partridge CA, Jeffrey JJ, Malik AB (1993) A 96-kDa gelatinase induced by TNF-α contributes to increased microvascular endothelial permeability. Am J Physiol 265:L438–L447
13. d'Ortho MP, Jarreau PH, Delacourt C et al (1994) Matrix metalloproteinase and elastase activities in LPS-induced acute lung injury in guinea pigs. Am J Physiol 266:L209–L216
14. Pardo A, Selman M, Ridge K, Barrios R, Sznajder JI (1996) Increased expression of gelatinases and collagenase in rat lungs exposed to 100% oxygen. Am J Respir Crit Care Med 154:1067–1075
15. Torii K, Iida KI, Miyazaki Y, et al (1997) Higher concentrations of matrix metalloproteinases in bronchoalveolar lavage fluid of patients with adult respiratory distress syndrome. Am J Respir Crit Care Med 155:43–46
16. d'Ortho MP, Clerici C, Yao PM, et al (1997) Alveolar epithelial cells in vitro produce gelatinases and tissue inhibitor of matrix metalloproteinase-2. Am J Physiol 273:L663–L675
17. Mulligan MS, Desrochers PE, Chinnaiyan AM, et al (1993) In vivo suppression of immune complex-induced alveolitis by secretory leukoproteinase inhibitor and tissue inhibitor of metalloproteinases 2. Proc Natl Acad Sci USA 90:11523–11527
18. Foda HD, Feldman J, George S, et al (1997) The synthetic matrix metalloproteinase (MMP) inhibitor BB-3031 attenuates oxidant-induced acute lung injury in rats. Am J Respir Crit Care Med 155:A652 (Abst)
19. Ricou B, Nicod L, Lacraz S, Welgus HG, Suter PM, Dayer JM (1996) Matrix metalloproteinases and TIMP in acute respiratory distress syndrome. Am J Respir Crit Care Med 154:346–352
20. Kossodo S, Gasche Y, Ricou B et al (1997) Do BAL fluid levels of metalloproteinases predict the development of ARDS? Am J Respir Crit Care Med 155:A90 (Abst)
21. Pugin J, Verghese G, Widmer MC, Matthay MA (1997) High levels of proinflammatory activity, IL-8, and gelatinase B in pulmonary edema fluid from patients in the early phase of ARDS. Am J Respir Crit Care Med 155:A390 (Abst)

Cardiocirculatory Alterations

Molecular Mechanisms of Action of Nitric Oxide in Heart Muscle

J. L. Balligand

Introduction

A growing body of evidence supports the functional role of nitric oxide (NO) in regulating cardiac function [1, 2]. Two constitutively expressed calcium-sensitive nitric oxide synthase (NOS) isoforms (neuronal isoform, or nNOS and endothelial isoform, or eNOS) and one inducible, calcium insensitive isoform (iNOS) catalyze the oxygen- and nicotinamide adenine dinucleotide phosphate (NADPH)-dependent oxidation of the cationic amino acid L-arginine with its subsequent conversion to L-citrulline and the production of NO. Numerous reports have recently described the expression of the three different isoforms of NOS in many cell types and tissues beyond the neurons, endothelial cells or monocytes where they were initially characterized.

There is now unequivocal evidence of the constitutive expression of eNOS in microvascular endothelial cells and myocytes comprising ventricular muscle from several animal species, including man [3, 4]. In addition, virtually all cells types within heart muscle express iNOS in response to exposure to inflammatory mediators, including cytokines [4]. NO produced endogenously by the constitutive or the inducible isoform has been shown to modulate cardiac contraction in response to autonomic stimuli in a variety of experimental preparations *in vitro* and also in animals and humans *in vivo* [1, 2]. Specifically, NO attenuates the positive inotropic effect of β1- and β2-adrenergic stimulation in ventricular myocytes isolated from adult rat hearts [5, 6], *in situ* dog hearts [7] and in patients with left ventricular dysfunction [8]. Large concentrations of NO produced by iNOS in models of sepsis also contribute to the blunting of the adrenergic responsiveness and contractile dysfunction of a variety of cardiac preparations [1, 2]. In addition, eNOS was shown to mediate the muscarinic cholinergic attenuation of adrenergically-increased L-type calcium current and contraction (the classical "accentuated antagonism") in atrial, atrioventricular and ventricular myocytes from rats and rabbits [3, 9, 10]. Finally, NO produced by the constitutively expressed eNOS in endocardial and microvascular endothelial cells acts paracrinally to increase diastolic relaxation and decrease oxygen consumption of adjacent myocytes in isolated guinea pig-hearts and dog hearts *in vivo*, respectively [11, 12, 13].

In view of these multiple functional effects both at the whole organ and single cell levels, it is likely that NO acts on a variety of intracellular effectors. To ensure a coordinated physiological effect, however, the intracellular action of NO must be tightly regulated. According to recent data on the subcellular localization of both constitutive and inducible isoforms of NOS in endothelial cells and cardiac myocytes [14], a plausible way of regulating NO's action would be through the targeting of each NOS isoform to specific effectors co-localized in the same subcellular compartment. In addition, NOS activity can be regulated through specific protein-protein interactions, e.g., with Ca^{++}/calmodulin [15] in specific cellular microdomains. The object of the following sections is to review the molecular targets of NO action that are relevant to cardiovascular biology and that probably mediate NO's effect on cardiac contractility.

Chemistry of Nitric Oxide Reactivity

Despite their apparently simple chemical nature, the rich redox chemistry of nitrogen oxides allows a complex interaction with molecular targets to mediate their physiologic effects, including oxidation events and covalent modification of proteins.

The presence of an unpaired electron after the combination of one atom of nitrogen with one atom of oxygen defines NO as a radical. Even though NO, as most radicals, has traditionally been regarded as highly reactive, this is not universally true in biological systems where pH and redox conditions greatly influence the reactivity of NO radical as well as its adducts. Biologically relevant chemicals reacting with NO radical include oxygen, superoxide anion and transition metals. Oxygen converts NO to nitrogen dioxide (NO_2) in a reaction which, in the aqueous phase, is slow, with a half-life of several hours at concentrations that exist in cells (equation 1) [16]

$$2 NO + O_2 \rightarrow 2 NO_2 \tag{1}$$

NO_2 subsequently reacts with water to give a mixture of nitrite and nitrate where nitrite is the predominant form in oxygenated water (equation 2)

$$2 NO_2 + H_2O \rightarrow HNO_2 + HNO_3 \tag{2}$$

This is the rationale for using the colorimetric assay for nitrite (known as the Griess test) as a measure of NO produced in biological systems.

S-Nitrosation Reactions

NO_2, in addition to the products of the reaction of NO with superoxide (O_2^-) and transition metals, supports additional nitrosative reactions at nucleophilic centers of acceptor molecules. Given their prevalence in the biological milieu, great attention has been given to thiols as potential nucleophils supporting the formation of S-nitrisothiols. Accordingly, naturally occuring endothelium-derived relaxing factor (EDRF) has been suggested to be a nitrosothiol, namely S-nitrocysteine, but a recent comparison of their physiological properties has shown that they are significantly different [17].

Nitrosothiols are found in human plasma, mainly as products of nitrosation of human serum albumin [18]. Even though nitrosothiols can be formed from each of the products of the reaction of NO with oxygen, metals and superoxide, as mentioned above, their biosynthesis under biologically relevant conditions is still a matter of controversy. They are not formed by the reaction of NO radical with thiol at a pH around 7. Nitrosothiols are produced from the reaction of NO_2 with thiols [19], but since the oxidation of NO_2 by oxygen is slow in aqueous solutions, this is an unlikely biosynthetic pathway. By contrast, the oxidized form of NO, the nitrosonium ion (NO^+) can support a number of electrophilic reactions, including nitrosothiol formation. However, highly reactive nitrosonium is a transient species in aqueous solution at pH 7 and its reaction with any nucleophile other than water is unlikely (equation 3):

$$NO^+ + H_2O \rightarrow HNO_2 + H^+ \tag{3}$$

Nitrosonium is the nitrosating species supporting nitrosothiol formation from nitrous acid in strongly acidic solution, where the reverse of equation 3 dominates, followed by equation 4:

$$HNO_2 + H^+ \rightarrow H_2O + NO^+$$

$$NO^+ + RSH \rightarrow RSNO + H^+ \tag{4}$$

Reaction (4) can also occur at much lower acidity and, more significantly from a biological point of view, the nitrosonium moiety can be transferred from a nitrosothiol to a second thiol or to another nucleophil [20, 21], through a process called transnitrosation (equation 5):

$$R_1SNO + R_2S^- \rightarrow R_1S^- + R_2SNO \tag{5}$$

In this way, although free nitrosonium cannot exist in a cell, nitrosothiols can be viewed as biological sources of nitrosonium for subsequent thiol nitrosation. This places nitrosothiols at a key point in NO signaling either as target sites for NO action, or as intermediate compounds supporting additional nitrosation of target molecules.

Functional Consequences of Protein Nitrosation

Several mechanisms can explain the regulation of protein function by S-nitrosylation, some of which have been examined in detail in proteins relevant to cardiovascular signaling. One such mechanism could be the alteration of intramolecular hydrogen bonding or electrostatic interactions by the NO group to produce structural alterations promoting the interaction of an enzyme with its substrate. Such a mechanism could be the basis of S-nitrosylation-induced activation of tissue plasminogen activator [19] or activation of pertussis toxin-sensitive G proteins and p21[ras] through an increase in the rate-limiting guanosine diphosphate (GDP) release [22]. Calcium-dependent potassium channels also contain a critical thiol residue probably mediating some of the NO-responsive control of blood vessel tone [23]. The observation that the NO group elicits an effect distinct from that of other thiol alkylators, however, suggests another mechanism than simple S-nitrosylation for the modulation of channel function, probably by the capacity of thiol nitrosylation to accelerate disulfide formation with another intramolecular thiol in the immediate vicinity of the molecule [21].

S-Nitrosation and Enzyme Inhibition

S-nitrosylation of critical cysteine residues at active sites of different classes of enzymes also induces inhibition of their enzymatic activities. Among the list of enzymes known to be inhibited by NO in this manner, glyceraldehyde-3-phosphate dehydrogenase (GAPDH) has recently received particular attention. S-nitrosylation of cysteine at position 149 (Cys[149]) is responsible for reversible inhibition of the enzyme [24]. In addition, transnitrosation from the active site nitrosothiol to the reduced nicotinamide ring of the enzyme co-factor NADH, appears to facilitate protein thiolate attack on the enzyme-bound co-factor, resulting in the attachment of the intact NADH molecule and irreversible enzyme inactivation [24]. This mechanism is consistent with the previous demonstration that both the ribose and nicotinamide moieties of NAD are incorporated by the enzyme [25], as opposed to simple adenosine diphosphate (ADP)-ribosylation. In this dual mechanism, S-nitrosylation may serve to protect GAPDH from oxidant inactivation in the setting of cytokine overproduction, and to regulate glycolysis. NADH attachment, by contrast, is more likely to be a pathophysiologic event associated with inhibition of gluconeogenesis [24].

S-nitrosylation may control the function of other proteins, including neutrophil NADPH oxidase. Inhibition of this enzyme by NO may serve to diminish injury at inflammatory sites by limiting superoxide anion production [26].

NO and Peroxynitrite

In the face of increased oxidant stress, such as muscle contraction or inflammatory reactions, NO chemistry may predominantly consist of nitrosative reactions with reactive oxygen intermediates (ROI), including super-oxide anion. The reaction of NO with superoxide yields peroxynitrite ($ONOO^-$), a powerful oxidant that in the presence of protons at physiological pH further decomposes to produce NO_2 and hydroxyl radicals (OH^-). This chain of reactions has been documented *in vivo* [27] and probably substantiates some of the cytotoxicity associated with NO and ROI, since hydroxyl radicals are known to be highly reactive and biologically destructive (equations 6 + 7):

$$NO + O_2^- \rightarrow ONOO^- \tag{6}$$

$$ONOO^- + H^+ \rightarrow NO_2 + OH^- \tag{7}$$

Peroxynitrite also oxidates protein thiols more effectively than other oxidants such as hydrogen peroxide (H_2O_2) [28].

The reactions described above may underly the dual role of NO, toxic or protective, in its interactions with reactive oxygen species. In circumstances where toxicity occurs predominantly from an excess of oxidant species, NO may limit damage by acting as a chain breaker "detoxifier" by focusing some of the oxidation reactions towards S-nitrosothiol formation, supported in part by the antioxidant glutathione. On the other hand, in biological systems where excessive NO production predominates, the reaction with oxygen species may be deleterious by promoting oxidative nitrosation reactions which destruct cellular functions by depletion of the endogenous thiol pool and exposure of other nucleophilic centers usually untouched under physiologic conditions, such as N-nitrosation of deoxyribonucleic acids (DNA) and nitration of tyrosine residues [29].

Eukaryotic cells submitted to an oxidant challenge also respond with up-regulation of specialized resistance genes such as manganese superoxide dismutase (SOD) [30], or glutathione S-transferase [31]. Expression of these genes is also a physiologic response to cytokines that induce the "high output" NOS [30], so that one could see the delayed expression of iNOS as an additional built-in regulatory mechanism to ensure that the natural defense network is in place within the NO producing cell when sustained NO production is invoked [21]. The formation of nitrosothiols may also be another way to channel NO production towards products which retain NO-like bioactivity but exhibit resistance to reactions with oxidants, including superoxide anion, leading to more toxic products [32].

NO and Iron

Another most significant property of NO in terms of its biological activity, is its reaction with iron in the centers of iron sulfur clusters and heme prosthetic groups which can lead to either a decline or an increase in protein activity. The irreversible destruction of the iron sulfer clusters by NO in the mitochondrial electron transport chain (complex I and complex II) which supports high energy phosphate metabolism, has been proposed as a mechanism of the cellular dysfunction following stimulation with inflammatory cytokines [33]. In the case of the tricarboxylic acid cycle enzyme, aconitase, the inactivating species seem to be superoxide anion and peroxynitrite instead of NO itself [34]. The inactivation of the iron sulfur center of cytosolic aconitase by NO adducts has also received much attention recently, given the role of this metal regulatory protein as the iron response element binding protein (IRE-BP). By promoting the release of iron, NO facilitates a thiol-dependent binding of apoaconitase to either the 5′ untranslated end of ferritin messenger ribonucleic acid (mRNA), or to the 3′ end of transferrin receptor mRNA, thereby implicating NO in the regulation of cellular iron homeostasis [35, 36].

NO and Heme Proteins

In contrast to the reaction of NO with iron sulfur clusters, which is irreversible, the reaction of NO with heme iron is a reversible process [37]; an essential requirement if NO is to act as a switch for the activity of several NO-responsive catalytic enzymes. When heme-containing proteins utilize the prosthetic group in catalysis, NO can inhibit enzyme activity. This is exemplified in the inhibition of cytochrome P450 enzymes [38] and NOS itself [39, 40]. Other heme proteins regulated by NO include myoglobin, hemoglobin, catalase, peroxidase, cytochrome C, and cyclooxygenase 1 and 2 [21, 41].

A prototypic enzyme which is reversibly activated by NO interaction with its heme prosthetic group is guanylyl cyclase (GC) which catalyzes the formation of cyclic guanosine monophosphate (cGMP) from guanosine triphosphate (GTP). The heme protein has been purified to homogeneity and its optical absorption spectrum is indicative of a 5-coordinate ferrous heme [42]. This is important in view of the fact that a major factor in heme-ligand coordination is the redox state of the heme iron. At physiological pH, ferric heme has a net unitary positive charge whereas ferrous heme is neutral and preferentially interacts with neutral ligands. The ligand strength with ferrous heme is also higher for NO than for carbon monoxide (CO) or oxygen [43]. That NO activates GC activity via direct interaction with the heme moiety was advanced by two groups [44, 45]. The catalytic activity of GC is increased by 10 to 100-fold in the presence of NO or NO-releasing compounds [46]. NO's interaction with heme may not be the only mechanism, however. Reports of marked activation of GC by glutathione under anaerobic conditions [47], for example, underscore the likely existence of additional redox modulatory sites.

Intracellular Pathways Activated by Cyclic GMP

The above considerations on the chemical activity of NO allow us to distinguish between direct intracellular reactions of NO involving covalent modifications of target proteins and indirect actions mediated by increases in intracellular cyclic GMP secondary to NO's activation of the soluble isoform of GC. Evidence provided from studies of several cell types have identified four main intracellular receptor proteins for cGMP, the relative importance of which will be reviewed in the specific context of the cardiovascular system. These include cGMP kinases, cGMP-regulated ion channels, and cGMP-binding cyclic nucleotide phosphodiesterases (PDE), to which ADP-ribosyl cyclase has recently been added following evidence extending its role in sea-urchin eggs to cGMP-dependent signaling pathways in eukaryotic cells.

Cyclic GMP Dependent Protein Kinases

Cyclic GMP kinases are serine/threonine protein kinases of which two general classes exist in eukaryotic cells. Type I cGMP kinase is a dimer of identical subunits each with a mass of approximately 71 kDa, which is widely distributed and isolated from the soluble fractions of tissues where it has been found. Two closely related isoforms (type Iα and Iβ) have been isolated from vascular tissue and are probably derived from alternatively spliced mRNAs [48, 49, 50].

Type II cGMP kinase is probably the product of a different gene and has been identified from intestinal epithelial cells [51]. Cyclic GMP kinases are selectively activated by low concentrations of cGMP *in vitro* (K_a: 0.05 to 1 μM), whereas higher concentrations of cyclic adenosine monophosphate (cAMP) are required to activate the enzyme *in vitro* (K_a: 5 to 10 μM). 8-substituted cyclic nucleotide analogs of cGMP (e.g 8-bromo-cyclic GMP) are more potent activators of the enzyme than the native nucleotide, especially for type Iα [49]. They do not, however, interact with the allosteric binding sites for cGMP on cGMP-regulated PDE, which is an important consideration for the interpretation of the functional effect of these analogs in several experimental settings.

The target proteins phosphorylated by cGMP kinases are also substrates for other protein kinases, including cAMP kinase [52, 53]. This may be explained in part by the fact that the canonical phosphorylation site for cAMP kinase also serves as a recognition motif for cGMP kinase [54]. It seems likely, however, that specificity determinants exist for cGMP kinase, such as phenylalanine residues in the COOH-terminal end of phosphorylated residues [55], or the stereochemistry of the phosphorylatable residue [56].

Perhaps the most thoroughly studied signaling events downstream from cGMP kinase are the regulation of intracellular calcium levels and the control of the contractile tone in vascular smooth muscle. Even though most of the evidence indicates that a reduction in intracellular free calcium levels is at least one of the mechanisms for cGMP-induced relaxation, a lot of uncertainty remains as to the exact mechanism of action for cGMP kinase. Putative target effectors in smooth muscle cells include calcium pumping ATPase at the plasma membrane or in the sarcoplasmic reticulum, the latter being activated through cGMP kinase-dependent phosphorylation of the regulatory protein phospholamban [57]. The latter mechanism may also be relevant in the regulation of intracellular calcium transients in cardiac muscle, since phosphorylation of phospholamban in response to β-agonists and elevation in cAMP is well known to mediate the sequestration of calcium into the sarcoplasmic reticulum and the shortening of systole [58]. Since the site of the phosphorylation of phospholamban by cGMP kinase is the same as for cAMP kinase, at least in aortic smooth muscle cells, this raises the question of how a single cell discriminates between the two signaling pathways. Potential mechanisms may include either additional specificity determinants for cGMP kinase, as mentioned above, or specific targeting of cGMP kinase co-localized with its substrate. The latter possibility is supported by the finding that in aortic smooth muscle cells, cGMP kinase is found associated with the sarcoplasmic reticulum, especially that in the perinuclear region of cells [59]. This area is also rich in intermediate filaments and other components of the cytoskeleton and it is possible that intracellular organelles such as the sarcoplasmic reticulum and cGMP kinase are bound to the cytoskeleton close to each other, in order to localize cGMP kinase near substrates. Considering that cGMP kinase is not an abundant protein, at least in heart muscle, and the affinities of substrates for protein kinases are not remarkable (micromolar in most cases), the co-localization mechanism would ensure that the appropriate signal, such as NO production, will lead to rapid and efficient protein phosphorylation by cGMP.

The same co-localization mechanism may underly some of the known effects of cGMP kinase on the phosphorylation state and function of membrane associated ion channels, many of which also have consensus cAMP kinase phosphorylation sequences. Cyclic GMP kinase-regulated ion channels may include calcium-activated potassium channels, which have been shown to be stimulated by NO in smooth muscle [60] or voltage operated calcium channels in heart myocytes [61]. In the latter, the involvement of cGMP kinase was demonstrated through perfusion of patch-clamped myocytes with a 65kDa catalytically active fragment of cGMP kinase, that was able to reverse the calcium current elevated by cAMP or its non-hydrolyzable analog, 8-Bromo-cAMP. These experiments did not clarify whether cGMP kinase affects I_{Ca} by directly phosphorylating the Ca^+ channel or some other regulatory proteins [61]. It should also be emphasized that although cGMP kinase has been shown to phosphorylate the α_1, and β subunits of skeletal muscle Ca^+ channels *in vitro* [53], experiments must clearly be extended to the cardiac Ca^+ channel and to more intact cell analyses in the future.

Cyclic GMP-Gated Ion Channels

Evidence for the occurrence of ion channels gated directly by cGMP was first provided by the study of retinal photoreceptors. The role for cGMP in mediating changes in the membrane polarity responsible for visual transduction in rod outer segments in the early eighties, was subsequently substantiated by the identification of a cation channel gated by the cyclic nucleotide [62]. Of note, there is a significant (30 to 50%) amount of homology between the cGMP-binding domain of the rod outer segment cation channel and the cGMP binding domain of cGMP kinase. The channel differs, though, by an unusually low binding affinity for the cyclic nucleotide, which probably plays a critical role in phototransduction since cGMP rapidly dissociates from the receptor enabling the hydrolysis of cGMP by the well-described transducin-cGMP PDE to induce rapid changes in membrane conductance [63].

Even though the distribution of the photoreceptor-type cGMP-gated cation channel is limited, other types of cGMP-binding ion channels have subsequently been identified. A similar channel protein has been cloned from olfactory epithelium and shown to have significant homology with the photoreceptor channel [64]. The renal epithelium also contains an amiloride-sensitive cation channel whose activity is inhibited by cGMP [65]. However, no ion channel gated directly by cGMP has been identified to date in heart myocytes of any species.

Cyclic GMP-Modulated Phosphodiesterases

Since the initial purification and characterization of PDE activity in the early sixties, accumulating evidence documenting the existence of a large number of different PDE isoenzymes widely distributed among various tissues stimulated interest in these molecules as regulators of intracellular cyclic nucleotide concentrations.

At least seven different families of cyclic nucleotide PDE are currently known to exist in mammalian tissue. Each family contains one, or more than one, gene product. Within each family, the PDEs are 65 percent or more homologous with each other when compared at the amino acid level. The similarity drops to less than 40 percent when the PDEs from different families are compared. All PDEs, however, contain a core of 217 highly conserved amino acids [66] which is probably part of the catalytic domain of the enzyme. Molecular characterization of PDEs has led to the realization that most PDE genes have more than one alternatively spliced mRNA transcribed from them. Furthermore, the alternative splicing appears to be highly cell-specific, which provides a mechanism for the selective expression of different isozymes in individual tissues and cell types. This probably explains the wide heterogeneity of kinetic data on PDE activity described in the early literature. On the other hand, characterization of the differential regulation between cell types is likely to unveil new important molecular mechanisms for the regulation of intracellular levels of cAMP and cGMP.

Among the different members of the seven families, members of PDE 1, 2, and 3 have clearly been shown to be expressed in heart tissue. Regulation of calcium/calmodul-independent PDE (PDE 1) and of the overall cyclic nucleotide concentration in a cell is expected to be complex because of competition for the active calcium/calmodulin co-factor between the PDEs and other calmodulin-binding proteins, some of which may, in turn, modulate cyclic nucleotide levels on their own. Examples include calcium/calmodulin activation of calcium/calmodulin-dependent protein phosphatases and of course, calcium/calmodulin-dependent constitutive NOS. Therefore, differences in the affinity for calmodulin of these enzymes, as well as the relative affinities for calmodulin of the PDEs versus the synthases will be determining factors in the overall cyclic nucleotide phenotype of the cell. One would, therefore, expect that the amplitude and the duration of the cAMP or cGMP signal will be directly determined by the specific isozymes of calmodulin-dependent phosphatase and PDE which are expressed, in addition to the isoform of NOS present within the same cell type expressing these proteins.

A distinctive feature of PDE2 members is that they contain a non-catalytic binding site with high specificity for cGMP. When cGMP binds to this site, it increases the affinity of the catalytic site by allosteric interaction. PDE2s, therefore, are known as cGMP-stimulated PDEs. The activity increase is transient, however, unless GMP synthesis is constantly elevated, since the enzyme hydrolyzes both cAMP and cGMP. Such a situation may be realized when iNOS is expressed within the same cell. In general, PDE2 isoforms have been found to be expressed in tissues in which the effects of cGMP are opposite to those of cAMP. The expression of an isoform of PDE2 in heart myocytes from several species, including the rat [67], is probably an illustration of this principle. Cyclic AMP is an important mediator of the positive inotropic effect of β-adrenergic agonist stimulation in cardiac myocytes, where the cyclic nucleotide increases the activity of cardiac L-type calcium channels through cAMP-dependent phosphorylation. The involvement of PDE activity in mediating the opposite effect of cGMP to decrease calcium channel activity was first demonstrated in cardiac myocytes from the frog [68]. The situation in the mammalian heart is much more complex, since multiple mechanisms for the effect of cGMP on calcium channel activity appear to operate [61, 69]. Some of the conflicting results in the literature may be explained by the different level of expression of various isoforms of PDE among species and even among different regions of the heart.

In platelets, PDE3A can be phosphorylated by cAMP-dependent protein kinase which activates the PDE [70]. Physiologically, this is likely to be an important part of the tachyphylaxis that occurs in response to continuous adenylyl cyclase stimulation in platelets and probably also in other tissues expressing this PDE isoform. In these instances, PDE3A appears as a key modulator not only of the amplitude of the cAMP signal but also of its duration. In the heart, inhibition of PDE3A by cGMP would initially potentiate the increase in intracellular cAMP, thereby producing a positive inotropic effect probably through an increase in L-type calcium current. In this regard, the effect of cGMP would be identical to those of the many selective inhibitors of PDE3 that have been (and still are being) used in clinical trials as cardiac inotropic agents [71]. The net result of cGMP increases in heart muscle cells, however, is more difficult to predict given the co-expression of both PDE2 and PDE3 isoforms in the same myocyte, at least in the rat species [67]. Factors probably concurring to produce either a potentiation or an attenuation of the cAMP effects in heart muscle cells include the relative differences in affinity and V_{max} for the same cyclic nucleotide between the two isoforms, and perhaps the localization of each isoform of PDE together with effector proteins for the cyclic nucleotide in the same subcellular compartment.

Cyclic GMP-Dependent Cyclic ADP-Ribose Signaling Pathway

The new messenger, cyclic ADP ribose (cADPR) was originally discovered in sea urchin eggs where it was shown to mobilize calcium from an intracellular store insensitive to inositol tris-phosphate (IP3) [72]. Even though the latter was known to be the messenger responsible for the opening of IP3 receptors, an analogous physiological regulator for the calcium release through the ryanodine receptor was not known. Recent evidence suggested that cADPR synthesized from βNAD^+ by the enzyme ADP ribosyl cyclase could activate the ryanodine receptor at least in reconstituted lipid bilayers [73, 74]. In addition, the level of cADPR in sea urchin eggs was shown to be regulated by cGMP [75], suggesting a link with the NOS pathway. Interestingly, studies on cardiac ryanodine receptors in planar lipid bilayers have shown that cADPR greatly increases the frequency of channel openings, while having no effect on type I ryanodine receptors of the skeletal muscle.

The messenger function of cADPR, therefore seems to be restricted to the cardiac-like type II receptors [74]. In a way similar to the co-agonist effect of IP3 and calcium in controlling calcium release by the IP3 receptor, cADPR potentiates the process of calcium-induced calcium release by sensitizing its target receptor to the stimulating action of calcium [76] (Fig. 1). Such a potentiating effect of NO-dependent cGMP and cADPR on calcium release from the intracellular stores might explain the ability of NO and cGMP to amplify gene transcription in neuronal cells induced by calcium-dependent signaling pathways such as the opening of voltage-operated calcium channels [77]. This amplification was apparent only if the two interacting pathways were activated within a narrow time window, suggesting that the cADPR control of calcium signaling may act in synergy with other calcium signaling pathways to generate complex calcium signals, such as calcium oscillations and calcium waves [78, 79], with very distinct spacial and temporal properties. In

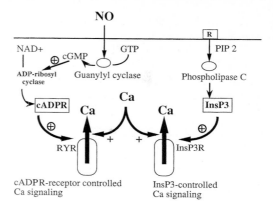

Fig. 1. Calcium-mobilizing second messengers. Two separate signaling pathways activate the ryanodine receptor (RYR) and the inositol triphosphate receptor (InsP₃R) respectively. cADPR, cyclic ADP ribose; NO, nitric oxide; PIP₂, phosphatidylinositol biphosphate

the context of a cardiac myocyte, the effect of cADPR in potentiating ryanodine receptor calcium release would have to be integrated with other known cGMP-dependent and GMP-independent effects of NO on other target proteins regulating calcium transients, including voltage operated calcium channels.

A second messenger role for cADPR requires that it mediates the intracellular actions of hormones or neurotransmitters in intact cells. This was recently shown by Galione's group who demonstrated that NO mobilizes calcium from intracellular stores via a pathway in part involving cGMP and leading to the activation of cADPR-sensitive calcium release mechanisms [80]. That a similar pathway is operative in intact cardiac myocytes with any functional effect on myocyte contractility is doubtful given the recently published negative evidence for the regulation of sarcoplasmic reticulum calcium release by cADPR in rat ventricular myocytes [81].

Potential Mechanisms by which NO Regulates Cardiac Function

In this last section we will review the evidence implicating any of the intracellular effectors reviewed above, in the functional effect of NO in modulating cardiac contractility (Fig. 2).

Cyclic GMP-Mediated Mechanisms

NO and cGMP have been shown to decrease cardiac myocyte L-type calcium current and contraction through the activation of phosphodiesterase type 2 in several species. The PDE stimulated by cGMP decreases intracellular AMP levels and the activity of protein kinase A, resulting in alterations in the phosphorylation state of several target proteins, including the alpha subunit of the L-type calcium channel. The involvement of PDE2 in the action of NO or cGMP to decrease myocyte contraction and/or L-type calcium current has been demonstrated in sino-atrial and atrio-ventricular myocytes from the rabbit [9], ventricular myocytes from the rat (all via muscarinic cholinergic activation of endogenous eNOS) [3, 10], and atrial myocytes

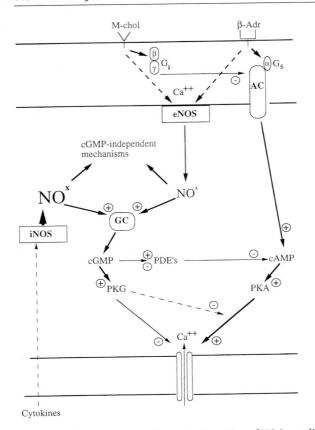

Fig. 2. Second-messenger pathways for the action of NO in cardiac myocytes. β-adrenergic receptor stimulation produces a positive inotropic effect through G protein α-s-coupled activation of adenylyl cyclase, leading to increases in intracellular cAMP levels. Subsequent activation of cAMP-dependent protein kinase leads to downstream phosphorylation of target proteins, including those on the L-type calcium channel. The resultant increased influx of Ca^{++} activates intracellular calcium-induced calcium release and enhances myofibrillar contraction. iNOS gene transcription and protein expression is induced in cardiac myocytes on exposure to cytokines or other inflammatory mediators. eNOS activation in cardiac myocytes occurs in response to both musarinic cholinergic or adrenergic receptor stimulation through unidentified mechanisms. NO produced by either eNOS or iNOS activates the soluble isoform of guanylyl cyclase to increase intracellular levels of cGMP, which oppose the positive inotropic effects of cAMP through (1) activation of the cGMP-stimulated phosphodiesterase (PDE type 2) to enhance the breakdown of cAMP (conversely cGMP may potentiate the effects of cAMP through inhibition of PDE (type 3); (2) activation of the cGMP-dependent protein kinase (PKG), leading to down-regulation of the L-type calcium current via either direct phosphorylation of the channel or phosphorylation of an intermediate protein opposing the effect of PKA; PKG also decreases myofilament sensitivity to calcium, thereby promoting relaxation (not shown). In addition, NO may affect myocyte contraction through mechanisms independent of cGMP elevation. Aside from stimulation of NO production, muscarinic cholinergic receptor stimulation results in G_i β,γ-mediated inhibition of adenylyl cyclase and activation of distinct K^+ channels (not shown), all of which variably participate in the parasympathetic inhibition of cardiac myocyte function depending on the species and region of heart. AC indicates adenylyl cyclase; M-chol, muscarinic cholinergic receptor; β-Adr, β-adrenergic receptor; GC, guanylyl cyclase; PDE, phosphodiesterase; PKG, cGMP-dependent protein kinase; and PKA, cAMP-dependent protein kinase

from the frog (the latter via perfusion with micromolar concentrations of the NO donor SIN-1) [69]. In all the studies mentioned above, an effect of NO was only observed when intracellular cAMP levels had been increased. NO had little, if any, effect on basal contractile state. NO was also unable to antagonize the effect of non-hydrolyzable analogs of cAMP or of cAMP in the presence of a PDE inhibitor, supporting the involvement of a cGMP-stimulated PDE.

However, there is considerable variability in the effect of NO according to the species used and the concentration of NO applied. For example, low concentrations of the NO donors SIN-1 (<100 nmol/l) and nitrosothiol-s-nitroso-N-acetyl-penicillamine (SNAP) (<100 mmol/l) potentiate the increases in cardiac myocyte contraction and L-type calcium current in frog atrial and adult rat ventricular myocytes [69, 82]. In these experiments, the effect of exogenous NO donors was mainly to accentuate the stimulatory effect of isoproterenol or cAMP through the inhibition of a cGMP-inhibited cAMP PDE (type 3PDE). Similar concentrations of SIN-1 had negligible effects on basal calcium current in frog cells [69], but increased calcium currents in human atrial myocytes, where basal cAMP levels might be higher. By contrast, higher concentrations of NO donors or cGMP analogs decrease calcium current intensity and contraction, in part through the activation of protein kinase G (PKG) [10, 61, 82, 83]. Again this effect has been identified mainly after initial stimulation of both calcium current and contraction following increases in cAMP. Aside from changes in calcium transients, activation of PKG by NO also decreases cardiac myocyte conctraction through a desensitization of cardiac myofilaments for calcium [84]. Preliminary evidence suggests that the latter effect may involve phosphorylation of troponin I by PKG [85] (unpublished observations).

Cyclic GMP-Independent Effects of Nitric Oxide

NO or a redox-derivative thereof, can regulate calcium channel function and cardiac contraction through mechanisms independent of elevations in cGMP. As mentioned above, peroxynitrite can interact with iron-sulfur clusters of key enzymes in the citric acid cycle, thereby impairing cellular engergy supplies [34]. NO in the form of the nitrosonium ion (NO^+) can S-nitrosylate enzymatic proteins such as GAPDH, the inactivation of which impedes glycolysis [24]. Muscle slices superfused with NO also exhibit a reduced oxygen consumption, that may result from inhibition of mitochondrial electron transfer through NO's inactivation of the heme moiety of cytochrome c-oxidase [85]. This effect has been reproduced in neonatal rat ventricular myocytes where iNOS had been induced on incubation with the cytokine IL-1β [86]. In isolated perfused hearts studied by ^{32}P nuclear magnetic resonance spectroscopy, perfusion with S-nitrosoacetylcysteine, an NO donor, blunted the positive inotropic effect of calcium, an effect that was accompanied by decreased ATP content but only a modest decline in phosphocreatine content. These effects of the NO donor have been attributed to nitrosylation of creatine kinase. Such nitrosylation could be reproduced with a purified creatine kinase exposed to NO *in vitro*, and resulted in inhibition of enzyme activity [87]. A similar enzyme inhibition *in vivo* would impede phosphoryl transfer from creatine phosphate to ATP, thereby impairing contractile reserve in cardiac muscle.

Conclusion

The complex biology of NO is reflected by the ever growing evidence for multiple mechanisms of intracellular action. A critical analysis of the literature reveals apparent discrepancies between the functional effects of NO supplied from exogenous NO donors or NO produced endogenously by the constitutive or inducible isoforms of NOS. Differences in the amount of NO generated by each of these two isoforms and exogenous NO donors may result in a different net effect on intracellular effectors. Oxidative modifications of target regulatory proteins are more likely to occur with the large quantities of NO produced by the "high output" enzyme, particularly in cells where superoxide anion production is additionally stimulated by cytokine exposure. Finally, the functional effect of NO may vary strikingly according to the differential regulation of downstream intracellular pathways from one species to another. The challenge for future work will be to re-evaluate the proposed molecular mechanisms of action of NO *in vivo*, in the light of recent information on the biochemistry of NO reactivity, as well as the subcellular localization of NOS isoforms that may target the NO produced to specific intracellular compartments and effector molecules.

References

1. Kelly RA, Balligand JL, Smith TW (1996) Nitric oxide and cardiac function. Circ Res 79:363–380
2. Balligand JL, Cannon PJ (1997) Nitric oxide synthases and cardiac muscle: autocrine and paracrine influences. Arteriosclerosis Thromb Vasc Bio (in press)
3. Balligand JL, Kobzik L, Han X, et al (1995) Nitric oxide-dependent parasympathetic signaling is due to activation of constitutive endothelial (type III) nitric oxide synthase in cardiac myocytes. J Biol Chem 270:14582–14586
4. Balligand JL, Smith TW (1997) Molecular regulation of NO synthase in the heart. In: Lewis M, Shah A (eds) Endothelial modulation of cardiac contraction. Harwood Acad Publishers (in press)
5. Balligand J, Kelly RA, Marsden PA, Smith TW, Michel T (1993) Control of cardiac muscle cell function by an endogenous nitric oxide signaling system. Proc Natl Acad Sci USA 90: 347–351
6. Balligand JL, Ungureanu D, Shussheim A, Maki T, Kelly RA, Smith TW (1993) Induction of nitric oxide synthase activity in ventricular myocytes reduces cAMP response to beta-adrenergic agonists. Circulation 88 (Suppl II):355–363
7. Keaney JF, Hare JM, Balligand JL, Loscalzo J, Smith TW, Colucci WS (1996) Inhibition of nitric oxide synthase augments myocardial contractile responses to beta-adrenergic stimulation. Am J Physiol 40:H2646–H2652
8. Hare JM, Loh E, Creager MA, Colucci WS (1995) Nitric oxide inhibits the positive inotropic response to beta-adrenergic stimulation in humans with left ventricular dysfuction. Circulation 92:2198–2203
9. Han X, Shimoni Y, Giles WR (1995) A cellular mechanism for nitric oxide-mediated cholinergic control of mammalian heart rate. J Gen Physiol 106:45–65
10. Han X, Kobzik L, Balligand JL, Kelly RA, Smith TW (1996) Nitric oxide synthase (NOS3)-mediated colinergic modulation of Ca^{2+} current in adult rabbit atrioventricular nodal cells. Circ Res 78:998–1008
11. Smith JA, Shah AM, Lewis MJ (1991) Factors released from endocardium of the ferret and pig modulate myocardial contraction. J Physiol 439:1–14
12. Grocott-Mason R, Fort S, Lewis MJ, Shah AM (1994) Myocardial relaxant effect of exogenous nitric oxide in isolated ejecting hearts. Am J Physiol 266:H1699–H1705

13. Xie YW, Shen W, Zhao G, Xu X, Wolin MS, Hintze TM (1996) Role of endothelium derived nitric oxide in the modulation of canine myocardial respiration in vitro. Circ Res 79:381–387

14. Feron O, Belhassen L, Kobzik L, Smith TW, Kelly RA, Michel T (1996) Endothelial nitric oxide synthase targeting to caveolae: specific interactions with caveolin isoforms in cardiac myocytes and endothelial cells. J Biol Chem 271:22810–22814

15. Michel JB, Feron O, Sacks D, Michel T (1997) Reciprocal regulation of endothelial nitric oxide synthase by Ca^{++} calmodulin and caveolin. J Biol Chem 272:15583–15586

16. Wink DA, Darbyshire JF, Nims RW, Saavedra JE, Ford PC (1993) Reactions of the bioregulatory agent nitric oxide in oxygenated aqueous media: determination of the kinetics for oxidation and nitrosation by intermediates generated in the NO/O_2 reaction. Chem Res Toxicol 6:23–27

17. Feelisch M, te Poel M, Zamora R, Deussen A, Moncaoda S (1994) Understanding the controversy over the identity of EDRF. Nature 368:62–65

18. Stamler JS, Simon DI, Osborne JA, et al (1992) S-nitrosylation of proteins with nitric oxide: synthesis and characterization of biologically active compounds. Proc Natl Acad Sci USA 89:444–448

19. Stamler JS, Simon DI, Jaraki O, et al (1992) S-nitrosylation of tissue-type plasminogen activator confers vasodilatory and antiplatelet properties on the enzyme. Proc Natl Acad Sci USA 89:8087–8091

20. Barnett DJ, Rios A, Williams DLH (1995) NO group transfer (transnitrosation) between S nitrosothiols and thiols. J Chem Soc Perkin Trans 27:1279–1282

21. Stamler JS (1994) Nitrosylation and related target interactions of nitric oxide. Cell 78:931–936

22. Lander HM, Sehajpal PK, Novogrodsyk A (1993) Nitric oxide signaling: a possible role for G proteins. Immunology 151:7182–7187

23. Bolotina VM, Najibi S, Palacino JJ, Pagano PJ, Cohen RA (1994) Nitric oxide directly activates calcium-dependent potassium channels in vascular smooth muscle. Nature 368:850–853

24. Mohr S, Stamler JS, Brüne B (1996) Posttranslational modification of glyceraldehyde-3-phosphate dehydrogenase by S-nitrosylation and subsequent NADH attachment. J Biol Chem 271:4209–4214

25. McDonald LJ, Moss J (1993) Stimulation by nitric oxide of an NAD linkage to glyceraldehyde-3-phosphate dehydrogenase. Proc Natl Acad Sci USA 90:6238–6241

26. Clancy RM, Leszcynska-Piziak J, Abramson SB (1992) Nitric oxide, an endothelial cell relaxation factor, inhibits neutrophil superoxide anion production via a direct action on the NADPH oxidase. J Clin Invest 90:1116–1121

27. Moro MA, Darley-Usmar VM, Goodwin DA, et al (1994) Paradoxical fate and biological action of peroxynitrite on human platelets. Proc Natl Acad Sci USA 91:6702–6706

28. Radi R, Beckman JS, Bush KM, Freeman BA (1991) Peroxynitrite oxidation of sulfhydryls. J Biol Chem 266:4244–4250

29. Haddad IY, Pataki G, Hu P, Galliani C, Beckman JS, Matalon S (1994) Quantitation of nitrotyrosine levels in lung sections of patients and animals with acute lung injury. J Clin Invest 94:2407–2413

30. Lewis-Molock Y, Suzuki K, Taniguchi N, Nguyen DH, Mason RH, White CW (1994) Lung manganese superoxide dismutase increases during cytokine-mediated protection against pulmonary oxygen toxicity in rats. Am J Respir Cell Mol Biol 10:133–141

31. Bergelson S, Pinkus R, Daniel V (1994) Intracellular glutathione levels regulate fos/jun induction and activation of glutathione S-transferase gene expression. Cancer Res 54:36–40

32. Gaston B, Reilly J, Drazen JM, et al (1993) Endogenous bronchodilator S-nitrosothiols in human airways. Proc Natl Acad Sci USA 90:10957–10961

33. Henry Y, Lepoivre M, Drapier MC, Ducrocq C, Boucher JL, Guissani AE (1993) PR characterization of molecular targets for NO in mammalian cells and organenes. FASEB J 7:1124–1134

34. Hausladen A, Fridovich I (1994) Superoxide and peroxynitrite inactivate aconitases, nitric oxide does not. J Biol Chem 269:29405–29408

35. Weiss G, Goosen B, Doppler W, et al (1993) Translational regulation via iron-responsive elements by the nitric oxide/NO-synthase pathway. EMBO J 12:3651–3657

36. O'Halloran TV (1993) Transition metals in control of gene expression. Science 261:715–730

37. Henry Y, Ducrocq C, Drapier JC, Servent D, Pellat C, Guissani A (1991) Nitric oxide, a biological effector. Electron paramagnetic resonance detection of nitrosyl-iron-protein complexes in whole cells. Eur Biophys J 20:1–15

38. Khatsenko OG, Gross SS, Rifkind AR, Vane JR (1993) Nitric oxide is a mediator of the decrease in cytochrome P450-dependent metabolism caused by immunostimulants. Proc Natl Acad Sci USA 90:11147–11151

39. Abu-Soud HM, Loftus M, Stuehr DJ (1995) Subunit dissociation and unfolding of macrophage NO synthase: Relationship between enzyme structure, prosthetic group binding, and catalytic function. Biochemistry 34:11167–11175

40. Hurshman AR, Marletta MA (1995) Nitric oxide complexes of inducible nitric oxide synthase: Spectral characterization and effect on catalytic activity. Biochemistry 34:5627–5634

41. Salvemimni D, Misko TP, Masferer JL, Seilbert K, Curri MG, Needleman P (1993) Nitric oxide activates cyclooxygenase enzymes. Proc Natl Acad Sci USA 90:7240–7244

42. Gerzer R, Böhme E, Hofmann F, Schultz G (1981) Soluble guanylate cyclase purified from bovine lung contains heme and copper. FEBS Lett 132:71–74

43. Tsai A (1994) How does NO activate hemeproteins? FEBS Lett 341:141–145

44. Ignarro LJ (1992) Haem-dependent activation of cytosolic guanylate cyclase by nitric oxide: a widespread signal transduction mechanism. Biochem Soc Trans 20:465–469

45. Traylor TG, Sharma VS (1992) Why NO? Biochemistry 31:2847–2849

46. Mulsch A, Gerzer R (1991) Purification of heme-containing soluble guanylyl cyclase. Methods Enzymol 195:377–383

47. Niroomand F, Rössle R, Mülsch A, Böhme E (1989) Under anaerobic conditions soluble guanylate cyclase is specifically stimulated by glutathione. Biochem Biophys Res Comm 161:75–80

48. Lincoln TM, Thompson M, Cornwell TL (1988) Purification and characterization of two forms of cyclic GMP-dependent protein kinase from bovine aorta. J Biol Chem 263:17632–17637

49. Wolfe L, Corbin JD, Francis SH (1989) Characterization of a novel isozyme of cGMP dependent protein kinase from bovine aorta. J Biol Chem 264:7734–7741

50. Francis SH, Woodford TA, Wolfe L, Corbin JD (1989) Types I alpha and I beta isozymes of cGMP-dependent protein kinase: alternative mRNA splicing may produce different inhibitory domains. Second Messengers Phosphoproteins 12:301–310

51. deJonge HR (1981) Cyclic GMP-dependent protein kinase in intestinal brush borders. Adv Cyclic Nucleotide Res 14:315–323

52. Raeymackers L, Hofmann F, Casteels R (1988) Cyclic GMP-dependent protein kinase phosphorylates phospholamban in isolated sarcoplasmic reticulum from cardiac and smooth muscle. Biochem J 252:269–273

53. Jahn H, Nastainczyk W, Rohrkasten A, Schneider T, Hofmann F (1988) Site-specific phosphorylation of the purified receptor for calcium-channel blockers by cAMP- and cGMP-dependent protein kinases, protein kinase C, calmodulin-dependent protein kinase II and casein kinase II. Eur J Biochem 178:525–542

54. Lincoln TM, Corbin JD (1977) Adenosine 3':5'-cyclic monophosphate- and guanosine 3':5'-cyclic monophosphate-dependent protein kinase: possible homologous proteins. Proc Natl Acad Sci USA 74:3239–3244

55. Colbran JL, Francis SH, Leach AB, et al (1992) A phenylalanine in peptide substrates provides for selectivity between cGMP-dependent and cAMP-dependent protein kinases. J Biol Chem 267:9589–9594

56. Wood JS, Yan X, Mendelow M, Corbin JD, Francis SH, Lawrence DS (1996) Precision substrate targeting of protein kinases. J Biol Chem 1271:174–179

57. Lincoln TM, Cornwell TL (1993) Intracellular cyclic GMP receptor proteins. FASEB J 7:328–338

58. Lindemann JP, Jones LR, Hathaway DR, Henry BG, Watanabe AM (1983) Beta-adrenergic stimulation of phospholamban phosphorylation and Ca^{2+}-ATPase activity in guinea pig ventricles. J Biol Chem 258:464–471

59. Cornwell TL, Pryzwansky KB, Wyatt TA, Lincoln TM (1991) Regulation of sarcoplasmic reticulum phosphorylation by localized cyclic GMP-dependent protein kinase in vascular smooth muscle cells. Mol Pharmacol 40:923–931

60. Thornbury KD, Ward SM, Dalziel HH, Carl A, Westfall DP, Sanders KM (1991) Nitric oxide and nitrocysteine mimic nonadrenergic noncholinergic hyperpolarization in canine proximal colon. Am J Physiol 261:G553–G557

61. Mery PF, Lohmann SM, Walter U, Fischmeister R (1991) Ca^{2+} current is regulated by cyclic GMP-dependent protein kinase in mammalian cardiac myocytes. Proc Natl Acad Sci USA 88:1197–1201

62. Cook NJ, Hanke W, Kaupp UB (1987) Identification, purification and functional reconstitution of the cyclic GMP-dependent channel from rod photoreceptors. Proc Natl Acad Sci USA 84:585–589

63. Gillespie PG (1990) Phosphodiesterases in visual transduction by rod and cones. In: Beavo J, Houslay MD (eds) Cyclic nucleotide phosphodiesterases: structure, regulation and drug action. Wiley, New York, pp 163–184

64. Ludwig J, Margalit T, Eismann E, Lancet E, Kaupp UB (1990) Primary structure of cAMP-gated channel from bovine olfactory epithelium. FEBS Lett 270:24–29

65. Morhmann M, Cantiello HF, Ausiella DA (1987) Inhibition of epithelial Na^+ transport by atriopeptin, protein kinase C and pertussis toxin. Am J Physiol 253:F371–F376

66. Charbonneau H (1990) Structure-function relationships among cyclic nucleotide phosphodiesterases. In: Beavo J, Houslay MD (eds) Cyclic nucleotide phosphodiesterases: Structure, function, regulation, and drug action. Wiley, New York, pp 267–298

67. Bode DC, Kanter JR, Brtulton LL (1991) Cellular distribution of phosphodiesterase isoforms in rat cardiac tissue. Circ Res 68:1070–1079

68. Fischmeister R, Hartzell HC (1987) Cyclic guanosine 3′5′-monophosphate regulates the calcium current in single cells from frog ventricle. J Physiol 387:453–472

69. Méry PF, Pavoine C, Belhassen L, Pecker F, Fischmeister R (1993) Nitric oxide regulates cardiac Ca^{2+} current. Involvement of cGMP-inhibited and cGMP-stimulated phosphodiesterases through guanylyl cyclase activation. J Biol Chem 268:26286–26295

70. Macfhee CH, Reifsnyder DH, Moore TA, Lerea KM, Beavo JA (1988) Phosphorylation results in activation of a cAMP phosphodiesterase in human platelets. J Biol Chem 263:10353–10358

71. Reeves ML, England PJ (1990) Cardiac phosphodiesterases and the functional effects of selective inhibition. In: Beavo JA, Houslay MD (eds) Cyclic nucleotide phosphodiesterases: Structure, regulation, and drug action. Wiley, New York, pp 299–316

72. Clapper DL, Walseth TF, Dargie PJ, Jee HC (1987) Pyridine nucleotide metabolites stimulate calcium release from sea urchin egg microsomes desensitized to inositol triphosphate. J Biol Chem 262:9561–9568

73. Galione A, Lee HC, Busa WB (1991) $Ca^{(2+)}$-induced Ca^{2+} release in sea urchin egg homogenates: modulation by cyclic ADP-ribose. Sciences 252:1143–1146

74. Meszaros LG, Bak J, Chu A (1993) Cyclic ADP-ribose as all endogenous regulator of the nonskeletal type ryanodine receptor Ca^{2+} channel. Nature 364:76–79

75. Galione A, White A, Willmott N, Turner M, Potter BV, Watson SP (1993) cGMP mobilizes intracellular Ca^{2+} in sea urchin eggs by stimulating cyclic ADP-ribose synthesis. Nature 365:456–459

76. Lee HC (1993) Potentiation of calcium- and caffeine-induced calcium release by cyclic ADP-ribose. J Biol Chem 268:293–299

77. Peunova N, Enikolopov G (1993) Amplification of calcium-induced gene transcription by nitric oxide in neuronal cells. Nature 364:450–453

78. Berridge MJ (1993) A tale of two messengers. Nature 365:388–389

79. Berridge MJ (1993) Inositol triphosphate and calcium signalling. Nature 361:316–325

80. Willmott N, Sethi JK, Walseth TF, Lee HC, White AM (1996) Nitric oxide induced mobilization of intracellular calcium via the cyclic ADP-ribose signaling pathway. J Biol Chem 271:3699–3705

81. Guo X, Laflamme A, Becker PL (1996) Cyclic ADP-ribose does not regulate sarcoplasmic reticulum Ca^{2+} release in intact cardiac myocytes. Cir Res 79:147–151

82. Kojda G, Kottenberg K, Nix P, Schluter KD, Piper HM, Noack E (1996) Low increase of cGMP induced by organic nitrates and nitrovasodilators improves contractile response of rat ventricular myocytes. Circ Res 78:91–101

83. Sumii K, Sperelakis N (1995) cGMP-dependent protein kinase regulation of the L-type Ca^{2+} current in rat ventricular myocytes. Circ Res 77:803–812

84. Shah AM, Spurgeon HA, Sollott SJ, Talo A, Lakatta EG (1994) 8-Bromo-cyclic GMP reduces the myofilament response to calcium in intact cardiac myocytes. Circ Res 74:970–978

85. Torres J, Darley-Usmar V, Wilson MT (1995) Inhibition of cytochrome c oxidase turnover by nitric oxide: Mechanism and implications for control of respiration. Biochem J 312:169–173
86. Oddis CV, Finkel MS (1995) Cytokine-stimulated nitric oxide production inhibits mitochondrial activity in cardiac myocytes. Biochem Biophys Res Commun 213:1002–1009
87. Gross SS, Wolin MS (1995) Nitric oxide: Pathophysiological mechanisms. Annu Rev Physiol 57:737–769

Development of Myocardial Tolerance to Ischemia/Reperfusion and Septic Injury

R. R. Nevière and W. J. Sibbald

Introduction

Myocardial resistance to ischemia/reperfusion (I/R) injury can be induced by pre-treating the myocardium with brief I/R episodes [1]. This protective effect of I/R pre-treatment is termed "pre-conditioning". Pre-conditioning can reduce I/R-induced infarct size, arrhythmias, and left ventricular contractile dysfunction [1–3]. This preconditioning-induced protection is much more potent than the protection afforded by other prophylactic interventions. The pre-conditioning-induced acute myocardial protection generally lasts only one to two hours after the initial I/R insult. Evidence is now emerging that another period of myocardial protection against I/R injury appears approximately twenty-four hours after the initial pre-conditioning period [4, 5]. This second window of protection (SWOP) has also been referred to as ischemic or oxidant tolerance [5]. Although this delayed form of protection has been extensively studied in the heart, there is evidence that the development of ischemic tolerance can also occur in organs such as the kidney, the skeletal muscle, the gut and the brain [6–9]. Finally, other unrelated stimuli such as hyperthermia, α1-adrenoreceptor stimulation, cytokine or endotoxin challenge also induce delayed cardioprotection after the conditioning stimulus [10–13]. This later phenomenon has been referred to as cross-tolerance to I/R.

This chapter summarizes the available literature showing that myocardial tolerance to I/R may be accomplished through both acute and delayed mechanisms. Also, the concept of cross tolerance to I/R is addressed. Finally, new information is presented which supports the hypothesis that prophylactic endotoxin exposure ameliorates sepsis-induced myocardial dysfunction.

I/R-Induced Ischemic Tolerance: An Acute and Delayed Phase of Protection

Acute Ischemic Pre-conditioning

Ischemic pre-conditioning was first described by Murry et al. [1] in 1986. Since this report, many investigators have demonstrated the remarkable protective effect that can be achieved by preceding a prolonged I/R episode with either a single I/R insult or a number of such I/R cycles [2, 3, 14]. In the initial study of Murry et al. [1], the protection was manifested as a reduction of infarct size in an open-chest anesthetized dog preparation. They showed that if dogs were subjected to brief (5 min) episodes of ischemia by complete coronary artery occlusion, each separated by brief periods of reperfusion, and were then subjected to a more prolonged (40 min) re-occlusion of the coronary artery, infarcts in these hearts were smaller, by up to 75% than those in controls. In similar experiments, the ratio of infarct size to the area at risk in pre-conditioned hearts was reduced from 30% in the controls to 4% in some animals subjected to pre-conditioning occlusion [14].

Pre-conditioning has since been demonstrated in a variety of species and both *in vivo* and *in vitro* models [15]. Such pre-conditioning has been found to elicit many cardioprotective effects including reduced infarct size, reduced incidence of ischemia or reperfusion induced arrhythmias and increased recovery of cardiac contractile function [15]. The protection from ischemic cell death induced by I/R pre-conditioning is considered the most powerful of any adjunct to reperfusion known to date.

Adenosine, ATP-sensitive Potassium (K_{ATP}) Channels, and Protein Kinase C Play Important Roles in Acute Pre-conditioning

Despite enormous interest in this acute protective phenomenon, the precise mechanism(s) involved in pre-conditioning-induced protection remains unresolved. The most likely explanation for the beneficial effects of pre-conditioning involves the release of pre-synthesized endogenous myocardial protective substance. A large body of evidence has demonstrated that adenosine acting on its A_1 receptor, myocardial adenosine triphosphate (ATP)-sensitive potassium (K_{ATP}) channels, and protein kinase C are three major factors involved in mediating ischemic pre-conditioning. It is generally accepted that adenosine mediates pre-conditioning via activation of the A_1 receptor, which is linked to the G_i protein pathway and has been proposed to open the K_{ATP} channel [16]. Adenosine stimulation of A_1 and A_3 adenosine receptors appears to be linked to protein kinase C in most species, which by phosphorylation of unknown targets provides reduction in infarct size during a subsequent ischemic period [17]. Linkage between these receptors and protein kinase C appears to involve, at least in some species, the K_{ATP} channels. K_{ATP} channels are present in cardiomyocytes and smooth muscle cells and these channels are coupled through G protein to adenosine A_1 receptors [18]. Inhibiting these channels inhibits vasodilation in response to hypoxia or ischemia and blocks pre-conditioning of myocytes. Stimulating these channels through the stimulation of muscarinic, bradykinin-B_2 and α_1-receptors can mimic pre-conditioning. Pre-conditioning also involves increasing ecto-5'-nucleotidase activity. The ecto-5'-nucleotidase enzyme in cardiomyocytes is partially responsible for adenosine production during myocardial ischemia and the reduction in infarct size during ischemia appears to be dependent on this adenosine release [19].

A Delayed Myocardial Protection Against I/R

Recent studies indicate that in addition to its early protective effects, ischemic pre-conditioning elicits a second, or late, phase of protection against myocardial infarction and myocardial stunning (SWOP or tolerance). This protection was discovered independently by two different laboratories while investigating the changes occurring in the transcription of stress protein and antioxidant genes in response to sublethal ischemia [5]. The development of I/R tolerance is gradual and of prolonged duration. For example, in the canine model used by Kuzuya et al. [20] the pattern of protection seen at 0, 3, 12 and 24 h after I/R insult supports the existence of an early (pre-conditioning), and late (tolerance), phase of protection. At 3 h, the early phase of protection has completely disappeared. By 12 h the later phase of protection was beginning to appear and by 24 h there was again a statistically significant reduction in infarct size. In a similar model, a 50% reduction in infarct size was seen 48 h after the initial I/R insult when compared with controls and even 72 h later there may be some infarct limiting effect [5]. Although delayed I/R tolerance has been most extensively studied in the heart, there is evidence that I/R tolerance occurs in organs such as kidney, skeletal muscle, gut and brain [6–9].

Mechanisms of Delayed Ischemic Oxidant Tolerance

Proposed mechanisms of delayed myocardial protection against I/R include the expression of pro-oncogenes, augmented stress protein synthesis, and increased antioxidant enzyme systems. Several lines of evidence have shown that delayed myocardial protection mechanisms involve changes in transcription of genes with subsequent translation of protective proteins. Specifically, the delayed phase of protection involves augmentation of heat shock proteins (HSP) and antioxidant proteins. For example, Hoshida et al. [21] reported that delayed I/R tolerance was associated with a significant increase in myocardial manganese superoxide dismutase (Mn-SOD), glutathione peroxidase and reductase. Further observations indicate that a brief burst of superoxide anion (O_2^-) production during the initial I/R insult activates the subcellular machinery leading to activation of myocardial antioxidant systems [5, 21]. Finally, studies in the gut indicate that this adaptation appeared to be specific for oxidant injury, since an initial I/R insult imposed 24 h earlier also protected against hydrogen peroxide (H_2O_2)-induced, but not acid- or ethanol-induced, barrier dysfunction [6]. Further experiments indicated that the initial I/R challenge induced an increase in antioxidant systems including catalase and glutathione peroxidase activities, and glutathione content, resulting in an increased resistance to a subsequent oxidant challenge [6].

Alternative mechanisms for the delayed protection may involve increased levels of HSP. A variety of stressful stimuli, including hyperthermia, ischemia, and anoxia, induce the synthesis of proteins, leading to the limitation of infarct size. In this scenario, the delayed pre-conditioning might induce the transcription of mRNA and subsequent synthesis of one or more HSP that would then protect the myocardium during sustained I/R [5, 22]. Elevation of myocardial HSP72 at 24 h after brief ischemia or heat stress was associated with resistance to ischemia. While a brief I/R period has been shown to induce HSPs possibly via accumulation of reactive free radicals such as O_2^-, it seems reasonable to state that the induction of HSPs may be a part of overall cellular defense mechanisms against the oxidant stress.

Another explanation for the delayed protection relates to the nitric oxide (NO) hypothesis recently proposed by Boli et al. [23]. These investigators have provided evidence that, in addition to its numerous other actions, NO plays a key role in the delayed myocardial adaptation to brief I/R stresses. In addition, Kim et al. [24] have recently shown in conscious dogs that a 10-minute coronary occlusion induces a delayed increase in the coronary flow response to endothelium-dependent vasodilators, as well as an increase in the cardiac production of NO. The enhanced NO production began at 6 h after I/R and peaked at 24 to 48 hours. Thus, these observations are compatible with a role of NO and NO synthase (NOS) in mediating the protective effects of the late phase (ischemic tolerance) of protection.

Sepsis-Induced Myocardial Tolerance to I/R (Cross Tolerance)

Potentially one of the most important experimental findings in the area of sepsis pathophysiology is the observation that long-term myocardial tolerance to I/R can develop after a single endotoxin challenge with protection observed up to 36 h after the challenge [10, 11]. In addition, mediators of endotoxin-induced systemic effects [interleukin-1 (IL-1) and tumor necrosis factor (TNF)] have been reported to independently induce similar, delayed cardioadaptive effects [12, 13]. Pre-treatment with endotoxin, or the endotoxin derivative monophosphoryl lipid A, before an I/R insult was shown to preserve left ventricular function, attenuate depletion of ATP, blunt creatine kinase release and reduce infarct size [10, 11, 25].

Endotoxin-induced cross tolerance to I/R was first described by Brown et al. [10] in 1989. Using a standard isolated and perfused rat heart model, they found that hearts from endotoxin-pretreated rats had increased catalase activity and decreased susceptibility to I/R injury. Since this report, many investigators have demonstrated the remarkable protective effect that can be achieved by preceding a prolonged I/R episode with exposure to endotoxin and endotoxin derivatives. For example, it has been demonstrated that hearts treated with a single dose of endotoxin given 24 hours prior to I/R resumed spontaneous contractive activity better and released less lactate than did the control hearts [11, 26]. This observation is consistent with increased myocardial antioxidant defenses as previous studies have shown that antecedent of sepsis induced by cecal ligation and perforation (CLP) induced protection to the effects of further myocardial oxyradical exposure [27], We [28] have recently reported that endotoxin exposure produces a dose-dependent improvement of post-I/R left ventricular developed pressure (LVDP) recovery: $30 \pm 6\%$ in sham, $78 \pm 9\%$ in 2.5 mg/kg, $93 \pm 8\%$ in 5 mg/kg, $107 \pm 10\%$ in 10 mg/kg endotoxin treated hearts. In this isolated and perfused heart model, the finding that endotoxin must be given 6 hours before heart isolation to be effective implies a slow process, possibly involving protein synthesis.

Based on these observations it has been suggest that noxious septic stimuli are sensed by the myocardium and it responds in an adaptational manner. Increases in antioxidant enzyme activities, i.e., catalase, SOD, glutathione peroxidase and reductase, have been associated with endotoxin-induced myocardial cross-tolerance to I/R injury [10, 12, 25]. While the mechanism of this form of myocardial protection is still poorly understood, these observations represent an important initial understanding of cardioadaptation with a potential for optimizing clinical myocardial protection.

Endotoxin-Induced Tolerance

While endotoxin has been used to induce cross tolerance to ischemia, it is reasonable to propose that endotoxin induces tolerance to other forms of injury. Adaptation or tolerance to endotoxin develops after repeated administration of small sublethal doses and is characterized by reduced systemic response to a subsequent challenge with a large dose of endotoxin [29, 30]. Endotoxin tolerance has been divided temporally into early-phase and late-phase tolerance. Early-phase tolerance occurs within the first days after exposure to endotoxin, is transient, and is not O-antigen specific. Late phase endotoxin tolerance is related to the production of anti-O-specific antibodies, occurs several weeks after the initial exposure to lipopolysaccharide (LPS), and persists for several weeks. Both *in vivo* and *in vitro* studies have demonstrated that the early phase endotoxin tolerance causes profound alterations in the release of pro-inflammatory cytokines and operates at the level of the macrophage/monocyte lineage [31]. Early phase tolerance develops to the lethal, metabolic and pyrogenic effects of endotoxin [30]. While *in vivo* studies have shown that tolerance can be induced to the cytotoxic effects of an endotoxin infusion, the impact of endotoxin-induced tolerance on the evolution of sepsis initiated by creating a focus of infection is unknown.

When a generalized infectious process develops, endotoxin tolerance may have two opposing effects. It may be detrimental when it alters the initial processes which serve to localize and control bacterial invasion, and to initiate repair of injured tissue [32]. On the other hand, it may be beneficial if endotoxin tolerance prevents the excessive cytokine production and subsequent organ dysfunction which occur when generalized infection develops. Consistent with previous observations [33], recent results from our laboratory show that endotoxin pre-treatment may decrease acute mortality from peritonitis induced by CLP. Our experiments also extend these observations by providing new information on the effects of endotoxin pre-treatment on heart and lung inflammation and dysfunction in a model of sepsis that reproduces many pathophysiologic features of human sepsis [34]. In these experiments, a schedule of endotoxin pre-treatment was able to reduce remote organ inflammation [heart and lung myeloperoxidase activity, bronchoalveolar lavage (BAL) leukocyte count] and dysfunction (BAL protein content and left ventricular contractility-relaxation).

Mechanisms of Endotoxin Induced Tolerance

In models of lethal endotoxin injection, endotoxin pre-treatment reduced the neutropenia and heart microcirculation leukocyte entrapment associated with endotoxemia [35]. Consequently, endotoxin pre-treatment may lower the number of activated leukocytes sequestered in different organs during the development of the sepsis process. The reduction of tissue leukocyte sequestration in tolerant animals is a key finding since a considerable body of evidence suggests that activated leukocytes are a major contributor to tissue injury and organ dysfunction in sepsis.

In addition, studies of endotoxin tolerance induced in *in vitro* and *in vivo* models have demonstrated a decrease in the production of cytokines such as TNF, IL-1 and IL-6 [29]. Tolerance does not lead to down-regulation of all inflammatory responses, as some genes are even increased in expression on secondary stimulation; these include p50 of nuclear factor-kappa B (NF-κB), TNF receptor type II and IL-10 [29]. The molecular events that regulate endotoxin tolerance are still poorly understood but result in repressed expression of cytokine genes and altered cytokine processing and secretion. Emerging results suggest that endotoxin induces many of its effects on cells by receptor coupled signaling of gene transcription involving NF-κB [36]. Proposed mechanisms of endotoxin tolerance include modification of the nuclear binding of nuclear transcriptional factors such as NF-κB [37]. For example, in our model of sepsis, myocardial nuclear binding of transcriptional factor NF-κB increased in CLP animals when compared with myocardium of sham animals. Endotoxin pre-treatment reduced the myocardial nuclear binding of NF-κB in CLP animals (unpublished observations).

Conclusion

Acute pre-conditioning of the heart with repetitive short periods of ischemia, separated by intermittent reperfusion, renders the myocardium more tolerant to subsequent I/R episodes, i.e., causes a reduction in infarct size, marked limitation of arrhythmias and ameliorates post-ischemic contractile dysfunction. Recently there have been reports of a new aspect of I/R-induced protection, namely a delayed phase of protection observed many hours after the initial I/R trigger and distinct from the classical pre-conditioning-induced protection. This delayed protection is due to a multifactorial stress response in the myocardium. Stimuli that are conventionally accepted to be deleterious to the myocardium, e.g., hyperthermia, ischemia, catecholamines, cytokines and endotoxin may actually induce a beneficial adaptation. The effects of endotoxin tolerance on sepsis-induced inflammation and dysfunction extends our knowledge concerning the inherent adaptative properties of the myocardium that may have real clinical relevance and offer the potential for therapeutic exploitation.

References

1. Murry CE, Jennings RB, Reimer KA (1986) Preconditioning with ischemia: A delay of lethal cell injury in ischemic myocardium. Circulation 74:1124–1136
2. Li GC, Vasquez JA, Gallager KP, Lucchesi BR (1990) Myocardial protection with preconditioning. Circulation 82:609–619
3. Liang BT (1996) Direct preconditioning of cardiac ventricular myocytes via adenosine A1 receptor and KATP channel. Am J Physiol 271:H1769–H1777
4. Kuzuya T, Hoshida S, Yamashita N (1993) Delayed effects of sublethal ischemia on the acquisition of tolerance to ischemia. Circ Res 72:1293–1299
5. Yellon DM, Walker DM (1995) A second window of protection or delayed preconditioning phenomenon: Future horizons for myocardial protection? J Mol Cell Cardiol 27:1023–1034

6. Osborne DL, Aw TY, Cepinskas G, Kvietys PR (1994) Development of ischemia reperfusion tolerance in the rat small intestine: An epithelium independent event. J Clin Invest 94: 1910–1918
7. Yoshika T, Bills T, Moore-Jarrett T, et al (1990) Role of intrinsic antioxidant enzymes in renal oxidant injury. Kidney Int 38: 282–288
8. Jerome SN, Akimitsu T, Gute DC, Korthuis RJ (1995) Ischemic preconditioning attenuates capillary no-reflow induced by prolonged ischemia and reperfusion. Am J Physiol 268: H2063–H2067
9. Kitogawa K, Matsumoto M, Kuwabara K, et al (1991) Ischemic tolerance phenomenon detected in various brain regions. Brain Res 561: 203–211
10. Brown JM, Grosso MA, Terada LS, et al (1989) Endotoxin pretreatment increases endogenous myocardial catalase activity and decreases ischemia reperfusion injury of isolated rat hearts. Proc Natl Acad Sci USA 86: 2516–2520
11. McDonough KH, Giaimo ME, Miller HI (1995) Effects of endotoxin on the guinea pig heart response to ischemia reperfusion. Shock 2: 139–142
12. Brown JM, White CW, Terada LS, et al (1990) Interleukin 1 pretreatment decreases ischemia reperfusion injury. Proc Natl Acad Sci USA 87: 5026–5030
13. Brown JM, Anderson BO, Repine JE, Shanley PF et al (1992) Neutrophils contribute to TNF induced-myocardial tolerance to ischemia. J Mol Cell Cardiol 24: 485–495
14. Liu Y, Downey JM (1992) Ischemic preconditioning protects against infarction in rat hearts. Am J Physiol 263: H1107–H1112
15. Cave AC (1995) Preconditioning induced protection against post-ischaemic contractile dysfunction: Characteristics and mechanisms. J Mol Cell Cardiol 27: 969–979
16. Downey JM, Liu GS, Thornton JD (1993) Adenosine and anti-infarct effects of preconditioning. Cardiovasc Res 27: 3–8
17. Ytrehus K, Liu Y, Downey JM (1994) Preconditioning protects ischemic rabbit heart by protein kinase C activation. Am J Physiol 35: H1145–H1152
18. Brooks G, Hearse DJ (1996) Role of protein kinase C in ischemic preconditioning: player or spectator? Circulation 79: 627–630
19. Kitakase M, Node K, Minamino T, et al (1996) Role of activation of protein kinase C in the infarct size-limiting effect of ischemic preconditioning through activation of ecto-5'-nucleotidase. Circulation 93: 781–791
20. Kuzuya T, Hoshida S, Yamashita N (1993) Delayed effects of sublethal ischemia on the acquisition of tolerance to ischemia. Circ Res 72: 1293–1299
21. Hoshida S, Kuzuya T, Fuji H, et al (1993) Sublethal ischemia alters myocardial antioxidant activity in canine heart. Am J Physiol 264: H33–H39
22. Nayeem MA, Hess ML, Qian YZ, et al (1997) Delayed preconditioning of cultured adult rat cardiac myocytes: role of 70- and 90-kDa heat stress proteins. Am J Physiol 273: H861–H868
23. Boli R, Bhatti ZA, Tang XL, et al (1997) Evidence that late preconditioning against myocardial stunning in conscious rabbits is triggered by the generation of nitric oxide. Circ Res 81: 42–52
24. Kim SJ, Ghaleh B, Kudej RK et al (1997) Delayed enhanced nitric oxide-mediated coronary vasodilation following brief ischemia and prolonged reperfusion in conscious dogs. Circ Res 81: 53–59
25. Nelson DW, Brown JM, Banerjee A, et al (1991) Pretreatment with a non toxic derivative of endotoxin induces functional protection against cardiac ischemia/reperfusion injury. Surgery 110: 365–369
26. McDonough KH, Causey KM (1994) Effects of sepsis on recovery of the heart from 50 min ischemia. Shock 6: 432–437
27. Davidson SB, Dulchavsky SA, Diebel LN, et al (1996) Effects of sepsis and 3,5,3'-triiodothyronine replacement on myocardial integrity during oxidant challenge. Crit Care Med 24: 850–854
28. Neviere R, Li FY, Singh T, Myers ML, Sibbald WJ (1997) Endotoxin depresses myocardial contractility but protects the myocardium against a subsequent ischemia reperfusion. Am J Respir Crit Care Med 155: A928 (Abst)
29. Ziegler-Heitbrock HWL (1995) Molecular mechanism in tolerance to lipopolysaccharide. J Inflam 45: 13–26
30. Greisman SE, Young EJ, Woodward WE (1996) Mechanisms of endotoxin tolerance. IV. Specificity of the pyrogenic refractory state during continuous intravenous infusion of endotoxin. J Exp Med 124: 983–1000

31. Ayala A, Chaudry IH (1996) Immune dysfunction in murine polymicrobial sepsis: Mediators, macrophages, lymphocytes and apoptosis. Shock 6: S27–S38
32. Keels M, Schregengerger N, Steckholzer U, et al (1996) Endotoxin tolerance after severe injury and its regulatory mechanisms. J Trauma 41: 430–438
33. Astiz ME, Dhanonjoy CS, Brooks K, et al (1993) Comparison of the induction of endotoxin tolerance in endotoxemia and peritonitis by monophosphoryl lipid A and lipopolysaccharide. Circ Shock 39: 194–198
34. Neviere R, Li FY, Myers ML, Kvietys PR, Sibbald WJ (1997) Endotoxin pretreatment attenuates sepsis-induced systemic inflammatory response and organ dysfunction in rats. Proceedings of ICU World Congress, Ottawa
35. Barroso-Aranda J, Schmid-Schonbein GW, Zweifach BW, et al (1991) Polymorphonuclear neutrophil contribution to induced tolerance to bacterial lipopolysaccharide. Circ Res 69: 1196–1206
36. Blackwell TS, Christman JW (1997) The role of nuclear factor-κB in cytokine gene regulation. Am J Respir Cell Mol Biol 17: 3–9
37. Zuckerman SH, Evans GF (1992) Endotoxin tolerance: *In vivo* regulation of tumor necrosis factor and interleukin-1 synthesis is at the transcriptional level. Cell Immunol 140: 513–519

Endothelial Cell Dysfunction in Septic Shock

B. Vallet and J. Leclerc

Introduction

Sepsis is a life-threatening syndrome that represents the host systemic response to an inflammatory focus. The systemic inflammatory response is triggered when circulating neutrophils encounter the stimulus that results in their activation. When this response provokes hypotension and organ dysfunction, it is called septic shock. A large number of vascular abnormalities have been described in patients with septic shock. The endothelial cell layer which represents a very large area in contact with blood is tightly involved in these alterations. Injury to the vascular endothelium is a critical and early event in the acute inflammatory response *in vivo*. In the activated state, neutrophils express increased adhesive properties that allow them to bind to endothelial cells. The target, i.e, the endothelial cell, then becomes an active participant in the injury process. Indeed, many of the inflammatory mediators that induce activation in neutrophils also influence endothelial cells and change their physiology.

Morphological and Cytological Injuries

Endothelium represents a very large area (700 m^2, 1.5 kg/70 kg body weight) in contact with blood elements. Endothelial cells have long been considered little more than a layer of nucleated cellophane and a passive bystander in their own injury. In fact, the endothelial cell is directly involved in the sepsis-associated inflammatory response.

There have been many studies assessing anatomical damage to the endothelium in endotoxic shock. Endotoxin-containing Gram-negative organisms are able to initiate the septic shock pathogenetic cascade in humans. In that way, injection of bacterial endotoxin (lipopolysaccharide, LPS) is often used experimentally as a simple animal model of septic shock. A single injection of LPS has long been demonstrated to be a non-mechanical technique of removing endothelium [1]. Vascular endothelial cell damage varies with the animal model, amount of LPS used, type of vessel and duration of LPS infusion. In a rat model of sepsis (single *Serratia marcescens* LPS injection, 200 µg/kg), Reidy and Schwartz [2] showed that LPS injection caused only cell detachment without any denudation. This was, however, associated with an increase in endothelial cell replication. These results tended to suggest that endothelial cell surface loss does not occur easily or rapidly.

Using scanning and/or transmission electron microscopy, various endothelial cell alterations have been reported following injury by endotoxin. Reidy and Bowyer [3] observed, one hour after LPS injection in rats (*E. coli* LPS, 3 mg/kg), that some aortic endothelial cells were curled up and spindle-shaped in appearance. They observed the presence of Weibel-Palade bodies, that correspond to Von Willebrand factor accumulation. In some areas, the endothelium was completely detached from the arterial wall, leaving large denuded zones. An abnormal relationship with the underlying subendothelial compartment was found by Young et al. [4]. These authors showed that endothelial cells were detached from the internal elastic lamina in a septic shock guinea pig model, with indication of subendothelial edema. Wang et al. [5] observed the same aspect 10 hours after the onset of sepsis in a cecal ligation and puncture (CLP) rat model. Lee et al. [6] gave *E. coli* LPS endotoxin to rabbits and rats and removed aortas for observation at intervals varying from 1 min to 4 hours after endotoxin. As early as 15 min after LPS injection, cellular injury was apparent in their model as evidenced by nuclear vacuolization, cytoplasmic swelling and protrusion, cytoplasmic fragmentation, and various degrees of detachment of the endothelium from its underlying layers. In a similar endotoxic rabbit model, we [7] demonstrated that endothelium denudation (as evidenced by platelet endothelial cell adhesion molecule-1 staining) was present at the level of the abdominal aorta and maximal at five days. It took around 21 days for the endothelial surface to recover. The de-endothelialized surface accounted for approximately 25% of the total surface.

Altered Anticoagulant and Anti-inflammatory Functions

Endothelial cells play an active role in maintaining the fluidity of blood. First of all, their presence prevents contact between blood constituents and the procoagulant subendothelium. Second, the outer membrane of the endothelial cell normally expresses various membrane components with anticoagulant properties. Among them are cell surface heparin-like molecules which may accelerate the inactivation of coagulation proteases by antithrombin III and represent a tissue factor pathway inhibitor reserve [8]. The cell surface also possesses a thrombin-binding protein, thrombomodulin, responsible for thrombin activity inhibition, and when bound to thrombin forms a potent protein C activator complex. Moreover, endothelium derived factors such as nitric oxide (NO) and prostacyclin (PGI_2) [9] have antiadhesive or tissue plasminogen activator-like properties. These properties are modified by sepsis.

It is well known that there is a close relationship between coagulant activity and the status of the endothelium. Inflammation and/or sepsis may change the anticoagulant phenotype of endothelial cells into a procoagulant phenotype. In septic shock, subendothelium exposure facilitates leukocyte and platelet aggregation. Tissue factor expression on endothelial cells is enhanced and associated with internalization of thrombomodulin. Moreover, endothelial cell production of mediators (NO, PGI_2) that control the vascular tone and platelet or neutrophil adhesion is impaired.

Recent studies performed in humans that were injected with small amounts of purified endotoxin showed that the initial procoagulant response to endotoxin was solely mediated by the extrinsic route of coagulation (for a review see [10]). Infusion of tumor necrosis factor (TNF)-α in human volunteers produced procoagulant responses that were identical to those responses observed after endotoxin challenge, but with a 45-min shorter delay after injection, which corresponds to the time gap between endotoxin administration and plasma peak TNF-α. This suggests that TNF-α is an important mediator of the procoagulant response to endotoxin. Regarding the cellular mechanisms of coagulation activation, there is some evidence favoring a role for monocytes. However, endothelial cells are likely to play a pivotal role in disseminated intravascular coagulation. Endotoxin, TNF-α and interleukin (IL)-1, induce tissue factor synthesis in endothelium, although at a slower rate than in monocytes. Given the large surface of the vascular endothelium, even minor tissue factor expression may be of critical importance. In addition, endothelial cells generate adhesion molecules during endotoxemia that bind neutrophils and monocytes and thus enhance local procoagulant reactions.

Inflammatory processes start at the microcirculatory level with an increase in granulocyte "sticking". Neutrophil margination occurs along the vascular endothelium, resulting in the release of many mediators and the migration of neutrophils into tissues. When stimulated, the leukocytes express various glycoproteins on their outer cell membrane, collectively termed the CD_{11}/CD_{18} complex. Meanwhile, the stimulation of endothelial cells induces the expression of cell surface adhesion molecules. Endothelial adhesion molecules include intercellular adhesion molecules (ICAMs), endothelial leukocyte adhesion molecules, platelet endothelial cell adhesion molecule-1, and vascular cell adhesion molecules. Many leukocyte and endothelial cell interactions are mediated by such glycoproteins. Monoclonal antibodies to these molecules have been shown to block leukocyte/endothelial cell interaction. Adhesion molecules enable circulating leukocytes to exert their destructive effects on the vessel wall. Leukocytes can then release active oxygen species, such as superoxide radicals, that can directly damage cells (for a review see [11]). Endothelial cell dysfunction has been found to involve a CD_{18}-dependent neutrophil adherence mechanism, and inhibition of neutrophil adherence to the endothelial cells exerts significant protective effects under those conditions [12]. Sessler et al. [13] measured blood levels of the adhesion molecule ICAM-1 as a potential marker of endothelial cell activation in septic adults and in healthy volunteers. They established a relationship between increased ICAM-1 levels and consequences of sepsis (i.e., multiple organ failure and death).

The systemic inflammatory response that occurs in sepsis leads to capillary leakage. The endothelial disruption allows inflammatory fluid and cells to shift from the blood into the vasculature. The pro-inflammatory cytokines including TNF-α, IL-1 and IL-6 increase the permeability of the endothelial cells in a process that may involve a "vascular permeability factor". The increased permeability is manifested approximately 6 hours after it is triggered and becomes maximal in 12–24 hours as the combination of cytokines exert potentiating effects [14].

Modified Endothelium-Derived Vasorelaxation

Endothelial cells act as a signaling pathway for blood messages to vascular smooth muscle cells. Furthermore, they synthesize and release various relaxing or contracting factors. Release of the short-lived vasodilatory agents PGI$_2$ and NO from endothelial cells plays a pivotal role in the regulation of local vascular tone.

NO release and/or endothelium derived relaxation may be used as indicators of endothelial cell function. Vascular endothelial cells possess receptors on their plasma membrane for numerous circulating factors that cause NO release. Endothelium-derived relaxation can be observed *in vitro* in isolated vascular rings in the presence of picomolar concentrations of acetylcholine [15]. An influx of calcium to the endothelial cell results from the receptor occupancy. The calcium-calmodulin complex triggers the activation of the endothelial constitutive enzyme NO-synthase (ecNOS). Influx of calcium can also be directly achieved by the calcium ionophore A23187. In physiological conditions, beside the basal release of NO from the endothelial cells, NO production is the result of shear stress and/or receptor activation. When NO is released, it diffuses to nearby smooth muscle cells and causes relaxation of the vascular smooth muscle via activation of the soluble smooth muscle cell guanylate cyclase (GC) and related increase in vascular smooth muscle cyclic guanosine monophosphate (cGMP) levels.

Endothelium-mediated vasorelaxation is impaired in septic shock vessels. Following *in vivo* endotoxemia, a number of investigators [16–18] have demonstrated attenuated acetylcholine-induced endothelium-dependent relaxation *in vitro* in vascular rings isolated from large arteries. Such studies suggest that this defect is due to impaired release of NO by the ecNOS isoform. One possible explanation is that ecNOS activity is impaired in the vascular endothelial cells of septic shock vessels. Pro-inflammatory cytokines such as TNF-α, as well as bacterial endotoxin, which are closely involved in the pathogenetic mechanisms of septic shock, have been found to downregulate *in vitro* endothelial cNOS mRNA activity in a dose and time-dependent manner (Fig. 1) by increasing the rate of mRNA degradation [19, 20]. Consistent with this Zhou et al. [21] recently demonstrated in a CLP rat

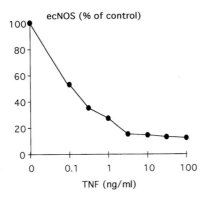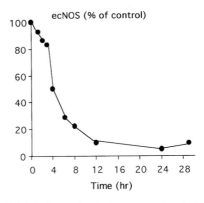

Fig. 1. Dose-response relation (left) and time course (right) of constitutively expressed endothelial nitric-oxide synthase (ecNOS) mRNA down-regulation by TNF-α. (From [18] with permission)

model of sepsis a decrease in the density of endothelial cNOS within endothelial cells.

However, this down-regulation of endothelial cNOS mRNA is certainly not the only mechanism involved in loss of endothelium-derived relaxation. We [7, 16] recently observed, that *in vitro* endothelial-dependent vascular relaxation was significantly depressed after low-dose LPS injection in rabbits. Indeed, a single and non-lethal injection of LPS (0.5 mg/kg) in rabbits was associated with a loss of acetyl-choline-induced relaxation, that was sustained for 5 days. Recovery was noticed at day 21 (Fig. 2). In parallel to abnormal endothelium-derived relaxation, we observed an increase in tissue factor expression in monocytes and endothelial cells. Increased tissue factor expression lasted longer (5 days) than observed abnormal disseminated intravascular coagulation (48 hours). Interestingly, in this model, A23187-induced relaxation was never altered, suggesting that endothelium-derived relaxation impairment in sepsis is much more related to a receptor-to-NOS coupling mechanism than to NOS dysfunction *per se*. These results confirm those of Parker et al. [17] whose observations were made in a canine model of sepsis.

More importantly, recent studies in the isolated perfused rabbit heart [22], auto-perfused rat cremaster [23], and rat mesentery [24, 25] have suggested that similar mechanisms may be operative in the microvasculature. Also, intravital microscopy on extensor digitorum longus muscle in rats made septic by CLP suggested [26] that sepsis was associated with a reduction in tissue perfused capillary density up to 36%. The spatial distribution of perfused capillaries was also more heterogeneous, and the mean intercapillary distance increased by 30%. Sepsis therefore seems to affect the ability of the skeletal muscle microcirculation to distribute red blood cells and consequently O_2 appropriately. Moreover, when using laser Doppler flowmetry to assess the functional hyperemic response of the muscle before and after a period

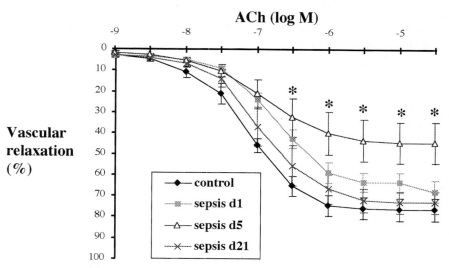

Fig. 2. Cumulative dose responses to various concentration of acetylcholine (Ach) in aortic rings from control rabbits and from rabbits one (sepsis d1), five (sepsis d5), or twenty-one days (sepsis d21) after endotoxin injection; * p < 0.05 vs control. (From [15] with permission)

of maximal twitch designed to increase O_2 demand, the authors [26] observed after contraction that the relative increase in red blood cell flux was less in CLP rats. They further concluded that sepsis affects the ability of the microcirculation to respond to increases in O_2 demand. In that respect, it is logical to consider that sepsis induces impaired O_2 extraction since evidence exists today that endothelial cells are involved in tissue O_2 extraction ability [27, 28].

In healthy volunteers, even a brief exposure to endotoxin or certain cytokines impairs endothelium-dependent relaxation for many days [29, 30]. This effect has been termed endothelial stunning. After recovery from the acute insult, the endothelium may remain dysfunctional ("stunned") for a long period of time before full recovery. Nevière et al. [31] have similarly shown that reactive hyperemia is attenuated in critically ill patients with septic shock despite normal or elevated whole-body oxygen delivery. Reactive hyperemia is a test of an organ's ability to increase flow on demand. The increased blood flow during reactive hyperemia results from an increase in flow in capillaries and by recruitment of additional capillaries. This response is the result of vasoactive factors that affect arteriolar smooth muscle directly as well as those that act via the arteriolar endothelium. Proposed mechanisms that explain blunted hyperemia in septic patients might therefore include impaired vascular reactivity and/or microvascular obstruction that limits the number of recruitable capillaries.

One may argue that despite down-regulation of ecNOS mRNA and dysfunction of receptor-NOS coupling, LPS and cytokines lead to expression of an inducible isoform of NOS (iNOS) that produces NO in larger quantities than ecNOS. Some data support the idea that increased production of NO by mediator-induced iNOS partially compensates for decreases in NO production by ecNOS under these conditions [32, 33, 34]. However, and this remains an important concern, iNOS does not contribute to agonist-induced endothelium-dependent relaxation since this enzyme is not responsive to increases in intracellular calcium. Therefore, selective spots of malperfusion with an abnormal response to increased O_2 demand might coexist with overperfusion due to overproduction of NO and global vasoplegia. In this context, it makes sense that inhibition of iNOS does not alter impaired O_2 extraction in endotoxemia, and is not able to improve survival in acute or chronic animal models of sepsis [33]. Moreover, when α-adrenergic drugs or NOS inhibitors just increase mean arterial pressure, β-adrenergic agents or other selective vasodilators may help to better restitute physiologic vasomotor tone and tissue perfusion during septic shock. The superiority of isoproterenol over phenylephrine in improving O_2 extraction capabilities in anesthetized dogs that received endotoxin was recently demonstrated [35].

Therapeutic Implications

Experimental studies have investigated a corrective approach to endothelial dysfunction associated with septic shock. However, because endothelial cell dysfunction can be investigated at different levels, it is difficult to summarize the effects of the various endothelial-directed treatments. Wang et al. [5] hypothesized, as others, that elevated plasma TNF-α levels were responsible, at least in part, for the endothelial

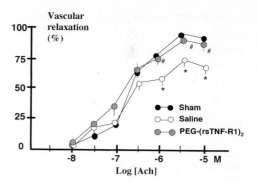

Fig. 3. Cumulative dose responses to various concentrations of acetylcholine (Ach) in aortic rings from animals that underwent sham-operation (Sham), cecal ligation and puncture (CLP) with normal saline (Saline), or CLP with the TNF inhibitor PEG-(rsTNF-R1)$_2$; * p<0.05 vs Sham; # p < 0.05 vs Saline (From [35] with permission)

dysfunction observed during septic shock. Using a TNF-α biological activity blocker they prevented vascular endothelial cell structure injury and dysfunction that occurs during CLP-associated septic shock (Fig. 3). Therefore, they suggested that pharmacological agents that inhibit TNF-α biological activity and/or production may be useful for protecting endothelial cells during sepsis. Interestingly, Polte et al. [36] recently demonstrated that NO protects endothelial cells from TNF-α-mediated cytotoxicity, presumably via a cGMP-dependent pathway. As conventional heparins are known to increase *in vitro* endothelial-NO synthesis, Morrisson et al. [37] tested heparin and the non-anticoagulant heparin GM1892 on sepsis-induced alterations in endothelium-derived relaxation. GM1892 and heparin maintained acetylcholine induced vascular relaxation in a rat CLP model of sepsis. In the same way, we used an angiotensin converting enzyme (ACE) inhibitor for its potential to interfere with the endothelial NO pathway. Indeed, we previously demonstrated that the ACE inhibitor perindopril allowed recovery of normal neoendothelium-derived relaxation after *in vivo* mechanical de-endothelialization [38]. This effect was suppressed by concurrent NOS inhibition. Likewise, in endotoxemic rabbits, we demonstrated that

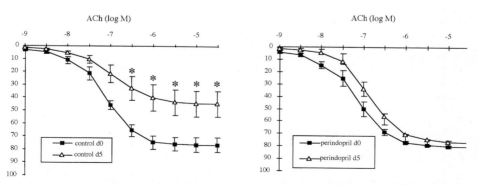

Fig. 4. Cumulative dose responses to various concentration of acetylcholine (Ach) in aortic rings from control rabbits (left) and perindopril treated rabbits (right) before (control d0, perindopril d0) and five days (control d5, perindopril d5) after endotoxin injection; * p < 0.05 vs d0

perindopril was able to prevent occurrence of endothelial-dependent relaxation impairment (unpublished results, Fig. 4). NOS inhibition also suppressed the effects of perindopril. However, the preventive effect of perindopril was not associated with a reduction in endothelial or monocyte tissue factor expression, suggesting that these sepsis-associated abnormalities are not strictly linked.

Conclusions

Several key endothelial cell functions are impaired during septic shock. One of these key functions involves endothelial cell NO production. Although the properties of NO include major protective effects on the endothelium, other important endothelial cell functions exist and do not involve the NO pathway. Endothelial-directed therapies might in the future involve these other aspects of endothelium function, such as, for example, inhibition of intravascular coagulation. Nevertheless, the decreased endothelium-derived NO production during sepsis appears to be deleterious. Therefore, administration of NOS inhibitors during sepsis does not seem particularly appropriate. Indeed, this type of treatment results in intrahepatic thrombosis, increased hepatic parenchymal damage, decreased kidney perfusion, and increased mortality in experimental animals [37, 39], despite correction of impaired vascular contractility.

Since endothelial cells are implicated in the pathophysiologic mechanisms of septic shock, their destruction and/or dysfunction might be, at least in part, involved in the occurrence of multiple organ failure syndrome. Endothelial cell dysfunction may also compromise sepsis recovery and patient outcome. Indeed, abnormal endothelium-derived vascular reactivity is involved as a prominent pathological feature in diseases such as hypertension, diabetes or atherosclerosis, and it is possible that this feature is partly responsible for the increased risk of death in septic patients following hospital discharge as found by Quartin et al. [40].

References

1. Gaynor E, Bouvier C, Spaet T (1958) Circulating endothelial cells in endotoxin-treated rabbits. Clin Res 16:535
2. Reidy MA, Schwartz SM (1983) Endothelial injury and regeneration. IV. Endotoxin: a nondenuding injury to aortic endothelium. Lab Invest 48:25–34
3. Reidy MA, Bowyer DE (1977) Scanning electron microscopy: morphology of aortic endothelium following injury by endotoxin and during subsequent repair. Atherosclerosis 26:319–328
4. Young JS, Headrick JP, Berne RM (1991) Endothelial-dependent and -independent responses in the thoracic aorta during endotoxic shock. Circ Shock 35:25–30
5. Wang P, Wood TJ, Zhou M, Ba ZF, Chaudry IH (1996) Inhibition of the biological activity of tumor necrosis factor maintains vascular endothelial cell function during hyperdynamic sepsis. J Trauma 40:694–701
6. Lee M, Schuessler G, Chien S (1988) Time dependent effects of endotoxin on the ultrastructure of the aortic endothelium. Artery 15:71–89
7. Leclerc J, Pu Q, Corseaux D, Jude B, Vallet B (1997) Prolonged blood vessel dysfunctions after single endotoxin injection in rabbit. Intensive Care Med 23 (Suppl I):S49 (Abst)
8. Bombeli T, Mueller M, Haeberli A (1997) Anticoagulant properties of the vascular endothelium. Thromb Haemost 77:408–423

9. Kirchhofer D, Tschopp TB, Hadvary P, Baumgartner HR (1994) Endothelial cells stimulated with tumor necrosis factor-alpha express varying amounts of tissue factor resulting in inhomogenous fibrin deposition in a native blood flow system. J Clin Invest 93:2073–2083
10. Ten Cate H, Brandjes D, Wolters H, Van Deventer S (1993) Disseminated intravascular coagulation: pathophysiology, diagnosis, and treatment. New Horizons 1:312–323
11. Varani J, Ward P (1994) Mechanisms of endothelial cell injury in acute inflammation. Shock 2:311–319
12. Ma X, Tsao P, Lefer A (1991) Antibody to CD-18 exerts endothelial cell and cardiac protective effects in myocardial ischemia and reperfusion. J Clin Invest 88:1237–1243
13. Sessler C, Windsor A, Schwartz M, et al (1995) Circulating ICAM-1 is increased in septic shock. Am J Respir Crit Care Med 151:1420–1427
14. Mantovani A, Bussolino F, Introna M (1997) Cytokine regulation of endothelial cell function: from molecular level to the bedside. Immunol Today 18:231–240
15. Furchgott R, Zawadzki J (1980) The obligatory role of endothelial cells in the relaxation of arterial smooth muscle by acetylcholine. Nature 288:373–376
16. Decoene C, Lebuffe G, Vallet B (1997) Endothelium-dependent relaxation is impaired after endotoxic shock in rabbits. Am J Respir Crit Care Med 155:A926 (Abst)
17. Parker J, Keller R, DeFily D, Laughlin M, Movotny M, Adams H (1991) Coronary vascular smooth muscle function in E. coli endotoxemia in dogs. Am J Physiol 260:H832–H842
18. Umans JG, Wylam ME, Samsel RW, Edwards J, Schumacker PT (1993) Effects of endotoxin *in vivo* on endothelial and smooth-muscle function in rabbit and rat aorta. Am Rev Respir Dis 148:1638–1645
19. Yoshizumi M, Perrella MA, John C, Burnett J, Lee M-E (1993) Tumor necrosis factor down-regulates an endothelial nitric oxide synthase mRNA by shortening its half-life. Circ Res 73:205–209
20. Lu J-L, Schmiege LM, Kuo L, Liao JC (1996) Downregulation of endothelial constitutive nitric oxide synthase expression by lipopolysaccharide. Biochem Biophys Res Comm 225:1–5
21. Zhou M, Wang P, Chaudry IH (1997) Endothelial nitric oxide synthase is downregulated during hyperdynamic sepsis. Biochim Biophys Acta 1335:182–190
22. Smith R, Palmer R, Moncada S (1991) Coronary vasodilatation induced by endotoxin in the rabbit isolated perfused heart is nitric oxide-dependent and inhibited by dexamethasone. Br J Pharmacol 140:5–6
23. Lübbe A, Garrison R, Cryer H, Alsip N, Harris P (1992) EDRF as a possible mediator of sepsis-induced arteriolar dilatation in skeletal muscle. Am J Physiol 262:H880–H887
24. Schneider F, Schott C, Stoclet J, Julou-Schaeffer G (1992) L-arginine induces relaxation of small mesenteric arteries from endotoxin-treated rats. Eur J Pharmacol 211:269–272
25. Wang P, Ba ZF, Chaudry IH (1995) Endothelium-dependent relaxation is depressed at the macro- and microcirculatory levels during sepsis. Am J Physiol 269:R988–R994
26. Lam C, Tyml K, Martin C, Sibbald W (1994) Microvascular perfusion is impaired in a rat model of normotensive sepsis. J Clin Invest 94:2077-2083
27. Vallet B (1994) Vascular reactivity and tissue oxygenation. In: Vincent JL (ed) Yearbook of intensive care and emergency medicine. Springer-Verlag, Berlin, Heidelberg, New York, pp 550–563
28. Curtis S, Vallet B, Winn M, Caufield J, Cain S (1995) Ablation of the vascular endothelium causes an oxygen extraction defect in canine skeletal muscle. J Appl Physiol 79:1352–1360
29. Bhagat K, Collier J, Vallance P (1996) Local venous responses to endotoxin in humans. Circulation 94:490–497
30. Bhagat K, Moss R, Collier J, Vallence P (1996) Endothelial "stunning" following a brief exposure to endotoxin: a mechanism to link infection and infarction? Cardiovasc Res 32:822–829
31. Nevière R, Mathieu D, Chagnon J-L, Lebleu N, Millien J, Wattel F (1996) Skeletal muscle microvascular blood flow and oxygen transport in patients with severe sepsis. Am J Respir Crit Care Med 153:191–195
32. MacNaul K, Hutchinson N (1993) Differential expression of iNOS and cNOS mRNA in human vascular smooth muscle cells and endothelial cells under normal and inflammatory conditions. Bichem Biophys Res Comm 196:1330–1334
33. Liu C, Adcock I, Old R, Barnes P, Evans T (1996) Differential regulation of the constitutive and inducible nitric oxide synthase mRNA by lipopolysaccharide treatment *in vivo* in the rat. Crit Care Med 24:1219–1225

34. Cobb JP, Danner RL (1996) Nitric oxide and septic shock. JAMA 275:1192–1196
35. Zhang H, De Jongh R, De Backer D, Checkaoui S, Vincent JL (1997) Effects of adrenergic agonists on hepatosplanchnic perfusion and oxygen extraction in endotoxic shock. Am J Respir Crit Care Med 155:A402 (Abst)
36. Polte T, Oberle S, Schröder H (1997) Nitric oxide protects endothelial cells from tumor necrosis factor-alpha-mediated cytotoxicity: possible involvment of cyclic-GMP. FEBS lett 409:46–48
37. Morrison AM, Wang P, Chaudry IH (1996) A novel nonanticoagulant heparin prevents vascular endothelial cell dysfunction during hyperdynamic sepsis. Shock 6:46–51
38. Van Belle E, Vallet B, Auffray JL, et al (1996) NO synthesis is involved in structural and functional effects of ACE inhibitors in injured arteries. Am J Physiol 270:H298–H305
39. Jourdain M, Tournoys A, Leroy X, et al (1997) Effects of Nomega-nitro-L-arginine methyl ester on the endotoxin-induced disseminated intravascular coagulation in porcine septic shock. Crit Care Med 25:452–459
40. Quartin AA, Schein RMH, Kett DH, Peduzzi PN (1997) Magnitude and duration of the effect of sepsis on survival. JAMA 277:1058–1063

Alterations of Important Regulators
of Macro- and Microcirculation in the Critically Ill

J. Boldt, D. Mentges, and B. Kumle

Introduction

Profound (peripheral) circulatory defect is the predominant cause of progressive organ failure, and ultimately, death in the critically ill [1]. Regulation of sufficient nutritive tissue blood flow is likely to be due to a balance between systemic and local regulators of blood flow. Maintenance of adequate circulation and fluid homeostasis is controlled through complex mechanisms, which include antidiuretic hormone (ADH), the renin-aldosterone-angiotensin system, and the autonomic nervous system. The principal actions of these systems are to restore water or intravascular volume deficit and to guarantee sufficient organ perfusion. Altered activity of these regulating systems is known to occur in stress situations, e.g., trauma, surgery, and critical illness (Table 1) [2, 3]. Several studies have shown a high incidence of postoperative complications in surgical patients as well as increased morbidity and mortality in intensive care patients with abnormal hormonal responses [5, 6]. Loss of (microregional) vascular control will result in some capillary regions being overperfused while others will be underperfused relative to oxygen needs [6]. In recent years, vasoactive substances released by the heart (atrial natriuretic peptide [ANP]) and produced by the endothelium (e.g. nitric oxide [NO], endothelin) have offered a new dimension when looking at regulators of the circulation [8, 9, 10]. It has been shown that endothelial-derived vasoactive factors are intimately involved in the pathophysiology of circulatory abnormalities and inadequate tissue perfusion [11]. Local endothelial cell injury results in the release of substances which may initiate or sustain derangements of microcirculatory hemodynamics, volume homeostasis, and blood pressure [12]. The function of some of these substances is not well understood, particularly in the critically ill. In the critically ill release of various vasoactive mediators may override normal autoregulation. The inability of tissues to

Table 1. Profile of vasoconstrictive substance during septic shock. (Modified from [41] with permission)

Substance	Concentration (control)	Onset of release	Magnitude of release
Vasopressin	4 pg/ml	15 min	× 500
Catecholamine	50–300 pg/ml	5 min	× 100–500
Angiotensin	100 µg/ml	20 min	× 60

extract adequate amounts of oxygen to meet their metabolic demands plays a key role in the development of multiple organ failure. Several mechanisms are involved in ineffective peripheral tissue oxygen extraction. The balance between these many, often opposing, humoral regulators of blood flow mainly determines (micro-) perfusion and thus organ function.

Circulating Catecholamines

Activation of vascular control is effected through nervous and humoral mechanisms. Activation of the sympathetic system involves a complex interaction of different stimuli including hypotension, hypovolemia, anxiety, and others [14]. In the critically ill, sympathetic activity is most likely elevated due to excitatory afferents from underperfused tissues and/or increased activity of baroreceptors. Renal hypoperfusion is one of the possible consequences of this increased sympathetic activity. This, however, may result in activation of the renin-angiotensin-system (RAS), which in turn enhances sympathetic activity. This induces the vicious cycle of vasoconstriction, organ dysfunction, volume retention, and cardiac decompensation. The increase in catecholamine plasma levels reflects the magnitude of the sympathetic nervous system response in this situation. An interplay with other regulators of circulation can additionally be assumed. Results from animal and human studies suggest that epinephrine stimulates ANP secretion, by which the negative effects of epinephrine on the (micro-) circulation may be compensated. Interestingly, changes in catecholamine plasma levels cannot always be correlated with hemodynamic parameters (e.g., mean arterial pressure, cardiac index, systemic vascular resistance). The lack of an adequate response to sympathomimetic vasoactive therapy is a common denominator of septic patients who die. It has been shown that mediators of sepsis may alter the normal response to (endogenous and exogenous) vasoactive substances. A "down-regulation" of the adrenoceptor system, counter-regulation by anti-vasoconstrictive hormones (e.g., ANP) or local substances released by the endothelium (e.g., NO) may account for this phenomenon.

The Renin-Angiotensin System

The RAS appears to play a pivotal role in the control of cardiovascular homeostasis and is markedly involved in the pathogenesis of various circulatory disorders [14, 15]. In the critically ill intensive care patient, activation of the RAS and the sympathetic nervous system is a compensatory mechanism to maintain peripheral perfusion. Initially this compensatory neurohumoral activation is beneficial, but with progress of the disease this mechanism becomes deleterious and may be associated with the development of multiple organ dysfunction syndrome (MODS).

The RAS is involved in short- as well as long-term blood pressure control by influencing sodium reabsorption, and by directly and indirectly influencing blood vessels. Angiotensin II appears to be of particular importance in this context because it is approximately 40 times as potent as norepinephrine [16]. In addition to its own vasoconstrictive properties, angiotensin II also influences vascular tone by indirect mechanisms, e.g., stimulation of the secretion of vasopressin and activation of the sympathetic nervous system [5]. The RAS not only mediates systemic hypertension, it also appears to be markedly involved in microcirculatory perfusion deficits. The gut and kidney are organs which are very susceptible to ischemia secondary to hypoperfusion. The gut is one of the organs first affected by impaired circulation in the critically ill [17, 18]. The increased gut mucosal permeability with the risk of bacterial translocation is most likely due to a decrease in splanchnic blood flow. It has been shown that the RAS plays an important role in mediating the disproportionate splanchnic hypoperfusion secondary to cardiogenic shock [18, 19].

Atrial Natriuretic Peptide (ANP)

In recent years, the discovery of ANP has added new insight into the regulation of blood pressure and volume homeostasis [20]. The exact role of ANP, however, has not yet been fully elucidated. ANP plays an important role in the control of blood pressure and blood volume [21]. It participates in the regulation of vasomotor tone either directly by its vasodilating actions or indirectly by its influence on hormone homeostasis: It has been reported to stop renin secretion in the kidney [22], and endothelin-1 has been shown to stimulate the release of ANP *in vivo* and *in vitro* [23, 24]. ANP plasma levels are related to atrial volume and pressure although the release of ANP seems to be more volume- than pressure-dependent [25, 26]. Relatively little is known about changes in ANP plasma levels in critical illness. In septic patients with acute respiratory failure, ANP was reported to be significantly elevated from normal [27], probably to prevent excess fluid retention in these patients who are developing (interstitial) pulmonary edema.

Endothelin

Recent evidence suggests that endothelial cells are markedly involved in the regulation of (micro-) circulatory perfusion. It has become obvious that substances released by the endothelium (prostaglandin I_2 [PGI_2], NO, angiotensin II) are intimately involved in the pathophysiology of macro- and microcirculatory abnormalities [11, 28–31]. Endothelin (ET-1, -2, -3) is one of the substances which has attracted attention. This 21-amino-acid peptide appears to have a greater vasoconstricting potency than any other known substance including vasopressin or catecholamines. ET seems to be involved in regional vasoconstriction followed by impaired organ blood flow. Increased shear stress, activated leukocytes, hypotension, low cardiac output, and an increase in circulating catecholamine levels are reported to increase ET plasma levels [24, 28]. In a study of 11 traumatized patients, the magnitude of ET plasma concentration correlated well with the extent of trauma [32]: All patients showed an elevated ET plasma level on admission to the intensive care unit (ranging from 0.9 to 2.3 fmol/ml), and the highest increase (4.8 fmol/l) was seen in patients with an injury severity score > 40. The interference of ET with other regulators of (micro-) circulation has not yet been clearly defined [12]. ET has been reported to stimulate the release of catecholamines and vasopressin [24], thus contributing to vasoconstriction and modifying blood flow at the microcirculatory level. ET also stimulates angiotensin-converting enzyme (ACE) activity thus elevating angiotensin II levels [33], by which the vasoconstricting properties of ET are potentiated. On the other hand, angiotensin II appears to induce ET release from endothelial cells [34]. It is of particular interest that the vasoconstrictive properties of ET are opposed by the release of other hormones including ANP and *vice versa* [24]. Plasma concentrations of ET-1 are likely to be higher at the interface of the endothelium than in the bloodstream [11]. Thus ET-1 is assumed to be a local rather than a systemic regulating factor.

Circulating Vasoactive Substances in Traumatized and Septic Patients

In a prospective study [35], plasma levels of important regulators of circulation were serially measured over 5 days in traumatized and septic patients. Septic patients

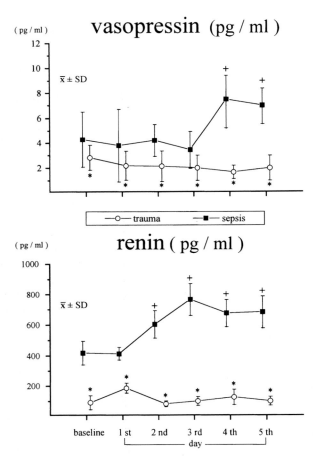

Fig. 1. Changes in plasma levels of vasopressin and renin in trauma and sepsis patients. * $p < 0.05$ different from the other group; $^+$ $p < 0.05$ different from baseline. (Modified from [35] with permission)

showed much more pronounced alterations in plasma levels of substances which are responsible for guaranteeing systemic and regional circulation, than the (non-septic) trauma patients (Figs. 1 and 2). Starting from already elevated baseline values, vasopressin (+75%), renin (+63%), epinephrine (+295%), norepinephrine (+248%), and ET (+193%) plasma levels further increased in the septic patients during the study period. The ongoing alterations in plasma levels of these regulators may sustain or even induce organ dysfunction in the septic patient.

The endocrine profile did not always parallel the hemodynamic changes. ANP plasma levels for example were markedly higher in the septic than in the traumatized patients, which can be explained only in part by the differences in loading pressures [e.g. pulmonary capillary wedge pressure (PCWP), central venous pressure (CVP)]. Other vasoactive substances may modify ANP plasma levels: Endothelin-1 has been shown to stimulate the release of ANP *in vivo* and *in vitro* [23, 24]. Both substances initiate important interactions at the vascular level: ANP appears to counteract the vasoconstrictive response to endothelin-1 [36]. ANP also influences plasma levels of other vasoactive substances [9, 25]: For example, it inhibits the release of renin from the juxtaglomerular apparatus. Although the effects of ANP on

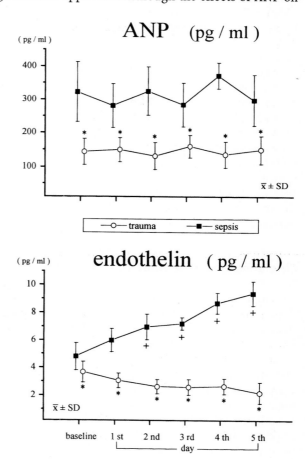

Fig. 2. Changes in plasma levels of atrial natriuretic peptide (ANP) and endothelin-1 in trauma and sepsis patients. * p < 0.05 different from the other group; + p < 0.05 different from baseline. (Modified from [35] with permission)

vasopressin release are not clearly defined, ANP appears to antagonize the vascular effects of vasopressin and the RAS [37].

ET-1 plasma levels were also significantly higher in the septic than in trauma patients [35]. This is in accordance with a study of 6 patients suffering from septic shock, in whom the ET-1 plasma concentration was significantly elevated (14.2 ± 5.2 pg/ml) [38]. In another study in septic patients, the greatest severity of disease paralleled with the highest level of ET-1 and an inverse relationship of ET-1 to cardiac index was found [39].

Differences in Circulating Vasoactive Substances between Survivors and Non-Survivors

It appears to be of particular interest whether survivors and non-survivors differ with regard to regulators of circulation. Thus plasma levels of important vasoactive substances were compared between surviving and non-surviving critically ill patients [40]. Plasma levels of renin (from 206 ± 40 to 595 ± 81 pg/ml) and vasopressin (from 5.78 to 7.97 pg/ml) increased significantly in the non-survivors. ANP plasma levels significantly increased also only in the non-survivors (from 188 ± 63 to 339 ± 55 pg/ml). ET-1 decreased in the survivors, whereas it significantly increased in the non-survivors (from 3.62 ± 0.68 to 9.37 ± 0.94 pg/ml) during the study period. Epinephrine and norepinephrine plasma concentrations were already elevated in the non-survivors at baseline and tremendously increased in these patients during the following days. Other authors have also shown that in patients whose clinical status improved, catecholamine plasma levels declined, whereas in patients who died, plasma levels (particularly norepinephrine) remained markedly elevated or even increased [41]. In survivors, plasma levels of important vasoactive substances almost normalized within the study period of 5 days. At the moment it can only be speculated whether these regulating systems were influenced by activation of various mediator cascades (e.g., coagulation system, various cytokines) or whether the vasoactives substances themselves influenced the negative outcome in the non-survivors.

Circulating Vasoactive Substances in Patients with Renal Failure

Development of acute renal failure (ARF) in intensive care patients is associated with a massive activation of sympathetic activity with secondary activation of the RAS. This aims to preserve perfusion pressure and glomerular filtration on the one hand, and to counteract the reduced renal blood flow secondary to the impaired circulation by the underlying disease on the other hand [42]. When ARF is established, alterations in regulators of circulatory homeostasis are also of interest, particularly when renal replacement therapy is used. Mortality of patients with ARF remains high in intensive care patients [44] in spite of sophisticated renal replacement techniques (dialysis, hemofiltration). The question thus arises how far (endocrine) regulators of the (micro-) circulation are influenced by continuous (pump-driven) veno-venous hemofiltration (CVVH). In a prospective study [44], changes in vaso-

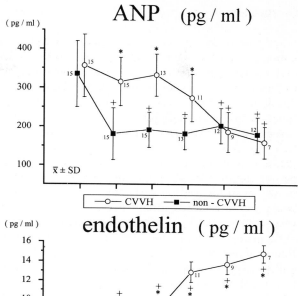

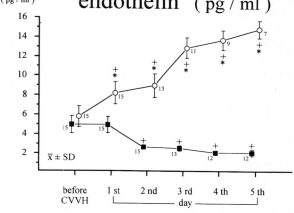

Fig. 3. Changes in plasma levels of atrial natriuretic peptide (ANP) and endothelin-1 in patients with acute renal failure undergoing continuous (pump-driven) veno-venous hemofiltration (CVVH) in comparison to a comparable group of patients without CVVH. Numbers indicate number of measured patients (baseline: n = 15; nonsurvivors in the CVVH group during the study period: n = 8). * $p < 0.05$ different from the other group; + $p < 0.05$ different from baseline. (Modified from [44] with permission)

active substances in critically ill patients with and without CVVH were serially monitored (Fig. 3). The renin plasma level was significantly higher already at baseline in the CVVH patients (907 ± 184 pg/ml) and further increased during CVVH (to 1,453 ± 186 pg/ml). Vasopressin increased only in the CVVH group (from 3.80 ± 0.66 to 11.85 ± 1.05 pg/ml). Plasma catecholamines were significantly elevated in the CVVH patients already at baseline (epinephrine: 5,011 ± 1,888 pg/ml; norepinephrine: 8,122 ± 2,011 pg/ml) and they further increased until the 5th day. ANP plasma levels were elevated in both groups at baseline (> 300 pg/ml). ANP decreased in the CVVH patients on the 4th and 5th days (to 190 ± 45 pg/ml). ET-1 plasma concentrations significantly increased only in the CVVH group (from 5.81 ± 1.07 to 14.8 ± 0.88 pg/ml). Changes in endocrine regulators did not reveal any relationship to the measured hemodynamic parameters. In patients undergoing pump-driven CVVH, plasma levels of important systemic and local vasoconstrictors increased significantly during CVVH. Disturbances in the balance of regulators of circulatory homeostasis may contribute to persisting organ failure, and the still high mortality in these patients.

Conclusion

Blood flow is usually regulated to match the tissues' metabolic needs. Several components are responsible for circulatory control at the central, regional and microregional levels including various vasoactive substances. Physiologic compensatory responses aim to maintain overall circulatory function and integrity. Abnormal distribution of blood flow is an important factor in the development of organ dysfunction in the critically ill [45]. Critical illness may lead to the release of potent vasopressors which can cause organ perfusion abnormalities. Splanchnic vasoconstriction results from the release of these vasoactive substances although there is a marked increase in the need for oxygen delivery in this situation. Therapeutic endpoints should attempt to prevent tissue hypoperfusion. In recent years interest has mostly been focused on activation of various mediator cascades and their circulatory and metabolic consequences. The extent to which these mediators influence vasoactive regulators or *vice versa* cannot be fully defined. Nevertheless, alterations of regulators of circulation may have important consequences for patient outcome. Interactions between positive and negative inotropic factors as well as vasodilating and vasoconstricting substances determine the cardiovascular profile of the critically ill. An imbalance of these regulatory systems may result in hemodynamic catastrophe. There is a complex interplay among these regulators, and an increase in any one may (directly or indirectly) interact with another. Whether (selectively) influencing these circulating vasoactive substances may improve the outcome of the critically ill warrants further study.

References

1. Thijs LG, Groneveld ABJ (1987) The circulatory defect in septic shock. In: Vincent JL, Thijs LG (eds) Septic shock – european view. Springer-Verlag, Berlin, Heidelberg, New York, pp 161–178
2. Bersten AD, Sibbald W (1989) Circulatory disturbances in multiple system organ failure. Crit Care Clin 5:233–254
3. Intaglietta M (1989) Objectives for the treatment of the microcirculation in ischemia, shock, and reperfusion. In: Vincent JL (ed) Update in Intensive Care and Emergency Medicine Vol 8. Springer-Verlag, Berlin, Heidelberg, New York, pp 293–298
4. Felicetta JV, Sowers JR (1987) Endocrine changes with critical illness. Crit Care Clin 5:855–869
5. van Zwieten PA, de Jong A (1986) Interaction between the adrenergic and the renin-angiotensin systems. Postgrad Med J 62 (suppl 1):23-27
6. Cain SM (1992) Tissue hypoxia in animal models of sepsis. In: Vincent JL (ed) Yearbook of Intensive Care and Emergency Medicine. Springer-Verlag, Berlin, Heidelberg, New York, pp 281–293
7. Lüscher TF (1992) Endothelin: Systemic arterial and pulmonary effects of a new peptide with biologic properties. Am Rev Respir Dis 146 (suppl 2):S56–S60
8. Rushkoaho H, Lang RE, Toth M, Ganten D, Unger T (1987) Release and regulation of atrial natriuretic peptide (ANP). Eur Heart J 8 (suppl B):99–109
9. Needleman P, Greewald JE (1986) Atriopeptin: a cardiac hormone intimately involved in fluid, electrolyte, and blood-pressure hemostasis. N Engl J Med 314:828–834
10. Underwood RD, Chan DP, Burnett JC (1991) Endothelin: An endothelium-derived vasoconstrictor peptide and its role in congestive heart failure. Heart Failure 4:50–58
11. Vane JR, Änggard EE, Botting RM (1990) Regulatory functions of the vascular endothelium. N Engl J Med 323:27–36

12. Brenner BM, Troy JL, Ballermann B (1989) Endothelium-dependent vascular responses. J Clin Invest 84:1373–1378
13. Turnbull AV, Little RA (1993) Neuro-hormonal regulation after trauma. Circulating cytokines may also contribute to an activated sympathetic-adrenal control. In: Vincent JL (ed) Update in Intensive Care and Emergency Medicine Vol 16. Springer-Verlag, Berlin, Heidelberg, New York, pp 574–581
14. Colson P (1993) Angiotensin-converting enzyme inhibition in cardiovascular anesthesia. J Cardiothorac Vasc Anesth 6:734–742
15. Fleetwood G, Boutinet S, Meier M, Wood JM (1991) Involvement of the renin-angiotensin system in ischemic damage and reperfusion arrhythmias in the isolated perfused rat heart. J Cardiovasc Pharmacol 17:351–356
16. Kostis JB, DeFelice EA, Pianko LJ (1987) The renin-angiotensin system. In: Kostis JB, DeFelice EA (eds) Angiotensin converting enzyme inhibitors. Alan R Liss, New York, pp 1–18
17. Richter C, Dousau MP, Guidicelli JF (1987) Systemic and regional hemodynamic profile of five angiotensin I converting enzyme inhibitors in the spontaneously breathing rat. Am J Cardiol 59:12D–17D
18. McNeill JR, Stark RD, Greeway CV (1970) Intestinal vaso-constriction after hemorrhage: roles of vasopressin and angiotensin. Am J Physiol 219:1342–1347
19. Bailey RW, Bulkley GB, Hamilton SR, Morris JB, Haglund U (1987) Protection of small intestine from nonoclusive mesenteric ischemic injury due to cardiogenic shock. Am J Surg 153:108–116
20. Flezzani P, McIntryre W, Xuan YT, Su YF, Leslie JB, Watkins WD (1988) Atrial natriuretic peptide plasma levels during cardiac surgery. J Cardiothorac Anesth 3:274–280
21. Athanassopoulos G, Cokkino DV (1991) Atrial natriuretic factor. Prog Cardiovasc Disease 5:313–328
22. Laragh JH, Atlas SA (1988) Atrial natriuretic hormone: a regulator of blood pressure and volume hemostasis. Kidney Internat 34 (suppl 25):S64–S71
23. Fukuda Y, Hirata Y, Yoshimi H (1988) Endothelin is a potent secretagogue for atrial natriuretic peptide in cultured rat atrial myocytes. Biochem Biophys Res Commun 155:167–172
24. Goetz KL, Wang BC, Madwed JB, Zhu JL, Leadley RJJ (1988) Cardiovascular, renal, and endocrine responses to intravenous endothelin in conscious dogs. Am J Physiol 255:R1064–R1068
25. Atlas SA (1986) Atrial natriuretic factor: a new hormone of cardiac origin. Recent Prog Horm Res 42:207–209
26. Bates ER, Shenker Y, Grekin RJ (1986) The relationship between plasma levels of immuno-reactive atrial natriuretic hormone and hemodynamic function in man. Circulation 73:1155–1161
27. Mitaka C, Nagura T, Sakaishi N, Tsunoda Y, Toyooka H (1990) Plasma alpha-atrial natriuretic peptide concentrations in acute respiratory failure with sepsis: prelimary study. Crit Care Med 18:1201–1207
28. Ganghi CR, Berkowitz DE, Watkins D (1994) Endothelins. Biochemistry and pathophysiologic actions. Anesthesiology 80:892–905
29. Dzau VJ (1988) Circulating versus local renin-angiotensin in cardiovascular homeostasis. Circulation 77 (suppl I):4–13
30. Palmer RM, Ashton DS, Moncada S (1988) Vascular endothelial cells synthesize nitric oxide from L-arginine. Nature 333:664–666
31. Lincoln J, Loesch A, Burnszock G (1990) Localization of vasopressin, serotonin and angiotensin II in endothelial cells of the renal and mesentric arteries in the rat. Cell Tissue Res 259:341–344
32. Koller J, Mair P, Wiser C, Pomaroli A, Puschendorf B, Herold M (1991) Endothelin and big endo-thelin concentration in injured patients. N Engl J Med 325:1518
33. Kawaguchi H, Sawa H, Yasuada H (1990) Endothelin stimulates angiotensin to angiotensin II conversion in cultured pulmonary artery endothelial cells. J Mol Cell Cardiol 22:839–842
34. Emori T, Hirata Y, Ohita K, et al (1991) Cellular mechanisms of endothelin-1. Release by angio-tensin and vasopressin. Hypertension 18:265–270
35. Boldt J, Wollbrück M, Menges T, Diridis K, Hempelmann G (1994) Regulators of circulatory homeostasis in the critically ill – a comparison between traumatized and septic patients. Clin Intensive Care 5:164–171

36. Marsden PA, Danthuluri NR, Brenner BM, Ballermann BJ, Brock TA (1989) Endothelin action on vascular smooth muscle involves inositol trisphosphate and calcium mobilization. Biochem Biophys Res Commun 158:86–93
37. Ballerman BJ, Brenner BM (1986) Role of atrial peptides in body fluid homeostasis. Circ Res 58:619–630
38. Voerman HJ, Stehouwer DA, van Kamp GJ, Strack van Schijndel JM, Groeneveld J, Thijs LG (1992) Plasma endothelin levels are increased during septic shock. Crit Care Med 20:1097–1101
39. Pittet JF, Morel DR, Hemsen A (1991) Elevated endothelin-1 concentrations are associated with severity of illness in patients with sepsis. Ann Surg 213:261–264
40. Boldt J, Menges T, Kuhn D, Diridis C, Hempelmann G (1995) Alterations in circulating vasoactive substances in the critically ill – a comparison between survivors and non-survivors. Intensive Care Med 21:218–225
41. Wilson MF, Brackett DJ (1983) Release of vasoactive hormones and circulatory changes in shock. Circ Shock 11:225–234
42. Mayer N, Zimpfer M (1988) Cardiocirculatory control mechanisms in health and disease. In: Vincent JL (ed) Update in Intensive Care and Emergency Medicine, Vol 5. Springer-Verlag, Berlin, Heidelberg, New York, pp 3–12
43. Schaefer JH, Jochimsen F, Keller F, Wegscheider K, Distler A (1991) Outcome prediction of acute renal failure in medical intensive care. Intensive Care Med 17:19–24
44. Boldt J, Wollbrück M, Menges T, Diridis K, Hempelmann G (1994) Changes in regulators of circulation in patients undergoing continuous pump-driven veno-venous hemodilution. Shock 2:157–163
45. Takala J, Ruokonen E (1991) Blood flow and adrenergic drugs in septic shock. In: Vincent JL (ed) Update in Intensive Care and Emergency Medicine. Vol 14, Springer-Verlag, Berlin, Heidelberg, New York, pp 144–152

Microvascular Regulation of Tissue Oxygenation in Sepsis

P. B. Anning, M. Sair, and T. W. Evans

Introduction

Sepsis and its related syndromes develop frequently in hospitalized patients, with an associated mortality of 10–20%. In the presence of circulatory failure, this figure rises to over 60% and may account for up to 200,000 deaths per annum in the USA alone [1]. Most patients succumb to a multiple organ dysfunction syndrome (MODS) rather than hypotension *per se* [2], but the reasons for this are not clear. Sepsis is known to disrupt microcirculatory flow and nutrient exchange, and an impaired response to endogenous and exogenous pressor agents is often reported [3]. Intravascular leukaggregation, abnormal red blood cell deformability, increased microvascular permeability, interstitial protein loss and tissue edema are frequently observed [4]. This systemic inflammatory response is promoted not only by reduced perfusion of nutrient vessels, but also from pro-inflammatory mediators released from activated, sequestered leukocytes, and activated macrophages, platelets and endothelial cells. It has been hypothesized that endothelial injury exacerbates maldistribution of regional blood flow leading to cellular hypoxia and vital organ dysfunction. Various injurious substances as well as several microbacteria toxins (e.g., peptoglycans from Gram-positive bacteria) may initiate this response. However, the most severe septic microvascular inflammatory responses are observed with Gram-negative bacteria, or more specifically the cell wall component, endotoxin.

Endotoxin and the Microvascular Inflammatory Response

Endotoxins are high molecular weight lipopolysaccharide (LPS) complexes which are integral components of the outer membranes of the cell walls of Gram-negative bacteria. These complexes are liberated from the bacteria when cell lysis occurs, with most of the toxic activity involving the lipid A moiety of the LPS component [5]. Both local or systemic Gram-negative infections can result in endotoxemia. Translocation of either endotoxin or Gram-negative bacteria across the wall of the gastrointestinal tract (GIT) into the circulation can also induce endotoxemia. This is usually due to increases in GIT permeability which occur in response to ischemia, stress, hemorrhage, trauma and abdominal surgery. However, even under healthy conditions, small quantities of endotoxin can be detected in portal blood [6, 7]. These small quantities of endotoxin are normally endocytosed by Kupffer cells in the liver, thereby preventing its build-up and any subsequent injurious effects in the systemic circulation [8]. Macrophages, neutrophils and monocytes located in other organs and tissues also contribute to the clearance of endotoxin.

Within the circulation, LPS combines with plasma components such as high-density lipoproteins or LPS binding protein (LBP) to form a LBP-LPS complex. This complex rapidly interacts with CD14, a high-affinity receptor for LPS expressed on monocytes/macrophages, resulting in the activation of these cells. The LBP-LPS complex can also interact with soluble CD14 in the blood, resulting in the stimulation of endothelial cells which do not themselves express CD14 [9]. The activation of these cell groups results in the implementation of a number of effector cascades and acute phase responses. These include the complement, coagulation, bradykinin/kinin, and hemopoietic systems, accompanied by the release of a large number of mediators. Of these, eicosanoids, nitric oxide (NO), cytokines, chemokines, adhesion molecules, reactive free radicals and platelet-activating factor all appear to be integral. Due to the intense interactions and potential synergistic effects of these systems and mediators, it is almost impossible to unravel the relevant importance of any one system or mediator. Further details of the biological activities of LPS are described in a number of review articles [10, 11].

Recently, the main thrust of clinical research in sepsis has involved the issue of adequate tissue oxygenation, especially in the microvasculature. This chapter outlines briefly the principal techniques used for assessing tissue oxygenation, whilst indicating relevant observations to sepsis.

Tissue Oxygenation

Systemic Tissue Oxygenation

In recent years, the principle technique for assessing tissue oxygenation has involved the measurement of the so called "Fick-derived variables", whole body oxygen delivery (DO_2) and oxygen consumption (VO_2) [12]. In health, DO_2 must be able to adapt to three or four fold increases in demand (e.g., during exercise). Tissue O_2 can be elevated by increasing cardiac output and DO_2, and also by increasing O_2 extraction. Above a certain critical value in DO_2 ($DO_{2\,crit}$), the level of VO_2 appears independent of changes in DO_2. Decreasing DO_2 in this region results in an increased O_2 extraction ratio and increased arterio-venous oxygen difference. Below $DO_{2\,crit}$, further reductions of DO_2 lead to a fall in VO_2 in a supply-dependent fashion. Initial observations of this biphasic relationship were made in animal studies and anesthetized human subjects. The observation of a single linear-phase relationship between these variables in patients admitted to the intensive care unit (ICU) led to the concept of pathological supply dependence and covert tissue oxygen debt. The discovery that survival was improved in high-risk surgical patients who achieved supranormal values of DO_2, VO_2, and cardiac index, led to the assertion that goal-directed therapy could reverse this tissue deficit and reduce mortality [13]. However, evidence to support this has been conflicting [14]. Studies using separate techniques to independently measure DO_2 and VO_2 have produced contradictory data. Furthermore, inotropes may exacerbate linkage by causing parallel increases in cardiac index and metabolic rate.

Impaired Vascular Reactivity

A decreased ability to extract O_2 has been observed in patients and in animal models of sepsis. During bacteremia or endotoxemia, regional changes in vascular tone are observed, suggesting that bacterial infection may induce redistribution of blood flow. Numerous studies have demonstrated impaired contractile responses to vaso-constrictors in vessels from endotoxemic animals [3, 15–17]. This effect was in-hibited by NO synthase (NOS) inhibitors [18], and was maintained in vessels in which the endothelium was removed, implying that the expression of inducible NOS (iNOS) in vascular smooth muscle is responsible for impaired contractile responses [15, 18]. However, the theory that excess NO production is solely responsible for the regional changes in blood flow is curbed by the observation that non-specific in-hibition of NOS fails to restore normal oxygen extraction in endotoxemia [19]. In addition, NOS inhibition produces mesenteric arteriolar vasoconstriction in con-trols, and exacerbates the microvascular changes in normotensive bacteremic rats [20]. Furthermore, treatment which increases α-adrenergic tone during sepsis, elevating perfusion pressure, does not improve oxygen extraction [21]. As oxygen extraction is supposedly the result of an equilibrium between vascular constriction and dilation, one explanation for the contrasting results above may be the presence of impaired vasodilator tone.

Numerous *in vitro* studies in dog, rabbit and rat have demonstrated impaired acetylcholine-induced endothelium-dependent relaxation in vascular rings follow-ing *in vivo* endotoxemia [16, 17]. This effect was attributed to impaired release of NO by the constitutive isoform of NOS (cNOS). Studies in rat microvascular mesenteric segment [22] and cremaster muscle [23] suggest that similar mechanisms are pre-sent in the microvasculature. In bacteremic, decerebrate rats, vasoconstriction of first and second order arterioles is accompanied by progressive dilation of locally regulated small, terminal pre-capillary arterioles [24, 25]. Studies using intravital microscopy in acutely septic rats have demonstrated a marked reduction in perfused diaphragmatic capillaries compared to hypovolemic controls with similar degrees of hypotension [26]. Observing microcirculatory changes using intravital microscopy in exteriorized ileum has also demonstrated vasoconstriction at all arteriolar levels in septic rats [27], despite preserved mesenteric arteriolar blood flow [28]. Further evidence that this reduction in capillary perfusion is independent of blood pressure is provided by skeletal intravital microscopy experiments in normotensive models of sepsis. One study [29] showed a 30% increase in mean intercapillary distance together with more than 250% increase in "stopped flow" capillaries in the digi-torum longus muscle of septic rats compared with controls. Specifically, a 30% reduction in perfused capillary density was observed in muscle with a marked in-crease in spatial heterogeneity [29], implying that sepsis affects the ability of the skeletal muscle microcirculation to distribute red blood cells and consequently O_2. Using laser Doppler flowmetry, the investigators also demonstrated that the func-tional hyperemic response of this muscle was impaired in the septic rats, implying that the ability of the microcirculation to respond to increases in O_2 requirements is defective in sepsis.

Intestinal Tissue Oxygenation

Experimental studies have demonstrated clearly the presence of gut mucosal hypoxia in sepsis, despite normal, or increased regional flow [30, 31]. This effect is probably due to impaired microvascular function, and a breakdown of microvascular flow regulation in the gut, resulting in an increase in muscle blood flow at the expense of the overlying mucosal layer. A number of *in vivo* studies have shown that inotropes, such as dopexamine can improve/reverse this flow imbalance by preferentially promoting blood flow to the mucosa [32, 33]. This effect appears to be mediated via dopamine-1 receptors. A recent study demonstrated that whilst both dopexamine and dopamine increased intestinal mucosal tissue oxygenation in a porcine model of endotoxemia, the β_1-agonist dobutamine, which has no dopaminergic actions, did not alter tissue oxygenation [34].

Gastric mucosal pH (pHi) levels are easily measured in patients using a nasogastric tonometer, and serve as a useful clinical indicator of the adequacy of splanchnic blood flow. pHi falls during sepsis as a result of hypoperfusion, with subsequent tissue hypoxia and acidosis [35]. This reduction in pHi is refractory to increases in systemic DO_2. Similar results have been observed in clinical investigations in septic patients with intramucosal acidosis. In one study [36], dopexamine was shown to increase gastric pHi in septic patients, with no corresponding changes in splanchnic blood flow, systemic DO_2 or cardiac output, indicating that the distribution of O_2 supply was improved at the microvascular level. Again, this was probably due to promotion of blood flow from the muscle to the mucosa. Another study [37] demonstrated that dobutamine induced an increase in systemic DO_2 and gastric pHi. Using laser Doppler flowmetry, the investigators observed an increase in gastric mucosal blood flow that was out of proportion to the parallel increase in systemic DO_2.

Microvascular Tissue Oxygenation

Tissue oxygenation can also be measured directly using microelectrodes which may be placed on the surface of, or implanted within tissue. The latter procedure has minimal effects on the microcirculation and causes little trauma [38]. Intramuscular polarographic needles can be left *in situ* to record local tissue PO_2 or advanced in a stepwise fashion enabling measurement of a tissue PO_2 profile.

Using this technique, a number of researchers have demonstrated marked reductions in tissue PO_2. In pigs with septic shock, impaired oxygenation appears to be a late manifestation of the condition [39], whilst in the rabbit, a marked reduction in tissue PO_2 is observed within 15 minutes of administration of endotoxin [40]. In a normodynamic model of rat sepsis, mean tissue PO_2 fell by almost 50% [41]. This was however, coupled with a significant fall in DO_2, and was prevented by fluid resuscitation in a treatment group. Conversely, other studies have demonstrated elevated tissue PO_2 in the endotoxemic rat bladder epithelium, indicating that changes in tissue oxygenation may be species and/or organ-specific [42, 43]. However, animals in these studies were also volume-resuscitated which has been shown to reverse falls in tissue PO_2 (see above and below). Depending on the duration and type of volume resuscitation, elevated tissue PO_2 might be expected in some studies. Our investigations have shown the presence of significant tissue hypoxia and abnormal microvascular regulation of tissue oxygenation in endotoxemic rats, despite apparently normal microcirculatory perfusion (Figs. 1 and 2). Although the tissue hypoxia observed was attenuated by volume resuscitation, our model of sepsis displayed a normodynamic circulation, suggesting that fluid deficit was limited to the peripheral microcirculation only [45]. By contrast, in control animals the non-specific NOS inhibitor, N^G-nitro-L-arginine methyl ester (L-NAME), caused significant tissue hypoxia similar to that observed in endotoxemia. Not surprisingly, L-NAME had no beneficial effect on tissue hypoxia in endotoxemic animals [46]. Moreover, administration of L-NAME together with volume resuscitation attenuated the beneficial effects of resuscitation alone on the endotoxemic-induced changes in tissue oxygenation described above (unpublished observations), indicating that L-NAME has detrimental effects on skeletal muscle tissue oxygenation.

PO$_2$ profiles have also been constructed in patients with sepsis using polarographic needle electrodes [47–49]. Initially, muscle PO_2 in patients with septic shock was shown to be lower than in controls [50]. By contrast, as with animal studies, others have demonstrated that mean tissue PO_2 in patients with sepsis/septic shock was significantly elevated compared with those with "limited infection" or cardiogenic shock [48]. However, neither investigator considered the effects of the administration of inotropic drugs, which are known to elevate tissue PO_2 [47, 51]. Despite this, the mean skeletal muscle PO_2 appeared directly proportional to the severity of the sepsis, adding weight to the concept of a primary O_2 utilization or extraction defect in resuscitated sepsis, rather than a delivery problem *per se.*

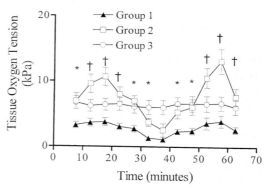

Fig. 1. *Experiment 1:* mean tissue oxygen tension response to changing inspired oxygen fraction (FiO$_2$). Group 1, endotoxemic rats in which the FiO$_2$ was altered every 10 minutes in the sequence 21% → 50% → 21% → 10% → 21% → 95% → 21% while continuous measurements of tissue PO_2 were made; group 2, sham-treated rats with identical FiO$_2$ protocol as *group 1*, and *group 3*, sham controls in which FiO$_2$ was constant at 21% throughout the experiment. Values are means ± SE. Significant differences between sham and endotoxemic ligation groups demonstrated using non-parametric ordinary ANOVA testing: *p < 0.05; †p < 0.01 (group 1 vs 2). (From [44] with permission)

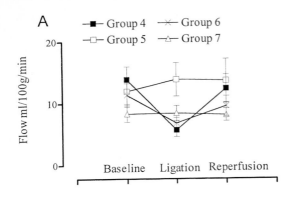

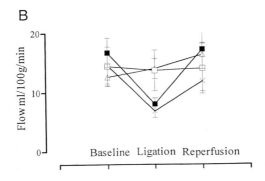

Fig. 2. *Experiment 2:* perfusion measurements. Group 4, endotoxemic ligation; group 5, endotoxemic control; group 6, sham ligation; and group 7, a sham control group. Non-parametric ordinary ANOVA did not demonstrate any differences between ligation groups. **A:** flow measured using H_2 clearance. **B:** flow measured using N_2O as the tracer gas. (From [44] with permission)

Conclusion

Both experimental and clinical data suggest that tissue hypoxia is a consequence of sepsis. Despite the availability of new experimental techniques for measuring tissue oxygen tension (e.g. microelectrodes), the phenomenon is poorly characterized. Results are conflicting, both elevated and decreased tissue oxygen tensions being observed. This can be partly attributed to a lack of uniformity with experimental protocols. Both our own data, and those of others have demonstrated that different interventions (e.g., volume resuscitation) can increase tissue oxygen tension in animal models of sepsis. Thus, this must be considered when assessing the severity of tissue hypoxia present, and its use accounted for if the pathophysiology of tissue hypoxia is being investigated. Similarly, patients are often given volume resuscitation and inotropes as treatment for sepsis. As both these interventions have been shown to increase tissue oxygen tension, they should be taken into account when interpreting results, especially when comparing different studies.

Further experiments are required to elucidate the exact mechanisms of sepsis-induced tissue hypoxia.

Acknowledgements. Dr. Peter Anning is supported by the British Heart Foundation.

References

1. Control CfD (1990) Increase in National Hospital discharge survey rates for septicemia – United States, 1979–1987. MMWR 39:31–34
2. St John RC, Dorinsky PM (1994) An overview of multiple organ dysfunction syndrome. J Lab Clin Med 124:478–483
3. Myers PR, Zhong Q, Jones JJ, Tanner MA, Adams HR, Parker JL (1995) Release of EDRF and NO in *ex vivo* perfused aorta: inhibition by *in vivo E. coli* endotoxemia. Am J Physiol 268:H955–H961
4. Curzen NP, Griffiths MJ, Evans TW (1994) Role of the endothelium in modulating the vascular response to sepsis. Clin Sci Colch 86:359–374
5. Raetz C (1990) Biochemistry of endotoxins. Ann Rev Biochem 59:129–170
6. Nolan J (1989) Intestinal endotoxins as mediators of hepatic injury – an idea whose time has come again. Hepatology 10:887–891
7. McCuskey R, Nishida J, Eguchi H (1995) Role of endotoxin in the hepatic microvascular inflammatory response to ethanol. J Gastroenterol Hepatol 10 (suppl 1):518–523
8. Ruiter D, van der Maulen J, Brouwer A, et al (1981) Uptake by liver cells of endotoxin following its intravenous injection. Lab Invest 45:38–45
9. Noel R, Sato T, Mendez C, Johnson M, Pohlman T (1995) Activation of human endothelial cells by viable or heat-killed gram-negative bacteria requires soluble CD14. Infect Immun 63:4046–4053
10. Ryan J, Morrison D (eds) (1992) Bacterial endotoxic lipopolysaccharides. II. Immunopharmacology and pathophysiology. CRC Press, Boca Raton
11. Szentivanyi E, Nowotny A, Friedman H (eds) (1986) Immunobiology and Immunopharmacology of bacterial endotoxins. Plenum Press, New York
12. Pallares LC, Evans TW (1992) Oxygen transport in the critically ill. Respir Med 86:289–295
13. Fiddian Green RG, Haglund U, Gutierrez G, Shoemaker WC (1993) Goals for the resuscitation of shock. Crit Care Med 21 (suppl 2):S25–S31
14. Hayes MA, Timmins AC, Yau EH, Palazzo M, Hinds CJ, Watson D (1994) Elevation of systemic oxygen delivery in the treatment of critically ill patients. N Engl J Med 330:1717–1722
15. McKenna TM (1988) Enhanced vascular effects of cyclic GMP in septic rat aorta. Am J Physiol 23:R436–R442
16. Parker JL, Keller RS, DeFily DV, Laughlin MH, Novotny MJ, Adams HR (1991) Coronary vascular smooth muscle function in *E. coli* endotoxemia in dogs. Am J Physiol 260:H832–H842
17. Umans JG, Wylam ME, Samsel RW, Edwards J, Schumacker PT (1993) Effects of endotoxin *in vivo* on endothelial and smooth muscle function in rabbit and rat aorta. Am Rev Respir Dis 148:1638–1645
18. Julou Schaeffer G, Gray GA, Fleming I, Schott C, Parratt JR, Stoclet JC (1990) Loss of vascular responsiveness induced by endotoxin involves L-arginine pathway. Am J Physiol 259:H1038–H1043
19. Schumacker PT, Kazaglis J, Connolly HV, Samsel RW, O'Connor MF, Umans JG (1995) Systemic and gut oxygen extraction during endotoxemia: role of nitric oxide synthesis. Am Rev Respir Crit Care Med 151:107–115.
20. Spain DA, Wilson MA, Bar Natan MF, Garrison RN (1994) Nitric oxide synthase inhibition aggravates intestinal microvascular vasoconstriction and hypoperfusion of bacteremia. J Trauma 36:720–725
21. Zhang H, De Jongh R, De Backer D, Checkaoui S, Vincent JL (1997) Effects of adrenergic agonists on hepatosplanchnic perfusion and oxygen extraction in endotoxic shock. Am J Resp Crit Care Med 155:A402 (Abst)
22. Wang P, Ba ZF, Chaudry IH (1995) Endothelium-dependent relaxation is depressed at the macro- and microcirculatory levels during sepsis. Am J Physiol 269:R988–R994
23. Lubbe AS, Garrison RN, Cryer HM, Alsip NL, Harris PD (1992) EDRF as a possible mediator of sepsis-induced arteriolar dilation in skeletal muscle. Am J Physiol 262:H880–H887
24. Cryer HM, Garrison RN, Kaebnick HW, Harris PD, Flint LM (1987) Skeletal microcirculatory responses to hyperdynamic *Escherichia coli* sepsis in unanesthetized rats. Arch Surg 122:86–92
25. Garrison RN, Cryer HMd (1989) Role of the microcirculation in skeletal muscle during shock. Prog Clin Biol Res 299:43–52

26. Boczkowski J, Vicaut E, Aubier M (1992) *In vivo* effects of *Escherichia coli* sepsis in unanaesthetized rats. J Appl Physiol 72:2219–2224
27. Steeb GD, Wilson MA, Garrison RN (1992) Pentoxifylline preserves small-intestine microvascular blood flow during bacteremia. Surgery 112:756–764
28. Theuer C, Wilson MA, Steeb GD, Garrison RN (1993) Microvascular vasoconstriction and mucosal hypoperfusion of the rat small intestine during bacteremia. Circ Shock 40:61–68
29. Lam C, Tyml K, Martin C, Sibbald W (1994) Microvascular perfusion is impaired in a rat model of normotensive sepsis. J Clin Invest 94:2077–2083
30. Hasibeder W, Germann R, Wolf H, et al (1996) Effects of short-term endotoxemia and dopamine on mucosal oxygenation in porcine jejunum. Am J Physiol 270:G667–G675
31. Ruokonen E, Takala J, Kari A, Saxen H, Mertsola J, Hansen E (1993) Regional blood flow and oxygen transport in septic shock. Crit Care Med 21:1296–1303
32. Cain S, Curtis S (1992) Systemic and regional oxygen uptake and lactate flux in endotoxic dogs resuscitated with dextran and dopexamine or dextran alone. Circ Shock 38:173–181
33. Shepherd A, Riedel G, Maxwell L, Kiel J (1984) Selective vasodilators redistribute intestinal blood flow and depress oxygen uptake. Am J Physiol 247:G377–G384
34. Germann R, Haisjackl M, Schwarz B, et al (1997) Inotropic treatment and intestinal mucosal tissue oxygenation in a model of porcine endotoxemia. Crit Care Med 25:1191–1197
35. Fiddian-Green R (1995) Gastric intramucosal pH, tissue oxygenation and acid base balance. Br J Anaesth 74:591–606
36. Smithies M, Yee T, Jackson L, Beale R, Bihari D (1994) Protecting the gut and liver in the critically ill: effects of dopexamine. Crit Care Med 22:789–795
37. Neviere R, Mathieu D, Chagnon JL, Lebleu N, Wattel F (1996) The contrasting effects of dobutamine and dopamine on gastric mucosal perfusion in septic patients. Am J Respir Crit Care Med 154:1684–1688
38. Greenbaum AR, Etherington PJ, Manek S, et al (1997) Measurements of oxygenation and perfusion in skeletal muscle using multiple microelectrodes. Muscle Res Cell Motil 18 (2):149–159
39. Kopp KH, Sinagowitz E, Muller H (1984) Oxygen supply of skeletal muscle in experimental endotoxic shock. Adv Exp Med Biol 169:467–476
40. Gutierrez G, Lund N, Palizas F (1991) Rabbit skeletal muscle pO_2 during hypodynamic sepsis. Chest 99:224–229
41. Astiz M, Rackow EC, Weil MH, Schumer W (1988) Early impairment of oxidative metabolism and energy production in severe sepsis. Circ Shock 26:311–320
42. Rosser DM, Stidwill RP, Jacobson D, Singer M (1995) Oxygen tension in the bladder epithelium rises in both high and low cardiac output endotoxemic sepsis. J Appl Physiol 79:1878–1882
43. Rosser DM, Stidwill RP, Jacobson D, Singer M (1996) Cardiorespiratory and tissue oxygen dose response to rat endotoxemia. Am J Physiol 271:H891–H895
44. Sair M, Etherington PJ, Curzen NP, Winlove CP, Evans TW (1996) Tissue oxygenation and perfusion in endotoxemia. Am Physiol 271:H1620–H1625
45. Sair M, Anning PB, Winlove CP, Evans TW (1997) Tissue oxygenation & cardiovascular effects of endotoxaemia: Effects of volume resuscitation. Intensive Care Med 23 (Suppl 1):S93 (Abst)
46. Sair M, Anning PB, Winlove CP, Evans TW (1997) Tissue oxygenation & cardiovascular effects of endotoxaemia: Effects of NOS inhibition. Intensive Care Med 23 (Suppl 1):S92 (Abst)
47. Naumann CP, Ruetsch YA, Fleckenstein W, Fennema M, Erdmann W, Zach GA (1992) pO_2-profiles in human muscle tissue as indicator of therapeutical effect in septic shock patients. Adv Exp Med Biol 317:869–877
48. Boekstegers P, Weidenhofer S, Kapsner T, Werdan K (1994) Skeletal muscle partial pressure of oxygen in patients with sepsis. Crit Care Med 22:640–650
49. Boekstegers P, Weidenhofer S, Pilz G, Werdan K (1991) Peripheral oxygen availability within skeletal muscle in sepsis and septic shock: comparison to limited infection and cardiogenic shock. Infection 19:317–323
50. Reinhart K, Bloos F, Konig F, Hannemann L, Kuss B (1990) Oxygen transport variables and muscle tissue oxygenation in critically ill patients with and without sepsis. Adv Exp Med Biol 277:861–864
51. Lund N, de Asla RJ, Cladis F, Papadakos PJ, Thorborg PA (1995) Dopexamine hydrochloride in septic shock: effects on oxygen delivery and oxygenation of gut, liver, and muscle. J Trauma 38:767–775

Selective Pharmacological Inhibition of Inducible Nitric Oxide Synthase in Experimental Septic Shock

L. Liaudet, M. D. Schaller, and F. Feihl

Introduction

In spite of major advances in the care of critically ill patients, septic shock remains a commonly fatal condition, with a mortality rate averaging 50% [1]. Recent progress in the understanding of the pathophysiology of septic shock has prompted an intense search for new therapeutic modalities. In particular, the recognition that an enhanced production of the vasodilator nitric oxide (NO) from an inducible isoform of NO synthase (iNOS) plays a major role in sepsis-induced hypotension, has suggested that the pharmacological inhibition of iNOS might be of great therapeutic value in this setting [2]. In this article, we will review the current state of knowledge regarding the inhibition of NO production in experimental septic shock, by focusing on the most recent data obtained with the newly developed selective inhibitors of iNOS.

Biosynthesis and Physiological Functions of NO

NO is synthesized from the terminal guanidino nitrogen of the amino acid L-arginine in a 5-electron oxidation reaction catalyzed by the enzyme NO synthase (NOS). The reaction consists of a two step oxygenation of L-arginine, yielding first hydroxyarginine and then NO and L-citrulline. Once produced, NO diffuses into adjacent cells where it activates guanylate cyclase (GC), leading to an increase in the intracellular concentration of cyclic guanosine monophosphate (cGMP), a pathway responsible for many, but not all, of the actions of NO [2]. Three distinct isoforms of NOS have been described so far, and their aminoacid and cDNA sequences determined [2]:

1) Brain NOS (bNOS or type I NOS), a constitutive, calcium-dependent isoform found in various populations of nervous cells. bNOS is involved in the regulation of cerebral blood flow, memory formation and the development of tolerance to opiates, as well as in non-adrenergic, non-cholinergic neurotransmission in the peripheral nervous system.

2) Endothelial cell NOS (ecNOS or type III NOS), a constitutive, calcium-dependent isoform which is activated in endothelial cells by various chemical (e.g., acetylcholine, bradykinin) and physical (e.g., shear-stress) stimuli. ecNOS-derived NO plays a major role in the regulation of arterial blood pressure and the distribution of regional blood flow and is involved in the inhibition of adhesion and aggregation of circulating blood cells (platelets and leukocytes) to the endothelium.

3) Inducible NOS (iNOS or type II NOS), a calcium-independent isoform normally not present under physiologic conditions and whose expression is induced in various cell types on stimulation by bacterial products (e.g. the lipopolysaccharide (LPS) of Gram-negative bacteria and the lipoteichoic acid of Gram-positive bacteria) and cytokines [tumor necrosis factor-α (TNF-α) interleukin 1β (IL-1β) and interferon (IFN)-γ]. The signal transduction events leading to the expression of iNOS are complex and not fully understood, and include the activation of tyrosine kinase and nuclear factor-kappa B (NF-κB) [2–4].

Role of NO in the Pathophysiology of Septic Shock

In recent years, evidence has emerged that an enhanced production of NO, related to diffuse iNOS expression, contributes to the pathophysiology of septic shock [4]. First, an increase in plasma nitrogen oxides (nitrite and nitrate), the stable oxidation products of NO, occurs both in experimental and human septic shock [5]. Second, the hyporeactivity of isolated blood vessels obtained from animals exposed to endotoxin, to vasoconstricting agents is largely mediated by NO overproduction in the vessel wall [4]. Third, various pharmacological inhibitors of NOS produce marked pressor effects in septic conditions when classical vasopressor agents fail to increase blood pressure [6]. Finally, mutant mice lacking the iNOS gene are conferred at least some protection against the lethal effects of LPS [7].

The enhanced NO synthesis occuring in vascular walls leads to a marked and sustained vasodilatation, associated with a decreased vascular reactivity to vasopressor agents, a fall in systemic vascular resistance (SVR) and the development of refractory hypotension. At the microcirculatory level, excess NO may play a role in the loss of microvascular control leading to maldistribution of tissue blood flows [2]. This NO-induced vasoplegia involves both cGMP-dependent and cGMP-independent mechanisms, such as inhibition of cellular bioenergetics (see below) and the activation of various membrane channels (e.g., ATP-sensitive K$^+$ channels) [4]. Excess NO may also contribute to the myocardial dysfunction observed during septic shock, but this point remains controversial [4].

High local concentrations of NO may be cytotoxic to host cells via different mechanisms [2–4]. Reaction of NO with the superoxide anion leads to the formation of peroxynitrite, which decays rapidly once protonated to the highly cytotoxic hydroxyl radical, initiating lipid peroxidation and irreversible cellular damage. Cytotoxic effects of NO also include NO-mediated DNA damage, inhibition of protein synthesis and complex interactions with the metabolic pathways involved in cellular energy production [2]. Indeed, NO inhibits the activity of key enzymes of the Krebs cycle (cis-aconitase) and the mitochondrial electron transport chain (NADH-ubiquinone reductase, NADH-succinate oxidoreductase), resulting in decreased cellular respiration and energy production. Furthermore, NO inhibits glyceraldehyde-3-phosphate deshydrogenase, a key enzyme in the glycolytic pathway, thus leading to decreased production of acetyl-coA and reducing equivalents. Finally, NO lowers cellular adenosine triphosphate (ATP) via an indirect route involving DNA repair processes. NO-mediated DNA strand breakage activates the nuclear enzyme poly-ADP-ribosyl-synthetase (PARS), which triggers a futile and energy consuming cycle of DNA repair depleting the cellular ATP stores. In addition, PARS cleaves NAD^+ into ADP ribose and nicotinamide, thus reducing the availability of NAD^+, leading to a further inhibition of glycolysis, electron transport and ATP formation [3, 4, 8]. According to recent evidence, this mechanism may involve peroxynitrite rather than NO itself [9]. It is important to emphasize that the cytotoxic effects of NO, while extremely hazardous when targeted against the host's own cells, may, on the contrary, be of paramount importance in the host defense against microorganisms [7].

Pharmacological Approaches to Limit NO Overproduction in Septic Shock

The recognition of NO as an important mediator of septic shock led to the proposal that reducing NO synthesis might be useful in the therapy of this condition. In principle, such a reduction may be achieved in two different ways: Inhibition of iNOS expression; or inhibition of NOS activity [3]. Molecules interfering with the mechanism of iNOS induction have been shown to produce beneficial effects in experimental models of septic shock. Examples of such molecules include glucocorticoids, dihydropyridine-type calcium channel antagonists, polyamines, cytokines (IL-4, IL-8, IL-10, IL-12) and transforming growth factor-β (TGF-β) [2–4]. However, the potential clinical utility of these agents is limited, since they must be administered preventatively to achieve their therapeutic benefit, which is obviously not feasible in the clinical setting. Therefore, this approach will not be further discussed, and we shall focus instead on the second therapeutic modality, which is that of NOS inhibition.

NOS Inhibition in Septic Shock

Several amino acids, substituted at the terminal guanidino nitrogen of L-arginine, act as competitive inhibitors of NOS. Agents from this class are represented by the L-arginine analogs N^G-monomethyl-L-arginine (L-NMMA), N^G-nitro-L-arginine (L-NA) and its methylester (L-NAME) as well as N^G-amino-L-arginine (L-NAA). All these compounds are non-selective NOS inhibitors, since they indiscriminately block all isoforms of NOS [4, 6].

Since the initial work by Kilbourn et al. [10, 11] and Thiemermann and Vane [12] in 1990, who showed that L-NMMA reversed the hypotension induced by TNF or endotoxin in dogs and rats, numerous investigators have reported that non-selective NOS inhibitors improve vascular reactivity and increase SVR and arterial blood pressure in experimental as well as human septic shock, lending support to the concept that NO overproduction plays a major role in the vascular dysfunction of this condition [6]. Unfortunately, treatment with these agents was also associated with numerous detrimental side effects, the most frequently reported being a fall in cardiac output (CO) [5], due either to a decreased venous return [13], or to an alteration in ventricular function related to coronary vasospasm [14] or increased left ventricular afterload [15]. Additional side effects included pulmonary hypertension [16], organ hypoperfusion [17], formation of microvascular thromboses [18], depression of tissue oxygenation [19] and enhancement of organ damage [20]. Regarding outcome, either no influence [21, 22] or a detrimental effect [23] of non-selective agents has been regularly reported. Although some of these negative results may have been favored by improper experimental conditions [4], they do not support the use of non-selective NOS inhibitors in the adjunctive therapy of septic shock.

The lack of discrimination between the different NOS isoforms represents the major limitation to the use of non-selective inhibitors in septic shock. Indeed, while targeting the iNOS-mediated NO overproduction might be useful, concomitant inhibition of ecNOS is likely to be counterproductive, by impairing essential functions of the endothelium such as agonist-stimulated vasodilation and down-regulation of activated blood cell adherence. The importance of ecNOS-derived NO in septic conditions has been emphasized by studies showing that the detrimental effects of non-selective inhibitors could be abbrogated by the co-administration of an NO donor, such as S-nitroso-N-acetyl-penicillamine (SNAP), to replace the loss of ecNOS-derived NO [24, 25]. Also, drugs preventing iNOS induction have proven beneficial in situations where non-selective NOS inhibitors were deleterious [25]. Finally, it is noteworthy that sepsis *per se* leads to endothelial dysfunction and reduces ecNOS expression (by transcriptional and posttranscriptional mechanisms) as well as ecNOS activity [3, 26]. In such conditions, further inhibition of ecNOS by nonselective inhibitors is likely to amplify the consequences of this endothelial dysfunction and to further impair microvascular homeostasis. These considerations imply that a more suitable approach to block NO overproduction in septic shock would be the use of agents able to selectively inhibit iNOS activity.

Selective Inhibitors of iNOS

The search for selective iNOS inhibitors has been a matter of considerable interest in the past few years, leading to the development of several compounds which have been tested *in vivo* in experimental septic shock. These agents can be categorized as amino acid-based and non-amino acid-based inhibitors. Amino acid-based iNOS inhibitors are the L-arginine analog L-canavanine [27] and the L-lysine analog L-N^6-(1-Iminoethyl)lysine [28]. L-canavanine is a relatively weak inhibitor of NOS, approximately 10 times more potent for iNOS than ecNOS or bNOS *in vitro*. L-N^6-(1-Iminoethyl)lysine has a much higher potency than L-canavanine and is at least 30 times more active on the inducible than on the constitutive isoforms. The recently developed non-amino acid-based compounds include amidines [29], guanidines [30], S-alkylisothioureas [31] and mercaptoalkylguanidines [32]. Some of these compounds are extremely potent and highly selective inhibitors of iNOS. Table 1 presents the major members of these different groups. For more detailed information, the interested reader is referred to a recent review on the pharmacology of these inhibitors [33].

Table 1. Selective pharmacological inhibitors of inducible nitric oxide synthase (see text for references)

Class	Group	Agent
Amino acid-based	L-arginine analog L-lysine analog	L-canavanine L-N⁶-(1-Iminoethyl)lysine
Non-amino acid-based	guanidines	aminoguanidine 1 -amino-2-hydroxy-guanidine 1-amino-2-methyl-guanidine
	amidines	2-iminopiperidine propionamidine 2-aminopyridine
	S-alkylisothioureas	S-methylisothiourea S-aminoethyl-isothiourea
	mercaptoalkylguanidines	mercaptoethylguanidine guanidinoethyldisulphide

Use of Selective iNOS Inhibitors in Experimental Septic Shock

The most frequently used model of septic shock in which the effects of selective iNOS inhibitors have been assessed is acute endotoxemia in the rat. In this model, administration of endotoxin is classically associated with a biphasic fall in arterial blood pressure, with early hypotension (1st hour), followed by transient recovery and then by a delayed hypotension, starting in the 3rd to 4th hour of endotoxemia. Both stages of hypotension are related to a fall in cardiac output (hypodynamic type of shock) associated with a marked depression of vascular reactivity to vasoconstrictor agents [34]. Early activation of ecNOS and delayed expression of iNOS have been shown to be the major pathophysiologic events responsible for this typical time-course of arterial blood pressure [2]. In addition to causing cardiovascular collapse, endotoxin administration in this model induces tissue hypoxia, multiple organ damage and dysfunction, thus reproducing most of the consequences of clinical septic shock [35]. Table 2 presents a summary of experimental studies using selective inhibitors of iNOS synthase in animal models of septic shock.

Cardiovascular Effects of Selective iNOS Inhibitors

All studies assessing the cardiovascular effects of selective iNOS inhibitors in endotoxic shock reported an improvement in arterial blood pressure and in the vascular reactivity to vasoconstrictors, as demonstrated by an increase in the pressor responses to norepinephrine administration [27, 28, 32, 36–45]. In contrast to nonselective NOS inhibitors, which increase vascular reactivity and arterial blood pressure at all stages of endotoxic shock, the effects of selective iNOS inhibitors were restricted to the delayed, iNOS-dependent stage of endotoxic shock. Also, when administered to normal rats, selective compounds did not elicit significant pressor

Table 2. Summary of experimental studies using selective inhibitors of inducible nitric oxide synthase (iNOS) in animal models of septic shock

Experimental model [reference]	iNOS inhibitor	Main effects
Anesthetized rats LPS [46]	aminoguanidine	Reduced hypotension; reduced liver, kidney and pancreatic dysfunction
Conscious rats LPS [47]	aminoguanidine	Reduced pulmonary transvascular flux
Conscious rats LPS [48]	aminoguanidine	Reduced intestinal mucosal damage; reduced bacterial translocation
Anesthetized rats Gram-positive cell wall components [37]	aminoguanidine	Reduced hypotension; increased pressor responses to norepinephrine; reduced metabolic acidosis and hypoxemia; reduced liver dysfunction
Anesthetized rats LPS [49]	aminoguanidine	Reduced hypotension; increased systemic vascular resistance; no effect on cardiac ouput and survival
Anesthetized rats LPS [50]	aminoguanidine	Increased survival time
Anesthetized rats LPS [38]	aminoguanidine	Reduced hypotension; increased pressor responses to norepinephrine
Conscious mice LPS [38]	aminoguanidine	Increased survival rate
Conscious rats LPS [51]	aminoguanidine	Reduced hypotension; reduced hindquarter and mesenteric blood flows
Anesthetized rats LPS [52]	aminoguanidine	Increased liver injury; impaired hepatic blood flow and oxygenation; reduced survival rate
Anesthetized rats LPS [44]	1-amino-2-hydroxy-guanidine	Reduced hypotension; increased pressor responses to norepinephrine; reduced metabolic acidosis; reduced liver and pancreas dysfunction
Anesthetized rats LPS [39]	guanidinoethyl-disulphide	Reduced hypotension; increased *ex vivo* vascular contractility to norepinephrine and relaxation to acetylcholine
Conscious mice LPS [39]	guanidinoethyl-disulphide	Increased survival rate
Anesthetized rats LPS [32]	mercaptoethyl-guanidine	Reduced hypotension
Conscious rats LPS [53]	S-methylisothiourea	Reduced liver and kidney dysfunction
Anesthetized rats LPS [36]	S-methylisothiourea	Reduced hypotension; increased cardiac output; reduced lactic acidosis; reduced renal dysfunction
Conscious rats LPS [47]	S-methylisothiourea	Reduced pulmonary transvascular flux
Conscious rats peritonitis [54]	S-methylisothiourea	Prolonged survival time
Conscious mice LPS [53]	S-methylisothiourea	Increased survival rate
Anesthetized rats LPS [40]	S-aminoethyl-isothiourea	Increased pressor responses to norepinephrine; reduced liver dysfunction
Anesthetizedrats LPS [32]	S-aminoethyl-isothiourea	Reduced hypotension

Table 2. (continued)

Experimental model [reference]	iNOS inhibitor	Main effects
Anesthetized rats LPS [55]	L-N⁶-(1-Iminoethyl-lysine)	Reduced hypotension; preservation of glomerular filtration rate and glomerular ecNOS activity
Anesthetized rats LPS [41]	L-canavanine	Reduced hypotension; increased pressor responses to norepinephrine; reduced lung and kidney damage
Anesthetized rats LPS [43]	L-canavanine	Reduced hypotension; increased survival rate
Anesthetized rats LPS [42]	L-canavanine	Reduced hypotension; increased pressor responses to norepinephrine
Anesthetized rats LPS [27]	L-canavanine	Reduced hypotension; increased cardiac output; reduced lactic acidosis
Anesthetized rats LPS [45]	L-canavanine	Reduced hypotension; increased cardiac output; increased mean systemic filling pressure
Anesthetized rats LPS [35]	L-canavanine	Increased liver, kidney, and intestine ATP levels; reduced liver and kidney dysfunction
Conscious mice LPS [22]	L-canavanine	Increased survival rate

responses, confirming a lack of ecNOS inhibition, at least when using low doses. Indeed, it must be stressed that selectivity is only relative and that these compounds may block all NOS isoforms when used at sufficiently high doses.

While the effects of selective agents on arterial blood pressure have been largely studied, data regarding their influence on CO are still limited. We have investigated the hemodynamic effects of L-canavanine in rats challenged with intravenous LPS and treated with a continuous infusion of L-canavanine (20 mg/kg/h) [27]. The effects of L-canavanine were compared with those of the non-selective NOS inhibitor L-NAME (5 mg/kg/h). Although both agents increased arterial blood pressure, the mechanisms underlying this effect were strikingly different. L-NAME acted through an intense vasoconstriction, as shown by a marked rise in SVR, at the cost of a severe reduction in CO, while L-canavanine increased CO, without affecting SVR (Fig. 1). In another study performed in endotoxemic rats, we obtained the same results with S-methylisothiourea, an iNOS inhibitor chemically unrelated to L-canavanine [36]. When infused in endotoxemic rats at a rate of 0.1 mg/kg/h, S-methylisothiourea increased blood pressure and CO without influencing SVR.

We have investigated the mechanisms by which selective iNOS inhibition improves CO in endotoxemic conditions [45]. We postulated that an enhanced production of NO in the venous side of the circulation might favor the pooling of blood in capacitance vessels, thereby decreasing venous return and hence CO. In rats challenged with endotoxin, we measured the mean systemic filling pressure (MSFP), a major determinant of venous hemodynamics, with and without L-canavanine treatment. After 6 hours of endotoxemia, blood pressure, CO, central venous pressure and MSFP were significantly reduced in the untreated rats, but maintained in those treated with L-canavanine, while blood volume was similarly expanded in both groups.

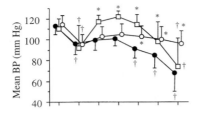

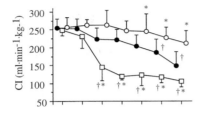

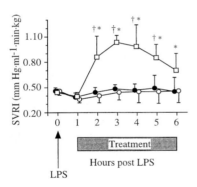

Treatment

Hours post LPS

LPS

Fig. 1. Hemodynamic effects of L-NAME and L-canavanine in endotoxemic rats. Anesthetized rats were
challenged at baseline with 10 mg/kg lipopolysaccharide (LPS) administered intravenously in 15 min. After
1 h, rats were randomly treated with a 5 h infusion of
either saline (2 ml/kg/h), L-canavanine (20 mg/kg/h)
or L-NAME (5 mg/kg/h). BP: blood pressure; CI: cardiac index; SVRI: systemic vascular resistance index.
● Saline; ○ L-canavanine; □ L-NAME. Values are
means ± SD. *P < 0.05 compared with saline treatment.
†P < 0.05 compared with values at baseline. (From [27]
with permission)

These effects indicated that (i) the main determinant of reduced cardiac ouptut in
endotoxic shock is relative hypovolemia, and (ii) selective iNOS inhibition with
L-canavanine is able to prevent these alterations, supporting the concept that an
enhanced NO production in capacitance vessels is an important pathophysiologic
event leading to venous pooling of blood in such conditions.

The current state of knowledge regarding the influence of selective iNOS inhibitors on regional perfusion is extremely limited. From a theoretical standpoint, the
influence of high local production of NO on regional blood flow may be two-fold.
On one hand, enhanced NO production may divert blood flow to the most vaso-
dilated vascular beds (putatively high NO production), at the expense of less vaso-
dilated vascular beds (putatively lower NO production). Alternatively, NO mediated
vasodilation may be fundamental for the maintenance of organ perfusion in conditions where the local and systemic production of vasoconstrictors is markedly in-

creased. The latter hypothesis appears confirmed in a recent study by Gardiner et al. [51], who investigated the effects of aminoguanidine on regional perfusion in a rat model of endotoxemia. Rats receiving a continuous infusion of endotoxin developed hypotension and hypoperfusion of the mesenteric and hindquarter vascular beds. Co-infusion of LPS and aminoguanidine prevented hypotension but exaggerated the fall in mesenteric and hindquarter blood flow. When aminoguanidine-treated rats were given an endothelin antagonist, the pressor effect and the vasoconstriction elicited by aminoguanidine were abolished, suggesting that iNOS inhibition unmasked the effects of endothelin, leading to decreased tissue blood flow. These results demonstrating a depressor effect of aminoguanidine on regional blood flow [51] are not entirely consistent with many studies indicating beneficial effects of selective iNOS inhibition in endotoxic shock (see above and below). This discrepancy cannot be explained at present, although the high dose of aminoguanidine used by Gardiner et al. [51] (45 mg/kg iv bolus, followed by 45 mg/kg/h) may have produced some inhibition of ecNOS.

Effects of Selective iNOS Inhibitors on Tissue Oxygenation

Abnormal tissue oxygenation plays an important role in the development of the multiple organ dysfunction syndrome (MODS) during septic shock. NO may contribute to these abnormalities in view of its well characterized effects on cellular energy metabolism (see above). There is indirect evidence that selective iNOS inhibition improves tissue oxygenation in experimental septic shock. Kengatharan et al. [37] found that aminoguanidine reduced the metabolic acidosis developing in rats challenged with lipoteichoic acid and peptidoglycan from *Staphylococcus aureus*. A similar observation was reported by Ruetten et al. [44] in endotoxemic rats treated with 1-amino-2-hydroxy-guanidine. Also, we found in 3 different studies that S-methylisothiourea and L-canavanine reduced lactic acidosis in rats challenged with endotoxin [27, 35, 36]. More direct evidence concerning the role of NO overproduction in the development of cellular dysoxia has come from measurements of ATP concentrations in various organs from endotoxemic rats. In this study [35], animals were challenged with endotoxin and treated after 1 hour with either saline or L-canavanine for a total of 4 hours. At the end of the experiments, ATP was measured in biopsies from the liver, small intestine and kidney. In these organs, endotoxin induced a severe fall in ATP which was largely attenuated (liver) or totally prevented (kidney, small intestine) by L-canavanine (Fig. 2).

These data are consistent with an improved state of oxidative metabolism following iNOS blockade, which is in striking contrast to the detrimental effects reported with non-selective inhibitors [19]. For instance, a direct comparison of the effects of L-NAME and L-canavanine showed that the compounds produced opposite effects on the endotoxin-induced lactic acidosis in anesthetized rats (Fig. 3) [27]. This difference, which probably reflects the negative effects of non-selective compounds on both systemic (decrease in cardiac output) and regional (excessive vasoconstriction) blood flow, emphasizes the ambivalent role of NO in septic shock: While cells may suffocate from excessive NO produced by iNOS, their oxygen supply might be critically dependent on NO-mediated vasodilatation.

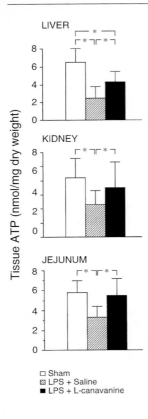

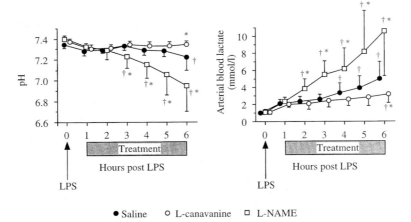

Fig. 2. Effects of L-canavanine on tissue ATP measured in biopsies from the liver, kidney and small intestine (jejunum). Anesthetized rats were challenged at baseline with an intravenous bolus of lipopolysaccharide (LPS, 5 mg/kg) and were treated after 1 h with a continuous infusion of either L-canavanine (20 mg/kg/h) or saline (2 ml/kg/h) given until the time of biopsies (5 h after baseline). Sham rats received saline in place of LPS and were treated after 1 h with a continuous infusion of saline until the end of experiments. Values are means ± SD. * P < 0.05. (From [35] with permission)

Fig. 3. Effects of L-NAME and L-canavanine on arterial blood pH and lactate concentration in endotoxemic rats. Anesthetized rats were challenged at baseline with 10 mg/kg lipopolysaccharide (LPS) administered intravenously in 15 min. After 1 h, rats were randomly treated with a 5 h infusion of either saline (2 ml/kg/h), L-canavanine (20 mg/kg/h) or L-NAME (5 mg/kg/h). Values are means ± SD. * P < 0.05 compared with saline treatment. † P < 0.05 compared with values at baseline. (From [27] with permission)

Effects of Selective iNOS Inhibitors on Tissue Damage and Multiple Organ Dysfunction

The cytotoxic potential of high local production of NO has been proposed as an important mechanism leading to organ injury and dysfunction in septic shock. To date there are only limited data regarding the effects of NOS inhibitors on these alterations. The non-selective compounds L-NMMA and L-NAME were found to enhance liver [20] and kidney [18] dysfunction in rodent models of endotoxic shock, by reducing perfusion and favoring the formation of microvascular thromboses. Alternatively, some studies reported that low doses of these inhibitors reduced liver injury in hypodynamic endotoxic shock [56] and improved renal function in hyperdynamic endotoxemia [57, 58]. Therefore, it appears that the effects of non-selective NOS inhibitors on organ damage and dysfunction are largely unpredictable, being in all likelihood critically dependent on the dose administered and the experimental model used. In contrast, more reproducible results were obtained in studies using selective iNOS inhibitors, which have generally been found to reduce organ damage in endotoxemic conditions.

Liver: Therapeutic administration of aminoguanidine [46], 1-amino-2-hydroxy-guanidine [44], aminoethyl-isothiourea [40], S-methylisothiourea [53] and L-canavanine [35] attenuated liver dysfunction and hepatocellular injury developing 4–6 hours after injection of endotoxin in the rat, as assessed by a reduction in the plasma levels of transaminases, alkaline phosphatase and bilirubin. One study reported opposite effects, i.e., a marked enhancement of endotoxin-induced liver injury in rats treated with a continuous infusion of aminoguanidine at 5 mg/kg/h, beginning at the time of endotoxin injection [52]. However, interpretation of these findings is difficult, as it is likely that non-specific effects of aminoguanidine, unrelated to NOS inhibition, contributed to these detrimental consequences. Indeed, when compared to L-NAME, the injurious effects of aminoguanidine on the liver were significantly more pronounced, while the level of NOS inhibition was similar (comparable reduction in plasma nitrate and nitrite). Also, 70% of the rats treated with aminoguanidine abruptly died after 4 hours, while there was no death in the L-NAME group. These unexpected differences emphasize the many pharmacological properties of aminoguanidine, which include inhibition of glycosylation, inhibition of polyamine catabolism, inhibition of histamine metabolism and inhibition of catalase [52].

Kidney: Several investigators have focused on the effects of selective iNOS inhibitors on endotoxin-induced renal failure. Treatment with aminoguanidine [46], 1-amino-2-hydroxy-guanidine [44] and aminoethyl-isothiourea [40], beginning 2 hours after endotoxin administration, neither improved nor worsened renal dysfunction in the rat. It has been suggested that this lack of influence was due to the fact that renal dysfunction develops very early in this model (i.e., during the first 2 hours of endotoxemia), so that treatment beyond this period is unlikely to produce any significant effect [3]. In contrast, a marked improvement in renal function was observed following treatment with L-canavanine [35] or S-methylisothiourea [36] initiated 1 hour after endotoxin injection, as well as with L-N$_6$-(1-iminoethyl)lysine, administered before and at the time of endotoxin [55]. Although these favorable effects might simply reflect an improved hemodynamic status, this is unlikely since in a study in which arterial blood pressure and CO were similarly improved with S-methyliso-thiourea or norepinephrine, only S-methylisothiourea was able to reduce renal dysfunction [36].

Two studies have shed some light on the potential mechanisms underlying the beneficial effects of selective iNOS inhibitors on renal function in endotoxic shock. Schwartz et al. [55], investigating the role of endothelial dysfunction in the development of renal failure in this setting, found that ecNOS activity was severely depressed in isolated glomeruli from endotoxemic rats, as evidenced by a marked inhibition of the cGMP response to the ecNOS agonist carbamylcholine. When treating rats with L-N^6-(1-iminoethyl)lysine, renal dysfunction was corrected (normalization of glomerular filtration rate), as was the cGMP response to carbamylcholine. These results were replicated when administering the agent 2,4-diamino-6-hydroxy-pyrimidine, an inhibitor of GTP cyclohydrolase, the rate limiting enzyme in the formation of the NOS co-factor tetrahydrobiopterin, which has been shown to selectively inhibit iNOS activity. In contrast, treatment with L-NAME further impaired both the fall in glomerular filtration rate and the endothelial dysfunction induced by endotoxin. These data might indicate that the enhanced NO production from iNOS is responsible for an NO-mediated inhibition of ecNOS activity, leading to renal vasoconstriction. This is consistent with the *in vitro* demonstration that NO exerts the capacity to autoinhibit NOS via specific binding sites on the enzyme [59]. Interestingly, the concentrations of NO required to block ecNOS (≈ 10 µM) were much lower than for iNOS ($\approx 50-100$ µM) [55]. Another possible explanation for the findings of Schwartz et al. [55] could be an NO-mediated down-regulation of GC activity and/or expression. Indeed, it has recently been shown that large concentrations of NO are able to decrease GC subunit mRNA stability via a transcription- and translation-dependent mechanism [60].

In another study [41], the effects of L-canavanine on the histological damage observed in the kidney of endotoxemic rats were investigated. Endotoxin resulted in severe endothelial disruption and the presence of platelets in the lumen of blood vessels, both changes which were markedly attenuated with L-canavanine. It is noteworthy that the opposite effect has heen associated with the administration of L-NAME, which severely increased the platelet deposits in the kidneys of endotoxemic rats [18]. Thus, it appears from these different studies that: (i) The selective inhibition of iNOS is beneficial to the integrity and the function of the glomerular endothelium in endotoxic shock, leading to improved perfusion and reduced activation of circulating blood cells; (ii) the non-selective inhibition of NOS further impairs endothelial dysfunction and amplifies the renal vasoconstriction and platelet activation induced by endotoxin.

Lung: Some studies have investigated the effects of selective iNOS inhibitors on the pulmonary dysfunction occuring in septic conditions. Kengatharan et al. [37] reported that aminoguanidine reduced hypoxemia developing in rats challenged with cell wall components of Gram-positive bacteria. This effect might reflect a decreased formation of pulmonary edema in aminoguanidine-treated rats, a hypothesis supported by a study from the group of Szabo [47], who showed that administration of either aminoguanidine or S-methylisothiourea to endotoxemic rats significantly reduced pulmonary transvascular flux, while reducing lung iNOS activity. An additional study [41] has investigated the effects of selective iNOS inhibition on endotoxin-induced lung injury. In this study, endotoxin induced a massive invasion of polymorphonuclear leukocytes (PMN) in lung capillaries, as well as marked endothelial cell swelling. When the rats were treated with L-canavanine, no PMN were seen in the lung, and there was a marked reduction in endothelial damage. Taken together, these results suggest that the enhanced NO production generated by iNOS in endotoxic shock causes a vascular leak in the lung, with infiltration of PMN and endothelial damage in the lung capillaries.

Intestine: Only one study has focused on the potential role of iNOS on the intestinal dysfunction observed in endotoxemia [48]. Rats challenged with endotoxin were treated with an infusion of saline or aminoguanidine at 500 mg/kg/day. 24 hours after endotoxin injection, the animals were killed and quantitative bacterial cultures were obtained from the peritoneal fluid, blood, mesenteric lymph nodes, liver and spleen, to assess the occurrence of bacterial translocation from the intestines. When compared with saline, aminoguanidine treatment was associated with significantly less intestinal mucosal damage and with fewer positive cultures, supporting an important pathophysiologic role of NO in the development of intestinal barrier failure in endotoxic shock. Indeed, previous studies reported that exogenous NO, or NO produced in response to cytokine induction of iNOS, was able to dilate gap junctions and increase epithelial permeability in intestinal epithelial cells [9, 61]. Some data also indicate that peroxynitrite formed from excess NO may be responsible for severe intestinal inflammation and a bioenergetic failure in intestinal epithelial cells [9]. It is noteworthy that, contrary to aminoguanidine, non-selective NOS inhibitors were found to enhance intestinal damage in endotoxic shock [24]. Therefore, although the inhibition of iNOS may limit intestinal dysfunction in this setting, the concomitant maintenance of ecNOS activity should also be regarded as critical.

Effects of Selective iNOS Inhibitors on Mortality

There are few data on the effects of NOS inhibitors on mortality in experimental septic shock. Teale and Atkinson [62] reported an improved survival in a murine model of bacterial peritonitis following the co-administration of the non-selective NOS inhibitor L-NMMA and the antibiotic imipenem. However, attempts to reproduce these results have been unsuccessful [21]. In other studies using nonselective compounds, either a lack of benefit [22] or a detrimental effect [23] were generally observed. Recently, the development of strains of mice lacking the iNOS gene has given the opportunity to more precisely delineate the pathogenic role of iNOS in septic shock, without the confounding consequences of ecNOS inhibition. To date, three studies have reported the consequences of endotoxin administration in such animals. Wei and co-workers [63] reported a significant improvement in the survival of iNOS-deficient mice, in contrast to the lack of any benefit reported by Laubach et al. [64]. In another study by MacMicking and colleagues [7], iNOS-knockout mice were conferred partial protection against the lethal effect of a high dose of endotoxin, while their survival was not influenced when challenged with sublethal doses.

An additional finding was an enhanced sensitivity to bacterial infection with intra-cellular pathogens in iNOS-deficient mice. Although these contrasting results are somewhat difficult to interpret, they suggest the following:

1) iNOS may play a role in endotoxin lethality, especially when high doses of endo-toxin are administered;
2) mechanisms independent from iNOS expression are involved in the lethal effects of endotoxin;
3) iNOS appears critical in the host defense mechanisms against at least some microorganisms.

From these data in transgenic mice, one might expect at least some protection to be conferred by treatment with selective iNOS inhibitors. Indeed, aminoguanidine [38], S-methylisothiourea [53] and guanidinoethyldisulphide [39] all improved short term survival in mice challenged with intraperitoneal endotoxin. We have also shown that therapeutic administration of L-canavanine 6 hours after endotoxin in-jection produced a significant reduction of mortality over a 7 day period [22], while treatment with L-NAME afforded no protection, but rather tended to accelerate the time of death (Fig. 4). One investigation evaluated the influence of selective iNOS inhibition on the mortality of Gram negative septic shock in the rat [54]. Septic rats were treated with antibiotics and received repeated doses of either S-methyliso-thiourea (5 mg/kg) or L-NAME (10 or 25 mg/kg) at 12 hour intervals. The main findings were that S-methylisothiourea prolonged survival time, while L-NAME had no effect at the low dose, and shortened survival time at the higher dose. These data are of major importance, since they provide evidence that treatment with a selective iNOS inhibitor prolongs survival in a clinically more relevant model of septic shock than acute endotoxemia.

In summary, the current state of knowledge regarding the influence of NOS in-hibitors on septic shock mortality is two-fold. First, a large body of evidence suggests that non-selective agents are detrimental and therefore should be avoided. Second,

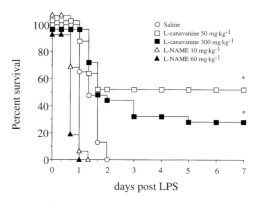

Fig. 4. Effects of L-NAME and L-canavanine on the survival from endotoxic shock in conscious mice. Mice were challenged with 70 mg/kg lipopolysaccharide (LPS) intraperitoneally at baseline and treated intraperitoneally 6 h later with either saline, 0.2 mL (n = 24), L-canavanine, 300 mg/kg (n = 25), L-canavanine, 50 mg/kg (n = 25), L-NAME, 60 mg/kg (n = 16), or L-NAME, 10 mg/kg (n = 15). * p < 0.05 compared with saline treatment. (From [22] with permission)

preliminary data on selective compounds, both in endotoxic and bacteremic models of septic shock, indicate that such agents might be useful adjuncts to antibiotic therapy.

Conclusion

An enhanced production of NO from L-arginine, following the diffuse expression of an inducible isoform of NOS, plays an important role in the pathophysiology of septic shock. Although iNOS inhibitors might be of great therapeutic value in this setting, the concomitant inhibition of the ecNOS with non-selective compounds has produced harmful consequences in experimental conditions. In contrast, preliminary information obtained with selective inhibitors of iNOS appears promising. The therapeutic usefulness of these agents should be promptly evaluated in clinically relevant models of septic shock.

References

1. Bone RC (1991) The pathogenesis of sepsis. Ann Intern Med 115:457–469
2. Szabo C (1995) Alterations in nitric oxide production in various forms of circulatory shock. New Horizons 3:2–32
3. Thiemermann C (1997) Nitric oxide and septic shock. Gen Pharmacol 29:159–166
4. Kilbourn RG, Traber DL, Szabo C (1997) Nitric oxide and shock. Disease-a-Month 43: 281–348
5. Cobb JP, Danner RL (1996) Nitric oxide and septic shock. JAMA 275:1192–1196
6. Kilbourn RG, Szabo C, Traber DL (1997) Beneficial versus detrimental effects of nitric oxide synthase inhibitors in circulatory shock: lessons learned from experimental and clinical studies. Shock 7:235–246
7. MacMicking JD, Nathan C, Hom G, et al (1995) Altered responses to bacterial infection and endotoxic shock in mice lacking inducible nitric oxide synthase. Cell 81:641–650
8. Salzman AL (1995) Nitric oxide and the gut. New Horizons 3:33–45
9. Szabo C (1996) DNA strand breakage and activation of poly-ADP ribosyltransferase: a cytotoxic pathway triggered by peroxynitrite. Free Rad Biol Med 21:855–869
10. Kilbourn RG, Gross SS, Jubran A, et al (1990) NG-methyl-L-arginine inhibits tumor necrosis factor-induced hypotension: implications for the involvement of nitric oxide. Proc Natl Acad Sci USA 87:3629–3632
11. Kilbourn RG, Jubran A, Gross SS, et al (1990) Reversal of endotoxin-mediated shock by N^G-methyl-L-arginine, an inhibitor of nitric oxide synthesis. Biochem Biophys Res Commun 172:1132–1138
12. Thiemermann C, Vane J (1990) Inhibition of nitric oxide synthesis reduces the hypotension induced by bacterial lipopolysaccharides in the rat *in vivo*. Eur J Pharmacol 182:591–595
13. Magder S, Vanelli G (1994) Venous circuit adaptations during high cardiac output sepsis in pigs. Am J Respir Crit Care Med 149:A654 (Abst)
14. Avontuur JAM, Bruining H, Ince C (1995) Inhibition of nitric oxide synthesis causes myocardial ischemia in endotoxemic rats. Circ Res 76:418–425
15. Cobb JP, Natanson C, Hoffman WD, et al (1992) N^ω-Amino-L-Arginine, an inhibitor of nitric oxide synthase, raises vascular resistance but increases mortality rates in awake canines challenged with endotoxin. J Exp Med 176:1175–1182
16. Robertson FM, Offner PJ, Ciceri DP, Bechker WK, Pruitt BA (1994) Detrimental hemodynamic effects of nitric oxide synthase inhibition in septic shock. Arch Surg 129:149–156
17. Spain DA, Wilson MA, Garison RN (1994) Nitric oxide synthase inhibition exacerbates sepsis-induced renal hypoperfusion. Surgery 116:322–331

18. Shultz P, Raij L (1992) Endogenously synthesized nitric oxide prevents endotoxin-induced glomerular thrombosis. J Clin Invest 90: 1718–1725
19. Statman R, Cheng W, Cunningham JN, et al (1994) Nitric oxide inhibition in the treatment of the sepsis syndrome is detrimental to tissue oxygenation. J Surg Res 57: 93–98
20. Harbrecht BG, Billiar TR, Stadler J, et al (1992) Nitric oxide synthesis serves to reduce hepatic damage during acute murine endotoxemia. Crit Care Med 20: 1568–1574
21. Evans T, Carpenter A, Silva A, Cohen J (1994) Inhibition of nitric oxide synthase in experimental Gram-negative sepsis. J Infect Dis 169: 343–349
22. Liaudet L, Rosselet A, Schaller MD, Markert M, Perret C, Feihl F (1998) Nonselective versus selective inhibition of inducible nitric oxide synthase in experimental endotoxic shock. J Infect Dis (In press)
23. Minnard EA, Shou J, Naama H, Cech A, Gallagher H, Daly JM (1994) Inhibition of nitric oxide synthesis is detrimental during endotoxemia. Arch Surg 129: 142–148
24. Boughton-Smith NK, Hutcheson IR, Deakin AM, Whittle BJR, Moncada S (1990) Protective effect of S-nitroso-N-acetyl-penicillamine in endotoxin-induced acute intestinal damage in the rat. Eur J Pharmacol 191: 485–488
25. Wright CE, Rees DD, Moncada S (1992) Protective and pathological roles of nitric oxide in endo-toxin shock. Cardiovasc Res 26: 48–57
26. Traber DL (1996) Presence and absence of nitric oxide synthase in sepsis. Crit Care Med 24: 1102–1103
27. Liaudet L, Feihl F, Rosselet A, Markert M, Perret C (1996) Beneficial effects of L-canavanine, a selective inhibitor of inducible nitric oxide synthase, during rodent endotoxemia. Clin Sci 90: 369–377
28. Moore WM, Webber RK, Jerome GM, Tjoeng FS, Misko TP, Currie MG (1994) L-N^6-(1-Iminoethyl)lysine: a selective inhibitor of inducible nitric oxide synthase. J Med Chem 37: 3886–3888
29. Southan GJ, Szabo C, O'Connor MP, Salzman AL, Thiemermann C (1995) Amidines are potent inhibitors of nitric oxide synthases: preferential inhibition of the inducible isoform. Eur J Pharmacol 291: 311–318
30. Misko TP, Moore WM, Kasten T, et al (1993) Selective inhibition of the inducible nitric oxide synthase by aminoguanidine. Eur J Pharmacol 233: 119–125
31. Southan GJ, Szabo C, Thiemermann C (1995) Isothioureas: potent inhibitors of nitric oxide synthases with variable isoform selectivity. Br J Pharmacol 114: 510–516
32. Southan GJ, Zingarelli B, O'Connor M, Salzman A, Szabo C (1996) Spontaneous rearrangement of aminoalkylisothioureas into mercaptoalkylguanidines, a novel class of nitric oxide synthase inhibitors with selectivity towards the inducible isoform. Br J Pharmacol 117: 619–632
33. Southan GJ, Szabo C (1996) Selective pharmacological inhibition of distinct nitric oxide synthase isoforms. Biochem Pharmacol 51: 383–394
34. Fink MP, Heard SO (1990) Laboratory models of sepsis and septic shock. J Surg Res 49: 186–196
35. Liaudet L, Fishman D, Markert M, Perret C, Feihl F (1997) L-canavanine improves organ function and tissue adenosine triphosphate levels in rodent endotoxemia. Am J Respir Crit Care Med 155: 1643–1648
36. Rosselet A, Feihl F, Markert M, Perret C, Liaudet L (1998) Selective iNOS inhibition is superior to norepinephrine in the treatment of rat endotoxic shock. Am J Respir Crit Care Med (In press)
37. Kengatharan KM, De Kimpe SJ, Thiemermann C (1996) Role of nitric oxide in the circulatory failure and organ injury in a rodent model of Gram-positive shock. Br J Pharmacol 119: 1411–1421
38. Wu CC, Chen SJ, Szabo C, Thiemermann C, Vane JR (1995) Aminoguanidine attenuates the delayed circulatory failure and improves survival in rodent models of endotoxic shock. Br J Pharmacol 114: 1666–1672
39. Szabo C, Bryk R, Zingarelli B, et al (1996) Pharmacological characterization of guanidinoethyl-disulphide (GED), a novel inhibitor of nitric oxide synthase with selectivity towards the in-ducible isoform. Br J Pharmacol 118: 1659–1668
40. Thiemermann C, Ruetten H, Wu CC, Vane JR (1995) The multiple organ dysfunction syndrome caused by endotoxin in the rat: attenuation of liver dysfunction by inhibitors of nitric oxide synthase. Br J Pharmacol 116: 2845–2851

41. Fatehihassanabad Z, Burns H, Aughey E, et al (1996) Effects of L-canavanine, an inhibitor of inducible nitric oxide synthase, on endotoxin-mediated shock in rats. Shock 6:194–200
42. Cai M, Sakamoto A, Ogawa R (1996) Inhibition of nitric oxide formation with L-canavanine attenuates endotoxin-induced vascular hyporeactivity in the rat. Eur J Pharmacol 295:215–220
43. Teale DM, Atkinson AM (1994) L-canavanine restores blood pressure in a rat model of endotoxic shock. Eur J Pharmacol 271:87–92
44. Ruetten H, Southan GJ, Abate A, Thiemermann C (1996) Attenuation of endotoxin-induced multiple organ dysfunction by 1-amino-2-hydroxy-guanidine, a potent inhibitor of inducible nitric oxide synthase. Br J Pharmacol 118:261–270
45. Fishman D, Liaudet L, Lazor R, Feihl F, Perret C (1997) L-canavanine, an inhibitor of inducible nitric oxide synthase, improves venous return in endotoxemic rats. Crit Care Med 25:469–475
46. Wu CC, Ruetten H, Thiemermann C (1996) Comparison of the effects of aminoguanidine and N-omega-nitro-L-arginine methyl ester on the multiple organ dysfunction caused by endotoxaemia in the rat. Eur J Pharmacol 300:99–104
47. Arkovitz MS, Wispé JR, Garcia VF, Szabo C (1996) Selective inhibition of the inducible isoform of nitric oxide synthase prevent pulmonary transvascular flux during acute endotoxemia. J Ped Surg 31:1009–1015
48. Sorrells DL, Friend C, Koltuksuz U, et al (1996) Inhibition of nitric oxide with aminoguanidine reduces bacterial translocation after endotoxin challenge *in vivo*. Arch Surg 131:1155–1163
49. Hock CE, Yin K, Yue G, Wong PYK (1997) Effects of inhibition of nitric oxide synthase by aminoguanidine in acute endotoxemia. Am J Physiol 272:H843–H850
50. Yen MH, Liu YC, Hong HJ, Sheu JR, Wu CC (1997) Role of nitric oxide in lipopolysaccharide-induced mortality from spontaneously hypertensive rats. Life Sci 60:1223–1230
51. Gardiner SM, Kemp PA, March JE, Bennett T (1996) Influence of aminoguanidine and the endothelin antagonist, SB 209670, on the regional haemodynamic effects of endotoxaemia in conscious rats. Br J Pharmacol 118:1822–1828
52. Huang TP, Nishida T, Kamiike W, et al (1997) Role of nitric oxide in oxygen transport in rat liver sinusoids during endotoxemia. Hepatology 26:336–342
53. Szabo C, Southan GJ, Thiemermann C (1994) Beneficial effects and improved survival in rodent models of septic shock with S-methylisothiourea sulfate, a potent and selective inhibitor of inducible nitric oxide synthase. Proc Natl Acad Sci USA 91:12472–12476
54. Aranow JS, Zhuang J, Wang H, Larkin V, Smith M, Fink MP (1996) A selective inhibitor of inducible nitric oxide synthase prolongs survival in a rat model of bacterial peritonitis: comparison with two nonselective strategies. Shock 5:116–121
55. Schwartz D, Mendonca M, Schwartz I, et al (1997) Inhibition of constitutive nitric oxide synthase (NOS) by nitric oxide generated by inducible NOS after lipopolysaccharide administration provokes renal dysfunction in rats. J Clin Invest 100:439–448
56. Nava E, Palmer RMJ, Moncada S (1991) Inhibition of nitric oxide synthesis in septic shock: how much is beneficial? Lancet 338:1555–1557
57. Meyer J, Traber LD, Nelson S, et al (1992) Reversal of hyperdynamic response to continuous endotoxin administration by inhibition of NO synthesis. J Appl Physiol 73:324–328
58. Meyer J, Lentz CW, Stothert JC, Traber LD, Herndon DN, Traber DL (1994) Effects of nitric oxide synthesis inhibition in hyperdynamic endotoxemia. Crit Care Med 22:306–312
59. Rengasamy A, Johns RA (1993) Regulation of nitric oxide synthase by nitric oxide. Mol Pharmacol 44:124–128
60. Filippov G, Bloch DB, Bloch KD (1997) Nitric oxide decreases stability of mRNAs encoding soluble guanylate cyclase subunits in rat pulmonary artery smooth muscle cells. J Clin Invest 100:942–948
61. Salzman AL, Menconi MJ, Unno N, et al (1995) Nitric oxide dilates tight junctions and deletes ATP in cultured Caco-2BBe intestinal epithelial monolayers. Am J Physiol 268:G361–G373
62. Teale DM, Atkinson M (1992) Inhibition of nitric oxide synthesis improves survival in a murine peritonitis model of sepsis that is not cured by antibiotics alone. J Antimicrob Chemother 30:839–842
63. Wei XQ, Charles IG, Smith A, et al (1995) Altered immune responses in mice lacking inducible nitric oxide synthase. Nature 375:408–411
64. Laubach VE, Shesely EG, Smithies O, Sherman PA (1995) Mice lacking inducible nitric oxide synthase are not resistant to lipopolysaccharide-induced death. Proc Natl Acad Sci USA 92:10688–10692

The Use of Dopamine and Norepinephrine in the ICU

A. R. J. Girbes and K. Hoogenberg

Introduction

The discovery and recognition of the pronounced effects of dopamine on renal function more than thirty years ago by the group of Goldberg [1], has contributed to the current extensive use of dopamine in the intensive care unit (ICU). Particularly in low-dose, dopamine is administered in the ICU for its presumed renal protective effects. According to a recent audit of 93 ICUs in the UK, 50% of all patients at risk of developing renal failure were on low-dose dopamine. Forty-three ICUs had a protocol for the use of dopamine in patients at risk [2]. The properties ascribed to the infusion of low-dose dopamine, i.e. enhancement or preservation of renal blood flow with an increase in urine output, have made it attractive for internists, anesthesiologists, cardiologists and intensivists to prescribe dopamine to the critically ill patient. Additionally, dopamine is used to reverse the effects of positive pressure ventilation with positive end-expiratory pressure (PEEP), i.e., a decrease in cardiac output and renal blood flow with a concomitant fall in urine output. Also, the positive inotropic properties of dopamine reverse the negative inotropic effects of anesthetics. Since the (hourly) diuresis of the critically ill patient is considered a good marker of (peripheral) tissue perfusion, the diuretic properties of dopamine are valued by the clinician.

On the contrary, the use of norepinephrine on renal function is ofter accompanied by fear of inducing a deterioration of renal function. This is mainly based on early experimental studies in the seventies with intra-arterial norepinephrine-induced acute renal failure [3, 4]. In these studies, relatively high doses of norepinephrine were used; up to 1.5 µg/kg/min. These results cannot and should not be extrapolated to the human pathophysiologic situation, e.g., septic shock, and do not sufficiently take into account the importance of restoring perfusion pressure to the kidney in patients with hypotension. Additionally, several recent reports on the use of norepinephrine in patients with sepsis show that norepinephrine is increasingly recognized as a valuable agent in the treatment of septic shock and can improve renal function [5, 6]. In this review we will appraise the available data from the literature on the use of dopamine and norepinephrine in the critically ill patient, focusing on renal function.

Physiology of Renal Hemodynamics

Arterial blood enters the kidney at the hilus through the renal artery, which divides into interlobar arteries, which in turn serially branch into arcuate and interlobular arteries. The interlobular arteries subdivide into numerous afferent arterioles, which deliver blood into the capillary networks: The glomeruli. Here filtration takes place and the blood remaining in the glomerulus leaves through an efferent arteriole into, sequentially, the peritubular capillaries, interlobular veins, arcuate veins, interlobar veins and finally the renal vein. The peritubular capillaries run in apposition to the adjacent tubules and the constitution of the fluid contained in these tubules is a determinant for reabsorption. As will be explained later this is related to the filtration fraction. Branches of the juxtamedullary glomeruli enter the medulla constituting the vasa recta capillaries. The glomerular capsule surrounds the glomerulus, like an inflated "chewing gum ball", wrapping up the glomerulus. In this "chewing gum ball", the capsular space, the (glomerular) ultrafiltrate is received: The primary urine, flowing down into the tubules. The amount of ultrafiltrate of plasma across the glomerulus is dependent on: (i) The permeability of the membrane and (ii) the net effect of hydraulic pressure and oncotic pressure gradients. Changes in the glomerular filtration rate (GFR) can therefore be produced by alterations in these factors or by the rate of renal plasma flow (RPF). A constriction of the afferent arteriole will decrease both RPF and GFR. A constriction of the efferent arteriole will tend to increase the GFR through a rise in intraglomerular pressure (Fig. 1). In this case the fraction of the amount of RPF that is filtered into the capsular space is increased, i.e., the filtration fraction (FF = GFR/RPF) is increased. A high filtration fraction, as seen in situations with a stimulated renin-angiotensin-aldosterone system (RAAS), and sympathetic nervous system (SNS) activity, such as hypotension, the hydrostatic pressure of the peritubular capillaries will fall and the oncotic pressure will rise. This results in an augmented tubular reabsorption with sodium and water retention. Renal vasodilation *per se* as induced by low doses of dopamine, however, induces natriuresis.

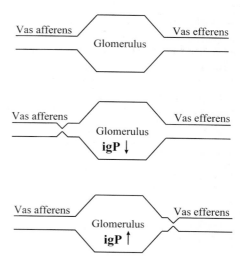

Fig. 1. Simplified representation of a glomerulus with afferent and efferent arteriole. Preglomerular vasoconstriction will result in a decrease in renal plasma flow (RPF), a fall in intraglomerular pressure (igP) and a subsequent fall in glomerular filtration rate (GFR). Postglomerular vasoconstriction will result in a rise in igP and a (relative) rise in GFR

Table 1. Counteracting systems on renal function

Vasoconstriction + Water/sodium retention	• Renin-angiotensin-aldosterone-system ↑ • Activation sympathetic nervous system • ADH (vasopressin) ↑ • Endothelin ↑
Vasodilation + Natriuresis	• Atrial natriuretic peptide • Endogenous dopamine • Prostaglandin E_2 (metabolites) • EDRF (NO)

The balance of afferent and efferent vascular tone with concomitant effects on renal hemodynamics and water- and sodium retention, is determined by the SNS and counteracting neurohumoral systems (Table 1). Prostaglandins are produced at various sites in the kidney and have important local functions but little systemic activity. Renal prostaglandins act as vasodilators, antagonize the water-retaining effect of antidiuretic hormone (ADH) and increase sodium excretion. The deleterious effects of prostaglandin synthesis inhibition by non-steroidal anti-inflammatory drugs in patients with shock can easily be derived from the actions of prostaglandins.

However, although the intraglomerular pressure is an important determinant of GFR, under physiological circumstances the GFR and RPF remain approximately constant, through so called autoregulation despite fluctuations of arterial pressure, provided the perfusion pressure, i.e., the mean arterial pressure, is sufficient. This underscores the importance of perfusion pressure in the maintenance of renal function, i.e., GFR.

Effects of Norepinephrine

Norepinephrine (NE), the effector component of the SNS, stimulates both α- and β-receptors (Table 2). After its release from the terminal nerve endings of the SNS, NE acts on local adrenoceptors in an autocrine fashion, while at the same time small amounts leak into the circulation [7]. This leaked NE is not an inert circulating neurotransmitter, but a hormonally active substance [8]. NE has a high binding affinity for α_1-adrenoceptors that cause vasocontriction in many vascular beds.

Table 2. The effects of dopamine and norepinephrine on adrenergic receptors. The amount of stimulation is graded from 0 (no stimulation) to 2 (potent stimulation). An asterisk indicates dose dependent effects, mainly observed at higher doses

	D1-like	D2-like	α_1	α_2	β_1	β_2
Dopamine	2	1	1–2*	0–1	1–2*	0–1*
Norepinephrine	0	0	2	1–2	1–2	1

The kidney is richly innervated by sympathetic nerves that terminate on both renal vasculature and discrete segments of the nephron [9]. α_1-adrenoceptors have been located along the interlobular, afferent and efferent glomerular arterioles, mesangial cells and tubular segments [10]. This distribution pattern suggests that NE may control glomerular blood flow, glomerular capillary pressure and renal sodium handling [7, 11]. Experimental studies on renal sympathetic nerves have shown that low frequency stimulation results in sodium retention and renin release, and high frequency stimulation in a fall in RPF and some decline in GFR [7,12]. Exogenous NE infusions have been documented to markedly reduce RPF without much change in GFR in animals [13]. These renal hemodynamic effects of NE are probably mediated via changes in glomerular arteriolar tone [11,13–15]. Studies of isolated renal vessels of rats and rabbits have shown that NE causes vasoconstriction of the interlobular renal arteries and of the afferent and efferent glomerular arterioles [14, 15]. The efferent arterioles are the major sites of flow resistance in the kidney and thus importantly determine renal blood flow, and are also involved in the control of intraglomerular pressure [11]. According to equation (1)

$$GFR = kf(\Delta Pc - \Delta\pi p) \tag{1}$$

glomerual ultrafiltration is determined by net hydraulic pressure (ΔPc), net oncotic pressure ($\Delta\pi$), filtration surface area and hydraulic permeability (kf) [11]. Under conditions of pressure equilibrium such as the hydropenic rat, changes in GFR are linearly related to changes in RPF [11]. This indicates that any decrease in RPF by NE will reduce GFR unless other factors like an increase in net hydraulic, e.g., intraglomerular, pressure compensate for a fall in GFR. Indeed, early micropuncture studies in the rat documented that the NE-induced fall in RPF was accompanied by an increase in intraglomerular pressure. The lack of change in GFR during NE infusion was explained by the increase in intraglomerular pressure offsetting the fall in RPF [13]. Interestingly, the glomerular vessel response was determined by the prevailing blood pressure. There was a predominant increase in efferent tone when blood pressure was kept unchanged, whereas both afferent and efferent glomerular resistance increased when blood pressure was allowed to increase [13]. Thus, in experimental studies exogenous NE has been recognized as an important renal vasoconstrictor that decreases RPF but without much change in GFR due to a rise in intraglomerular pressure.

In the human situation the precise effects of NE on afferent and efferent glomerular vasoconstriction and intraglomerular pressure are unknown, and it is uncertain to what extent intrarenal α-adrenoceptor distribution differs from species like rats and rabbits. Nonetheless, renal hemodynamic responses to NE infusion show obvious similarities with animal data. Intravenous infusion of NE lowers RPF but has little effect on GFR [16–21]. Even with high NE infusion rates that decreased RPF up to 40 to 50% in healthy volunteers, we have not noted any deleterious effect on GFR [20]. Consequently, NE raises the filtration fraction (i.e., the quotient of GFR and RPF), which may reflect a change in pressure profile along glomerular arterioles. Moreover, NE infusion augments proteinuria in nephrotic patients [19] and increases microproteinuria in healthy subjects and diabetic patients in conjunction with a large rise in blood pressure [20, 21]. Taking the rise in filtration fraction and the proteinuria promoting effects of NE, it is plausible that NE also increases intra-glomerular pressure in man. The finding that GFR is independent from a wide range of NE-induced reductions in RPF, could also imply that glomerular blood flow is not the most important determinant of human ultrafiltration. It therefore seems that the dependency of GFR on RPF is not operative in adequately hydrated humans, unlike the hydropenic rat [11]. The notion that RPF is a determinant of human GFR is, in fact, only based on observations that GFR is highly correlated with RPF in man [22]. Moreover, it has been outlined that an increase in filtration fraction concomitantly with a fall in RPF, does not necessarily reflect a predominant increase in efferent over afferent glomerular arteriolar resistance and thus an increase in intraglomeru-lar pressure [23]. In fact, the filtration rises to some extent with a proportional in-crease in afferent and efferent glomerular arteriolar tone. Thus, the lack of a decre-ase in GFR during NE infusion in humans could also indicate a large functional RPF reserve in man.

NE infusions are associated with an anti-natriuretic effect in healthy subjects in most but not all studies which is in accordance with experimental nerve stimulation studies [7, 16–18]. The sodium retaining effect of NE is ascribed to direct stimula-tion of proximal tubular sodium reabsorption. In addition, intrarenal angiotensin II generation by NE has been proposed to play a contributory role. This is supported by the finding that angiotensin converting enzyme (ACE) inhibitors blunt NE-induced anti-natriuresis in healthy man [24]. The physiological importance of the NE effects of renal sodium handling under normal circumstances are not well known, but it is evident that pressure natriuresis is not a feature of NE-induced rises in blood press-ure. This indicates that exogenous infusions of NE may reset renal sodium handling towards sodium retention.

NE is a potent vasoconstrictor substance that is increasingly reported to be a very effective agent to restore blood pressure and tissue perfusion in patients with septic shock [5, 6, 25]. However, fear of renal function loss with NE infusions is common. This is in fact only based on studies in animals in which relatively high doses of intra-arterially administered NE produced renal ischemia and insufficiency [3, 4]. No data are available on the exact renal hemodynamic effects as measured by ap-propriate clearance methods in the critically ill. Using indirect measures such as urine output and/or creatinine values, it has been shown that NE is able to quickly reverse oliguria in septic patients [5, 6, 25, 26]. From these observations it can be inferred that the benefits of NE are due to restoration of perfusion pressure e.g., intraglomerular pressure, which is generally conceived to be the driving force of the human glomerular ultrafiltration process [22]. It has been suggested, therefore, that the NE-induced reduction in RPF is of limited importance in patients with septic shock and does not deteriorate renal function. In contrast, renal vasoconstriction by NE may increase perfusion pressure and thus improve renal function (i.e., GFR), provided adequate fluid resuscitation has been established.

Effects of Dopamine

Dopamine has a complicated influence on the cardiovascular and renal system. This is due to the fact that dopamine stimulates different types of adrenergic receptors:

not only α- and β-adrenergic but also specific dopamine receptors [27, 28], each of which can be divided into two subtypes according to the effects occurring when stimulated (Table 2). Dopamine has various indications depending on the dose given. This is due to the amount of stimulation and the change in the balance of these receptor effects for different doses. Dopamine receptors are present at various sites in the body, not only in the central nervous system (CNS), but also outside the CNS, the so called peripheral dopamine receptors. These receptors are divided into two types; postsynaptic D1-like, and (presynaptic) D2-like receptors. D1-like receptors are located in blood vessels and in the (mainly proximal) tubule of the kidney [29]. Stimulation induces vasodilation and natriuresis. The D2-like receptors are situated prejunctionally on sympathetic nerve terminals and in the adrenal gland. Stimulation of D2-like receptors results in inhibition of norepinephrine release and inhibition of aldosterone secretion [28, 29].

Dopamine is known to increase cardiac output (CO) at lower doses due to β- and α-receptor stimulation, without change or with a slight fall, in systemic vascular resistance [27, 30, 31]. In patients with low or depressed CO dopamine can be used to increase CO. In conditions with total body fluid overload the diuretic properties (mainly D1-like receptor stimulation) of dopamine are of additional value [32]. At higher doses (>10 µg/kg min) systemic vascular resistance will increase. For this reason dopamine is often used in critically ill patients with septic (hyperdynamic) shock, which in the early phase is characterized by a high CO and low systemic vascular resistance.

Low-dose dopamine (<4 µg/kg/min), still wrongly nicknamed by many clinicians as "renal dose" suggesting only renal effects, increases renal blood flow by preferential postglomerular vasodilation, and increases CO [29, 31]. The renal vasodilation together with direct tubular effects will lead to an increase in natriuresis and diuresis [28]. In a recent study we [31] also demonstrated a decrease in plasma aldosterone concentration in postoperative mechanically ventilated patients, which would contribute to the natriuretic effect of dopamine. However, the effects of dopamine on renal plasma flow are dependent on the GFR. Effects are significantly blunted or even absent in cases of a low GFR [33].

An increase in mesenteric flow has been observed in anesthetized preoperative patients at a dopamine dose of 4 µg/kg/min [34] and in patients undergoing elective spinal cord surgery [35]. Additionally, in animal studies improved oxygenation of the jejunal mucosa has been observed [36]. The different studies describing the effects of dopamine on the systemic and local circulation make it attractive for use in the ICU and operating room. Since effects on blood flow are considered to be beneficial, dopamine is often used as a drug for preservation of regional blood flow, and is given for prevention of impairment of cardio-renal function and protection of splanchnic flow. Additionally, dopamine in this context is suitable for different types of shock and its effects can be modified by simply increasing the dose. However, the studies on splanchnic flow are not conclusive: A study by Segal et al. [37], showed an indication of earlier onset of gut ischemia with dopamine use in a porcine model of hemorrhagic shock. Hemmer and Suter [38] demonstrated that the 20% fall in CO and oxygen delivery (DO_2) and the 47% decrease in creatinine clearance during mechanical ventilation with 20 cm PEEP could be reversed by dopamine. Similarly, cardiovascular depression due to anesthetic agents is counteracted by dopamine [30,

39]. Furthermore, the hypertension observed in patients undergoing general anesthesia without thoracic epidural analgesia, was neutralized by dopamine, making the patient more "stable" during anesthesia [40]. In a study by Flancbaum et al. [41] it was shown that some critically ill oliguric patients respond to dopamine administration with a > 50% increase of diuresis. However, prospective controlled studies using more appropriate endpoints are scarce and disappointing for those who expect a favorable effect of dopamine to be demonstrated. In a prospective double-blind placebo controlled study by Myles et al. [42] the effect of 3 μg/kg/min dopamine on renal function following cardiac surgery was examined in 49 patients with a previous serum creatinine value < 300 mmol/l. Dopamine did not improve renal creatinine clearance, although systemic hemodynamics were ameliorated by dopamine during the operation [42]. In a prospective double-blind placebo controlled study [43] in 60 patients undergoing renal transplantation, with pair-wise randomization of both kidneys of one donor, no beneficial effect of 3 μg/kg/min of dopamine could be detected. Dopamine was started 10 minutes before the release of the vascular clamps and continued until 48 hours after the transplantation. Outcome after 3 months was identical in both groups [43].

The use of dopamine in septic patients has been questioned as several studies now show that norepinephrine is more efficacious in restoring blood pressure in these patients, thereby establishing a better perfusion pressure [6]. Furthermore, it has been suggested that dopamine causes an uncompensated increase in splanchnic oxygen requirements in septic patients [43].

Cardiac failure with extensive fluid retention might remain a special indication for dopamine since it both increases CO, renal blood flow and sodium excretion, which will result in relief of the symptoms of dyspnea. Studies comparing treatment with diuretics and dobutamine versus dopamine are lacking, but, in general as any clinician can confirm, such patients show rapid improvement.

Conclusion

The widespread use of dopamine in the ICU is by no means supported by the literature. Until now, all studies on low-dose dopamine have failed to demonstrate a renal protective effect in any patient group. Clinicians confuse an increase in diuresis with preservation or improvement of renal function. So why do clinicians still administer low-dose dopamine to mechanically ventilated, but otherwise stable patients? Perhaps because they feel happier with a patient with a diuresis of 100 ml/hr than with the same patient with a diuresis of 30 ml/hr. However, the question should be whether this patient is better off in the end with a (temporary) increase in diuresis? Low-dose dopamine does increase CO and exerts positive inotropic and chronotropic effects by β_1-receptor agonist activity. It therefore increases intracellular Ca^{2+} which can lead to arrhythmias. Vasoactive drugs should never be considered harmless and only be given when an indication is present. Fear of NE use comes from animal studies using high doses of intra-arterial NE or dehydrated animals. The misconception that renal blood flow is equal to renal function also contributes to this fear. GFR is the most important determinant of renal function and is independent of (a wide range of) renal blood flow. Evidence now exists that NE improves renal function in patients with septic shock, provided adequate fluid resuscitation has been achieved [5, 25]. Additionally, studies have now shown that NE is more efficacious at restoring the blood pressure of septic patients after fluid resuscitation than dopamine [6]. Prevention of renal failure with low-dose dopamine is disappointing, since no human study has shown evidence of such an effect. However, it should be acknowledged that in clinical practice dopamine can be used in patients with shock in whom the diagnosis is not yet established, if it improves the hemodynamic status. We should accept of course that well controlled prospective studies are not always available and even not always necessary. Although a prospective controlled study of the efficacy of a parachute is lacking, no one would doubt its usefulness …!

It can be concluded, however, that routine administration of low-dose dopamine should be banned and the role of dopamine in the ICU should be reassessed. NE is a pharmacologically rational choice in patients with septic shock and can be safely given provided an adequate fluid status is present.

References

1. McDonald Jr RH, Goldberg LI, McNay JL, Tuttle Jr EP (1964) Effects of dopamine in man; augmentation of sodium excretion, glomerular filtration rate and renal plasma flow. J Clin Invest 43:1116–1124
2. Casement J, Irgin SM, Manji M (1997) Audit of the use of renal dose dopamine in intensive care units in the UK. Intensive Care Med 23:S91 (Abst)
3. Knapp R, Hollenberg NK, Busch GJ, Abrams HL (1972) Prolonged unilateral acute renal failure induced by intra-arterial norepinephrine infusion in the dog. Invest Radiol 7:164–173
4. Baehler RW, Kotchen TA, Ott CE (1978) Failure of chronic sodium chloride loading to protect against norepinephrine-induced acute renal failure in dogs. Circ Res 42:23–27
5. Martin C, Eon B, Saux P, Aknin P, Gouin F (1990) Renal effects of norepinephrine used to treat septic shock patients. Crit Care Med 18:282–285
6. Martin C, Papazian L, Perrin G, Saux P, Gouin F (1993) Norepinephrine or dopamine for the treatment of hyperdynamic septic shock? Chest 103:1826–1831
7. DiBona GF, Kopp UC (1997) Neural control of renal function. Physiol Rev 77:75–197
8. Silverberg AB, Shah SD, Haymond MW, Cryer PE (1978) Norepinephrine: hormone and neurotransmitter in man. Am J Physiol 234:E252–E256
9. Barajas L (1978) Innervation of the renal cortex. Fed Proc 37:1192–1201
10. Stephenson JA, Summers RJ (1986) Autoradiographic evidence for a heterogeneous distribution of alpha 1-adrenoreceptors labelled by [3H] prazosin in rat, dog and human kidney. J Auton Pharmacol 6:109–116
11. Maddox DA, Brenner BM (1996) Glomerular ultrafiltration. In: Brenner BM, Rector FC (eds) The kidney. WB. Saunders Co, Philadephia, pp 286–333
12. Kon V, Ichikawa I (1983) Effector loci for renal nerve control of cortical microcirculation. Am J Physiol 245:F545–F553
13. Myers BD, Deen WM, Brenner BM (1975) Effects of norepinephrine and angiotensin II on the determinants of glomerular ultrafiltration and proximal tubule fluid reabsorption in the rat. Circ Res 37:101–110
14. Edwards RM (1983) Segmental effects of norepinephrine and angiotensin II on isolated renal microvessels. Am J Physiol 244:F526–F534
15. Ito S, Arima S, Ren YL, Juncos LA, Carretero OA (1993) Endothelium-derived relaxing factor/ nitric oxide modulates angiotensin II action in the isolated microperfused rabbit afferent but not efferent arteriole. J Clin Invest 91:2012–2019
16. Smythe M, Nicke JF, Bradley SE (1952) The effect of epinephrine (usp), 1-epinephrine, and 1-norepinephrine on glomerular filtration rate, renal plasma flow and the urinary excretion of sodium, potassium and water in normal man. J Clin Invest 31:499–506

17. Richer M, Robert S, Lebel M (1996) Renal hemodynamics during norepinephrine and low-dose dopamine infusions in man. Crit Care Med 24:1150–1156
18. Hoogenberg K, Smit AJ, Girbes ARJ (1998) Effects of low dose dopamine on renal and systemic haemodynamics during incremental norepinephrine infusion in healthy volunteers. Crit Care Med (in press)
19. Lathem W (1965) Renal circulatory dynamics and urinary protein excretion during infusions of l-norepinephrine in patients with renal disease. J Clin Invest 35:1277–1285
20. Hoogenberg K, Sluiter WJ, Van Haeften TW, Smit AJ, Reitsma WD, Dullaart RPF (1996) No difference in renal haemodynamic and albuminuric response to noradrenaline in IDDM and healthy subjects. Diabetol 39:294a (Abst)
21. Hoogenberg K, Navis GJ, Dullaart RPF (1997) Norepinephrine-induced blood pressure rise and renal vasoconstriction is not attenuated by enalapril in microalbuminuric IDDM. Neph Dial Transplant (in press)
22. Brenner BM, Humes HD (1977) Mechanics of glomerular ultrafiltration. N Engl J Med 297:148–154
23. Carmines PK, Perry MD, Hazelrig JB, Navar LG (1987) Effects of preglomerular and postglomerular vascular resistance alterations on filtration fraction. Kidney Int Suppl 20:S229–S232
24. Lang CC, Rahman AR, Balfour DJ, Struthers AD (1993) Enalapril blunts the antinatriuretic effect of circulating noradrenaline in man. J Hypertens 11:565–571
25. Meadows D, Edwards JD, Wilkins RG, Nightingale P (1988) Reversal of intractable septic shock with norepinephrine therapy. Crit Care Med 16:663–666
26. Redl-Wenzl EM, Armbruster C, Edelmann G, et al (1993) The effects of norepinephrine on hemodynamics and renal function in severe septic shock states. Intensive Care Med 19:151–154
27. Goldberg LI (1972) Cardiovascular and renal actions of dopamine; potential clinical applications. Pharmac Rev 24:1–24
28. Smit AJ (1989) Dopamine and the kidney. Neth J Med 34:47–58
29. Girbes ARJ, Van Veldhuisen DJ, Smit AJ (1992) Nouveaux agonistes de la dopamine en thérapie cardiovasculaire. Presse Med 21:1287–1291
30. Raner C, Biber B, Lundberg J, Martner J, Winso O (1994) Cardiovascular depression by isoflurane and concomitant thoracic epidural anesthesia is reversed by dopamine. Acta Anaesthesiol Scand 38:136–143
31. Girbes ARJ, Lieverse AG, Smit AJ, et al (1996) Lack of specific renal haemodynamic effects of different doses of dopamine after infrarenal aortic surgery. Br J Anaesth 77:753–757
32. Ramdohr B, Schüren KP, Biamino G, Schröder R (1973) Der Einfluss von Dopamine auf Haemodynamik und Nierenfunktion bei der schweren Herzinsuffizienz des Menschen. Klin Wschr 51:549–556
33. Wee PM ter, Smit AJ, Rosman JB, Sluiter WJ, Donker AJM (1986) Effect of intravenous infusion of low-dose dopamine on renal function in normal individuals and in patients with renal disease. Am J Nephrol 6:42–46
34. Lundberg J, Lundberg D, Norgren L, Ribbe E, Thorne J, Werner O (1990) Intestinal hemodynamics during laparotomy: effects of thoracic epidural anesthesia and dopamine in humans. Anesth Analg 71:9–15
35. Aono J, Mamiya K, Ueda W, Manabe M (1994) Effect of dopamine administration on ICG-disappearance rate during prone position anesthesia. Masui 43:1857–1860
36. Germann R, Haisjackl M, Hasibeder W, et al (1994) Dopamine and mucosal oxygenation in the porcine jejunum. J Appl Physiol 77:2845–2852
37. Segal JM (1992) Low-dose dopamine hastens onset of gut ischemia in a porcine model of hemorrhagic shock. J Appl Physiol 73:1159–1164
38. Hemmer M, Suter PM (1979) Treatment of cardiac and renal effects of PEEP with dopamine in patients with acute respiratory failure. Anesthesiol 50:399–403
39. Trekova NA, Dementyeva II, Dzemeshkevich SL, Asmangulyan YeT (1994) Blood oxygen transport function in cardiopulmonary bypass surgery for acquired heart valvular diseases. Int Surg 79:60–64
40. Lundberg J, Lundberg D, Norgren L, Werner O (1990) Dopamine counteracts hypertension during general anesthesia and hypotension during combined thoracic epidural anesthesia for abdominal aortic surgery. J Cardiothorac Anesth 4:348–353

41. Flancbaum L, Choban PS, Dasta JF (1994) Quantitative effects of low-dose dopamine on urine output in oliguric surgical intensive care unit patients. Crit Care Med 22:61–68
42. Myles PS, Buckland MR, Schenk NJ, et al (1993) Effect of "renal-dose" dopamine on renal function following cardiac surgery. Anaesth Intensive Care 21:56–61
43. Kadieva VS, Friedman L, Margolius LP, Jackson SA, Morell DF (1993) The effect of dopamine on graft function in patients undergoing renal transplantation. Anesth Analg 76:362–365

Oxygen Carriers

The Red Blood Cell: New Ideas About an Old Friend

O. Eichelbroenner, C. G. Ellis, and W. J. Sibbald

Introduction

With the introduction of the microscope in the early 1600s, scientists observed "red particles" in circulating fluid. Borel (1620–1689) and Kircher (1602–1680), both pioneer microscopists, descibed these objects as "animals of the shape of whales or dolphins swimming in a red ocean … formed to consume the depraved elements of the blood" and as "worms floating in the blood stream and causing diseases". The most detailed description at this time, however, was included in a letter to a friend by Leewenhoek, who mentioned that "blood taken from his hand consists of red globules, also floating about in a crystalline fluid". He then speculated about their properties: "Those sanguineous globules must be very flexible and pliant if they shall pass through the capillary arteries and veins, and an their passage they change into an oval figure reassuming their roundness when they come into a larger room ", and mentioned the possibility of shape and deformability alterations of these cells after their exposure to different substances [1].

In the 19th century, the function of blood to carry oxygen (O_2) was considered likely when Stokes associated reduction and oxidation with changes in the visible spectrum, and reported that these processes were reversible. In the early 20th century, Huefner applied the law of mass action to the reversable hemoglobin-oxygen binding and predicted a rectangular curve. Shortly thereafter, however, Bohr, Roberts and Barcroft proved that the O_2 dissociation curve had a sigmoid shape, and the effect of carbon dioxide (CO_2) on the oxyhemoglobin dissociation curve (Bohr effect) was then described by Krogh in 1907. Although significant progress was made in understanding the steps of O_2 binding to a four-site molecule in the 1920s, it took another 30 years for Gibson and Roughton to prove the kinetic heme-heme interaction at the final stage of the reaction of hemoglobin with O_2 or CO_2. Subsequently, Chanutin and the Benesches demonstrated the effect of 2,3-diphosphoglycerate (2,3-DPG) and congeners on the O_2 affinity of hemoglobin, and Perutz and Kendrew unraveled hemoglobin's three-dimensional structure and its conformational changes between the oxy and deoxy state [2]. Realizing the need to be able to store red cells, Robertson developed a solution in 1918 which extended the storage of erythrocytes up to 21 days [3]. This expansion in storage time initiated the development of transfusion medicine with the red blood cell (RBC) being its leading performer.

The early view of RBCs has thus generally been one in which they were considered as "hemoglobin containing red balloons", exclusively for the purpose of transporting O_2 and CO_2. Such a limited view, however, neglects the fact that nature tends to think and plan in a complex, comprehensive and evolutionary manner. Erythrocytes represent nearly 50% of the blood volume, carry O_2, and exhibit an ability to routinely access every area in the body. To some, it was therefore logical to assume that nature has created additional and as yet undescribed tasks for the red cell.

The objective of this chapter is to introduce the reader to newer concepts about other functions of the red blood cell and its possible roles in illnesses relevant to critical care.

Erythrocyte – Endothelial Cell Interactions

Cell-cell interactions are a crucial aspect in the process of inflammation. Activated neutrophils, monocytes, platelets and endothelial cells communicate and act by releasing cytokines, lipid mediators and oxygen derived radicals. These mediators propagate the inflammatory process by accentuating adhesion between these blood borne cells and the endothelium [4]. While there is a substantial and comprehensive literature about the adhesion process between neutrophils and the endothelium, knowledge about erythrocyte-endothelial cell interaction in critical illness is rudimentary, but probably no less important. There are a number of conditions where RBCs demonstrate adhesive interactions with endothelial cells, including diabetes, malaria, sickle cell disease and, as shown recently, after exposure to endotoxin. By reviewing knowledge from the study of these conditions, insight and further research themes in the interaction of RBCs and microcirculatory dysfunction in the pathophysiology of sepsis may be explored.

Diabetes Mellitus

Diabetes mellitus is associated with a high prevalence of microvascular disease and rheologic abnormalities, including a loss of RBC deformability and an increase in RBC adhesivness. Wautier et al. [5] found that diabetic RBCs stuck to endothelial cells *in vitro* twice as frequently as RBCs from control subjects. Additionally, a significant correlation was noted between the rate of RBC-endothelial adhesion and clinical vascular complications in diabetic patients. In a subsequent study, Zoukourian et al. [6, 7] reported that an accumulation of AGE (advanced glycation end products) on the RBC membrane mediated their adhesion with endothelial cells through RAGE35, a specific receptor for AGE expressed on endothelium (Fig. 1). In the same study, iloproust (a prostacyclin analog) treatment significantly reduced surrogate markers of oxidative stress in the endothelial cells, such as an increase in permeability of the cell layer to albumin, production of thiobarbituric acid reactive substances (TBARS), and release of interleukin-6 (IL-6).

In summary, these data of the RBC-endothelial interaction in diabetes show that: (i) RBC-endothelial adhesion in diabetes has been correlated with the extent and severity of diabetic microvascular and atherosclerotic disease and diabetic vasculopathies, and (ii) abnormalities in blood rheology and RBC properties may trigger

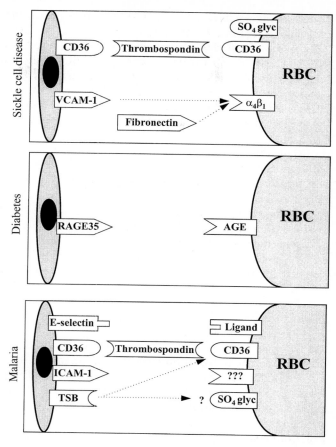

Fig. 1. Principal mechanisms responsible for erythrocyte-endothelial cell interactions in different pathologies. RBC: red blood cell; VCAM: vascular cell adhesion molecule; AGE: advanced glycation end products; ICAM: intercellular adhesion molecule

and/or perpetuate inflammation-like processes which can provide a milieu for adhesive interactions between RBCs and endothelium.

Malaria

During infection with *Plasmodium falsiparum,* parasitized RBCs adhere to endothelial cells and accumulate in the microcirculation of various organs. Research has now shown that this phenomenon requires the expression of adhesion molecules on the endothelium (Fig. 1). Ockenhouse et al. [8] incubated tumor necrosis factor-α (TNF-α) activated endothelial cells with infected RBCs and found these RBCs were bound by the activated endothelial cells and the RBC-endothelial adhesion could be partially inhibited by E-selectin and vascular cell adhesion molecule (VCAM) antibodies. Using soluble E-selectin and VCAM they also showed that these adhesion molecules were bound to the RBC surface.

In studies from Cooke et al. [9], the role of intercellular adhesion molecules (ICAM-1), CD36 and thrombospondin in rolling and stationary cytoadhesion of infected RBCs to the endothelium was demonstrated. These data showed that the adhesion molecules mediated sticking of infected RBCs and endothelium at shear stresses within the physiological range. The majority of RBCs formed rolling rather than static attachment via ICAM-1, whereas static adhesion predominated with CD36 and thrombospondin [29]. Subsequently, Cooke's group [10] added another to the list of adhesive molecules, chondroitin sulfate A, a glycosaminoglycan associated with the endothelial surface which immobilizes RBCs under conditions of flow. Furthermore, serum levels of TNF-α are consistently elevated during acute malaria infection and correlate both with the level of peripheral parasitemia and the severity and prognosis of disease [11].

These findings point out that: (i) adhesion of red blood cells to endothelium via adhesion molecules is important in the pathogenesis of malaria and (ii) the adherence of RBCs to microvascular endothelial cells is accentuated by cytokine mediators that are believed to play a key role in the pathogenesis of sepsis.

Sickle Cell Disease

Recurring episodes of vaso-occlusion in sickle crises cause tissue hypoxia [12], and may include anomalies in both the vessel wall and in the RBC. Measurements performed under both static [13] and dynamic [14] conditions demonstrate that sickled RBCs have a sticky surface and adhere more readily than normal RBCs to cultured endothelial cells. Recent investigations have started to unravel the molecular structures responsible for the adhesion of sickled RBCs to endothelium (Fig. 1). All RBCs, but especially those from patients with the sickle trait, carry integrin α4β1 on their surface which can bind to both fibronectin and VCAM [15]. These two molecules are expressed on the endothelium during inflammation. In addition, both normal RBCs and sickled RBCs express CD36 (which is also located on the surface of endothelial cells), a non-integrin adhesive receptor which binds to collagen and thrombospondin. Soluble plasma thrombospondin excreted by activated platelets is postulated to bridge these CD36 receptors present on endothelium and RBCs [16–19], thus encouraging firm adhesion of sickled RBCs to endothelial cells. Setty and Stuart [12] investigated the role of hypoxia on sickled RBC-endothelial adherence and showed that VCAM is responsible for hypoxia-induced adhesion, but not for basal adherence, while ICAM-1 has no effect on either basal or hypoxia-induced adhesion.

Healthy RBCs do not usually activate endothelial cells in any form by contact. However, abnormal RBCs, such as sickled RBCs, have also been reported to activate naive endothelial cells. Exposure of healthy endothelial cells to sickled RBCs initiated a five fold increase in formation of TBARS, an activation of transcription factor nuclear factor-kappa B (NF-κB) and increased surface expression of ICAM-1, E-selectin and VCAM-1 [20].

These studies investigating the pathomechanisms of sickle cell disease confirmed (i) the importance of adhesion molecules in the attachment of RBCs to endothelium and (ii) also indicated that the adherence of sickled RBCs to the endothelium may lead to cell injury by causing an oxidative stress.

Endotoxin Infusion

Lipopolysaccharide (LPS) infusion will initiate a systemic inflammatory response syndrome by promoting the release of early cytokines such as TNF-α and IL-1. Alone or in combination, these mediators prime immunologically active cells circulating in blood and also activate vascular endothelial cells to express molecules for cell-cell interaction. As a result, leukocytes, monocytes and macrophages bind to endothelial cells during LPS infusion, thereby causing tissue injury by obstructing nutrient microcirculatory flows and/or emigrating into the extravascular space and releasing mediators such as reactive oxygen species.

Van Patot et al. [4] reported that LPS induced adhesion of bovine RBCs to bovine pulmonary artery endothelial cells in a static non-flowing assay. The extent of this abnormal adhesion depended on the LPS concentration and the presence of divalent cations such as Ca^{2+} and Mg^{2+}. Cytokines such as TNF-α and IL-1 also triggered the adhesion of RBCs to endothelium, but platelet activating factor (PAF) had no effect. The addition of antioxidants exhibited unexpected results. In contrast to their effects on leukocyte adhesion where they decrease adhesion, antioxidants (superoxide dismutase, catalase, dimethyl sulfoxide) increased the adherence of RBC to endothelial cells. Only phosphatidylserine, an aminophospholipid which is usually confined to the inner leaflet of the RBC bilayer membrane, reduced adhesion. The presence of phosphatidylserine in the outer leaflet of the membrane may be a consequence of oxidative stress and lipid peroxidation which impair the normal asymmetric phospholipid distribution in the membrane [21, 30].

While there is no doubt that the static assays have made important contributions to our understanding of cytoadhesion, they neglect the fact that adhesive interactions between these cells occur in the dynamic environment of the microcirculation. They also ignore numerous important issues concerning qualitative and quantitative aspects of adhesion. For example, the influence of shear forces generated by the flow of blood in the vasculature must be considered in any attempt to assess the pathological importance of cytoadhesion [10]. We therefore used a dynamic flow system and human tissues for our studies. We [22] found that endotoxin significantly increases RBC adhesion to cultured human umbilical vascular endothelial cells in the presence of shear stress. However, increases in flow rate reduced adhesion of LPS-treated RBC to baseline levels. In contrast, when intermittent flow, as is present

Table 1. Adhesion of RBCs to endothelium

	CON	ETX1	ETX2	IMF
Number of RBCs/mm² endothelial cells	71 ± 8	172 ± 25^a	89 ± 20	$274 \pm 35^{a,b}$

CON: naive cells; ETX1: flow = 0,65ml/min; ETX2: flow = 1,3ml/min; IMF: intermittent flow; [a] $p < 0.05$ (to baseline); [b] $p < 0.05$ (to ETX1)

in the septic microcirculation [23], was introduced, RBC adhesion was significantly elevated (Table 1). Preliminary data from subsequent studies in our laboratory show that adhesion is more pronounced when endothelial cells are primed by LPS, although adhesion of primed RBCs to naive endothelium is still higher than in the control experiments.

Summary: Erythrocyte-Endothelial Cell Interactions

The RBC membrane is an immunologically active and interactive surface involved in the inflammatory process in the microcirculation of various diseases. While the role of leukocytes has been extensively investigated in the pathophysiology of sepsis, the role of abnormal RBC-endothelial interactions in this syndrome has not been the subject of any in depth analysis. However, the findings previously reviewed about the interaction of RBCs with endothelium in diabetes, malaria and sickle cell disease lead to the speculation that abnormal RBC-endothelial interactions in sepsis contribute to the microvascular dysfunction that is typical of this condition.

The Red Blood Cell and its Relations with Nitric Oxide

The binding of oxygen in the lungs, carrying it through the macrocirculation and finally releasing it in the tissues is a fine tuned and sophisticated process determined by the tetrameric structure of hemoglobin, by cooperation within the molecule and the cooperation between several mechanisms, such as conformational adaptations by 2,3 DPG to optimize uptake and release at different anatomical sites under extreme conditions. Recently, a novel theory was reported by Stamler et al. [24] who postulated that nitric oxid (NO)-hemoglobin interactions are crucial components for mircocirculatory blood flow and oxygen transport.

Classic View

The traditional understanding of RBCs is that they transport O_2 from the lungs to the tissue where O_2 is released in arterioles and capillaries. In exchange for O_2, they load metabolic waste products such as CO_2 and H^+ and displace them in the lungs for elimination. The matching of O_2 need with supply is well-regulated by the metabolic requirements of the tissues. Thus, tissue hypoxia increases, while hyperoxia decreases nutritive blood flow. These dogmas are thought to be significantly mediated by NO released from endothelial cells in the tissues [25].

Novel Theory

Recently, it has been suggested that RBCs play a far more active role in the regulation of blood flow within and between tissues and that the respiratory circle involves three, instead of two, major gases transported by hemoglobin: O_2, CO_2 and NO [24].

This latter model assumes a dynamic circle in which O_2 and NO are bound by hemoglobin in the lungs and delivered to the microcirculation where NO, originating from hemoglobin, modulates vascular tone [26] while the endothelium-derived NO is considered to play only a secondary role in the autoregulation of blood flow.

The Hemoglobin-Oxygen-NO Circle

Hemoglobin exists in two alternative allosteric conformations, the R-state (R for relaxed, high oxygen affinity state) and the T-state (T for tense, low oxygen affinity state) (Fig. 2). On its journey between the lungs and the microcirculation, hemoglobin switches back and forth between these two shapes either to take up (R-state) or release (T-state) O_2 and NO. When hemoglobin enters the lungs, it is still in the T-state, carries two to three molecules of O_2 and is partially nitrosylated, with the NO group bound to the metal group (heme) of the hemoglobin ($Hb[Fe^{++}]NO =$ nitrosyl$[Fe^{++}]$-hemoglobin). In the presence of high oxygen tensions (PO_2) hemoglobin saturates the open binding sites and changes into the R-state. Simultaneously, NO is picked up and bound to the highly reactive sulfhydryl group (SH) of the cysteine 93 in the β-chains (Cysβ93) forming SNO-oxyhemoglobin (SNO-$Hb[Fe^{++}]O_2$). This R-state hemoglobin loaded with O_2 and NO now enters the arte-

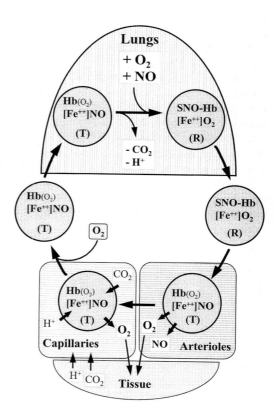

Fig. 2. The hemoglobin-oxygen nitric oxide (NO) circle

rial circulation. In the precapillary arterioles a significant amount of O_2 is released before the RBCs travel into the capillaries. This loss of O_2 in the precapillary resistance vessels effects an allosteric transition in the hemoglobin (change from R to T-state), which liberates NO from the Cysβ93 residues. These NO fractions, set free from the hemoglobin-molecule, dilate vessels and thereby improve blood flow [24]. Finally, the hemoglobin travels through the capillary bed and further releases oxygen according to the tissue needs. On its way back through the postcapillary venules hemoglobin picks up one or two of the extra O_2 diffused across from the precapillary arterioles or areas with high PO_2 and is loaded with CO_2 and H^+ for elimination in the lungs where the circle starts over again.

A series of experiments provides *in vitro* and *in vivo* evidence supporting the importance of RBC-NO interactions in the circulation. First, Craescu et al. [27] and Garel et al. [28] reported that oxygenation of hemoglobin is associated with allosteric changes which increase the activity of Cysβ93. Jia et al. [26] observed that the rate of S-nitrosylation of hemoglobin (transfer of NO to SH) depends on the conformational state, with a higher rate of S-nitrosylation in the oxy (R) than in the deoxy (T) state. Furthermore, the rate of S-nitrosylation was accelerated for both conformtions at increased pH which exposes the Cysβ93 residue to the surface that is otherwise covered. Similiar conditions are present in the lungs where elimination of CO_2 and H^+ induce a slight increase of blood pH. These findings suggest that the increased SH-reactivity in the oxy-hemoglobin is favored by improved access to the Cysβ93 residue in the oxy-conformation of the hemoglobin molecule.

To determine whether SNO-Hb is naturally occuring in the blood in mammals and if so, what its distribution is between arterial and venous blood, Jia et al. [26] measured the concentrations of S-nitroso-Hb (NO bound to SH of cysteine) and nitrosyl-(Fe^{++})Hb (NO bound to the heme) in rat arterial and venous blood. They found that arterial blood contained higher levels of S-nitroso-Hb than nitrosyl-(Fe^{++})Hb (311 ± 55 vs. 32 ± 14 nM). When they infused N^G-nitro-monomethyl-L-arginine (L-NMMA), to block NO synthesis, SNO-Hb was depleted as well as total Hb-NO (80 and 50%, respectively). Also, the arterial-venous distribution of nitrosyl-Hb revealed an inverse relationship as the concentration of nitrosyl-(Fe^{++})Hb was higher in the venous than in the arterial blood (894 ± 126 vs. 536 ± 99 nM).)

In experiments to verify biological activity and relevance, the same group compared the effects of free SNO-Hb and nitrosyl-Hb infusions, and infusions of RBC containing the different fractions of hemoglobion on blood pressure and blood flow.

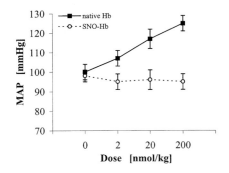

Fig. 3. *In vivo* effects of cell-free hemoglobin (Hb) and SNO-Hb on mean arterial pressure (MAP). Bolus administration of 2–200 nmol/kg of Hb(Fe^{++})O_2 increased mean arterial pressure (mal) in a dose dependant manner (solid squares). The same doses of SNO-Hb did not change (open circle) blood pressure. (Modified from [26] with permission)

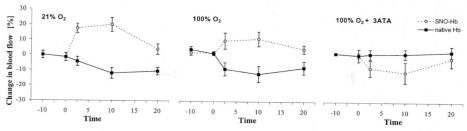

Fig. 4. Effects of hemoglobin and SNO-Hb on local cerebral blood flow in the caudate putamen nucleus at different O_2 concentrations. SNO-Hb increased blood flow both at 21% and 100% inspiratory oxygen and reduced flow at overpressure combined with 100% oxygen. In contrast, hemoglobin decreased blood flow at 21% and at 100% O_2. At 100% O_2 + 3ATA flow was not different between the two hemoglobin fractions. (Modified from [24] with permission)

As expected, infusion of native hemoglobin induced an increase in blood pressure, while SNO-Hb did not affect the blood pressure (Fig. 3). The experiments measuring the effects of different hemoglobins on blood flow revealed that only SNO-Hb increased or maintained regional blood flow at different inspiratory oxygen fractions (Fig. 4). These findings were interpreted that SNO-Hb appropriately increased blood flow in relatively hypoxic tissues [24]. In further experiments, they were able to show that low molecular R-SNO is formed within the RBCs which mediates the SNO interactions with the vessel wall by export from the RBC (possibly supported by the close contact of the RBC and endothelium in the microcirculation).

Overall, these data establish the endogenous erythrocytic origin of SNO-Hb and its bioactivity *in vivo*. Its interactions with blood flow and blood pressure indicate an active role of the RBC on oxygen transport and circulatory dynamics.

Conclusion

This review shows that the role of the RBC goes far beyond the pure transport of the oxygen molecule from the lungs to the tissue. Its bilayer membrane represents an immunologically active surface in a variety of diseases with enhanced RBC-endothelium interactions after exposure to endotoxin which may contribute to the microvascular injury in sepsis. The ability of the red cell to scavenge NO at the heme and to transport NO as SNO-Hb assigns a dual role to the RBC both acting as a sink and a donor of NO depending on the local milieu. This ambiguity of the RBC towards NO may allow the RBC to actively regulate microcirculatory blood flow according to tissue oxygen needs.

References

1. Bessis M, Delpech G (1981) Discovery of the red blood cell with notes on priorities and credit of discoveries, past, present and future. Blood Cells 7:447–480
2. Antonini E (1979) History and theory of the oxyhemoglobin dissociation curve. Crit Care Med 9:360–367

3. Chin-Yee I, Arya N, d Almeida M (1998) The red cell storage lesion and its implication for transfusion. Transfusion Science (in press)

4. van Patot MC, Mackenzie S, Tucker A, Voelkel N (1996) Endotoxin-induced adhesion of red blood cells to pulmonary artery endothelial cells. Am J Physiol 270: L28–L36

5. Wautier JL, Paton RC, Wautier MP, et al (1981) Increased adhesion of erythrocytes to endothelial cells in diabetes mellitus and its relation to vascular complications. N Engl J Med 305: 237–242

6. Zoukourian C, Wautier MP, Chappey O, et al (1996) Endothelial cell dysfunction secondary to the adhesion of diabetic erythrocytes. Modulation by iloprost. Int Angiol 15: 195–200

7. Wautier JL, Wautier MP, Schmidt AM, et al (1994) Advanced glycation end products (AGEs) on the surface of diabetic erythrocytes bind to the vessel wall via a specific receptor inducing oxidant stress in the vasculature: a link between surface-associated AGEs and diabetic complications. Proc Natl Acad Sci USA 91: 7742–7746

8. Ockenhouse CF, Tegoshi T, Maeno Y, et al (1992) Human vascular endothelial cell adhesion receptors for Plasmodium falciparum-infected erythrocytes: roles for endothelial leukocyte adhesion molecule 1 and vascular cell adhesion molecule 1. J Exp Med 176: 1183–1189

9. Cooke BM, Rogerson SJ, Brown GV, Coppel RL (1996) Adhesion of malaria-infected red blood cells to chondroitin sulfate A under flow conditions. Blood 88 (10): 4040–4044

10. Cooke BM, Berendt AR, Craig AG, MacGregor J, Newbold CI, Nash GB (1994) Rolling and stationary cytoadhesion of red blood cells parasitized by Plasmodium falsiparum: separate roles for ICAM-1, CD-36 and thrombospondin. Br J Hematology 87: 162–170

11. Cooke BM, Coppel RL (1995) Cytoadhesion and Falciparum malaria: Going with the flow. Parasitology Today 11 (8): 282–287

12. Setty BN, Stuart MJ (1996) Vascular cell adhesion molecule-1 is involved in mediating hypoxia-induced sickle red cell adherence to endothelium: potential role in sickle cell disease. Blood 88: 2311–2320

13. Hebbel PR, Yamada O, Moldow CF, Jacob HS, White JG, Eaton JW (1980) Abnormal adherence of sickle erythrocytes to cultured vascular endothelium: a possible mechanism for microvascular occlusion in sickle cell disease. J Clin Invest 65: 154–160

14. Barabino GA, McIntire LV, Eskin SG, Sears DA, Udden M (1987) Endothelial cell interaction with sickle cell, sickle trait mechanically injured and normal erythrocytes under controlled flow. Blood 70: 152–157

15. Bunn HF (1997) Pathogenesis and treatment of sickle cell disease. N Engl J Med 337: 762–769

16. Sugihara K, Sugihara T, Mohandas N, Hebbel RP (1992) Thrombospondin mediates adherence of CD36$^+$ sickle reticulocytes to endothelial cells. Blood 80: 2634–2642

17. Brittain HA, Eckman JR, Swerlick RA, Howard RA, Wick TM (1993) Thrombospondin from activated platelets promotes sickle erythrocytes adherence to human microvascular endothelium under physiologic flow. Blood 81: 2137–2143

18. Joneckis CC, Ackley RL, Orringer EP, Wayner EA, Parise LV (1993) Integrin a4bl and glycoprotein IV (CD36) are expressed on circulating reticulocytes in sickle cell anemia. Blood 82: 3548–3555

19. van Schravendijk MR, Handunetti SM, Barnell JW, Howard RJ (1992) Normal erythrocytes express CD36, an adhesion molecule of monocytes, platelets and endothelial cells. Blood 80: 2105–2114

20. Kalra VK, Rattan V, Sultana C, Shen Y, Johnson C, Meiselman HH (1997) Sickle red cell interaction with endothelial cells augments the expression of adhesion molecules and transendothelial migration of monocytes. Microcirculation 4: 130–136

21. Schlegel RA, Prendergast TW, Williamson P (1985) Membrane phospholipid asymmetry as a factor in erythrocyte-endothelial cell interactions. J Cell Physiol 123: 215–218

22. Eichelbrönner O, Cepinskas G, Kvietys P, Chin-Yee I, Sibbald WJ (1998) Adhesion of human erythrocytes to human endothelial cells is increased by endotoxin. Crit Care Med (in press)

23. Madorin S, Martin CM, Potter RF, Sibbald WJ (1996) Dopexamine attenuates flowmotion of ileal mucosal arterioles in septic rats. Intensive Care Med 22 (suppl 3): S442 (Abst)

24. Stamler JS, Jia L, Eu JP, et al (1997) Blood flow regulation by S-nitrosohemoglobin in the physiological oxygen gradient. Science 276: 2034–2037

25. Park KH, Rubin LE, Gross SS, Levi R (1992) Nitric oxide is a mediator of hypoxic coronary vasodilatation. Relation to adenosine and cyclooxygenase-induced metabolites. Circ Res 71: 992–1001

26. Jia L, Bonaventura J, Stamler JS (1996) S-nitrosohaemoglobin: a dynamic activity of blood involved in vascular control. Nature 380:221–226

27. Craescu CT, Poyart C, Schaeffer C, Garel MC, Kister J, Beuzard Y (1986) Covalent binding of glutathione to hemoglobin. II. Functional consequences and structural changes reflected in NMR spectra. J Biol Chem 261:14710–14716

28. Garel MC, Beuzard Y, Thillet J, et al (1982) Binding of 21 thiol reagents to human hemoglobin in solution and in intact cells. Eur J Biochem 3:513–519

29. Ockenhouse CF, Ho M, Tandon NN, et al (1991) Molecular basis of sequestration in severe and uncomplicated Plasmodium falciparum malaria: differential adhesion of infected erythrocytes to CD36 and ICAM-1. J Infect Dis 164:163–169

30. Zwaal RF, Schroit AJ (1997) Pathophysiologic implications of membrane phospholipid asymmetry in blood cells. Blood 89:1121–1132

Transfusion Requirements in Critical Care: A Multicenter Controlled Clinical Trial

P. C. Hébert

Introduction

Anemia is common in the critically ill and results in the frequent use of red cell transfusions [1, 2]. For decades, an arbitrary transfusion threshold of 100 g/L has been employed widely in clinical medicine including the management of critically ill patients [3]. Recently, a re-evaluation of this practice was prompted both by the fear of transfusion-related infections such as aquired immune deficiency syndrome (AIDS), and the prospect of an ever decreasing blood supply [4–6]. These concerns also resulted in the formulation of red cell transfusion guidelines by a number of organizations for the use of red cells [7–10]. However, published guidelines, for the most part, have not addressed how red cells should be administered in critically ill patients.

This patient population is affected by complex metabolic, respiratory and cardio-vascular pathophysiologic processes which predispose then to the adverse consequences of anemia such as the potential risk of myocardial infarction and death. It is also possible that critically ill patients are at increased risks of adverse consequences from allogeneic red cell transfusions, particularly the immunosuppressive [11–16] and microcirculatory [17–19] effects of red cells.

Despite the intense public scrutiny of transfusion practice and the conflicting rationale for different approaches to the administration of red cells (Table 1), there remain very few well controlled clinical trials evaluating transfusion practice. In a recent systematic review of transfusion practice [20], six randomized controlled

Table 1. Theoretical reasons supporting the restrictive or the liberal use of allogeneic red cells in normovolemic critically ill patients

Rationale supporting the liberal use of red cells
1) Augmenting oxygen delivery may improve survival
2) Increased risk of cororary ischemia due to increased demand
3) Age, disease severity and drugs may interfere with adaptation to anemia
4) Improved safety margin if further blood loss

Rationale supporting the restrictive use of red cells
1) Red cell transfusions impair microcirculatory flow
2) Pathologic supply dependency is rare
3) Risks of viral infections
4) Immunodepression causing increased infections following transfusion
5) Cardiac consequences of red cells less important

clinical trials (RCT) identified and contrasted two transfusion strategies (Table 2) [21–26]. The only large RCT was undertaken to determine if red cell transfusions prevent sickle cell crisis. Other more relevant studies were too small to provide clinically useful inferences in critically ill patients. Transfusion decisions in critically ill patients are therefore based on studies evaluating adaptive responses to anemia [27] and transfusions or observational studies and poorly controlled clinical trials [20]. In order to better elucidate the risks and benefits of transfusions, we conducted a large RCT to determine if mortality rates and organ dysfunction, as well as a number of secondary outcomes, were equivalent following a restrictive versus liberal transfusion strategy in normovolemic critically ill patients. In this article, the background outlining the divergent risks and benefits of a restrictive and a liberal approach to the transfusion of allogeneic red cells, the study design implemented in the Transfusion Requirements in Critical Care (TRICC) trial and the preliminary results will be discussed.

Transfusion Practice Variation in Critical Care

As an initial step in the planning of a large RCT, the TRICC trial investigators agreed that significant practice variation was a necessary precondition for a large RCT contrasting two existing approaches to the administration of red cells. Two observational studies, a survey of critical care physicians and a large cohort study, were conducted to determine individual and hospital practice variation.

In a 1992 Canadian survey of critical care practitioners [28], we documented that 35% of respondents identified 90 g/L as the minimum concentration and an additional 40% selected 100 g/L. Overall baseline transfusion thresholds ranged from a low of 50 g/L to 120 g/L. Thresholds were significantly different ($p < 0.001$) between scenarios (Table 2). All clinical characteristics evaluated, except congestive heart failure ($p > 0.05$), significantly ($p < 0.0001$) changed transfusion thresholds of Canadian critical care practitioners. We also noted significant differences between four clinical scenarios and a number of potential risk factors. There was a significant association between having an academic affiliation and transfusion practice across all scenarios ($p < 0.0001$). Physicians with an academic affiliation transfused red cells at a lower transfusion threshold than non-academics. When grouped into four major geographic locations (West, Ontario, Quebec, East), with no more than five academic centers per region, we noted that there was a statistically significant difference ($p < 0.01$) for baseline transfusion thresholds across all scenarios. In a second study [29] involving a cohort of 4 470 patients, we also documented a significant variation in nadir hemoglobin levels prior to transfusion amongst six academic intensive care units (ICU) using multivariate techniques adjusting for the influence of diagnosis, disease severity, patient age and transfusion status ($p < 0.0001$). Both studies provide compelling evidence of significant individual, institutional and regional variation in critical care transfusion practice indicating uncertainty regarding optimal hemoglobin levels and a need for further study.

Table 2. Randomized clinical trials of transfusion practices

Authors/Year Published	Level of Evidence	No. of Patients	Study Population	Interventions	Outcomes	Comments
Weisel et al. [21] (1984)	II	27	CABG	Crystalloid alone (n = 14) vs. Blood or colloid solutions (n = 13)	- [Hb] lower in crystalloid group 20 h postoperation (p = 0.01) - Reduction in blood utilization in the crystalloid group - No difference in pulmonary edema and hemodynamic parameters (cardiac index and filling pressures)	- Small sample size - No difference in mortality or myacardial infarction rates - Delayed recovery of myocardial extraction in a small number of patients in the crystalloid group
Johnson et al. [22] (1992)	II	38	CABG	Conservative group Hct maintained at 25% (n = 20) v. liberal group Hct maintained at 32% (n = 18)	- Conservative group transfused with fewer units than the liberal group (p = 0.012) - Mean cardiac index same for both group in the OR and 1 day postop - Mean postop LOS: 7.6 ± 1.9 days (liberal), 7.9 ± 4.3 days (conservative) - No difference in fluid requirement, hemodynamic parameters or hospital complications - No relation between exercise tolerance on the 5th and 6th days and Hct	- Small sample size - No postoperative deaths reported - No difference in ischemic event
Blair et al. [26] (1986)	II	50	GI hemorrhage	At least 2 units of PRCs (immediate) (n = 24) v. no transfusion unless [Hb] < 80 g/L (delayed) (n = 26)	- Decreased transfusions in delayed group (2.6 v 4.6 units/patient, p < 0.05) - The number of re-bled patients was greater in the immediate transfusion group (9 v. 1, p < 0.01)	- Small sample size - Study design included a pilot study - Laboratory and clinical measurement available - No detailed data related to operative interventions and mortality rate - Prolonged clotting time and higher re-bleeding rate due to blood transfusions in the first 24 hours

Table 2. (continued)

Authors/Year Published	Level of Evidence	No. of Patients	Study Population	Interventions	Outcomes	Comments
Fortune et al. [23] (1987)	II	25	Adult trauma	Hct = 30% (n = 12) v. Hct = 40% (n = 13)	– 5 units of PRC more in Hct = 40% groups – No difference in hemodynamic parameters – Higher intrapulmonary shunt in Hct = 40% group	– Small sample size – Physiologic outcome measurement only – No data on mechanisms and type of traumatic injury – No data on clinical outcomes
Hébert et al. [24] (1995)	II	69	ICU	Restrictive group: [Hb] = 70–90 g/L (n = 33) v. liberal group: [Hb] = 100–120 g/L (n = 36)	– Average daily [Hb] = 90 g/L v.109 g/L ($p < 0.001$) – Number of units transfused 48% less in restrictive group (2.5 v. 4.8 units/patient) – No difference in mortalily and organ failures ($p > 0.05$) – No difference in ICU and hospital LOS ($p > 0.05$)	– Small sample size – Pilot unable to detect difference in clinically important outcomes
Vichinsky et al. [25] (1995)	I	604	Sickle cell disease in surgery	Aggressive (n = 303) v. conservative (n = 301) regimens	– No difference in life-threatening complication rates but more transfusion associated complications, i.e. hemolytic reactions and alloantibodies in the aggressive group	– Total of 551 patients undergoing 604 operations – Randomized procedures not patients – Study in a specific population – Only 1 patient died in all procedures

[Hb] = hemoglobin concentration, Hct = hematocrit, CABG = coronary artery bypass grafting, GI = gastrointestinal

Evidence for Restrictive and Liberal Approaches to Transfusions

The liberal use of red cells in critically ill patients may be justified based on the theory that oxygen delivery should be increased or maintained at high levels in critically ill patients because of the possibility of ongoing tissue damage from ischemia. Disease processes such as sepsis and acute respiratory distress syndrome (ARDS) [30–48] have been hypothesized to induce tissue hypoxia by producing an abnormally elevated anaerobic threshold. Below this threshold or critical level of oxygen delivery, oxygen consumption decreases as oxygen delivery decreases. This abnormal linear relationship is often referred to as "pathologic supply dependence". The resultant tissue hypoxia may eventually contribute to the evolution of irreversible multiple system organ failure followed by death. Indeed, two prospective observational studies [36, 40] found a significant association between mortality and the finding of pathologic supply dependence.

A number of clinical trials [49–51] have attempted to define optimal levels of oxygen delivery in critically ill and high risk perioperative patients. All seven randomized open-labeled clinical trials [49–55] evaluated therapeutic interventions other than red cells to augment oxygen delivery. A recent meta-analysis combining results from these studies suggested greater benefit from augmented oxygen delivery in the perioperative setting [56]. However, there is still very limited consensus as to which patients are most likely to benefit from increased oxygen delivery and which intervention or approach is superior (i.e. fluids, red cells, inotropic agents or some combination of these interventions). It is also important to note that all published RCTs maintained hemoglobin values greater than 100 g/L, hence inferences regarding optimal red cell transfusion strategies were not possible.

In addition to RCTs, we identified 13 before and after trials (Table 3) evaluating the impact of red cell transfusions on oxygen kinetics. Oxygen delivery uniformly increased but oxygen consumption was observed to change in only 5 of the studies. The lack of change in oxygen consumption reflects either methodologic errors [57] or patients who did not have an elevated anaerobic threshold, rather than an indication that red cells were unnecessary as suggested by one of the studies [58]. In summary, the liberal administration of allogeneic red cells using a threshold of at least 100 g/L may be justified based on the presence of pathologic supply dependency in the critically ill patient [3, 59, 60].

Critical care practitioners may opt to transfuse more liberally in patients considered at risk of coronary artery disease or having established cardiac disease. Two large cohort studies documented that increasing degrees of anemia were associated with a disproportionate increase in mortality rate in the subgroup of patients with cardiac disease. Critically ill patients with cardiac disease had a trend towards an increased mortality when hemoglobin values were <95 g/L (55% versus 42%, $p=0.09$) as compared to anemic patients with other diagnoses [1]. Patients with anemia, a high APACHE II score (>20) and a cardiac diagnosis had a significantly lower mortality rate when given 1 to 3 or 4 to 6 units of allogeneic red cells (55% (no transfusions) versus 35%(1 to 3 units) or 32% (4 to 6 units) respectively, p=0.01). In Jehovah's Witness patients undergoing surgical interventions, the adjusted risk of death increased from 2.3 (95% Cl of 1.4 to 4.0) to 12. 3 (95% Cl of 2.5 to 62.1) as preoperative hemoglobin values decreased from a range of 100–109 g/L to 60–69 g/L in patients with cardiac disease [61]. In non-cardiac patients with comparable levels of anemia, there was no impact of anemia on mortality. Even though both studies were observational in nature and may not have controlled for a number of important confounders, it appears that anemia increases the risk of death in patients with cardiac disease. As a corollary, moderate levels of anemia may be safely tolerated in critically ill patients with other diagnoses.

A more conservative approach to the administration of red cells in the perioperative setting has been advocated by many clinical practice guidelines [7, 9]. Most of these guidelines highlight the risks associated with the transmission of viruses such as human immunodeficiency virus (HIV) and hepatitis through transfusions as an important concern. In addition to the direct transmission of viruses, critically ill patients may also be at increased risks of adverse consequences from allogeneic red cell transfusions, particularly the immunosuppressive and microcirculatory effects of red cells. In a bibliographic search of the literature, we identified 6 RCTs examining the role of transfused red cells in immune modulation [11–16]. There were mixed results from these studies. Only three studies, comparing either leukodepleted red cells [13, 14] or autologous transfusions [16], to allogeneic transfusions demonstrated decreased rates of postoperative infections. If allogeneic red cells result in clinically important immune suppression, this may result in significant increases in the rates of nosocomial infections, multisystem organ dysfunction and death, given that infections are a major cause of morbidity and mortality in the ICU.

While the effect of hemoglobin levels (hematocrit) on systemic oxygen transport in the central circulation has been well studied, it remains unclear how raising hematocrit levels might impact on oxygen delivery in the microcirculation [62–64]. There are many storage-related changes in red cells [5, 65–74] and changes caused by diseases such as sepsis [17–19, 75, 76] that decreases red cell deformability and the ability to off-load oxygen in the microcirculation. In conjunction with significant systemic microcirculatory dysfunction observed in many critically ill patients, the decrease in red cell deformability may dramatically affect tissue oxygen delivery in many critically ill patients [17–19, 75]. Therefore, there is evidence to suggest that red cell transfusions increase systemic oxygen delivery but may have adverse effects on microcirculatory oxygen delivery to the tissues.

As described previously, we only identified six RCTs attempting to contrast all of these benefits, risks, harms and costs of red cell transfusion in a total of 813 patients. The only level I RCT was conducted in patients with sickle cell disease [25]. One of the studies enrolled otherwise healthy patients with a gastrointestinal hemorrhage. The study documented an increase in coagulation abnormalities following the use of a more liberal transfusion strategy. Patients undergoing coronary revascularization were included in two studies [21, 22]. Johnson et al. [22] randomized 39 patients to receive either a liberal transfusion strategy (maintaining hematocrit levels of 32% or hemoglobin concentrations of 105 g/L) or a conservative approach (maintaining hematocrit levels of 25% or hemoglobin concentrations of 82 g/L). There was no difference in postoperative complication rates in the conservative group even though the conservative group experienced a significant decrease in total postoperative blood use. A second RCT, carried out by Weisel et al. [21], assessed day five exercise tolerance as well as hemodynamic and myocardial metabolic response following normovolemic hemodilution in 27 patients. Patients received either red cells if their

Table 3. Thirteen studies examining oxygen delivery, oxygen consumption and lactate levels before and after red cell tranfusion

Author & Pub. Year	Study population	No. of patients	Average amount of transfusion	Changes in measurements post-transfusion				
				↑HgB	↑DO₂	↑VO₂	↑Lactate	Comments
Ronco et al. [32] (1990)	PCP Pneumonia	5	1.5 units	Yes	Yes	Yes	NA	All patients had ↑ lactate baseline. Thermodilution used for DO₂/VO₂ measurements.
Fenwick et al. [33] (1990)	ARDS	24	1.5 units	Yes	Yes	No	No	Normal lactate (n=1) were compared to high lactate (n=13) group.
				Yes	Yes	No	Yes	Used hemodilution catheter for all measurements. Significant increases in VO₂ in response to transfusion in high lactate group.
Ronco et al. [30] (1991)	ARDS	17	1.5 units	Yes	Yes	No	NA	Normal lactate (n=7) compared to high lactate group (n=10). No relationship between VO₂ and DO₂ when VO₂ directly measured with expired gases.
Shah et al. [81] (1982)	Posttrauma	8	1 or 2 units	Yes	Yes	Yes	NA	1 RBC unit (n=5) or 2 units (n=3) given to patients. Thermodilution used for DO₂/VO₂ measurements.
Steffes et al. [82] (1991)	Postoperative + Posttrauma	21	1–2 units	Yes	Yes	Yes	No	27 measurement sets in 21 patients. Thermodilution used for DO₂ and VO₂ measurements. Increased lactate values did not predict VO₂ response.
Babineau et al. [58] (1992)	Postoperative	31	328 ± 9 ml	Yes	Yes	No	NA	32 or 33 transfusions were single units. Thermodilution used for DO₂/VO₂ measurements. 58% of transfusions did not increase VO₂.
Gilbert et al. [34] (1988)	Septic	17	Δ 20 g/L (1)	Yes	Yes	No	No	33 measurement sets in 31 patients. 10 of 17 patients had increased lactate. VO₂ significantly increased in high group only.

Table 3. (continued)

Author & Pub. Year	Study population	No. of patients	Average amount of transfusions	Changes in measurements posttransfosion				
				↑ HgB	↑ DO_2	↑ VO_2	↑ Lactate	Comments
Dietrich et al. [83] (1990)	Medical shock (septic/cardiac)	32	577 ml	Yes	Yes	No	No	36 measurement sets in 32 patients. No change in VO_2 after transfusion. Thermodilution used for DO_2/VO_2 measurements.
Conrad et al. [31] (1990)	Septic shock	19	△ 30 g/L (1)	Yes	Yes	No	No	Normal lactate (n = 8) compared to high lactate (n = 11) group. No increase in VO_2 with transfusion in either group. Thermodilution used for DO_2/VO_2 measurements.
Marik et al. [84] (1990)	Septic	23	3 units	Yes	Yes	No	No	DO_2 measured independently of VO_2. Using gastric tonometry, patients receiving old red cells developed evidence of gastric ischemia.
Lorento et al. [85] (1993)	Septic	16	2 units	Yes	Yes	No	NA	Dobutamine significantly increased VO_2 while red cells did not. Thermodilution used for DO_2/VO_2 measurements.
Mink et al. [86] (1990)	Septic shock 2 mo – 8 yrs	8	8–10 ml/kg × 1–2 h	Yes	Yes	No	NA	In pediatric patients, VO_2 did not increase with red cells. Thermodilution used for DO_2, VO_2 measurements.
Lucking et al. [87] (1990)	Septic shock 4 mo – 15 yrs	7	10–15 ml/kg × 1–3 h	Yes	Yes	Yes	NA	8 measurement sets in 7 patients. Thermodilution used for DO_2/VO_2 measurements.

↑DO_2: increased O_2 delivery; ↑VO_2: increased O_2 consumption; NA: not available. (1) Authors only indicated average hemoglobin change not number of units transfused

hemoglobin concentrations fell below 120 g/L in addition to colloids in one group (n = 13), versus crystalloids and allogeneic red cells only if hemoglobins fell below 70 g/L (n = 14). Though patients in the low hemoglobin trigger group received significantly less red cell transfusions than the other group, there were no differences in morbidity, mortality or exercise tolerance. In a small subset of patients (n = 6), there were differences in the rate of myocardial lactate recovery in the low hemoglobin trigger group suggesting increased myocardial ischemia from anemia. Hébert et al. [24] randomly allocated 69 critically ill patients to a restrictive red cell transfusion strategy (hemoglobin concentrations between 70 g/L–90 g/L) or a liberal strategy (hemoglobin concentrations between 100 g/L–120 g/L), in order to evaluate the impact of the treatments on mortality rates, organ dysfunction scores and other markers of morbidity. The results showed that neither mortality nor the development of organ dysfunction were affected by the transfusion strategy. However, the maintenance of hemoglobin concentrations between 70 and 90 g/L decreased the average number of units transfused from 4.8 to 2.5 units (a 48% reduction, p < 0.001). Finally, a clinical trial in critically ill trauma victims [23] randomly allocated 25 patients to allogeneic red cell transfusions once hematocrit levels reached either 30% or 40%. The authors concluded that there were no discernible differences in oxygen transport variables between both transfusion strategies. In summary, five of the six studies enrolled too few patients to make significant inferences regarding important outcomes from red cell transfusions and the one remaining large RCT only documented the effects of transfusions using a disease-specific outcome in sickle cell disease.

From this review, it is apparent that an optimal and safe lower limit to the transfusion threshold has not been established in critically ill patient populations [77]. There is therefore a need for further randomized controlled clinical trials.

The Transfusion Requirements in Critical Care (TRICC) Trial

Overview

The TRICC trial is a randomized clinical trial designed to answer whether conservative and liberal transfusion strategies are equivalent in usual clinical ICU practice. We believe that a clinical trial should demonstrate that both strategies are equally safe and effective (equivalent). If the treatment approaches are found to be equivalent, then a lower threshold may be recommended in critically ill patients. In addition, the analysis of subgroups using secondary outcomes planned in this study will permit a detailed evaluation of the intervention where clinically relevant.

In the planning phase of this trial, we have chosen to implement a study design that reflects a compromise between the "efficacy" and "effectiveness" approaches (Table 4). Study characteristics are frequently quite dissimilar between both approaches. Efficacy trials will generally opt for restricted eligibility, rigorous treatment protocols and disease-specific outcomes responsive to the potential benefits of the experimental intervention. A similar study attempting to determine effectiveness would implement liberal eligibility criteria, loosely defined treatment protocols, and outcomes which represent patients' overall response to an intervention.

Table 4. Comparison of study characteristics using either an efficacy or an effectiveness approach when designing a study

Study characteristics	Efficacy trial	Effectiveness trial
Research question	Does the intervention work under ideal conditions?	Will the intervention result in more good than harm under usual practice conditions?
Setting	Restricted to centers of excellence	Open to all institulions
Patient selection	Specifc diseases in well-defined patients	Wide range of patients identified using broad eligibility criteria
Study design	Small single or multicenter study	Very large multicenter clinical trial
Baseline assessment	Elaborate and detailed	Simple and clinician friendly
Intervention	Tightly controlled Optimal therapy under optimal study conditions	Less controlled Therapy administered according to usual care
Treatment protocols	Rigorous and detailed Compliance essential	Very general Non compliance tolerated
Endpoints	Disease-related Related to biologic effect "Surrogate" endpoints (e.g. allogeneic exposure)	Patient-related (e.g. All-cause mortality or quality of life)
Analysis	By treatment received Non-compliers excluded	Intention-to-treat All patients included
Data management – Data collection – Data monitoring*	Elaborate Detailed and rigorous	Minimal and simple Minimal

* Data monitoring refers to the review of source documents and adjudication/verification of outcomes

Patient Selection

In this study, we enrolled all patients admitted to one of the 26 tertiary level ICU between November 1st, 1994 and November 14th, 1997 who were considered eligible for this study.

We included patients who:
1) were expected to stay more than 24 hours;
2) had a hemoglobin value less than or equal to 90 g/L within 72 hours of ICU admission; and
3) were considered volume resuscitated or normovolemic by the attending staff.

Patients were excluded for any of the following reasons:
1) less than 16 years of age;
2) enrollment in another interventional study;
3) unable to receive blood products;
4) active blood loss at the time of enrollment, defined as a 30 g/L decrease in hemoglobin in the preceding 12 hours or requiring at least 3 units of packed red cells during the same period;

5) Chronic anemia defined as at least one hemoglobin value ≤ 90 g/L documented more than one month prior to hospital admission;
6) pregnancy ascertained by history, physical examination or confirmed using βHCG;
7) brain dead or not expected to survive more than 24 hours;
8) moribund and not expected to survive more than 24 hours;
9) expected length of stay in ICU less than 24 hours;
10) a lack of commitment from attending staff to continue active treatment of the patient; and
11) admitted following routine cardiac surgical interventions.

The protocol was approved by the research ethics board of each participating institution. Informed consent was obtained from either the patient or the closest family member.

Treatment Protocols

Transfusion guidelines for both the restrictive and liberal treatments were developed through a consensus building process involving the TRICC trial executive committee, the Canadian critical care trials group and faculty of the University of Ottawa, clinical epidemiology unit and information from the national survey of Canadian critical care practioners [28] and a pilot study [24]. Once randomized, a study patient's hemoglobin level was maintained using allogeneic red cell transfusions as required. Patients allocated to the restrictive strategy had their hemoglobin levels maintained between 70 and 90 g/L, with a transfusion trigger at 70 g/L. Patients allocated to a liberal transfusion strategy had their hemoglobin levels maintained between 100 and 120 g/L, with a transfusion trigger at 100 g/L. Physicians in both groups were advised to transfuse red cells one unit at a time and to measure hemoglobin concentrations after each unit. The study interventions were only required during the ICU stay. On discharge from the study, a copy of the ACP guidelines [7] were placed in the patient's medical record. Compliance with the transfusion protocols was monitored by examination of hemoglobin concentrations and transfusion records sent to the study coordinating center on a monthly basis. Individual centers were given regular feedback as to their ability to maintain hemoglobin levels in the target range.

Outcome Measures

The primary outcome measure in this study will be 30 day all cause hospital mortality. The 30-day monitoring interval was chosen because:

1) 30-day mortality is the primary outcome in most interventional trials in critically ill patients at this time;
2) The critical care community at large considers that 30-day all cause hospital mortality is a clinically relevant end point; and

3) Major government agencies such as the National Institute of Health (NIH) and the Food and Drug Administration support 28–30 day mortality as the primary outcome in ICU trials.

Secondary outcomes include other mortality rates such as ICU mortality, hospital mortality and survival times, different measures of organ failure and dysfunction [40, 78, 79], related morbidities such as lengths of ICU and hospital stay, and infectious complications defined as the rates of nosocomial pneumonia, line sepsis and bacteremia.

Conclusions

Around the world, issues related to blood safety from the transmission of viruses have resulted in devastating health consequences and major changes to the blood delivery system of many countries. This same fear continues to fuel a multi-billion dollar industry aiming to develop new technologies to replace red cells (e.g., oxygen carriers) or minimize patient exposure (e.g., drugs such as erythropoeitin and aprotinin, techniques such as hemodilution and perioperative autologous transfusion). In the perioperative setting, drugs such as erythropoeitin and aprotinin decrease allogeneic exposure by one to two red cell units on average [80], often costing several thousand dollars without any evidence documenting their overall effectiveness. In contrast, the transfusion requirements in critical care (TRICC) trial pilot study [24] demonstrated that maintaining hemoglobin levels between 70 and 90 g/L decreased the average number of units transfused from 4.8 to 2.5 units (a 48% reduction, $p < 0.001$). In the present study, we hope to demonstrate that such a simple and cheap intervention is not only efficacious in decreasing allogeneic red cell use but is also safe in high risk patients.

Acknowledgements. I wish to thank the Transfusion Requirements in Critical Care (TRICC) trial Executive Committee members for their wisdom and ongoing support, the TRICC investigators for their commitment to the study and its ideals.

References

1. Hébert PC, Wells G, Tweeddale M, et al (1997) Does transfusion practice affect mortality in critically ill patients? Am J Respir Crit Care Med 155: A20 (Abst)
2. Corwin HL, Parsonnet KC, GeffingerA (1995) RBC transfusion in the ICU. Is there a reason? Chest 108: 767–771
3. Cane RD (1990) Hemoglobin: how much is enough? Crit Care Med 18: 1046–1047
4. Phillips TF, Soulier G, Wilson RF (1987) Outcome of massive transfusion exceeding two blood volumes in trauma and emergency surgery. J Trauma 27: 903–910
5. Welch HG, Meehan KR, Goodnough LT (1992) Prudent strategies for elective red blood cell transfusion. Ann Intern Med 116: 393–402
6. Surgenor DM, Wallace EL, Hale SG, Gilpatrick MW (1988) Changing patterns of blood transfusions in four sets of United States hospitals, 1980 to 1985. Transfusion 28: 513–518
7. American College of Physicians (1992) Practice strategies for elective red blood cell transfusion. Ann Intern Med 116: 403–406

8. Petz LD, Tomasulo PA (1987) Red cell transfusion. In: Kolins J, McCarthy LJ (eds) Contemporary transfusion practice. American Association of Blood Banks, Arlington, pp 1–26
9. Consensus Conference (National Institutes of Health) (1988) Perioperative red blood cell transfusion. JAMA 260:2700–2703
10. Expert Working Group (1997) Guidelines for red blood cells and plasma transfusion for adults and children. Can Med Assoc J 156:S1–S24
11. Houbiers JGA, Brand A, van de Watering LMG ,et al (1996) Randomised controlled trial comparing transfusion of leucocyte-depleted or buffy-coat-depleted blood in surgery for colorectal cancer. Lancet 344:573–578
12. van de Watering LMG, Houbiers JGA, Hermans J, et al (1996) Leukocyte depletion reduces postoperative mortality in patients undergoing cardiac surgery. Br J Haematol 93:312
13. Jensen LS, Andersen AJ, Christiansen PM, et al (1992) Postoperative infection and natural killer cell function following blood transfusion in patients undergoing elective colorectal surgery. Br J Surg 79:513–516
14. Jensen LS, Kissmeyer-Nielsen P, Wolff B, Qvist N (1996) Randomised comparison of leucocyte-depleted versus buffy-coat-poor blood transtusion and complications after colorectal surgery. Lancet 348:841–845
15. Busch ORC, Hop WCJ, Hoynck van Papendrecht MAW, Marquet RL, Jeekel J (1993) Blood transfusions and prognosis in colorectal cancer. N Engl J Med 328:1372–1376
16. Heiss MM, Memple W, Jauch K, et al (1993) Beneficial effects of autologous blood transfusion on infectious complications after colorectal cancer surgery. Lancet 342:1328–1333
17. Hurd TC, Dasmahapatra KS, Rush BF, Machiedo GW (1988) Red blood cell deformability in human and experimental sepsis. Arch Surg 123:217–220
18. Langenfeld JE, Livingston DH, Machiedo GW (1991) Red cell deformability is an early indicator of infections. Surgery 110:398–404
19. Baker CH, Wilmoth FR, Sutton ET (1986) Reduced RBC versus plasma microvascular flow due to endotoxin. Circ Shock 20:127–139
20. Hébert PC, Schweitzer I, Calder L, Blajchman M, Giulivi A (1997) Review of the clinical practice literature on allogeneic red blood cell transfusion. Can Med Assoc J 56:S9–S26
21. Weisel RD, Charlesworth DC, Mickleborough LL et al (1984) Limitations of blood conservation. J Thorac Cardiovasc Surg 88:26–38
22. Johnson RG, Thurer RL, Kruskall MS, et al (1992) Comparison of two transfusion strategies after elective operations for myocardial revascularization. J Thorac Cardiovasc Surg 104:307–314
23. Fortune JB, Feustel PJ, Saifi J, Stratton HH, Newell JC, Shah DM (1987) Influence of hematocrit on cardiopulmonary function after acute hemorrhage. J Trauma 27:243–249
24. Hébert PC, Wells GA, Marshall JC, et al (1995) Transfusion requirements in critical care. A pilot study. JAMA 273:1439–1444
25. Vichinsky EP, Haberkern CM, Neumayr L, et al (1995) A comparison of conservative and aggressive transfusion regimens in the perioperative management of sickle cell disease. N Engl J Med 333:206–213
26. Blair SD, Janvrin SB, McCollum CN, Greenhalgh RM (1986) Effect of early blood transfusion on gastrointestinal haemorrhage. Br J Surg 73:783–785
27. Hébert PC, Hu LQ, Biro GP (1997) Review of physiologic mechanisms in response to anemia. Can Med Assoc J 156:S27–S40
28. Hébert PC, Schweitzer I, Wells GA, et al (1994) A survey of red cell transfusion practices in Canadian critical care practitioners. Clin Invest Med 17:B22 (Abst)
29. Hébert PC, Wells G, Schweitzer I, et al (1995) Red cell transfusion practices in the critically ill: the Canadian experience. Clin Invest Med 18:B29 (Abst)
30. Ronco JJ, Phang PT, Walley KR, Wiggs B, Fenwick JC, Russell JA (1991) Oxygen consumption is independent of changes in oxygen delivery in severe adult respiratory distress syndrome. Am Rev Respir Dis 143:1267–1273
31. Conrad SA, Dietrich KA, Hebert CA, Romero MD (1990) Effect of red cell transfusion on oxygen consumption following fluid resuscitation in septic shock. Circ Shock 31:419–429
32. Ronco JJ, Montaner JSG, Fenwick JC, Ruedy J, Russell JA (1990) Pathologic dependence of oxygen consumption on oxygen delivery in acute respiratory failure secondary to AIDS-related *Pneumocystis carinii* pneumonia. Chest 98:1463–1466

33. Fenwick JC, Dodek PM, Ronco JJ, Phang PT, Wiggs B, Russell JA (1990) Increased concentrations of plasma lactate predict pathologic dependence of oxygen consumption on oxygen delivery in patients with adult respiratory distress syndrome. J Crit Care 5:81–86

34. Gilbert EM, Haupt MT, Mandanas RY, Huaringa AJ, Carlson RW (1986) The effect of fluid loading, blood transfusion, and catecholamine infusion on oxygen delivery and consumption in patients with sepsis. Am Rev Respir Dis 134:873–878

35. Powers SR, Jr., Mannal R, Neclerio M, et al (1973) Physiologic consequences of positive end-expiratory pressure (PEEP) ventilation. Ann Surg 178:265–272

36. Gutierrez G, Pohil RJ (1986) Oxygen consumption is linearly related to O_2 supply in critically ill patients. J Crit Care 1:45–53

37. Vincent J-L, Roman A, De Backer D, Kahn RJ (1990) Oxygen uptake/supply dependency. Effects of short-term dobutamine infusion. Am Rev Respir Dis 142:2–7

38. Vincent J-L, Roman A, Kahn RJ (1990) Dobutamine administration in septic shock: addition to a standard protocol. Crit Care Med 18:689–693

39. Silverman HJ, Slotman G, Bone RC, et al (1990) Effects of prostaglandin E1 on oxygen delivery and consumption in patients with the adult respiratory distress syndrome. Chest 98:405–410

40. Bihari D, Smithies M, Gimson A, Tinker J (1987) The effects of vasodilation with prostacyclin on oxygen delivery and uptake in critically ill patients. N Engl J Med 317:397–403

41. Bihari CJ, Tinker J (1988) The therapeutic value of vasodilator prostaglandins in multiple organ failure associated with sepsis. Intensive Care Med 15:2–7

42. Kaufman BS, Rackow EC, Falk JL (1984) The relationship between oxygen delivery and consumption during fluid resuscitation of hypovolemic and septic shock. Chest 85:336–340

43. Haupt MT, Gilbert EM, Carlson RW (1985) Fluid loading increases oxygen consumption in septic patients with lactic acidosis. Am Rev Respir Dis 131:912–916

44. Wolf YG, Cotev S, Perel A, Manny J (1987) Dependence of oxygen consumption on cardiac output in sepsis. Crit Care Med 15:198–203

45. Kariman K, Burns SR (1985) Regulation of tissue oxygen extraction is disturbed in adult respiratory distress syndrome. Am Rev Respir Dis 132:109–114

46. Kruse JA, Haupt MT, Puri VK, Carlson RW (1990) Lactate levels as predictors of the relationship between oxygen delivery and consumption in ARDS. Chest 98:959–962

47. Russell JA, Ronco JJ, Lockhat D, Belzberg A, Kiess M, Dodek PM (1990) Oxygen delivery and consumption and ventricular preload are greater in survivors than in nonsurvivors of the adult respiratory distress syndrome. Am Rev Respir Dis 141:659–665

48. Dorinsky PM, Costello JL, Gadek JE (1988) Relationships of oxygen uptake and oxygen delivery in respiratory failure not due to the adult respiratory distress syndrome. Chest 93:1013–1019

49. Gattinoni L, Brazzi L, Pelosi P, et al (1995) A trial of goal-oriented hemodynamic therapy in critically ill patients. N Engl J Med 333:1025–1032

50. Boyd O, Ground M, Bennett D (1993) A randomized clinical trial of the effect of deliberate perioperative increase of oxygen delivery on mortality in high-risk surgical patients. JAMA 270:2699–2707

51. Hayes MA, Timmins AC, Yau EHS, Palazzo M, Hinds CJ, Watson D (1994) Elevation of systemic oxygen delivery in the treatment of critically ill patients. N Engl J Med 330:1717–1722

52. Tuchschmidt J, Fried J, Astiz ME, Rackow E (1992) Elevation of cardiac output and oxygen delivery improves outcome in septic shock. Chest 102:216–220

53. Shoemaker WC, Appel PL, Kram HB, Waxman K, Lee T-S (1988) Prospective trial of supranormal values of survivors as therapeutic goals in high-risk surgical patients. Chest 94:1176–1186

54. Yu M, Levy MM, Smith P, Takiguchi SA, Miyasaki A, Myers SA (1993) Effect of maximizing oxygen delivery on morbidity and mortality rates in critically ill patients: a prospective, randomized, controlled study. Crit Care Med 21:830–838

55. Yu M, Takanishi D, Myers SA, et al (1995) Frequency of mortality and myocardial infarction during maximizing oxygen delivery: a prospective, randomized trial. Crit Care Med 23:1025–1032

56. Heyland DK, Cook DJ, King D, Kernerman P, Brun-Buisson C (1996) Maximizing oxygen delivery in critically ill patients: a methodologic appraisal of the evidence. Crit Care Med 24:517–524

57. Russell JA, Wiggs BR (1990) Oxygen kinetics: pitfalls in clinical research revisited. J Crit Care 5:213–217

58. Babineau TJ, Dzik WH, Borlase BC, Baxter JK, Bistrian BR, Benotti PN (1992) Reevaluation of current transfusion practices in patients in surgical intensive care units. Am J Surg 164:22–25
59. Czer LSC, Shoemaker WC (1978) Optimal hematocrit value in critically ill postoperative patients. Surg Gynecol Obstet 147:363–368
60. Crosby ET (1992) Perioperative haemotherapy: I. Indications for blood component transfusion. Can J Anesth 39:695–707
61. Carson JL, Duff A, Poses RM. et al (1996) Effect of anaemia and cardiovascular disease on surgical mortality and morbidity. Lancet 348:1055–1060
62. Messmer KFW (1987) Acceptable hematocrit levels in surgical patients. World J Surg 11:41–46
63. Messmer K, Kreimeier U, Intaglietta M (1986) Present state of intentional hemodilution. Eur Surg Res 18:254–263
64. Messmer K, Sunder-Plassmann L, Klovekorn WP, Holper K (1972) Circulatory significance of hemodilution: rheological changes and limitations. Adv Microcirc 4:1–77
65. Kennedy AC, Valtis DJ (1954) The oxygen dissociation curve in anemia of various types. J Clin Invest 33:1372–1381
66. Sugerman HJ, Davidson DT, Vibul S, Delivoria-Papadopoulos M, Miller LD, Oski FA (1970) The basis of defective oxygen delivery from stored blood. Surg Gynecol Obstet 137:733–741
67. Race D, Dedichen H, Schenk WGJ (1967) Regional blood flow during dextran-induced normovolemic hemodilution in the dog. J Thorac Cardiovasc Surg 53:578–586
68. Collins J (1976) Massive blood transfusion. Clinics Hematol 5:201–222
69. Sohmer PR, Dawson RB (1979) Transfusion therapy in trauma: a review of the principles and techniques used in the M.I.E.M.S. program. Ann Surg 45:109–125
70. McConn R, Derrick JB (1972) The respiratory function of blood: transfusion and blood storage. Anesthesiology 36:119–127
71. Jesch F, Webber LM, Dalton JW, Carey JS (1975) Oxygen dissociation after transfusion of blood stored in ACD or CPD solution. J Thorac Cardiovasc Surg 70:35–39
72. Haradin AR, Weed RJ, Reed CF (1969) Changes in physical properties of stored erythrocytes: relationship to survival *in vivo*. Transfusion 9:229–237
73. LaCelle PL (1969) Alteration of deformability of the erythrocyte membrane in stored blood. Transfusion 9:238–245
74. Longster GH, Buckley T, Sikorsky J, Touey LAD (1972) Scanning electron microscope studies of red cell morphology: changes occurring in red cell shape during storage and post transfusion. Vox Sang 22:161–170
75. Mollitt DL, Poulos ND (1991) The role of pentoxyfilline in endotoxin-induced alterations of red cell deformability and whole blood viscosity in the neonate. J Pediatr Surg 26:572–574
76. Powell RJ, Machiedo GW, Rush BFJ, Dikdan G (1991) Oxygen free radicals: effect on red blood cell deformability in sepsis. Crit Care Med 19:732–735
77. Crosby ET (1992) Perioperative haemotherapy: II. Risks and complications of blood transfusion. Can J Anesth 39:822–837
78. Hébert PC, Drummond AJ, Singer J, Bernard GR, Russell JE (1993) A simple multiple system organ failure scoring system predicts mortality of patients who have sepsis syndrome. Chest 104:230–235
79. Marshall JC (1994) A scoring system for multiple organ dysfunction syndrome. In: Reinhart K, Eyrich K, Sprung C (eds) Sepsis. Current perspectives in pathophysiology and therapy. Springer-Verlag, Berlin, Heidelberg, New York, pp 38–49
80. Forgie M, Wells PS, Ferguson D (1996) A meta-analysis of the efficacy of preoperative autologous donation of blood. Blood 88:529A (Abst)
81. Shah DM, Gottlieb ME, Rahm RL, et al (1982) Failure of red blood cell transfusion to increase oxygen transport or mixed venous PO_2 in injured patients. J Trauma 22:741–74
82. Steffes CP, Bender JS, Levison MA (1991) Blood transfusion and oxygen consumption in surgical sepsis. Crit Care Med 19:512–517
83. Dietrich KA, Conrad SA, Hebert CA, Levy GL, Romero MD (1990) Cardiovascular and metabolic response to red blood cell transfusion in critically ill volume-resuscitated nonsurgical patients. Crit Care Med 18:940–944
84. Marik PE, Sibbald WJ (1993) Effect of stored-blood transfusion on oxygen delivery in patients with sepsis. JAMA 269:3024–3029

85. Lorente JA, Landin L, De Pablo R, Renes E, Rodriguez-Diaz R, Liste D (1993) Effects of blood transfusion on oxygen transport variables in severe sepsis. Crit Care Med 21:1312–1318
86. Mink RB, Pollack MM (1990) Effect of blood transfusion on oxygen consumption in pediatric septic shock. Crit Care Med 18:1087–1091
87. Lucking SE, Williams TM, Chaten FC, Metz RJ, Mickell JJ (1990) Dependence of oxygen consumption on oxygen delivery in children with hyperdynamic septic shock and low oxygen extraction. Crit Care Med 18:1316–1319

Artificial Oxygen Carriers

D. R. Spahn

Introduction

Artificial oxygen (O_2) carriers aim at improving O_2 transport and O_2 unloading to the tissues. Artificial O_2 carriers thus may be used as an alternative to allogeneic blood transfusions or to improve tissue oxygenation and function of organs with marginal O_2 supply. The aim of the present article is to describe the currently evaluated artificial O_2 carriers, to summarize their efficiency and to discuss potential side effects.

Currently evaluated artificial O_2 carriers can be grouped into modified hemoglobin solutions and fluorocarbon emulsions (Table 1). The native human hemoglobin molecule needs to be modified in order to decrease O_2 affinity and to prevent rapid dissociation of the native α_2-β_2 tetramer into α-β dimers. This has been reviewed in detail previously [1].

The O_2 transport characteristics of modified hemoglobin solutions and fluorocarbon emulsions are fundamentally different (Fig. 1). The modified hemoglobin solutions exhibit a sigmoidal O_2 dissociation curve similar to blood. In contrast, the fluorocarbon emulsions are characterized by a linear relationship between O_2 partial pressure and O_2 content. Modified hemoglobin solutions thus provide O_2 transport and unloading capacities similar to blood. This means that already at a relatively low arterial O_2 partial pressure substantial amounts of O_2 are being transported. In contrast, relatively high arterial O_2 partial pressures are necessary to maximize the O_2 transport capacity of fluorocarbon emulsions. Despite these fundamental differences, the efficiency of both groups of artificial O_2 carriers has been proven in a variety of experimental conditions (see below).

Table 1. Artificial oxygen (O_2) carriers. The modified hemoglohin solutions are grouped by the source of the hemoglobin.

Modified hemoglobin solutions
- Outdated human blood
- Bovine hemoglobin
- Human recombinant hemoglobin
- - E. coli [28]
- - Transgenic tabacco [29]

Fluorocarbon emulsions
- Perflubron

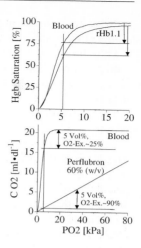

Fig. 1. *Top:* O_2 dissociation curve of native human blood (Blood) and human recombinant hemoglobin version 1.1 (rHb1.1). Note the greater O_2 unloading capacity for rHb1.1 compared with native blood indicated by the arrows, when assuming a mixed venous PO_2 of 5.3 kPa (modified from [28] with permission). *Bottom:* O_2 carrying capacity of native human blood (Blood) and perflubron. Note that 5 Vol% of O_2 can be unloaded by blood as well as by perflubron. With perflubron, however, higher arterial PO_2 values are required. Note also, that perflubron transported O_2 is more completely unloaded than blood transported O_2 resulting in approximate O_2 extraction (O_2-Ex.) ratios of 90% and 25%. CO_2 denotes O_2 content and PO_2 denotes O_2 partial pressure. (Modified from [21] with permission)

Hemoglobin Solutions

The efficiency of hemoglobin solutions to transport and unload O_2 has been shown in a variety of shock models and at extreme hemodilution (referenced in [1]). In a whole animal sheep model, Vlahakes et al. [2] showed that extreme hemodilution to a hematocrit of $2.4 \pm 0.5\%$ was only tolerated when a polymerized bovine hemoglobin solution was used but not in animals treated with hydroxyethyl starch devoid of O_2 carrying capacity. All animals surviving acute hemodilution also survived the following 25 days without evidence of renal or hepatic dysfunction [2].

More recently, Siegel at al. [3] found in dogs that infusion of human recombinant hemoglobin (rHb1.1) resulted in a more rapid reversal of O_2 debt after progressive hemorrhage, a more uniform reperfusion and a more complete wash-out of acids accumulated during build-up of the O_2 debt during hemorrhage compared with treatment with a mixture of autologous blood and colloid.

In a rat model of hemorrhage and surgical trauma, Xu et al. [4] furthermore demonstrated that treatment with α-α-diaspirin cross linked hemoglobin improved wound healing, enhanced hepatic cell proliferation and most importantly, decreased splanchnic bacterial translocation when compared with transfusion of fresh autologous blood. It is of particular interest that treatment with α-α-diaspirin cross linked hemoglobin induced a more favorable response to trauma and hemorrhage than transfusion of fresh autologous blood considering the fact that the efficiency of blood transfusions in improving O_2 consumption and aerobic metabolism is not exactly defined [5]. In fact, only fresh blood (3 days old) but not 28 day old blood was recently shown to partially correct the decrease in O_2 consumption induced by extreme hemodilution [6]. It is therefore particularly noteworthy that α-α-diaspirin was even more efficient than transfusion of fresh autologous blood which was not stored at all [4].

Bovine polymerized hemoglobin was also more efficient in restoring muscle PO_2 after extreme hemodilution to a hematocrit of 10% in dogs, than fresh (day of experiment) or old (21 days) autologous blood [7]. Likewise, muscle PO_2 was better restored with bovine polymerized hemoglobin than hydroxyethyl starch in a dog model of hemodilution (hematocrit of 23–27%) and 95% arterial stenosis [8].

Thus, modified hemoglobin solutions are indeed very promising in improving O_2 transport and tissue oxygenation to a physiologically relevant degree. Without the need for cross matching these solutions thus hold great promise as an alternative to allogeneic blood transfusions, and as O_2 therapeutics which might be of great value in the prehospital resuscitation of trauma victims or in specific situations in intensive care medicine.

Since the breakdown of the native α_2-β_2 hemoglobin tetramer into α-β dimers is largely prevented by genetic modification or chemical modification, nephrotoxicity is no longer a potential side effect of these solutions [9]. Simultaneously also, intravascular half life is prolonged. Interestingly, intravascular half life increases with increasing dose [10] (for α-α-diaspirin cross linked hemoglobin) and increases with achieved plasma hemoglobin concentration [9] (human recombinant hemoglobin, rHb1.1). Although there are no definitive data available on the intravascular half live of the various modified hemoglobin solutions in man, a dose related increase in intravascular half life could be very advantageous for the clinical use of these substances.

Vasoconstriction resulting in an increase in systemic and pulmonary artery pressures has been observed with all modified hemoglobin solutions evaluated so far. The mechanisms involved include nitric oxide (NO) scavenging [1, 11–13], endothelin release [14] and a sensitization of peripheral α-adrenergic receptors [15]. NO scavenging has been the subject of a variety of studies [1, 11, 13]. NO produced by the endothelial cells is intended to react with the Fe^{2+} in the guanylate cyclase located in the smooth muscle cells of the vessel wall to modulate the vascular tone towards vasodilatation. In the presence of free hemoglobin, NO may react with the Fe^{2+} of the heme and also with the highly reactive (sulfhydryl) SH group of the cysteine on position 93 of the β chain [11]. In fact S-nitrosylation of the hemoglobin molecule prevented an increase in mean arterial pressure in rats [11]. Furthermore, NO donors such as nitroglycerin and L-arginine could decrease hemoglobin induced hypertension [16]. An increase in mean arterial pressure due to hemoglobin infusion could also be prevented with endothelin receptor antagonists [14]. Thus there are ways to prevent or treat hemoglobin mediated vasoconstriction.

Hemoglobin induced vasoconstriction may be regarded as an untoward side effect. This view may be correct when relatively small volumes of hemoglobin solutions are being given to patients with a reduced cardiac contractility and a normal or elevated mean arterial pressure. In such patients a hemoglobin infusion may induce increases in systemic and pulmonary vascular resistances high enough to cause a reduction in cardiac output [12]. In contrast, in a previously healthy trauma victim suffering from severe hypovolemia due to massive hemorrhage, the combined effects of volume replacement, increased O_2 transport capacity and a certain vasoconstriction due to the infusion of a modified hemoglobin solution, may be very beneficial indeed. Very important in this regard is the recent observation that the vasoconstriction due to α-α-diaspirin cross-linked hemoglobin is not distributed evenly throughout the body. Dietz et al. [13] found that vasoconstriction was most pronounced in the femoral artery supplying mainly skeletal muscles but no

Table 2. Hemoglobin solutions: PROs and CONs

PROs:	Carries and unloads O_2
	Sigmoidal O_2 dissociation curve
	100% FiO_2 is not mandatory for maximal potency
	Easy to measure
CONs:	Side effects
	– Vasoconstriction
	– Interference with colorimetric laboratory methods

vasoconstriction was observed in the mesenteric vasculature and a distinct vaso-dilatory effect was observed in the coronary arteries.

Other aspects of hemoglobin solutions deserve mentioning. Since hemoglobin solutions are colored, the potential exists that some colorimetric laboratory measurement methods may be disturbed. There is also one report in dogs, in which infusion of human recombinant hemoglobin induced an increase in liver enzymes as well as amylase [3]. However, in other studies in which even larger quantities of bovine hemoglobin have been given, no hepatic dysfunction was observed during 25 days after near complete exchange transfusion [2]. The advantages and disadvantages of these solutions are summarized in Table 2.

Fluorocarbon Emulsions

Fluorocarbons are carbon-fluorine compounds characterized by a high gas dissolving capacity (O_2, carbon dioxide and other gases), low viscosity, and chemical and biologic inertness [1, 17]. Fluorocarbons are virtually not miscible with water. The first generation fluorocarbons, such as Fluosol® (Green Cross Corp., Japan), used a poloxamer type Pluronic F-68 as an emulsifier, which, however, has the potential to cause anaphylaxis [17]. The second generation fluorocarbons use egg-yolk phospholipid as emulsifier, which is well tolerated except in patients with an egg allergy [1, 17].

Manufacturing an emulsion with very specific characteristics is a great technologic challenge, because only droplets of a very specific size (around 0.2 µm diameter) are well tolerated. The spectrum of side effects also critically depends on the size distribution of the droplets; the narrower the distribution around the target size, the less, in general, are the side effects. With the development of a stable 60% (58% perfluorooctyl bromide and 2% perfluorodecyl bromide) emulsion there is now a relatively highly concentrated emulsion which is clinically well tolerated [17, 18]. After intravenous application, the droplets of the emulsion are taken up by the reticulo-endothelial system (RES). This uptake determines the intravascular half life [1, 17]. No exact data are yet available on the intravascular half life in humans. After the initial uptake of the fluorocarbon emulsion into the RES, the droplets are slowly broken down, the fluorocarbon molecules are taken up in the blood again (bound to blood lipids) and transported to the lungs, where the unaltered fluorocarbon molecules are finally excreted via exhalation. The metabolism of fluorocarbon molecules in humans remains unknown [1, 17].

The ability of fluorocarbon emulsions to transport and efficiently unload O_2 is unndisputed. Young et al. [19] showed, in patients undergoing coronary angioplasty, that distal coronary perfusion with oxygenated Fluosol® largely blunted myocardial lactate release during balloon inflation and prevented major regional wall motion abnormalities resulting in a far better preserved left ventricular ejection fraction. The ischemia preventing effect of distal coronary perfusion with Fluosol® was confirmed by Kent et al. [20], again demonstrating by echocardiography that wall motion was far better preserved during balloon inflation in transluminal coronary angioplasty and that patients experienced significantly less angina. Perflubron has been assessed in a variety of hemodilution studies. Keipert et al. [21] applied perflubron in dogs after acute normovolemic hemodilution at a hematocrit of 10%. During hemodilution the expected increase in cardiac output was observed [1, 21]. With the application of perflubron, cardiac output tended to increase further and a massive rise in mixed venous O_2 partial pressure and mixed venous saturation was observed. The percentage of metabolized O_2 originating from endogenous hemoglobin decreased dramatically with the application of perflubron indicating that the O_2 transported by perflubron is preferentially metabolized, most likely due to the excellent O_2 unloading characteristics of this fluorocarbon emulsion [21]. Furthermore, Holman et al. [22] tested perflubron in severely hemodiluted dogs undergoing cardiopulmonary bypass. Without using catecholamines, dogs treated with increasing doses of perflubron survived cardiopulmonary bypass progressively better than control animals. Perflubron may also be beneficial as an adjunct to resuscitation. In a porcine model of near fatal hemorrhage, perflubron treatment in addition to standard resuscitation decreased mortality from 43% to 13% [23]. Although this difference did not reach statistical significance due to a low number of observations (n = 15 total) it was felt by the authors that the added and readily available O_2 provided by perflubron was beneficial. Also in a dog model of ventricular fibrillation the additional direct infusion of oxygenated perflubron into the aortic arch improved the chances of spontaneous return of the circulation and if so, this was achieved earlier as with standard resuscitation [24].

Perflubron has also been used in humans [18]. Acute normovolemic hemodilution to a hemoglobin concentration of approximately 9 g/dL was performed preoperatively. During surgery, perflubron (0.9 g/kg) was administered when a blood transfusion was deemed necessary by the anesthesiologist which occurred at a hemoglobin concentration of approximately 8 g/dL. Mixed venous oxygen tension and mixed venous oxygen saturation both increased significantly after perflubron administration and cardiac output was stable. Although only relatively little O_2 was transported by perflubron (approximately 1%), 5% of the metabolized O_2 originated from perflubron transported O_2, again indicating that perflubron transported O_2 is preferentially metabolized [18, 21].

Fluorocarbon emulsions also have side effects. Volunteers experienced mild 'flu-like symptoms with myalgia and light fever and an approximately 15% decrease in platelet count 3 days post-dosing returning to normal by day 7 [17, 25]. Traditional coagulation tests including bleeding time, however, were unaffected by perflubron [25]. With a modification of the fluorocarbon emulsion, these side effects were blunted and thus do not represent a relevant clinical problem any more. The advantages and disadvantages of fluorocarbon emulsion are summarized in Table 3.

Table 3. Fluorocarbon emulsions: PROs and CONs

PROs:	Carries and unloads O_2
	Few and mild side effects
	No known organ toxicity
CONs:	100% FiO_2 is mandatory for maximal potency
	Additional colloid often necessary with potential side effects

Comparison Between Hemoglobin Solutions and Fluorocarbon Emulsions

The direct comparison between hemoglobin solutions and fluorocarbon emulsions is difficult. To a large extent this is related to the fact that there are no comparative studies, neither between different hemoglobin solutions, nor between hemoglobin solutions and fluorocarbon emulsions. Despite the lack of such direct comparisons, there are several aspects in which these substances can be compared. In this comparison, qualitatively similar properties of the different hemoglobin solutions are assumed, knowing that this assumption may not be correct.

Hemoglobin solutions are isooncotic or even hyperoncotic colloidal volume expanders. Infusion of these solutions thus not only provides additional O_2 carrying and unloading capacity, these solutions will also correct hypovolemia. In contrast, the volume of fluorocarbon emulsions infused is relatively small with the doses currently used. Therefore, additional volume expanders have to be infused to correct hypervolemia. The more liberal use of additional volume expanders may render their side effects more clinically relevant. Among these side effects, the effect on blood coagulation may be particularly important. Egli et al. [26] have recently demonstrated that blood coagulation may become compromised during advanced hemodilution and that there are differences between gelatin, albumin and hydroxyethyl starch volume expanders.

Another clinical issue is monitoring of the effectiveness of artificial O_2 carriers. This may seem to be particularly difficult for the fluorocarbon emulsions because there is no bedside fluorocarbon concentration or fluorocrit measurement available. In contrast, with hemoglobin solutions, such a problem seems not to exist because regular laboratory measurement techniques measure total hemoglobin, i.e. the sum of endogenous hemoglobin (within red blood cells) and exogenous hemoglobin (in the plasma) correctly. However, since we should not go by hemoglobin concentration alone in our decision regarding blood transfusions [27], the above difference may not be as relevant. However, daily practice in many institutions is still to transfuse blood primarily based on institutional guidelines in which the hemoglobin concentration may be a crucial parameter.

The recourse used for the production of these solutions may also be of importance for certain groups of physicians and patients, such as Jehovah's Witnesses.

Conclusion

Public knowledge about both categories of artificial O_2 carriers is not sufficient to favor one over another solution at present time. Hemoglobin solutions as well as fluorocarbon emulsions have both been proven in many situations to efficiently transport and unload O_2. Furthermore, it is expected that modified formulations will be developed which serve this purpose even better in the future. Artificial O_2 carriers are thus very promising substances which will enter clinical medicine within the next 5 years.

References

1. Spahn DR, Leone BJ, Reves JG, Pasch T (1994) Cardiovascular and coronary physiology of acute isovolemic hemodilution: a review of nonoxygen-carrying and oxygen-carrying solutions. Anesth Analg 78:1000–1021
2. Vlahakes GJ, Lee R, Jacobs EE, LaRaia PJ, Austen WG (1990) Hemodynamic effects and oxygen transport properties of a new blood substitute in a model of massive blood replacement. J Thorac Cardiovasc Surg 100:379–388
3. Siegel JH, Fabian M, Smith JA, Costantino D (1997) Use of recombinant hemoglobin solution in reversing lethal hemorrhagic hypovolemic oxygen debt shock. J Trauma 42:199–212
4. Xu L, Sun L, Rollwagen, et al (1997) Cellular responses to surgical trauma, hemorrhage, and resuscitation with diaspirin cross-linked hemoglobin in rats. J Trauma 42:32–41
5. Hébert PC, Hu LQ, Biro GP (1997) Review of physiologic mechanisms in response to anemia. Can Med Ass J 156:S27–S40
6. Fitzgerald RD, Martin CM, Dietz GE, Doig GS, Potter RF, Sibbald WJ (1997) Transfusing red blood cells stored in citrate phosphate dextrose adenine-1 for 28 days fails to improve tissue oxygenation in rats. Crit Care Med 25:726–732
7. Standl T, Horn P, Wilhelm S, et al (1996) Bovine haemoglobin is more potent than autologous red blood cells in restoring muscular tissue oxygenation after profound isovolaemic haemodilution in dogs. Can J Anaesth 43:714–723
8. Horn EP, Standl T, Wilhelm S, et al (1997) Bovine hemoglobin increases skeletal muscle oxygenation during 95 percent artificial arterial stenosis. Surgery 121:411–418
9. Viele MK, Weiskopf RB, Fisher D (1997) Recombinant human hemoglobin does not affect renal function in humans: analysis of safety and pharmacokinetics. Anesthesiology 86:848–858
10. Przybelski RJ, Daily EK, Kisicki JC, et al (1996) Phase I study of the safety and pharmacologic effects of diaspirin cross-linked hemoglobin solution. Crit Care Med 24:1993–2000
11. Jia L, Bonaventura J, Stamler JS (1996) S-nitrosohaemoglobin: a dynamic activity of blood involved in vascular control. Nature 380:221–226
12. Kasper SM, Walter M, Grüne F, Bischoff A, Erasmi H, Buzello W (1996) Effects of a hemoglobin-based oxygen carrier (HBOC-201) on hemodynamics and oxygen transport in patients undergoing preoperative hemodilution for elective abdominal aortic surgery. Anesth Analg 83:921–927
13. Dietz NM, Martin CM, Beltrandelrio AG, Joyner MJ (1997) The effects of cross linked hemoglobin on regional vascular conductance in dogs. Anesth Analg 85:265–273
14. Gulati A, Sharma AC, Singh G (1996) Role of endothelin in the cardiovascular effects of diaspirin crosslinked and stroma reduced hemoglobin. Crit Care Med 24:137–147
15. Gulati A, Rebello S (1994) Role of adrenergic mechanisms in the pressor effect of diaspirin cross-linked hemoglobin. J Lab Clin Med 124:125–133
16. Schultz SC, Grady B, Cole F, Hamilton I, Burhop K, Malcolm DS (1993) A role for endothelin and nitric oxide in the pressor response to diaspirin cross-linked hemoglobin. J Lab Clin Med 122:301–308
17. Riess JG (1992) Overview of progress in the fluorocarbon approach to *in vivo* oxygen delivery. Biomater Artif Cells Immobil Biotechnol 20:183–202

18. Wahr JA, Trouwborst A, Spence RK, et al (1996) A pilot study of the effects of a perflubron emulsion, AF0104, on mixed venous oxygen tension in anesthetized surgical patients. Anesth Analg 82:103–107

19. Young LH, Jaffe CC, Revkin JH, McNulty PH, Cleman M (1990) Metabolic and functional effects of perfluorocarbon distal perfusion during coronary angioplasty. Am J Cardiol 65:986–990

20. Kent KM, Cleman MW, Cowley MJ, et al (1990) Reduction of myocardial ischemia during percutaneous transluminal coronary angioplasty with oxygenated Fluosol. Am J Cardiol 66:279–284

21. Keipert PE, Faithfull NS, Bradley JD ,et al (1994) Oxygen delivery augmentation by low-dose perfluorochemical emulsion during profound normovolemic hemodilution. Adv Exp Med Biol 345:197–204

22. Holman WL, Spruell RD, Ferguson ER, et al (1995) Tissue oxygenation with graded dissolved oxygen delivery during cardiopulmonary bypass. J Thorac Cardiovasc Surg 110:774–785

23. Stern SA, Dronen SC, McGoron AJ, et al (1995) Effect of supplemental perfluorocarbon administration on hypotensive resuscitation of severe uncontrolled hemorrhage. Am J Emerg Med 13:269–275

24. Manning JE, Batson DN, Payne FB, et al (1997) Selective aortic arch perfusion during cardiac arrest: enhanced resuscitation using oxygenated perflubron emulsion, with and without aortic arch epinephrine. Ann Emerg Med 29:580–587

25. Keipert PE, Faithfull NS, Roth DJ, et al (1996) Supporting tissue oxygenation during acute surgical bleeding using a perfluorochemical-based oxygen carrier. Adv Exp Med Bio 388:603–609

26. Egli GA, Zollinger A, Seifert B, Popovic D, Pasch T, Spahn DR (1997) Effect of progressive hemodilution with hydroxyethyl starch, gelatin and albumin on blood coagulation. An in vitro thrombelastography study. Br J Anaesth 78:684–689

27. A report by the American Society of Anesthesiologists Task Force on Blood Component Therapy (1996) Practice guidelines for blood component therapy. Anesthesiology 84:732–747

28. Looker D, Abbott-Brown D, Cozart P, et al (1992) A human recombinant haemoglobin designed for use as a blood substitute. Nature 356:258–260

29. Dieryck W, Pagnier J, Poyart C, et al (1997) Human haemoglobin from transgenic tobacco. Nature 386:29–30

Epidemiology and Markers of Sepsis – Clinical Trials

Do We Really Know the Epidemiology
and Clinical Course of Sepsis?

L. Ilkka, I. Parviainen, and J. Takala

Introduction

Sepsis can be defined as the systemic inflammatory response to infection. It is an important cause of morbidity and mortality in hospitalized patients and a predominant cause of prolonged intensive care. The vast majority of intensive care resources is used to treat these patients with sepsis-related states. Despite this, the epidemiology and especially the clinical course of sepsis have not been well described.

In the past, the term "sepsis" has been used quite variably to indicate bacteremia, clinical impression of infection, and verified localized or systemic infections combined with biochemical and clinical signs and symptoms (Table 1) [1–9]. The selection of the criteria confounds any epidemiological and clinical data. From the clinical and pathophysiologic point of view a definition of sepsis should take into account the obvious link between serious infection, and its systemic manifestations, including organ dysfunction.

Verification of infection is fundamental. Since microbiologic cultures may remain negative despite obvious infection, especially in bacteremia, new radiologic findings consistent with infection as well as demonstration of gross infectious foci and pus have also been used. A systemic response closely resembling or even identical to sepsis may also be induced by non-infectious factors, including ischemia, major burns, or pancreatitis.

Patients with "suspected sepsis", without positive cultures, are treated in daily practice without great problems of definition. This term may include very heterogeneous patient populations, and is heavily influenced by differences between clinicians and clinical practice, and is therefore not suitable for research purposes. It is unlikely that one single definition would be practical for all purposes. For clinical routine, a low threshold of suspicion and aggressive search for infectious foci is vital, whereas therapeutic trials should preferably use more strict criteria. In this review, we use the term sepsis to indicate the systemic response to infection.

A North American consensus conference published the recommendations for the definitions of sepsis and related clinical conditions in 1992 [10]. Sepsis was defined as a systemic inflammatory response in the presence of infection, with two to four clinical manifestations (Table 2). Systemic inflammatory response syndrome (SIRS) was introduced to indicate an evident systemic inflammatory response in the absence of a verified infection. When these consensus conference definitions were subsequently tested prospectively, it became evident that SIRS as an entity is too

Table 1. Examples of various definitions or criteria of sepsis

Ref.	Evidence of infection	Clinical signs
[1]	Bacteremia, other positive cultures	Not precisely defined
[2]	Positive blood cultures, body fluid cultures, or unmistakable evidence of a septic process	Not precisely defined
[3]	Microbiological event inducing some host response or the presence of these microorganisms in a normally sterile tissue	Not precisely defined
[4]	Not precisely defined	Manifestations related to the systemic response to infection (tachycardia, tachypnea, alterations in temperature, and leukocytosis), and those related to organ-system dysfunction (cardiovascular, respiratory, renal, hepatic, and hematologic abnormalities)
[5]	Clinical evidence suggestive of infection	Tachypnea, tachycardia, hyperthermia or hypothermia
[6]	Not precisely defined	A toxic clinical picture, including fever or hypothermia, tachycardia, tachypnea, and mental obtundation
[7]	The presence of microorganisms or their products invading normally sterile host tissues	Alterations in one or more of temperature, white blood cell count, and mentation in association with a hyperdynamic hypermetabolic state
[8]	Known or suspected (Gram-negative in this study)	Fever or hypothermia, tachycardia and tachypnea, and either hypotension or two of the following six signs of systemic toxicity or peripheral hypoperfusion: unexplained metabolic acidosis, arterial hypoxemia, acute renal failure, elevated prothrombin or partial-thromboplastin time or reduction of the platelet count, sudden decrease in mental acuity, and elevated cardiac index with low systemic vascular resistance
[9]	Known or suspected (Gram-negative in this study)	Fever or hypothermia, tachycardia, tachypnea, plus at least one of these signs of organ dysfunctions: hypoxemia, increased serum lactate concentration, oliguria, altered mentation, new coagulopathy

sensitive and non-specific both for research and clinical practice [3, 11, 12]. The majority of intensive care unit (ICU) patients and many hospitalized patients occasionally fulfill the criteria of SIRS. SIRS alone has little clinical relevance or value for guiding treatment or predicting outcome. Some SIRS patients develop sepsis or even septic shock. The criteria of SIRS do not help to detect these patients from a large population. Due to the sensitivity and non-specificity the rather arbitrary criteria of SIRS should probably be considered with other criteria if they are used for including patients in prospective clinical or epidemiologic studies.

Table 2. The definitions of the ACCP/SCCM consensus conference [10]

Infection	Microbial phenomenon characterized by an inflammatory response to the presence of microorganisms or the invasion of normally sterile host tissue by those organisms.
Bacteremia	The presence of viable bacteria in the blood.
SIRS	The systemic inflammatory response to a variety of several clinical insults. The response is manifested by two or more of the following conditions: temperature $> 38\,°C$ or $< 36\,°C$, heart rate > 90 beats/min, respiratory rate > 20 breaths/min or $PaCO_2 < 32$ torr (< 4.3 kPa), and WBC $> 12\,000$ cells/mm^3 or < 4000 cells/mm^3 or $> 10\%$ immature (band) forms.
Sepsis	The systemic response to infection. This systemic response is manifested by two or more of the following conditions as a result of infection: temperature $> 38\,°C$ or $< 36\,°C$, heart rate > 90 beats/min, respiratory rate > 20 breaths/min or $PaCO_2 < 32$ torr (< 4.3 kPa), and WBC $> 12\,000$ cells/mm^3 or < 4000 cells/mm^3 or $> 10\%$ immature (band) forms.
Severe sepsis	Sepsis associated with organ dysfunction, hypoperfusion, or hypotension. Hypoperfusion and hypotension abnormalities may include, but are not limited to lactic acidosis, oliguria, or acute alteration in mental status.
Septic shock	Sepsis with hypotension despite adequate fluid resuscitation, along with presence of perfusion abnormalities that may include, but are not limited to lactic acidosis, oliguria, or acute alteration in mental status. Patients who are on inotropic or vasopressor agents may not be hypotensive at the time that perfusion abnormalities are measured.
Hypotension	A systolic BP < 90 mmHg or a reduction of > 40 mmHg from baseline in the absence of other causes of hypotension.
Multiple organ dysfunction syndrome	Presence of altered organ function in a acutely ill patient such that homeostasis cannot be maintained without intervention.

Epidemiology

Prospective epidemiologic studies of sepsis with sufficient patient samples and clearly defined criteria have been published only recently. Since the population characteristics of hospitalized patients has probably changed over the last decades, older epidemiologic data may not be relevant today. Two large prospective epidemiologic studies of SIRS and sepsis-related states were published in 1995. Rangel-Frausto et al. [11] studied 3700 patients admitted to three critical care units and three wards. SIRS was very common and 20% of patients with SIRS subsequently progressed to septic shock. Positive blood cultures, end-organ dysfunction, and mortality increased when the severity of the systemic inflammatory response increased. In the Italian sepsis study [12] with 1100 patients SIRS was also common at the time of admission. The mortality was related to the severity of sepsis, but SIRS alone had little prognostic value. None of these studies allow evaluation of the true incidence of sepsis, since it is unclear how well the populations in the studies represent ICU patients in general.

Two prospective studies evaluated the prevalence and incidence of ICU-acquired infections and sepsis. Nearly half of the patients were infected during their ICU stay in a European 1-day cross-sectional prevalence study of about 10 000 patients [13].

Severe sepsis has been observed in nearly 10% of ICU admissions. The difficulties related to obtaining positive cultures is probably a contributing factor in the observation that only three of four patients presenting clinical sepsis had documented infection [14].

ICU patients are at increased risk for nosocomial infections The need for intensive care may increase the risk of nosocomial infections by two to three fold. Less than 10% of hospitalized patients are treated in ICUs. In contrast, about one fourth of all nosocomial infections are in intensive care patients [15]. The prevalence of nosocomial infection in hospitalized patients is between 5 and 17% [13], and in intensive care patients varies from 15 to 40% [16]. Both the increasing length of stay in the ICU and the use of invasive devices increase the risk of nosocomial infection.

The pathogens responsible for infections in ICUs have changed during the last decades [15]. Today Gram-positive bacteria have become more common as compared to the 1960s and 1970s when Gram-negative pathogens were predominantly causative. Nosocomial infections due to coagulase-negative staphylococci, methicillin-resistant *Staphylococcus aureus*, and enterococci have increased worldwide. Gram-positive and Gram-negative bacteria represent roughly equal proportions. The number of anaerobic bacteremias has decreased with *Bacteroides fragilis* the most common microbe in anaerobic infections [17]. Fungal infections, especially caused by *Candida* species [17, 18], have become much more common. *Candida* species cause less than 10% of positive blood cultures, but the mortality in these cases is over 50%.

Changes in medical practice and the availability of intensive care probably contribute to the changing profile of infectious foci [15]. In ICUs respiratory tract infections are the most common, whereas in general wards urinary tract infections predominate. Blood stream infections now cover more than 10% of hospital infections and 15% of ICU infections. More than 40% of these infections are catheter-related. Pneumonia and other respiratory tract infections cover about half of infections in ICU patients. Urinary tract is the source in about 10–20%. Infections of surgical wound, upper airway infections and gastrointestinal or central nervous system infections account for about one fourth of infections [13–15].

The severity of sepsis, the type of infection and bacterial etiology affect mortality. The crude mortality of infected patients varies from 10 to 80%, depending on the type of the ICU and, once again, the definition of sepsis [16]. The mortality increases from SIRS and sepsis to severe sepsis and septic shock [11]. Less than 10% of SIRS-patients have died in one month, whereas half of the patients progressing to septic shock died within one month [11]. When sepsis is due to pneumonia and bacteremia the mortality increases about two to three fold [13, 19]. Late-onset pneumonias with high-risk pathogens, such as *Acinetobacter* or *Pseudomonas* species, increase the risk to several fold [19]. Multiresistant organisms, for example vancomycin-resistant enterococci or methicillin-resistant *Staphylococcus aureus* greatly increase risk of death. Gram-negative organisms and coagulase-negative staphylococci seem to carry a lesser risk than other organisms. Septic patients with multiple foci have a poor prognosis [16]. With late-onset infections, it is difficult to distinguish between patients dying because of infection and those dying with infection.

Clinical Course of Sepsis

Although the clinical progress of sepsis is not well known, the duration of ICU stay and hospitalization, and the incidence of organ failures progressing after sepsis have been somewhat better established. Sepsis prolongs both ICU-stay and hospitalization. Matched case-control studies have assessed the extra length of hospitalization due to infection [19]. The excess length of stay in these ICU patients varies between one and two weeks. Bacteremic ICU patients stayed in the hospital for a median of 40 days as compared to 26 days for matched control patients without infections [19]. In patients with other foci, the excess length of stay has been reported to be around one week. 56% of all patients with sepsis were already septic on the day of admission in the study of Rangel-Frausto et al. [11]. Similarly, 42% of all patients with severe sepsis and 29% of patients with septic shock fulfilled the criteria during the day of admission. The time interval for progressing from one category to another varied and was independent of the presence of confirmed infection. The 28-day mortality was 9%, but the increased death rate continued throughout the six months following discharge from the ICU. In severe sepsis, the median length of ICU stay was over one week and the 28-day mortality over 50% [14]. Due to early deaths, the length of ICU stay was markedly different between survivors and nonsurvivors, 34 days versus 4 days, respectively. One third of patients stayed in the ICU for more than two weeks.

In patients with sepsis end-organ dysfunctions are common. At first multiple organ failure (MOF) was thought to be caused by uncontrolled or undiagnosed infection [8]. Later, the concept that organ dysfunction can develop and progress in the absence of uncontrolled infection has become accepted. It is also clear that the treatment of infection may fail to prevent the development of MOF. End-organ failure rates increase with the number of SIRS criteria [11]. The attack rates of acute respiratory distress syndrome (ARDS), disseminated intravascular coagulation (DIC), acute renal failure (ARF), and shock were comparable in SIRS and sepsis patients (about 4, 16, 13 and 21%, respectively). Patients with severe sepsis and septic shock had increased rates of these organ dysfunctions (Table 3).

The acute hemodynamic effects of sepsis and septic shock have been described in much detail, but the pathogenesis is still poorly understood. The hyperdynamic circulatory status, tachycardia, increased cardiac output, and decreased systemic vascular resistance characteristic to sepsis were first described in 1965 [20]. The type of micro-organism seems to have no effect on this clinical picture. In a study by Parker et al. [21] a decrease in heart rate (HR) and cardiac index (CI) or an increase in systemic vascular resistance (SVR) during the first 24 hours of septic shock were reported to be indicators for better prognosis. The hemodynamic profile of survivors and non-survivors may differ already before the onset of shock [22]. We analyzed the hemodynamics of 14 patients with septic shock, six survivors and eight non-survivors, during the seven hours before onset of the clinical manifestation of shock i.e. the start of vasopressor treatment. Survivors had a higher HR and CI, and lower SVR index than the non-survivors (Fig. 1 and 2). Periods of hypotension not requiring vasopressors were observed more frequently in the survivors before shock (Fig. 3). The other hemodynamic or oxygen transport parameters were not different between the two groups. Better cardiovascular reserves and the ability to maintain a hyperdynamic circulation seem to contribute to a better prognosis.

Table 3. Attack rates for end-organ dysfunction in the study of Rangel-Frausto et al. [11]

Syndrome	No of patients	ARDS (%)	DIC (%)	ARF (%)	Shock (%)
SIRS with 2 criteria		2	8	9	11
SIRS with 3 criteria		3	15	13	21
SIRS with 4 criteria	Total in SIRS 2527	6	19	19	27
Positive culture sepsis	649	6*	16*	19*	20*
Negative culture sepsis	892	3	20	5	27
Severe sepsis with positive cultures	467	8	18	23*	28*
Severe sepsis with negative cultures	527	4	17	16	22
Septic shock with positive cultures	110	18	38	51	100
Septic shock with negative cultures	84	18	38	38	100

* = p value < 0.05 between culture positive and culture negative stages

Myocardial depression is common in septic shock [23]. The pathogenesis of this phenomenon is not clear, but some circulating humoral substance may be responsible [24]. Cytokines, especially tumor necrosis factor (TNF), and endotoxin have been implicated, since when given intravenously they produce symptoms similar to septic shock [25, 26]. Nevertheless identification of any single substance responsible for the myocardial depression in clinical sepsis has not been confirmed. Numerous cytokines appear in the circulation during septic states. In fact, the myocardial depression in sepsis may be multifactorial. The role of cytokines in the pathogenesis of

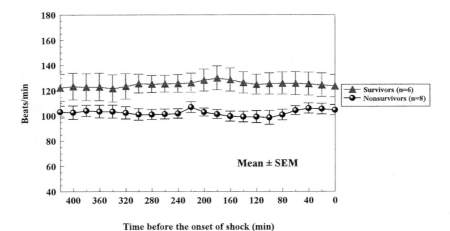

Fig. 1. Heart rate of survivors and non-survivors preceding septic shock. Area under the curve: p = 0.05. (From [22] with permission)

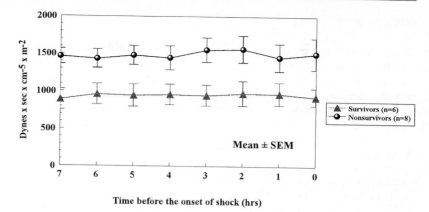

Fig. 2. Systemic vascular resistance index of survivors and non-survivors preceding septic shock. Two-way ANOVA: p = 0.03

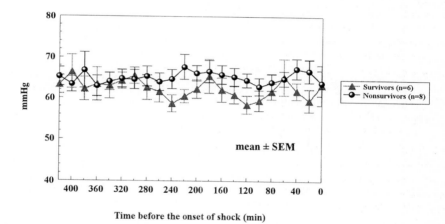

Fig. 3. Mean systemic arterial pressure of survivors and non-survivors preceding septic shock. Area under the curve: p = 0.25 for whole period, p = 0.002 for hypotension periods

sepsis and as treatment targets in sepsis and septic shock remains highly controversial. So far, despite many promising results of anti-cytokine or anti-cytokine receptor therapies in animal models, none of these therapies have been effective in humans. Since cytokines work as a complex network, the idea of treating sepsis by modulating single cytokines is clearly simplistic. Despite increased blood concentrations, some mediators may be epiphenomena rather than pathogenetically important. Nitric oxide (NO) may be responsible for some cardiovascular abnormalities in sepsis, especially hypotension [27]. As for anti-cytokine therapies, promising results of studies treating the hypotension in sepsis by blocking the synthesis of NO have been published [28]. Large clinical trials assessing the effect of NO synthase in sepsis are now ongoing.

Conclusion

Sepsis is an important cause of morbidity and mortality in ICU patients. Despite the vast amount of resources used for its treatment and in the search of new therapies, the epidemiology and clinical course of sepsis remain poorly documented. In order to better understand the pathophysiology and the develop of new therapies, a more defined description of this syndrome and its clinical course is needed.

References

1. Wiles JB, Cerra FB, Siegel JH, Border JR (1980) The systemic septic response: does the organism matter? Crit Care Med 8:55–60
2. Shoemaker WC, Appel PL, Kram HB, Bishop MH, Abraham E (1993) Sequence of physiologic patterns in surgical septic shock. Crit Care Med 21:1876–1889
3. Vincent J-L (1997) Dear SIRS, I'm sorry to say that I don't like you ... Crit Care Med 25:372–374
4. Parrillo JE (1993) Pathogenetic mechanisms of septic shock. N Engl J Med 328:1471–1477
5. Bone RC (1991) Sepsis, the sepsis syndrome, multi-organ failure. A plea for comparable definitions. Ann Intern Med 114:332–333
6. Rackow EC, Astiz ME, Weil MH (1988) Cellular oxygen metabolism during sepsis and shock. The relationship of oxygen consumption to oxygen delivery. JAMA 259:1989–1993
7. Marshall JC, Sweeney (1990) Microbial infection and the septic response in critical surgical illness. Sepsis, not infection, determines outcome. Arch Surg 125:17–25
8. Ziegler EJ, Fisher CJ, Sprung CL, et al (1991) Treatment of Gram-negative bacteremia and septic shock with HA-1A human monoclonal antibody against endotoxin. A randomized, double-blinded, placebo-controlled trial. N Engl J Med 324:429–436
9. Bone RC, Balk RA, Fein AM, et al (1995) A second large controlled clinical study of E5, a monoclonal antibody to endotoxin: Results of a prospective, multicenter, randomized, controlled trial. Crit Care Med 23:994–1006
10. American College of Chest Physicians/Society of Critical Care Medicine Consensus Conferences (1992) Definitions for sepsis and organ failure and guidelines for the use of innovative therapies in sepsis. Crit Care Med 20:864–874
11. Rangel-Frausto MS, Pittet D, Costigan M, Hwang T, Davis C, Wenzel RP (1995) The natural history of the systemic inflammatory response (SIRS). A prospective study. JAMA 273:117–123
12. Salvo I, de Cian W, Musicco M, et al (1995) The Italian sepsis study: Preliminary results on the incidence and evolution of SIRS, sepsis, severe sepsis and septic shock. Intensive Care Med 21 (suppl 2):S244–S249
13. Vincent J-L, Bihari DJ, Suter PM, et al (1995) The prevalence of nosocomial infection in intensive care units in Europe. Results of the European prevalence of infection in intensive care (EPIC) study. JAMA 274:639–644
14. Brun-Buisson C, Doyon F, Carlet J, et al (1995) Incidence, risk factors, and outcome of severe sepsis and septic shock in adults. A multicenter prospective study in intensive care units. JAMA 274:968–974
15. Wildmer A (1994) Infection control and prevention strategies in the ICU. Intensive Care Med 20 (suppl 1):S7–S11
16. Pittet D, Brun-Buisson C (1996) Nosocomial infections and the intensivist. Curr Opinion Crit Care 2:345–346
17. Goldstein EJC (1996) Anaerobic bacteremia. Clin Infect Dis 23:S97–S101
18. Pfaller M, Wenzel R (1992) Impact of the changing epidemiology of fungal infections in the 1990s. Eur J Clin Microbiol Infect Dis 11:287–291
19. Girou E, Brun-Buisson C (1996) Morbidity, mortality, and the cost of nosocomial infections in critical care. Curr Opinion Crit Care 2:347–351
20. Wilson RF, Thal AP, Kindling PH, Grifka T, Ackerman E (1965) Hemodynamic measurements in septic shock. Ann Surg 91:121–129

21. Parker MM, Shelhamer JH, Natanson C, Alling DW, Parrillo JE (1987) Serial cardiovascular variables in survivors and nonsurvivors of human septic shock: Heart rate as an early predictor of prognosis. Crit Care Med 15:923–929
22. Ilkka L, Takala J (1996) Hemodynamic pattern preceding septic shock. Intensive Care Med 22 (suppl 2):S329 (Abst)
23. Parker MM, Shelhamer JH, Bacharach SL, et al (1984) Profound but reversible myocardial depression in patients with septic shock. Ann Intern Med 100:483–490
24. Parrillo JE, Burch C, Shelhamer JH, Parker MM, Natanson C, Schuette W (1985) A circulating myocardial depressant substance in humans with septic shock. J Clin Invest 76:1539–1553
25. Natanson C, Eichenholz PW, Danner RL, et al (1989) Endotoxin and tumor necrosis factor challenges in dogs simulate the cardiovascular profile of human septic shock. J Exp Med 169: 823–832
26. Danner RL, Elin RJ, Hosseini JM, Wesley RA, Reilly JM, Parrillo JE (1991) Endotoxemia in human septic shock. Chest 99:169–175
27. Lorente JA, Landin L, Renes E, et al (1993) Role of nitric oxide in the hemodynamic changes of sepsis. Crit Care Med 21:759–767
28. Takala J, Guntupalli K, Donaldson J, Watson D (1997) Multicentre, placebo-controlled, double-blind study of the nitric oxide synthase inhibitor 546C88 in patients with septic shock: effect on early non-cardiovascular organ function. Intensive Care Med 23 (suppl 1):S51 (Abst)

Prognostic Markers in Sepsis

A. Rhodes, P. J. Newman, and E. D. Bennett

Introduction

Sepsis remains one of the leading causes of death on the intensive care unit (ICU). Despite a greater understanding of the pathophysiologic state, there is still no specific treatment that has been proven to improve outcome. The increased awareness of the mechanisms behind the septic state, has led to an appreciation of a variety of factors that may either influence or be related to the severity of the illness or the eventual patient outcome. As these prognostic markers become better understood, new treatment strategies can be directed towards a "high risk" group of patients, who have the greatest potential for improvement. This paper attempts to discuss a variety of these factors which may influence, and/or be used to identify, outcome in sepsis.

Hemodynamic Measurements

Sepsis is a complex pathophysiologic state associated with profound hemodynamic disturbances, which can lead to multiple organ dysfunction and death. The association of hypotension with peripheral vasodilatation and a hyperdynamic circulation is almost pathomnemonic of sepsis. A number of studies have shown that survival from sepsis is associated with an increase in mean arterial blood pressure [1], systemic vascular resistance [2], cardiac index [3] and left ventricular stroke work index [4] (Table 1). The values of these variables at baseline, do not seem to differ between survivors and non-survivors. However the two groups have dramatically different responses to resuscitation and treatment [5].

Table 1. Hemodynamic variables of predictive value in sepsis

Predictive variable	Reference
Increase of mean arterial blood pressure from baseline	[1]
Increase in systemic vascular resistance from baseline	[2]
Increase in cardiac index in response to fluid resuscitation	[3]
Increase in left ventricular stroke work index	[4]
Increase in both oxygen delivery and consumption	[3]
Increase in oxygen consumption in response to dobutamine	[7, 8]

The identification of a pathologic oxygen supply dependency relationship by an oxygen flux test, has previously been thought to have been related to covert tissue hypoxia and thus a poor outcome [6]. Recent studies now seem to question this theory, with the realization that survival is associated with a greater degree of physiologic reserve, i.e., the ability to increase the cardiac index and so oxygen delivery (DO_2) and oxygen consumption (VO_2) [3, 7, 8]. This association between outcome and increased DO_2 and VO_2 has been noted in other patient groups, including trauma [9], acute respiratory distress syndrome [10] and high risk surgical patients [11].

Hayes et al. [3] have demonstrated that although the therapeutic targeting of cardiac index, DO_2 and VO_2 in a mixed group of critically ill patients was not associated with an improved outcome, those patients who were able to increase their VO_2 following resuscitation, had a lower mortality than those who could not. When they then analyzed the subgroup of those patients with sepsis, they were able to show that the survivors were characterized by the ability to raise both DO_2 and VO_2 following resuscitation, whereas non-survivors had no change in VO_2 despite an increase in DO_2, inferring a reduction in oxygen extraction [3].

This association between raised VO_2 and good outcome has been reported in other studies. Vallet et al. [8] demonstrated that following an infusion of dobutamine (an oxygen flux test) to patients with the sepsis syndrome, but not septic shock, survival was associated with a significant increase in VO_2. This has been confirmed in patients with severe sepsis or septic shock by Rhodes et al. [7], who demonstrated an 11.1% mortality for patients who could increase their VO_2 by greater than 15%, as compared to a mortality of 87.5% for patients who could not, when given an infusion of dobutamine at 10 mcg/kg/min. The presumption behind this is that an increase in resting energy expenditure is required by these patients for survival. Patients whose cells are unable to increase their oxidative metabolism or oxygen extraction, possibly due to an overwhelming septic insult, do badly.

Gastric Intramucosal pH and the CO_2 Gap

Ischemia and/or hypoperfusion of the splanchnic beds are thought to be pivotal in the development of multiorgan failure. Routine clinical parameters such as heart rate, blood pressure or urine output provide information about the general state of organ perfusion, whereas whole body hemodynamics can provide information about oxygen delivery and oxygen consumption. The idea that a relatively non-invasive catheter, "the gastric tonometer" could provide data relating directly to the state of the gastric beds would seem attractive.

Over the last few years, the gastric tonometer has thus been suggested as a measure of splanchnic perfusion and mesenteric ischemia. Measurement of carbon dioxide tension in the fluid (or air) of the balloon of the tonometer, when combined with the arterial bicarbonate concentration, allows an estimation of the pH of the gastric mucosa (pHi). A lower pHi indicates increasing acidosis of this region and suggests reduced splanchnic perfusion and/or increasing anaerobic metabolism [12]. Patients most likely to benefit from tonometry, are those who may have covert tissue hypoxia, for whom a low pHi is a sensitive predictor of a poor outcome [13].

In critically ill patients who have a systemic acidosis, however, the pHi is closely correlated with data that can be obtained from routine blood gas analysis [14]. These findings are not unexpected, as the equations for the derivation of arterial pH and pHi contain the same variable (arterial bicarbonate concentration). In order to get around the problems of utilizing this monitor in the presence of acidemia, it is now suggested that the gap between the gastric intramucosal and arterial carbon dioxide tensions, could be a better estimate of mesenteric ischemia [12].

Recent papers have demonstrated the usefulness of the gastric tonometer in identifying patients who are at high risk of a poor outcome. Fiddian-Green et al. [15] demonstrated the usefulness of this tool in patients with massive hemorrhage from stress ulceration, and subsequently this same effect has been shown during cardiac surgery [16] and in other heterogeneous groups of critically ill patients [13,17]. Most researchers have used a cut off point of pHi <7.32 as the marker of increased mortality [18, 19], however Maynard's group [13] demonstrated that the best marker was a pHi <7.32 at 24 hours, presumably relating to the degree of physiologic derangement post resuscitation. Recent work has suggested that although pHi could distinguish survivors from non-survivors for emergency intensive care admissions, neither the CO_2 gap nor the arterial pH to pHi gradient could be used for this purpose [20]. Despite this effect on heterogenous populations, there have been only a few studies published on septic patients. Joynt et al. [21] compared serum lactate to gastric pHi, and found that lactate was a better overall marker, and that the pHi could not predict outcome until 48 hours. This contrasts with Marik [22], who investigated the predictive value of pHi and other hemodynamic values within 24 hours of the development of sepsis and found that the pHi was significantly lower in the non-survivors and was the best predictor of outcome.

In summary, in septic patients it seems that pHi is not consistently able to distinguish between survivors and non-survivors, until after 24 hours, thus its use as either a marker of severity or as a guide to resuscitation is limited. The value of the CO_2 gap as a predictive marker, overcomes some of the limitations of pHi, but so far there has been very little published literature on the use of CO_2 gap in sepsis.

Cytokines

Cytokines are a group of small signaling proteins produced by a large variety of cells which act on cell surface receptors to regulate and modify cell growth, maturation and repair, as well as the acute phase response to inflammation [23]. Although these cytokines have an important role in homeostasis, excessive production and release initiate widespread tissue injury which can result in organ dysfunction. Proinflammatory cytokines are undoubtedly involved in the pathophysiology of severe sepsis, where an overwhelming systemic derangement is caused by release of pro-inflammatory cytokines into the circulation. The recent ability to measure and quantify cytokine levels, has led to a number of studies where levels of different cytokines have been correlated with severity of illness and eventual patient outcome [24–27]. Four cytokines, tumour necrosis factor-α (TNF-α), interleukin (IL)-1β, IL-6, and IL-8 have been associated with the sepsis syndrome and assessed as prognostic tools (Table 2).

Table 2. Cytokines that have been demonstrated to show predictive value in sepsis

Cytokines	References
TNF-α	[24–29, 32]
IL-1β	[29, 34–36]
IL-6	[24, 29, 36–38]
IL-8	[29, 40]

TNF-α can be detected in the plasma of many patients with sepsis, although the correlation of actual levels with severity of illness remains contentious. TNF-α production is rapidly induced by endotoxin, and itself then activates a number of other mediators, including IL-1β, IL-6, IL-8 and a number of cytokine neutralizing molecules, the p55 and p75 TNF receptors. Various authors have reported an association of elevated TNF-α levels with a poor outcome [26, 27] whilst others have demonstrated that rather than an initial high level, it is the persistence of high levels which is important [24, 28]. Friedland et al. [29], who measured TNF-α, IL-1β, IL-6, and IL-8 levels in a mixed group of intensive care patients, found that TNF-α bioactivity, but not absolute concentrations, was the only cytokine measurement that had an independent predictive effect on outcome, although this effect was relatively small. They [29] also found no difference in levels at the time of admission when comparing survivors to non-survivors which is in contrast to other studies [30, 31]. A possible explanation for this is that TNF-α receptors exert a possible beneficial protective *in vitro* and *in vivo* effect, thus making the measurement of bioactivity more relevant than absolute levels. When they studied the patients in a longitudinal manner they discovered only two patients who had persistently raised TNF-α levels and they both died. However the majority of patients had raised TNF-α levels for only a transient period, which was similar to findings by Marano et al. [25]. The disparity between results in the studies on TNF-α may be a result of both the timing of the assays and also the specific assay used. TNF-α levels usually seem to be raised in patients with sepsis, however, persistently raised concentrations or activity may be a better predictor of activity than a single measurement [32].

IL-1β is a mediator produced by endotoxin-stimulated human monocytes and can be detected in the plasma of septic animals. Infusion of IL-1β causes fever, hemodynamic abnormalities, anorexia, malaise and neutrophilia [33]. Like TNF-α, IL-1β causes release of further cytokines including TNF-α, IL-6, and IL-8. There have been a number of studies assessing whether IL-1β can be used as a predictive marker for sepsis, which show that initial levels of IL-1β correlate with the severity of sepsis but there is no association with mortality [34–36]. Casey et al. [36] demonstrated that 37% of patients with sepsis had initially detectable concentrations of IL-1β, but that these levels could not predict outcome. These findings were confirmed by Friedland et al. [29], who demonstrated that IL-1β levels on admission were higher in those patients who died in intensive care, although the relationship did not hold when looking at overall hospital mortality. This study [29] also showed, however, no association between levels of IL-1β and physiological derangement and severity of illness for critically ill patients.

Together with TNF-α and IL-1β, IL-6 is one of the mediators of the acute phase response. In addition, IL-6 can activate the coagulation system and function as a pyrogen [32]. Although the precise role of IL-6 in sepsis is unclear, circulating levels of this cytokine seem to correlate well with outcome. Various studies have demonstrated a correlation in sepsis between peak IL-6 levels, APACHE II scores and death [24, 36–38]. Not all studies have confirmed this, and Marecaux et al. [39] demonstrated that lactate could predict outcome better than either TNF-α or IL-6 for patients with septic shock. Friedland et al. [29] confirmed that IL-6 levels on admission were higher for non-survivors than survivors, correlated with disease severity, but that IL-6 was not an independent predictor of death. IL-6 concentrations seem to correlate more closely than other cytokines with severity and outcome of human sepsis, and it may be that it acts as a marker for activation of the cytokine cascade, thus reflecting disease severity [32].

IL-8 is a potent chemotactic agent for neutrophils, and may be important for mediating some of the organ dysfunction and acute lung injury associated with the sepsis syndrome. IL-8 levels are elevated in patients with sepsis and these higher concentrations are correlated with increasing physiologic derangement, organ dysfunction and death [29, 40].

In summary, the relationship between deranged physiology, poor outcome and fluctuating plasma pro-inflammatory cytokine concentrations is complex. TNF-α, IL-1β, IL-6, and IL-8 levels are all frequently elevated in sepsis and have all been correlated with disease severity and outcome in certain studies. The specific nature of all these molecules, however, requires complex specific assays which have to be performed at specific time points in disease progression to maintain reliable results. At present the implication from this, is that these are not practicable tools for monitoring disease progression or severity in the intensive care setting.

Type 1-Prophospholipase A₂ Propeptide (PROP)

Phospholipids form a major part of cell membranes. The phospholipid moiety is constructed from a glycerol molecule, with two fatty acyl chains esterified to each of the first and second carbon atoms and phosphoric acid esterified to the third. Cell membranes consist of phospholipid bilayers, whose stability results from the hydrophobic interactions between the two fatty acyl chains. If one of these chains is cleaved off by an enzyme such as phospholipase A_2, the membrane is destabilized and cell lysis occurs. This action of phospholipase A_2 on phospholipids causes the release of the second fatty acyl chain, known as arachidonic acid, and lysophosphatidic acid which forms platelet activating factor (PAF). The catalytic activities of phospholipase A_2 therefore influence two short pathways, both of which rapidly lead to the formation of molecules which are potent participants in the inflammatory process.

Recently an assay has been developed to determine the degree of activation of phospholipase A_2 [41]. Like many other enzymes, phospholipase A_2 is stored in an inactive form and is activated by the cleavage of a short aminoterminal propeptide. Determining the concentration of this activation propeptide by an enzyme-linked immunosorbent assay (ELISA), then gives an estimation of the concentration of the activated form of phospholipase A_2. The name given to this test for the activation propeptide released from type 1-prophospholipase A_2, is the PROP assay. The PROP assay appears to be a highly specific marker of granulocyte activation [42]. In an initial series of intensive care patients by Rae et al. [43], the PROP assay predicted the onset of acute respiratory distress syndrome (ARDS) and multi-organ dysfunction with a sensitivity of 100% and a specificity of 93%. Once the propeptide was detected in the plasma, the signal remained until recovery or death. Where early samples were available, the PROP assay was able to predict the onset of ARDS by up to 36 hours before the clinical criteria for the syndrome were established. Although this study was on a mixed group of intensive care patients, the likelihood is that the results would be similar for septic patients, and further studies are at present underway.

Procalcitonin

Procalcitonin (PCT), which is the key precursor of calcitonin, has been reported to be a specific marker of bacterial sepsis [44]. High serum levels have been documented in a variety of conditions, including medullary cell carcinoma of the thyroid, neoplastic diseases, acute and chronic inflammation of the lung, pancreatitis, renal failure and meningococcemia [44]. Release of PCT into the circulation has been demonstrated 3–6 hours after endotoxin injection, and there is then a steady increase in levels for up to 24 hours [45]. The source of the release of the PCT in sepsis remains unclear, but there is not a concomitant rise in the concentration of calcitonin unlike in medullary cell carcinoma of the thyroid, and the release of PCT has been demonstrated in septic patients even after they have undergone a thyroidectomy [45].

The concentrations of PCT during sepsis have been shown to correlate with the severity of the sepsis, levels greater than 200 ng/mL only being found in septic shock [44]. The presence of localized infection or a viral illness only leads to a mildly raised titre of PCT, and appropriate treatment with antimicrobial therapy has been shown to be associated with a rapid reduction in serum concentrations [46]. Monneret et al. [46] compared the levels of PCT and C-reactive protein (CRP) in neonatal sepsis and found that PCT had an earlier increase and return to baseline, and a wider variation in levels with deterioration as compared to CRP. More recently it has been shown that PCT can accurately differentiate between the fever of rejection and that of sepsis in post liver transplant patients [47].

At present, PCT seems to be a sensitive predictor of the severity of sepsis. False positive results may occur however, especially in combination with other conditions, for example acute lung injury [46]. At present there are few studies demonstrating the correlation between disease severity and PCT levels, and more work is needed if this assay is to be used as a prognostic tool for outcome or as a method of directing therapy.

Conclusion

There are many prognostic markers which help to identify outcome in sepsis. They encompass both biochemical tests such as cytokines or PROP, and also the physiological response to sepsis i.e., the ability to extract oxygen or the gastric intramucosal pH. At present our treatment strategies for established sepsis are poor and there is a high mortality associated with this disease process. If we were able to identify those patients who were likely to progress to severe sepsis by using these prognostic markers, we may be better able to direct resources or new treatment strategies towards this group and therefore stand a better chance of improving outcome.

References

1. Metrangolo L, Fiorillo M, Friedman G, et al (1995) Early hemodynamic course of septic shock. Crit Care Med 13:1971–1975
2. Parker MM, Shelhamer JH, Natanson C, Alling DW, Parrillo JE (1987) Serial cardiovascular variables in survivors and nonsurvivors of human septic shock: heart rate as an early predictor of prognosis. Crit Care Med 15:923–929
3. Hayes MA, Timmins AC, Yau EH, Palazzo M, Watson DH, Hinds CJ (1997) Oxygen transport patterns in patients with sepsis syndrome or septic shock: influence of treatment and relationship to outcome. Crit Care Med 25:926–936
4. D'Orio V, Mendes P, Saad G, Marcelle R (1990) Accuracy in early prediction of prognosis of patients with septic shock by analysis of simple indices: prospective study. Crit Care Med 18:1339–1345
5. Wray GM, Hinds CJ (1997) Determinants of outcome from sepsis and septic shock. In: Vincent JL (ed) Yearbook of intensive care and emergency medicine. Springer-Verlag, Berlin, Heidelberg, New York, pp 168–179
6. Bihari D, Smithies M, Gimson A, Tinker J (1987) The effects of vasodilation with prostacyclin on oxygen delivery and uptake in critically ill patients. N Engl J Med 317:397–403
7. Rhodes A, Malagon I, Lamb FJ, Newman PJ, Grounds RM, Bennett ED (1996) Failure to increase oxygen consumption is a predictor of mortality in septic patients. Intensive Care Med 22:S274 (Abst)
8. Vallet B, Chopin C, Curtis SE, et al (1993) Prognostic value of the dobutamine test in patients with sepsis syndrome and normal lactate values: a prospective, multicenter study. Crit Care Med 21:1868–1875
9. Bishop MH, Shoemaker WC, Appel PL, et al (1995) Prospective, randomized trial of survivor values of cardiac index, oxygen delivery, and oxygen consumption as resuscitation endpoints in severe trauma. J Trauma 38:780–787
10. Yu M, Levy MM, Smith P, Takiguchi SA, Miyasaki A, Myers SA (1993) Effect of maximizing oxygen delivery on morbidity and mortality rates in critically ill patients: a prospective, randomized, controlled study. Crit Care Med 21:830–838
11. Boyd O, Grounds RM, Bennett ED (1993) A randomized clinical trial of the effect of deliberate perioperative increase of oxygen delivery on mortality in high-risk surgical patients. JAMA 270:2699–2707
12. Rhodes A, Boyd O, Bland JM, Grounds RM, Bennett ED (1997) Routine blood gas analysis and gastric tonometry: a reappraisal. Lancet 350:413–420
13. Maynard N, Bihari D, Beale R, et al (1993) Assessment of splanchnic oxygenation by gastric tonometry in patients with acute circulatory failure. JAMA 270:1203–1210
14. Boyd O, Mackay CJ, Lamb G, Bland JM, Grounds RMB, Bennett ED (1993) Comparison of clinical information gained from routine blood-gas analysis and from gastric tonometry for intramural pH. Lancet 341:142–146

15. Fiddian-Green RG, McGough E, Pittenger GR, Rothman E (1983) Predictive value of intramural pH and other risk factors for massive bleeding from stress ulceration. Gastroenterology 85:613–620
16. Fiddian-Green RG, Baker S (1987) Predictive value of the stomach wall pH for complications after cardiac operations: comparison with other monitoring. Crit Care Med 15:153–156
17. Gutierrez G, Palizas F, Doglio G, et al (1992) Gastric intramucosal pH as a therapeutic index of tissue oxygenation in critically ill patients. Lancet 339:195–199
18. Gutierrez G, Bismar H, Dantzker DR, Silva N (1992) Comparison of gastric intramucosal pH with measures of oxygen transport and consumption in critically ill patients. Crit Care Med 20:451–457
19. Gys T, Hubens A, Neels H, Lauwers LF, Peeters R (1988) Prognostic value of gastric intramural pH in surgical intensive care patients. Crit Care Med 16:1222–1224
20. Gomersall CD, Joynt GM, Ho KM, Young RJ, Buckley TA, Oh TE (1997) Gastric tonometry and prediction of outcome in the critically ill. Arterial to intramucosal pH gradient and carbon dioxide gradient. Anaesthesia 52:619–623
21. Joynt GM, Lipman J, Gomersall CD, Tan J, Scribante J (1997) Gastric intramucosal pH and blood lactate in severe sepsis. Anaesthesia 52:726–732
22. Marik PE (1993) Gastric intramucosal pH. A better predictor of multiorgan dysfunction syndrome and death than oxygen-derived variables in patients with sepsis. Chest 104:225–229
23. Sheeran P, Hall GM (1997) Cytokines in anaesthesia. Br J Anaesth 78:201–219
24. Pinsky MR, Vincent JL, Deviere J, Alegre M, Kahn RJD, Dupont E (1993) Serum cytokine levels in human septic shock. Relation to multiple-system organ failure and mortality. Chest 103:565–575
25. Marano MA, Fong Y, Moldawer LL, et al (1990) Serum cachectin/tumor necrosis factor in critically ill patients with burns correlates with infection and mortality. Surg Gynecol Obst 170:32–38
26. Girardin E, Grau GE, Dayer JM, Roux-Lombard P, Lambert PH (1988) Tumor necrosis factor and interleukin-1 in the serum of children with severe infectious purpura. N Engl J Med 319:397–400
27. Waage A, Halstensen A, Espevik T (1987) Association between tumour necrosis factor in serum and fatal outcome in patients with meningococcal disease. Lancet 1:355–357
28. Martin C, Saux P, Mege JL, Perrin G, Papazian L, Gouin F (1994) Prognostic values of serum cytokines in septic shock. Intensive Care Med 20:272–277
29. Friedland JS, Porter JC, Daryanani S, et al (1996) Plasma proinflammatory cytokine concentrations, Acute Physiology and Chronic Health Evaluation (APACHE) III scores and survival in patients in an intensive care unit. Crit Care Med 24:1775–1781
30. Beutler B, Grau GE (1993) Tumor necrosis factor in the pathogenesis of infectious diseases. Crit Care Med 21:S423–S435
31. Strieter RM, Kunkel SL, Bone RC (1993) Role of tumor necrosis factor-alpha in disease states and inflammation. Crit Care Med 21:S447–S463
32. Blackwell TS, Christman JW (1996) Sepsis and cytokines: current status. Br Anaesth 77:110–117
33. Dinarello CA (1991) Interleukin-1 and interleukin-1 antagonism. Blood 77:1627–1652
34. Goldie AS, Fearon KC, Ross JA, et al (1995) Natural cytokine antagonists and endogenous antiendotoxin core antibodies in sepsis syndrome. The Sepsis Intervention Group. JAMA 274:172–177
35. McAllister SK, Bland LA, Arduino MJ, Aguero SM, Wenger PN, Jarvis WR (1994) Patient cytokine response in transfusion-associated sepsis. Infect Immun 62:2126–2128
36. Casey LC, Balk RA, Bone RC (1993) Plasma cytokine and endotoxin levels correlate with survival in patients with the sepsis syndrome. Ann Intern Med 119:771–778
37. Moscovitz H, Shofer F, Mignott H, Behrman A, Kilpatrick L (1994) Plasma cytokine determinations in emergency department patients as a predictor of bacteremia and infectious disease severity. Crit Care Med 22:1102–1107
38. Damas P, Ledoux D, Nys M, Vrindts Y, De Groote DF, Lamy M (1992) Cytokine serum level during severe sepsis in human: IL-6 as a marker of severity. Ann Surg 215:356–362
39. Marecaux G, Pinsky MR, Dupont E, Kahn RJ, Vincent JL (1996) Blood lactate levels are better prognostic indicators than TNF and IL-6 levels in patients with septic shock. Intensive Care Med 22:404–408

40. Hack CE, Hart M, van Schijndel RJ, et al (1992) Interleukin-8 in sepsis: relation to shock and inflammatory mediators. Infect Immun 60:2835–2842
41. Gudgeon AM, Patel G, Hermon-Taylor JH, Bowyer RC, Jehanli AM (1991) Detection of human pancreatic pro-phospholipase A_2 activation using an immunoassay for the free activation peptide DSGISPR. Ann Clin Biochem 28:497–503
42. Rae D, Sumar N, Beechey-Newman N, Gudgeon MH (1995) Type 1-prophospholipase A_2 propeptide immunoreactivity is released from activated granulocytes. Clin Biochem 28:71–78
43. Rae D, Porter J, Beechey-Newman N, Sumar N, Bennett D, Hermon-Taylor J (1994) Type 1-pro-phospholipase A_2 propeptide in acute lung injury. Lancet 344:1472–1473
44. Assicot M, Gendrel D, Carsin H, Raymond J, Guilbaud J, Bohuon C (1993) High serum procalcitonin concentrations in patients with sepsis and infection. Lancet 341:515–518
45. Gendrel D, Assicot M, Raymond J, et al (1996) Procalcitonin as a marker for the early diagnosis of neonatal infection. J Pediatrics 128:570–573
46. Monneret G, Labaune JM, Isaac C, Bienvenu F, Putet G, Bienvenu J (1997) Procalcitonin and C-reactive protein levels in neonatal infections. Acta Paediatrica 86:209–212
47. Kuse ER, Langefeld I, Jaeger J, et al (1997) Procalcitonin differentiates infection and rejection after solid organ transplantation. Intensive Care Med 23 (suppl 1):S62 (Abst)

Procalcitonin – An Indicator of Sepsis

W. Karzai, A. Meier-Hellmann, and K. Reinhart

Introduction

Sepsis is defined as a systemic inflammatory response to severe infections. However a similar systemic inflammatory response may also be triggered by other insults such as pancreatitis [1], major trauma [2], and burns [3]. Common clinical signs of systemic inflammation such as changes in body temperature, leukocytosis, and tachycardia may therefore have an infectious or non-infectious etiology and are neither specific nor sensitive for sepsis. It is, thus, frequently difficult to distinguish patients with systemic infection from those who appear septic but have no evidence of infection. Bacteriologic evidence of infection also has drawbacks because it may not develop concurrently with clinical signs of sepsis, and a negative bacteriologic result does not exclude the presence of infection or of sepsis [4]. Since these common clinical and laboratory parameters lack sensitivity and specificity, others are needed to provide an early marker of the infectious etiology of a generalized inflammatory response and thus allow early diagnosis and the application of more specific therapeutic interventions. Furthermore, new parameters may also help identify subgroups of septic patients who may benefit from pro- or anti-inflammatory therapies. One such parameter, procalcitonin (PCT), has recently drawn attention as a possible marker of the systemic inflammatory response to infection.

Biology of Procalcitonin

PCT is the propeptide of calcitonin which consists of 116 amino acids with a molecular weight of 13 kD [5, 6], and under normal circumstances, is produced in the C-cells of the thyroid glands. A specific protease then cleaves PCT to calcitonin, katacalcin, and a N-terminal residue [5]. In contrast to the short half-life of calcitonin (10 minutes) PCT has a long half-life of 25-30 hours [7] in serum. PCT levels are undetectable (<0.1 ng/ml) in healthy humans but increase to over 100 ng/ml during severe infections (bacterial, parasitic and fungal) with systemic manifestations.

During severe systemic infections, PCT is mostly produced by extra-thyroid tissues. Thus, patients who have previously undergone a total thyroidectomy can still produce high levels of PCT (without secretion of calcitonin) during a severe infectious episode [8]. The exact site of PCT production during sepsis is, however, uncertain. One investigator, using katacalcin antibodies, has identified PCT-like activity in human leukocytes [9], while others suggest neuroendocrine cells and the lungs [10–12] as possible sites of production. Remarkably, the large amounts of PCT produced during infections do not lead to an increase in plasma calcitonin levels or activity [8] and calcium levels seems to be independent of PCT-like activity.

Procalcitonin is measured with an immunoluminometric assay (B.R.A.H.M.S. Diagnostika, Berlin). This assay is specific in that it uses two antibodies that bind to two sites (calcitonin and katacalcin) of the PCT molecule thus ruling out cross-reactivity. The detection limit of the assay is 0.1 ng/ml and PCT levels of healthy subjects are usually <0.1 ng/ml [13]. Previously, some investigators had found increases in serum "calcitonin-like" activity in patients with infections [14] or with lung disease [10, 11]. However, those methods did not discriminate between calcitonin and PCT although some of the "calcitonin-like" activity in these studies may well have been attributable to increases in PCT levels.

Procalcitonin During Infections

Severe generalized bacterial, parasitic or fungal infections with systemic manifestations are associated with increased PCT serum levels. In contrast, severe viral infections or inflammatory reactions of non-infectious origin do not, or only moderately increase PCT levels. In a well-documented study [8], 79 children with suspected infections displayed PCT levels which were either very low (<0.1 ng/ml) in those with no infection, or very high (6–53 ng/m) in those with severe infection. Antibiotic therapy in those with severe infection led to a resolution of the infection and to decreases in PCT levels. Localized bacterial infections without systemic manifestations, and viral infections, produced only small to modest increases in PCT (0.3–1.5 ng/ml). Calcitonin was undetectable in these patients regardless of how high PCT levels were. Because of these properties, PCT has been proposed as an indicator of severe generalized infections or sepsis [8,13].

Specificity and Sensitivity of PCT

The specificity of PCT for infections increases with increasing PCT values i.e., patients with PCT values above 1.5 ng/ml are more likely to have a severe infection (sensitivity 100%, specificity 72%) than patients with PCT values above 0.1 ng/ml (sensitivity 100%, specificity 35%) [15]. However, since the number of patients in such studies are limited, both high and low cut-off values of PCT have been used to predict infectious complications in patients with an underlying active inflammatory disease. In patients with pancreatitis, PCT levels greater than 1.8 ng/ml predicted infectious complications with a diagnostic accuracy of 87% which was comparable to that of fine-needle aspiration (84%) [16]. The diagnostic accuracy improved if increases in PCT levels (>1.8 ng/ml) occurred at least twice during the observation period. In contrast, the cut-off value which was used to predict bacterial infection in patients with underlying active lupus erythematosis was merely 0.5 ng/ml (unpublished observations) with a sensitivity of 1.00 and a specificity of 0.84. These findings suggest that levels of PCT which best differentiate between infectious and non-infectious states in patients with underlying inflammatory syndrome may depend on the characteristics of the patient population studied.

PCT and Infectious Versus Non-Infectious Causes of Severe Systemic Inflammation

PCT has been used to differentiate between infectious and non-infectious causes of severe inflammatory states. Preliminary results suggest that PCT helps differentiate infectious (cholangitis by bile duct obstruction) from non-infectious (ethanol) pancreatitis [17], infectious from non-infectious causes of the acute respiratory distress syndrome (ARDS) in adults, and systemic fungal [18] and bacterial infections from episodes of graft rejection [19] in patients after organ transplantation. Although small patient populations and inadequate use of statistics makes it difficult to interpret the results of these studies, they do suggest that PCT levels may help identify non-viral infection as a cause of the systemic inflammatory response.

PCT and Severity of Infection

PCT levels increase with increasing severity of the inflammatory response to infection. A recent study [15] compared PCT values in patients with bacterial pneumonia and septic shock. PCT values were moderately increased in patients with bacterial pneumonia (mean: 2.4 ng/ml) but were markedly increased in patients with septic shock (means: 72–135 ng/ml) (Fig. 1). Preliminary results of other studies [20–22] suggest that once the PCT level is increased, it may then reflect the severity of the inflammatory/infectious response. When patients were categorized into systemic inflammatory response syndrome (SIRS), sepsis, severe sepsis, and septic shock using the ACCP/SCCM consensus conference criteria [23]. PCT levels were especially elevated in patients with severe sepsis and septic shock (Table 1).

On the other hand, PCT levels are not, or are only moderately, increased in the systemic inflammatory response to viral or to non-infectious stimuli (infections other than viral). In neonates and children, those with bacterial meningitis had sig-

Table 1. Procalcitonin, TNF-α, and IL-6 values in various stages of the inflammatory/infectious response.

	TNF-α (pg/ml)	IL-6 (pg/ml)	PCT (ng/ml)
SIRS	24± 4	269± 22	1.3±0.2
Sepsis	51± 9*	435± 52*	2.0±0.0*
Severe sepsis	59±17	969±168*	8.7±2.5*
Septic shock	118±18	996± 57	38.6±5.9*

Values are expressed as mean ± SEM. TNF-α = tumor necrosis factor-alpha; IL-6 = interleukin-6; PCT = procalcitonin; SIRS = systemic inflammatory response syndrome
* $p < 0.05$ as compared to preceding value. (From [21] with permission)

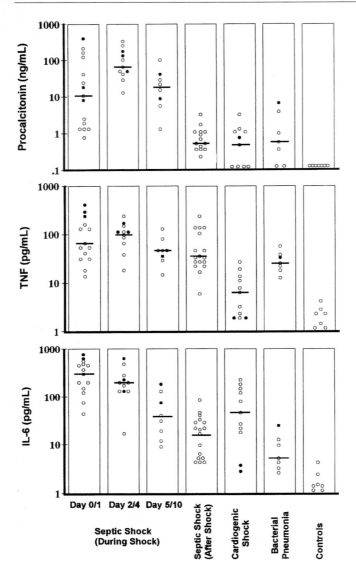

Fig. 1. Concentrations of tumor necrosis factor (TNF)-α, interleukin-6 (IL-6), and procalcitonin in the plasma of patients with septic shock, cardiogenic shock, bacterial pneumonia, and in normal volunteers. *Open circles:* survivors, *closed circles:* non-survivors. (Modified from [15] with permission)

nificantly higher levels of PCT (mean: 57.9 ng/ml) than those with viral meningitis (mean: 0.3 ng/ml) (unpublished data). In patients infected with human immunodeficiency virus (HIV), PCT levels were increased only in those with bacterial sepsis, whereas HIV-infection alone, even in the late stages of disease, did not lead to increases in PCT levels [24].

PCT and Severity of Disease

PCT values in cardiogenic shock are only moderately increased (mean 1.4 ng/ml) in comparison to the large increases in patients with septic shock (means: 72–135 ng/ml) [15] (Fig. 1). This finding shows that increases in PCT during septic shock are due to the inflammatory reaction to infection and not due to poor organ perfusion. Thus, although the severity of the systemic response to infection is reflected in corresponding increases in PCT levels, even severe disease of non-infectious etiology does not necessarily lead to corresponding increases in PCT levels.

Prognostic Value of PCT

Since PCT levels increase with increasing severity of the inflammatory response to infection they may be of prognostic value and may help to judge therapeutic efficacy. In patients with melioidosis, infection with *Pseudomonas pseudomallei*, a fatal outcome was associated with significantly higher levels of PCT than that seen in patients who survived [25]. In a study performed at our institution [26], PCT values obtained on the day sepsis was diagnosed were significantly higher in non-survivors of sepsis than in survivors. Furthermore, PCT levels increased during the course of disease in non-survivors whereas they decreased in surviving patients. In pediatric patients, PCT levels fell after successful antibiotic treatment [8]. Therefore, therapies effective in controlling infections and reducing severity of disease may lead to reductions in PCT levels.

PCT and C-reactive Protein

C-reactive protein (CRP) is also a useful clinical tool in assessing the severity of the inflammatory response to infections. CRP has been successfully used to differentiate between true pneumonia and endotracheal infections in patients with chronic obstructive lung disease [27], to increase diagnostic accuracy in patients with appendicitis [28], to detect post-operative sepsis in infants [29], as an indicator of the resolution of sepsis, and to differentiate between bacterial and viral infections [30]. In a recent study [31], CRP and PCT were simultaneously measured in children with infectious disease. PCT increased earlier and returned to the normal range more quickly than CRP. Our clinical experience suggests that CRP may be an important marker in infections without systemic manifestations where PCT concentrations are usually low. PCT, however, may be a superior marker during infections with systemic manifestations. More studies are needed to determine whether PCT is superior to CRP in differentiating between inflammation of infectious and non-infectious origin.

PCT and Cytokines

Cytokines have been implicated in the pathogenesis of severe infections and sepsis. Like PCT, cytokines such as tumor necrosis factor (TNF), interleukin-1 (IL-1) and IL-6 are frequently elevated in patients with severe bacterial infections (sepsis) [32, 33]. Healthy volunteers injected with *Escherichia coli* endotoxin developed symptoms of systemic manifestation such as fever, myalgia, and chills 1–3 hours later [34]. PCT levels, undetectable at baseline, started to rise 4 hours after endotoxin and plateaued at 4 ng/ml at 8–24 hours. TNF and IL-6 levels peaked 2–3 hours after endotoxin and were undetectable at 24 hours (Fig. 2). That the same kinetics can be expected to occur in human septic shock has been recently described in a rare and interesting case [35]. A hemodialysate of calf blood contaminated with *Acineto-bacter baumanii* was injected in a 76 year old patient leading, within hours, to septic shock. TNF was detectable in serum at 1.5 hours, peaked at 3 hours, and declined thereafter. PCT was first detectable at 3 hours, peaked 14 hours after the injection (300 ng/ml), and remained increased for more than 24 hours. Thus, in response to endotoxin or to live bacteria, increases in circulating PCT levels occur shortly after cytokines have peaked. Differences in the half-lives of PCT (25–30 hours) and the cytokines measured may explain why PCT is detectable longer, or cytokines released after endotoxin administration might induce PCT production. Unpublished observations show that in cancer patients, TNF or IL-2 infusions lead to increases in PCT levels. These reports, if substantiated, could better explain the described kinetics of PCT and cytokines.

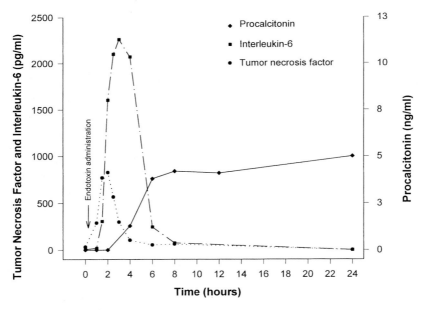

Fig. 2. Serial procalcitonin (PCT), tumor necrosis factor (TNF-α), and interleukin-6 (IL-6) values after endotoxin administration in humans. (From [34] with permission)

The chances of detecting elevated cytokine levels during severe infections are limited by their short half-lives. In contrast, PCT remains detectable in blood much longer and correlates more readily with the clinical presentation of the patient. In a study at our institution [20], when compared to TNF and IL-6, PCT best discriminated the severity of the inflammatory infectious response (Table 1). Further, both TNF and IL-6 may decline despite persistence or even increased severity of sepsis, but PCT levels remain elevated or may increase. The same cytokines are also frequently elevated in patients with (inflammatory) autoimmune disease (rheumatoid arthritis, lupus erythematosis), in which PCT remains undetectable [7]. Increases in cytokine levels are not confined to the intravascular space and during infections, cytokine levels in body compartments (pleural fluid, bronchoalveolar fluid, cerebro-spinal fluid, ascites) often exceed cytokine levels in the intravascular space. In contrast, increased PCT levels are mostly confined to the intravascular space and PCT is either undetectable or markedly low in other body compartments [36].

Open Questions Regarding the Biology and Use of PCT

Biology of PCT

Despite numerous observational studies, it is still not clear which cells produce PCT during infectious episodes, which stimuli prompt these cells to produce PCT, and what purpose high PCT levels serve during severe infections.

Clinical use of PCT

Although many clinical studies have been published on PCT, the questions as to whether PCT is a marker of (bacterial, fungal, or parasitic) infection or of the inflammatory response (to infectious or non-infectious stimuli) are not satisfactorily answered. Clearly, PCT is not a marker of infection as such, since localized infections or infections with no systemic manifestation may not cause any appreciable increase in PCT levels [37]. For example, with some exceptions, PCT levels only increase a modest 1–2.4 ng/ml during community acquired pneumonia [15, 37]. In patients with localized infections without signs of systemic manifestation, therapeutic measures such as antibiotics or surgical intervention may be necessary despite normal PCT levels. Although elevated PCT values during severe infections may decrease to very low levels with appropriate therapy, this does not always indicate complete eradication of the infection but merely that generalization of the infection or the septic response is under control. Continuation of antibiotic therapy or surgical measures may be necessary until all clinical signs of infection have disappeared.

PCT levels may also be elevated during non-infectious inflammatory states. Patients after major trauma or surgery [38, 39], and patients after cardiopulmonary bypass [40] may present with increased PCT levels without any evidence of severe infections. In high-risk cardiac surgery patients, PCT was not helpful in differentiating between the inflammatory reaction to infection or to surgery as such [41]. In addition, patients with C-cell carcinoma of the thyroid gland [42] and small-cell carcinoma of the lung [43] without underlying infection may also have increased PCT levels.

Conclusion

PCT may prove to be a valuable indicator capable of identifying the presence and intensity of severe systemic non-viral infections. PCT monitoring may be useful in patients likely to develop a systemic inflammatory response of infectious origin, such as intensive care unit (ICU) patients after major surgery or trauma, ICU patients with nosocomial infections which may lead to sepsis, and immunocompromised patients. Abrupt increases in, or high PCT values in these patients justify a search for a source of infection. PCT measurements may also be helpful in differentiating between infectious or non-infectious causes in patients presenting with SIRS. PCT monitoring may, therefore, be used during pancreatitis (differentiating infectious-cholestatic versus alcohol-toxic), ARDS (differentiating infectious versus non-infectious), and after transplantation (differentiating rejection reaction versus infections). Further, PCT measurements may differentiate between viral and bacterial infections (with systemic manifestation).

References

1. Steinberg W, Tenner S (1994) Acute pancreatitis. N Engl J Med 330:1198–1205
2. Moore FA, Haenel JB, Moore EE, Whitehill TA (1992) Incommensurate oxygen consumption in response to maximal oxygen availability predicts postinjury multiple organ failure. J Trauma 33:58–67
3. Saffle JR, Sullivan JJ, Tuohig GM, Larson CM (1993) Multiple organ failure in patients with thermal injury. Crit Care Med 21:1673–1683
4. Gramm H-J, Reinhart K, Goecke J, Bülow JV (1989) Early clinical, laboratory, and hemodynamic indicators of sepsis and septic shock. In: Reinhart K, Eyrich K (eds) Sepsis – an interdisciplinary challenge. Springer-Verlag, Berlin, Heidelberg, New York, pp 45–57
5. Le Moullec JM, Jullienne A, Chenais J, et al (1984) The complete sequence of preprocalcitonin. FEBS 167:93–97
6. Jacobs JW, Lund PK, Potts JT, Bell HH, Habener JF (1981) Procalcitonin is a glycoprotein. J Biol Chem 256:2803–2807
7. Meissner M (1996) PCT-Procalcitonin. A new and innovative parameter in diagnosis of infections. B.R.A.H.M.S. Diagnostica, Berlin, pp 14–60
8. Assicot M, Gendrel D, Carsin H, Raymond J, Guilbaud J, Bohuon C (1993) High serum procalcitonin concentrations in patients with sepsis and infection. Lancet 341:515–518
9. Oberhoffer M, Vogelsang H, Meier-Hellmann A, Jäger L, Reinhart K (1997) Anti-katacalcin-antibody reaction in different types of human leukocytes indicates procalcitonin content. Shock 7 (suppl 1):A487 (Abst)
10. Nylen ES, Snider RH, Thompson KA, Rohatgi P, Becker KL (1996) Pneumonitis-associated hypercalcitoninemia. Am J Med Sci 312:12–18
11. Becker KL, O'Neill W, Snider RH, et al (1993) Hypercalcitoninemia in inhalation burn injury: A response of the pulmonary neuroendocrine cell? Anatomic Record 236:136–138
12. Cate CC, Pettingill OS, Sorensen GD (1986) Biosynthesis of procalcitonin in small cell carcinoma of the lung. Cancer Res 46:812–818
13. Gendrel D, Bohuon CJ (1997) Procalcitonin, a marker of bacterial infection. Infection 133–134

14. Mallet E, Lanse X, Devaux AM, Ensel P, Basuyau JP, Brunelle P (1983) Hypercalcitoninemia in fulminant meningococcaemia in children. Lancet 1 : 294–299
15. De Werra I, Jaccard C, Corradin SB, et al (1997) Cytokines, nitrite/nitrate, soluble tumor necrosis factor receptors, and procalcitonin concentrations: Comparisons in patients with septic shock, cardiogenic shock, and bacterial pneumonia. Crit Care Med 25 : 607–613
16. Rau B, Steinbach G, Gansauge F, Mayer JM, Grünert A, Beger HG (1997) The potential role of procalci-tonin and interleukin-8 in the prediction of infected necrosis in acute pancreatitis. Gut 41 : 832–840
17. Brunkhorst FM, Forycki ZF, Wagner J (1995) Frühe Identifikation der biliären akuten Pankreatitis durch Procalcitonin-Immunreaktivität – vorläufige Ergebnisse (Early identification of acute biliary pancreatitis with procalcitonin immunoreactivity – preliminary results). Chir Gastroenterol 11 : S47 (Abst)
18. Gerard Y, Hober D, Petitjean S, et al (1995) High serum procalcitonin level in a 4-year-old liver transplant recipient with a disseminated candidiasis. Infection 23 : 310–311
19. Staehler M, Hammer C, Meiser B, Reichart B (1997) Procalcitonin: a new marker for differential diagnosis of acute rejection and bacterial infection in heart transplantation. Transplant Proc 29 : 584–585
20. Oberhoffer M, Bögel D, Meier-Hellmann A, Vogelsang H, Reinhart K (1996) Procalcitonin vs immunological markers in infection/inflammation. Br J Anaesth 76 : A352 (Abst)
21. Oberhoffer M, Bitterlich A, Hentschel T, Meier-Hellmann A, Vogelsang H, Reinhart K (1996) Procalcitonin (ProCt) correlates better with the ACCP/SCCM consensus conference definitions than other specific markers of the inflammatory response. Clin Intensive Care 7 : 46 (Abst)
22. Al-Nawas B, Krammer I, Shah PM (1996) Procalcitonin in the diagnosis of severe infections. Eur J Med Res 1 : 331–333
23. Reith HB, Mittelkötter U, Kamen S, Beier W, Dohle J, Kozuschek W (1998) Langenb Arch Chir (in press)
24. Gerard Y, Hober D, Assicot M, et al (1997) Procalcitonin as a marker of bacterial sepsis in patients infected with HIV 1. J Infect 35 : 41–46
25. Smith MD, Suputtamongkol Y, Chaowagul W, et al (1995) Elevated serum procalcitonin levels in patients with melioidosis. Clin Infect Dis 20 : 641–645
26. Oberhoffer M, Bögel D, Meier-Hellmann A, Vogelsang H, Reinhart K (1996) Procalcitonin is higher in non-survivors during course of sepsis, severe sepsis, and septic shock. Intensive Care Med 22 : A245 (Abst)
27. Smith RP, Lipworth BJ (1995) C-reactive protein in simple community acquired pneumonia. Chest 107 : 1028–1031
28. Erikson S, Grantström L, Olander BJ, Wretlind B (1995) Sensitivity of interleukin-6 and C-reactive protein concentrations in the diagnosis of acute appendicitis. Eur J Surg 161 : 41–45
29. Chwals WJ, Fernandez ME, Jamie AC, Charles BJ, Rushing JT (1994) Detection of postoperative sepsis in infants with the use of metabolic stress monitoring. Arch Surg 129 : 437–442
30. Shaw AC (1991) Serum C-reactive protein and neopterin concentrations in patients with viral or bacterial infection. J Clin Pathol 44 : 596–599
31. Monneret G, Labaune JM, Isaac C, Bienvenu F, Putet G, Bienvenu J (1997) Procalcitonin and C-reactive protein levels in neonatal infections. Acta Paediatr 86 : 209–212
32. Leser H-G, Gross V, Scheibenbogen C, et al (1991) Elevation of serum interleukin-6 concentration precedes acute phase response and reflects severity in acute pancreatitis. Gastroenterology 101 : 782–785
33. Kragsberbjer P, Holmberg H, Vikefors T (1995) Serum concentrations of interleukin-6, tumor necrosis factor-alpha, and C-reactive protein in patients undergoing major operations. Eur J Surg 161 : 17–22
34. Dandona P, Nix D, Wilson MF, et al (1994) Procalcitonin increase after endotoxin injection in normal subjects. J Clin Endocrinol Metab 79 : 1605–1608
35. Brunkhorst FM, Forycki ZF, Wagner J (1997) Release and kinetics of procalcitonin (PCT) after gram-negative bacterial injection in a healthy subject. Shock 7 : 124 (Abst)
36. Brunkhorst FM, Forycki ZF, Wagner J (1996) Identification of immunactivation of infectious origin by procalcitonin-immunreactivity in different body fluids. Clin Intensive Care 7 : 41 (Abst)

37. Gramm H-J, Dollinger P, Beier W (1995) Procalcitonin-A new marker of host inflammatory response. Longitudinal studies in patients with sepsis and peritonitis. Chir Gastroenterol 11 (Suppl 2):51–54
38. Gramm H-J, Zimmermann J, Quedra N, Wegscheider K (1997) The procalcitonin (PROCT) response in severe sepsis is closely correlated to cytokine kinetics. Shock 7 (suppl 1):A489 (Abst)
39. Marnitz R, Gramm H-J, Zimmermann J (1997) Elaboration of mediators of inflammatory response after major surgery. Shock 7:124 (Abst)
40. Meisner M, Tschaikowsy K, Schmidt J, Schüttler J (1996) Procalcitonin (PCT) – Indications for a new diagnostic parameter of severe bacterial infection and sepsis in transplantation, immunosuppression, and cardiac assist devices. Cardiovasc Eng 1:67–76
41. Pilz G, Kreuzer E, Appel R, Werdan K (1997) Procalcitonin (PCT) serum levels in the early postoperative period of cardiac surgical patients at high risk for sepsis. Shock 7 (suppl 1):A491 (Abst)
42. Bertagna XY, Nicholson WE, Pettengill OS, Sorensen GD, Mount CD, Orth DN (1978) Ectopic production of high molecular weight calcitonin and corticotropin by human small cell carcinoma cells in tissue culture: evidence for separate precursors. J Clin Endocrinol Metab 47:1390–1393
43. Raue F, Blind E, Grauer A (1992) PDN-21 (katacalcin) and chromogranin A: tumor markers for medullary thyroid carcinoma. Henry Ford Hosp Med J 40:296–298

Is There a Role for Surrogate Markers in the Evaluation of Sepsis Trials?

J. Cohen

Introduction

The successive failure of a number of clinical trials of experimental agents in sepsis or septic shock is now an all too familiar theme, and one which has generated much discussion. Many investigators have given considerable thought to possible explanations, including incorrect reasoning (i.e., poor basic science), ineffective drugs, and poor trial design. One aspect is the question of endpoints, and the use of 28-day mortality as the "gold standard" of success or failure of a new drug. Many have questioned the wisdom of this approach, arguing that death is too blunt a tool, and that we may be missing potentially useful therapies by demanding too much efficacy, too soon. The way to avoid this problem, they say, is to accept surrogate markers as valid endpoints, i.e., to find a more amenable measurement than death. In this paper, I will discuss some of the issues raised by this proposal, and show some of the advantages, and disadvantages, that it might offer.

What They Are – and What They Are Not

A "surrogate" is a replacement, or substitute for something else, and in the setting of clinical trials, it is used to mean (usually) a biological measurement that reflects the effect of an intervention. Here is a useful definition [1]: "… a surrogate endpoint of a clinical trial is a laboratory measurement or a physical sign used as a substitute for a clinically meaningful endpoint that measures directly how a patient feels, functions or survives. Changes induced by a therapy on a surrogate endpoint are expected to reflect changes in a clinically meaningful endpoint."

For instance, we can use the plasma glucose to see how good an anti-diabetic therapy is, or the blood pressure to evaluate an anti-hypertensive drug. It is also important to have a clear understanding of what is meant by clinical efficacy, which has been defined as something which "unequivocally reflects tangible benefit to the patient" [2]. Thus, to be potentially useful, surrogate markers should:

1) Be a measure of a biological effect (because these are most likely to reflect an important – and therefore meaningful – process)
2) Be of sufficient magnitude to be measured easily. Clearly, it is not much help if the assay is working at the very limit of its sensitivity. Furthermore, it is advantageous if the parameter has a relatively wide range, and ideally, a steep dose-response curve, all factors which will help with the precision of the test.

3) Occcur relatively early in the disease process, so as to provide the maximum benefit from the information.

A key distinction is between a correlate and a surrogate; they are not the same thing. One of the most familiar examples is in the field of anti-human immunodeficiency virus (HIV) therapy. It was learnt some years ago that a falling CD4 count was correlated with advancing disease and an increased risk of the symptomatic complications of acquired immune deficiency syndrome (AIDS), but it does not follow that if a treatment induces changes in the CD4 count that this will necessarily predict better treatment-related outcomes. In fact, we now know that the CD4 count is not a very satisfactory surrogate marker of the effects of nucleoside analogs, for instance, and we use viral load measurements instead (although some have argued that they too have their limitations [3]).

Surrogate markers are also not the same as scores, such as the APACHE score. These scores are in general designed to evaluate risk, i.e., the likelihood that a given patient will suffer a specific outcome, such as acute respiratory distress syndrome (ARDS) or death, and they are calculated at a particular point in time, usually when the patient first presents to the hospital, or is admitted to the intensive care unit (ICU). They can be used to compare observed and expected mortality between two groups in a therapeutic trial, but here they are acting as comparators of risk, not surrogate markers.

More recently, several investigators have been developing the idea of "organ failure scores", in which numerical values are used to quantify the extent of organ dysfunction [4]. A variation on this is the concept of "failure free days" to designate the ability of the investigational drug to reduce morbidity due to organ dysfunction (personal communication). It is possible to argue that these scores could be used as alternatives to death as the endpoint of a clinical trial, but that is not the same as a surrogate marker of death. Indeed, it does not necessarily follow that a reduction in morbidity because of fewer (or less severe) organ failures is necessarily associated with a reduction in mortality.

Limitations of Surrogate Markers

As de Gruttola et al. [3] have pointed out, surrogate markers work best when the pathogenesis of the disease is well understood. They cite the example of bacterial endocarditis, in which the attainment of negative blood cultures is an important and useful surrogate marker of the efficacy of the antibiotic treatment. However, this also provides a useful illustration of one of the limitations of surrogate markers, that is, that they can only ever reflect a proportion of the total treatment effect. For instance, negative blood cultures give us no information about the residual damage to the heart valves, or about drug toxicity. In fact, it is possible to derive equations which show the extent to which changes in the surrogate marker accurately represent changes in the endpoint of interest (e.g., in-patient survival). Worryingly, apparently beneficial changes in the surrogate can conceal unanticipated harmful effects on unrelated mechanisms of death [3], and great care must be taken to remain alert to this possibility, particularly when testing novel agents with complex mechanisms of action.

Why do we need them?

As noted above, the current gold standard for trials examining the efficacy of novel agents in sepsis is a significant reduction in all-cause 28-day mortality. There is of course an important debate which needs to be resolved around the issue of what is meant by "significant", and the distinction between biological relevance and statistical significance (without mentioning the important philosophical and ethical issues here). Nevertheless, for the time being let us simply consider the validity of death as an endpoint. It has much to commend it:
1) It is easy to diagnose.
2) It is unambiguous (life "unequivocally reflects tangible benefit to the patient", to re-state the definition above [2]).

However, for all its apparent simplicity, there are problems.
1) It is a discrete (rather than continuous) variable, so with an intervention of even modest benefit there will usually need to be a relatively large number of observations to show a difference.
2) It is a non-specific endpoint, in that it does not reflect a specific mechanism of action.
3) It has many causes, and therefore poor sensitivity (in essence, the old problem of "attributable mortality").
4) Its definition is imprecise: Do we mean time to death, deaths within a certain period (3 days, 7 days, 28 days, longer?); deaths while on the ICU, deaths before hospital discharge? And how do we deal with the question of withdrawal of life-support?

Some familiar examples illustrate the problems. The NORASEPT I study of monoclonal anti-tumor necrosis factor (TNF) antibody, for instance, found a statistically significant reduction in 3-day and 7-day mortality between placebo and the treatment arms, but this difference was not seen at 28 days, the prospectively defined endpoint [5]. However, these findings were not reproduced by a parallel study with the same antibody, INTERSEPT [6], and a third study, NORASEPT II, failed to show any benefit at all (personal communication).

On the other hand, the requirement of a significant reduction in 28-day mortality could conceal a potentially important biological effect, especially if (as many people feel) we will ultimately need to use combination therapy. Consider the theoretical situation where a drug A has a significant survival advantage over the first 3 days, but the final effect on mortality is not significant (Fig. 1). Now consider a second drug, B, which has a different mode of action from A and acts later, at a different stage in the process and on a rather different population to drug A. When B is given alone it has no effect, but when the two drugs are used together there is a significant survival advantage over 28 days. Clearly, we would never know about this combined effect because drug A would have been discarded as yet another failure.

For these, and other reasons, valid surrogate markers would be an attractive option for sepsis studies, in that they may allow us to capture a biologically important effect more easily and without the problems, and perhaps some of the costs, associated with trials based on 28-day survival.

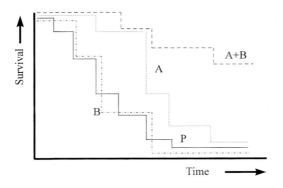

Fig. 1. A Kaplan-Meier plot illustrating the survival curves of patients in a sepsis trial which was studying two imaginary drugs, A and B, given alone or in combination (A + B), versus placebo (P). Drug A has some early survival advantage but that is lost by the endpoint (e.g., 28 days) when the survival is not different to the placebo group. Drug B on its own has no effect. When both drugs are used together there is a significant survival advantage

Surrogate Markers – Some Candidates

Cytokines are obvious candidates for surrogate markers and TNF has been studied extensively. Many investigators have examined the correlation between TNF levels and outcome, and in some circumstances (e.g., meningococcal disease [7]) this is quite strong. Furthermore, there may be correlates between TNF and relevant biological markers: For instance, my colleagues and I have had the opportunity to examine a very large cohort of samples in relation to the INTERSEPT study [8], and we found that TNF levels correlated well with the duration and severity of shock, and with serum lactate. However, there is no evidence that TNF can act as a surrogate marker for the efficacy of treatment, even an anti-TNF treatment. For instance, in the trial of the type II, p75 soluble TNF-receptor fragments there was a statistically significant adverse outcome in the high-dose treatment group, based on 28-day all-cause mortality [9]. Detailed information about TNF levels is not provided in that manuscript, but it is noted that there were no differences in TNF levels between the groups, perhaps because of the "stabilizing" effect of the TNF-TNF receptor complex. Whatever the reason, TNF levels were clearly not informative.

Another cytokine which has been proposed as a surrogate marker is interleukin-6 (IL-6). Many studies have documented a correlation between IL-6 levels and outcome, but of particular interest was a report by Reinhart et al. [10] that the IL-6 level at trial entry could predict the response to MAK 195F, an anti-TNF antibody fragment which they had studied. In a phase II study, 122 patients received placebo or one of several doses of the antibody. There were no significant differences in outcome between the groups, but in a retrospective analysis they found that patients with an IL-6 level > 1000 pg/mL at trial entry appeared to benefit from MAK 195F in a dose dependent fashion [10]. Furthermore, IL-6 levels decreased during the first 24 hours in the anti-TNF treated groups but not in the placebo group. Based on this experience, these investigators proceeded to a phase III trial to test the hypothesis prospectively, but unfortunately the trial proved unsuccessful and an IL-6 level of 1000 pg/mL did not prove to be a helpful predictor of outcome (personal communication).

Several other cytokines have been studied but they show no particular advantage. For instance, levels of both IL-1 receptor antagonist (IL-1ra) and IL-10 are elevated in patients at risk of ARDS, but in neither case does measurement of the levels help in predicting which patients will actually develop the disease [11]. Procalcitonin has recently been the subject of considerable interest as a possible marker of sepsis; it seems to be a good means of detecting infection (as opposed to other causes of inflammation) [12] but at present there is no evidence that it can be used as a marker of treatment responses in sepsis. E-selectin levels are rather more interesting because, at least in one report, there was a correlation between elevated levels and hemodynamic status [13], but once again, we have no evidence that changes in E-selectin levels can be used to measure treatment effect.

Finally, what of endotoxin levels? Endotoxin has some attraction as a potentially useful marker: It is clearly related to the disease process; it is a bacterial, rather than a host product; and there are data that show endotoxin levels correlate with hemodynamic changes and outcome [14]. However the drawbacks are obvious: Plasma endotoxin measurements are difficult and expensive to do; and there are wide inter- and intra-assay variations. Finally, this approach is probably restricted to Gram negative infections, or at the very least, to interventions specifically targeted at endotoxin, either being designed to prevent its entry from the gut or to neutralize it in the circulation. For the moment at least, it is not a feasible option.

Conclusion

Death has many disadvantages as an endpoint for clinical trials, and by insisting on demonstrating a survival benefit in 28-day all-cause mortality we may be needlessly hampering our ability to find a new approach to the treatment of a serious disease with a high mortality. For these reasons, surrogate markers might offer significant advantages. However, as I have shown in this paper, surrogate markers have limitations: They only reflect a proportion of the treatment effect, and they may conceal important adverse events. Although there are many markers which correlate with outcome measures in sepsis, there are none which have yet been shown to be good surrogates. That is not to say that other endpoints should not be considered: Variables such as reversal of shock; number of organ failures, ventilator-free days etc.; may all be suitable measures of outcome. For the moment, however, a true surrogate marker for use in sepsis studies, analogous to viral load measurements in anti-HIV trials, remains elusive.

References

1. Fleming TR, DeMets DL (1996) Surrogate end points in clinical trials: are we being misled? Ann Intern Med 125:605–613
2. Fleming TR (1994) Surrogate markers in AIDS and cancer trials. Stat Med 13:1423–1435
3. De Gruttola V, Fleming T, Lin DY et al (1997) Perspective: validating surrogate markers – are we being naive? J Infect Dis 175:237–246
4. Marshall JC, Cook DJ, Sibbald WJ, Roy PD, Christou NV (1995) Multiple organ dysfunction score: a reliable descriptor of a complex clinical outcome. Crit Care Med 23:1638–1652
5. Abraham E, Wunderink R, Silverman H, et al (1995) Efficacy and safety of monoclonal antibody to human tumor necrosis factor a in patients with sepsis syndrome. A randomized, controlled, double-blind, multicenter clinical trial. JAMA 273:934–941

6. Cohen J, Carlet J, INTERSEPT Study Group (1996) INTERSEPT: An international multicentrer placebo-controlled trial of monoclonal antibody to human TNF-α in patients with sepsis. Crit Care Med 24:1431–1440

7. Waage A, Halstensen A, Shalaby R, et al (1989) Local production of tumor necrosis factor alpha, interleukin 1, and interleukin 6 in meningococcal meningitis. Relation to the inflammatory response. J Exp Med 170:1859–1867

8. Lemm G, Carlet J, Cohen J, et al (1995) Cytokine levels in patients with the sepsis syndrome treated with a monoclonal antibody to human TNF a (INTERSEPT trial). Clin Intensive Care 6:68 (Abst)

9. Fisher Jr CJ, Agosti JM, Opal SM, et al (1996) Treatment of septic shock with the tumor necrosis factor receptor: Fc fusion protein. N Engl J Med 334:1697–1702

10. Reinhart K, Wiegand-Löhnert C, Grimminger F, et al (1996) Assessment of the safety and efficacy of the monoclonal anti-tumor necrosis factor antibody-fragment, MAK 195F, in patients with sepsis and septic shock: a multicenter, randomized, placebo-controlled, dose-ranging study. Crit Care Med 24:733–742

11. Parsons PE, Moss M, Vannice JL, et al (1997) Circulating IL-1ra and II-10 levels are increased but do not predict the development of acute respiratory distress syndrome in at-risk patients. Am J Respir Crit Care Med 155:1469–1473

12. de Werra I, Jaccard C, Corradin SB, et al (1997) Cytokines, nitrite/nitrate, soluble tumor necrosis factor receptors, and procalcitonin concentrations: comparisons in patients with septic shock, cardiogenic shock, and bacterial pneumonia. Crit Care Med 25:607–613

13. Cummings CJ, Sessler CN, Beall LD, et al (1997) Soluble E-selectin levels in sepsis and critical illness. Correlation with infection and hemodynamic dysfunction. Am J Respir Crit Care Med 156:431–437

14. Danner RL, Elin RJ, Hosseini J, et al (1991) Endotoxemia in human septic shock. Chest 99:169–175

Discourse on Method:
Measuring the Value of New Therapies in Intensive Care

D. C. Angus

Introduction

The intensive care unit (ICU) is a favorite rotation among our final year medical students at the University of Pittsburgh. Because time is so short, we aim to teach them only the very basic elements of multiorgan failure and the principles of organ support and resuscitation. We do not currently focus on teaching them how to read and interpret our literature. Our fellows on the other hand spend a minimum of one year with us. This allows us to expose them in much greater detail to the underlying mechanisms of critical illness and the clinical management of critically ill patients. We spend a few hours in the year teaching them how to read and interpret our literature. During these hours, we wax semi-eloquently about the advantage of prospective studies, randomization, blinding, and adequate sample size, but we quickly move on to much more exciting things like the latest cell adhesion molecule implicated in the sepsis cascade. I suspect we are not so very different from many other universities.

Why do we spend so little time discoursing over our methods? In part because we believe them to be somewhat static – we know how to conduct a trial, and we know when we have a positive result. The scholars of the early 1600s similarly relied on well established rules and writings for the conduct of scientific inquiry. In his "Discourse on methods," published in 1637, Descartes challenged the existing methods of the day, stating that they relied too much on existing assumptions and, as such, were biased, inaccurate, and unhelpful [1]. Descartes suggested revisions were flawed in many ways but his passion for methodology and his desire to promote discussion of methodology among the general public was notable.

Today, as in the early 1600s, we are making many great discoveries, gaining knowledge at a ferocious pace. Yet assimilating that knowledge is difficult; we are overburdened with often contradictory information and it is difficult to form a clear picture of the changes around us. Indeed, we may relate to Descartes' comment: "For I was assailed by so many doubts and errors that the only profit I appeared to have drawn from trying to become educated, was progressively to have discovered my ignorance" [1]. Undoubtedly, today our methodology is in better condition than that of the early 1600s. But we are perhaps paying less attention to it than we should. In particular, the nature of clinical research is changing rapidly and there are many issues today about the questions we ask that challenge the abilities of our existing methodologies. Though there are no easy solutions to these issues, open discourse and involvement of physicians will be critical.

Physicians place considerable faith in the results of randomized clinical trials (RCTs) [2, 3]. This faith is placed with good reason: Randomization remains perhaps our most elegant solution to avoid misinterpreting the effect of a therapy in the presence of confounding variables [4]. However, RCTs are expensive, difficult, and sometimes unethical to conduct with the consequence that less than 20% of clinical policies are based on their results [5]. Moreover, many important questions, such as determining the optimal timing of a new therapy, cannot practically be studied by RCTs.

The field of intensive care has particularly unique problems today with regard to the use of RCTs. Over the last twenty years, multiple RCTs of new therapies in the "ICU diseases," such as sepsis and acute respiratory distress syndrome (ARDS), have failed to demonstrate benefit despite advances in both the development of new therapies and trial design [6–8]. Some have argued that this is because we do not yet have enough understanding of the underlying mechanisms of sepsis and organ dysfunction and that consequently more basic research is required [7–11]. While this is no doubt true, others have also emphasized the need to further examine and improve the design of RCTs in intensive care [7, 8, 10]. In particular, attention has been focused on which patients should be selected, whether the process of care should be standardized, and whether the choice of end points is correct.

Added to these problems, there is now increasing attention on the impact a new therapy will have on health care practice and spending. The effect size measured under the rigorous conditions of a tightly controlled trial (efficacy) is being criticized as unrepresentative of the likely effect in the real world (effectiveness). Reasons for effectiveness falling short of efficacy include differences in patient selection, timing and dosing of therapy, and use of concomitant therapies, all of which represent the realities of the world we live in. Furthermore, as rising health care costs put increasing pressure on us to consider the costs and benefits of new therapies, we begin to qualify the value we place on new therapies. Where previously a therapy would be deemed valuable purely on the basis of its effect, value is now seen more as a trade-off of the costs incurred per effects gained [12]. Yet how should we best measure cost and what are the implications of considering cost and effectiveness, as opposed to efficacy, for experimental design in future intensive care studies?

In this paper, I will review some of the methodologic issues currently under debate in RCT design, discuss briefly the role of observational outcomes studies as alternatives to RCTs, and explore the implications that the consideration of cost has on RCT design as we attempt to judge the value of new therapies in intensive care.

Determining Sample Size

It is well known, and indeed generally well accepted, that the patients enrolled in sepsis or ARDS RCTs vary widely in both their demographic characteristics and underlying diseases. The reason this variance has been tolerated is the underlying premise that the sepsis or organ failure, and not the underlying disease, is the principal threat to short term outcome. However, each patient brings with them a constellation of features that contribute to their risk of short-term survival, including age, co-morbid illnesses, presence of concomitant complications and infectious agent. Since many of these features pose a risk that cannot be diminished by a new therapy targeted at reversing the sepsis, or respiratory failure, the ability of a new anti-sepsis strategy to decrease mortality may be less than might have been anticipated during the design of the study (Fig. 1).

When determining the sample size for an RCT, we generate an estimate of the effect that ought to be both clinically relevant and plausibly achievable. Clinical relevance is clearly important but is exceedingly subjective and difficult to consider in isolation from other influencing factors. Such factors include prior beliefs and assumptions regarding the anticipated cost and side-effects of the therapy, the nature of the underlying clinical problem, the availability of health care resources, the difficulty inherent in conducting a study to detect small changes, the available funding for the study, and the competing philosophies of deontologic versus pluralistic health care. Consequently, there is no consistent standard adopted by researchers and the determination of clinical relevance seems to vary widely between studies.

The recent global use of strategies to open occluded coronary arteries (GUSTO) III study of alternative tissue plasminogen activators in the treatment of acute myocardial infarction (AMI) was powered to detect only a $\geq 20\%$ relative change in mortality [13]. In their editorial, Ware and Antman [2] commented that this effect size was well regarded as the appropriate margin to support replacing standard therapy with an innovative therapy. In 1993, the GUSTO investigators published their results demonstrating the superiority of tissue plasminogen activator (tPA) over streptokinase in the treatment of AMI [14]. This study was powered to detect an absolute change of 1% (from 8% to 7%) which is a relative change of 12.5%. The results of that study have led to widespread use of tPA, suggesting 12.5% was clinically relevant.

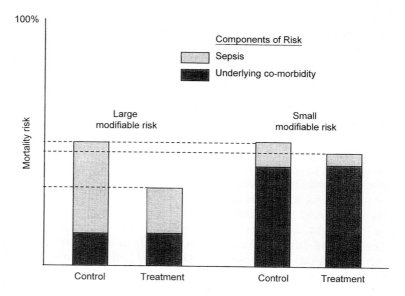

Fig. 1. Alternative scenarios for sepsis study with therapy that has strong effect on sepsis process

This is especially striking since the absolute rate is only 1% (implying one hundred patients must be treated to save one additional life) and several other trials have failed to demonstrate efficacy [15]. Thus, clinical relevance seems to be defined somewhat arbitrarily and interpreted variably depending on extenuating circumstances.

To estimate the effect size the therapy might plausibly achieve, investigators must adopt a Bayesian consideration of prior evidence [16]. When designing a cardiology trial, investigators can look to size and design characteristics of the many successful prior studies. When designing a sepsis or ARDS trial, investigators have no such reference to call upon: Our trials have all failed to demonstrate effect. Consequently, the effect size thought achievable is usually estimated from the results of the therapy seen in animal studies. Human data is usually only available for phase I studies of healthy volunteers or for phase II studies designed principally to evaluate the safety, toxicity and dosing of the therapy. Such studies are not powered to measure effect. Yet, as pointed out by Piper et al. [17], most animal studies are conducted on animals who are well prior to the induction of sepsis or acute organ injury. Thus, their short-term survival is principally linked to the acute process and, consequently, potentially changeable by a therapy that has a beneficial effect on that process. In clinical situations we should be less optimistic that a new therapy would have the same effect on survival. Indeed, in the few studies conducted on animals in which chronic illness was induced prior to inducing sepsis or acute organ dysfunction, mortality was much higher and much less open to manipulation by otherwise promising therapies [17, 18].

The implications for sample size in RCTs are profound. The typical RCT in sepsis and ARDS has been conducted on less than 1 500 patients and often on only several hundred patients. Typically, these studies are designed with the assumption that septic patients have a hospital mortality of around 40% and that the therapy under consideration will reduce that mortality by 25%, an absolute change of 10%, to 30%. When constructed to have 80% power, this would require 750 patients, and, at 90% power, 1200 patients. The GUSTO study, on the other hand, to detect a 12.5% relative difference (1% absolute difference) at 90% power, required 40 000 patients. If we apply the same relative change to a sepsis trial (i.e., to drop mortality from 40% to 35%), we need 3 000 patients at 80% power and 3 700 at 90% power. A sepsis study designed to detect a similar absolute change (i.e., a 1% drop from 40% to 39%) would require 76 000 patients at 80% power and 100 000 patients at 90%.

Even with the more aggressive assumption of a 12.5% relative change, we would be required to perform a RCT that may be practically or financially impossible in intensive care. First, at current enrollment rates, it would take many, many years to conduct such a study. The large cardiology trials have enrolled patients much faster than sepsis and ARDS trials. Second, the costs of performing the study might not be justified by the relatively small market the therapy would garner after approval. This is quite different from studies of AMI, an event which occurs considerably more often in the population than ARDS, and perhaps also severe sepsis, and which may require not only immediate treatment but therapy for many years thereafter. Of interest, recent work has highlighted that the decision whether to conduct an RCT, weighing its likely costs against the benefits derived from the information it would yield, can be modeled using simulation techniques [16]. Such decision-making models might better quantitate which trials we can, and cannot, afford to do.

Assuming we are limited by some upper sample size that falls short of those used in large cardiology trials, can we attempt to choose our patients better in order to conduct smaller yet adequately powered studies that enroll only patients with the maximum likelihood of responding to therapy?

Identifying the Right Patients

Currently, entry criteria used to identify patients for sepsis and ARDS studies consist of a constellation of clinical and laboratory data thought likely to identify the disease in question [19–21]. Though standardization of such criteria, through mechanisms such as consensus conferences, may have enhanced the reliability with which we identify these diseases, there remain significant problems with the accuracy and validity of our definitions [22, 23].

The problem can be illustrated by looking again at the field of cardiology. AMI develops acutely and is relatively easy to confirm early in the disease process [using serum enzymes and electrocardiogram (EKG)]: The AMI is the major cause of morbidity and mortality, and the extent of the infarction is both easy to measure (by serum markers, EKG, and cardiac imaging studies) and correlated with outcome. Thus, studies of therapies aimed at the treatment of AMI can be performed on a patient group that is easy to define and stratify, where the definition and severity is based on an underlying pathophysiologic event, and the subsequent outcomes are closely related to the management of, and recovery from, that event.

When we compare this scenario to sepsis, our problem is clearly evident. Sepsis is a vague term and it is unclear at what point a patient can be said to have switched from a non-septic to a septic state. There is no clear set of diagnostic tests to confirm the event. Furthermore, the subsequent course and outcome of the patient is not necessarily correlated with the management of, and recovery from, the event. Many patients sick enough to develop septic shock die despite resolution of the infection. And those who die while apparently still septic cannot clearly be said in many instances to have "died of", as opposed to "died with", the sepsis. The same is true for ARDS and multisystem organ failure.

In an attempt to improve the selection process, authors have suggested using a score that predicts risk of outcome to better screen and stratify patients [24]. The premise of such an approach is that, by selecting only patients in a medium range of risk (e.g., 30–80% risk of hospital mortality), patients will be sick enough to respond but not too sick as to have no meaningful chance to respond. However, current scoring systems still fail to distinguish between the relative contribution to that risk of factors which can and cannot be modified by the therapy under evaluation. Work by others to measure the burden of acute illness at enrollment using organ failure scores may help by characterizing different elements of a patient's disease process but further exploration is required [25, 26].

Others have also argued that we need to identify patients sooner if we are to maximize the chance of eliciting a significant effect. Intuitively, early intervention is more likely to work and certainly the most promising results in animal sepsis models are from studies where animals are pre-treated before being given a septic challenge [17]. This has prompted several epidemiologic studies in the last few years of the prevalence of infection and sepsis in the ICU and in hospital wards in an attempt to better determine the prodrome for sepsis [27–29]. For several years this prodromal period has been known as SIRS, the systemic inflammatory response syndrome, and studies have suggested that a large number of patients with SIRS do indeed go on to develop sepsis and organ failure.

Unfortunately, several problems remain with this concept. First, SIRS as an early marker of sepsis is both insensitive and non-specific [30]. Second, SIRS, similar to both sepsis and ARDS, is based on a rather broad set of criteria of clinical and laboratory data, not closely linked to an underlying physiologic event [30]. Third, perhaps as a consequence of the broadness of its definition, different studies of the prevalence and outcome of SIRS have reported different estimates of mortality and the rate at which sepsis, severe sepsis and septic shock occur [27–29, 31, 32]. Fourth, there is increasing evidence that SIRS is only one of several clinical presentations in patients at risk of developing sepsis and organ failure [33]. Finally, RCTs that enroll patients with pre-organ failure or pre-septic clinical conditions will presumably enroll many patients who would never have gone on to either develop sepsis or die from the process. Such patients neither need, nor will benefit from, the intervention under study, leading to a further increase in sample size and, consequently, cost and logistic problems for the RCT.

The problem is no better with ARDS. The American-European consensus conference attempted to define an early, milder phase of ARDS known as acute lung injury (ALI) [21]. However, there exists no good evidence that the two conditions are linked temporaneously. Indeed, those with acute respiratory failure who are not "sick enough" to meet ARDS criteria still seem to incur very high mortality rates.

Thus, it seems that the two major paths by which we can better delineate which patients to study will be: 1) Identification of rapid tests that allow a more accurate determination of the specific underlying pathophysiologic process; or 2) Development of better risk stratification that separates the different components contributing to risk into those that are modifiable and those that are not modifiable by the therapy under study. Such risk models might include, for example, the response of physiologic parameters to standard therapy.

Controlling the Process of Care

The high mortality of many of the ICU diseases has led to several alternative approaches to patient care, even with existing and approved therapies. In ARDS, for example, it is unclear whether the patient should be managed "wet" or "dry", prone or supine, and with high or low intrathoracic pressures. Similarly, the decision whether to use pressors or fluids in the management of septic hypotension is made differently by different clinicians. With the multiple therapies required in the care of a critically ill patient, and with the wide variation in the application of these therapies, the subsequent "noise" may quickly obliterate any "signal" of effect from the therapy under study.

In response to this "signal-to-noise" problem, Morris et al. [34] propose reducing noise through the use of computerized protocols that specify the same response to a given set of clinical characteristics. Developed initially to control for differences in ventilator management of ARDS patients managed with and without extracorporeal carbon dioxide removal, these protocols are computer driven and react to ventilator and arterial blood gas data to offer instructions for oxygen and ventilation management [35]. While this approach has proven to be both feasible and able to reduce signal to noise ratios, it is difficult to initiate, requires sophisticated computerization of ICUs, significant clinician training and acceptance, and still only controls one portion of the clinical management, the ventilator. We remain a long way away from complete management of the critically ill patient by protocol but the Morris approach certainly has lit the path.

It must be appreciated, however, that the use of such protocols moves the care of the patient further away from that which happens in many day-to-day environments. Thus, we may better be able to determine the efficacy of a new therapy with such an approach but at the same time reduce our ability to determine effectiveness. Thus, the extent to which we wish to control the process of care will be very dependent on the question we ask.

In addition, the use of certain protocols may contaminate our dependent variables. For example, in weaning trials where the dependent variable is length of mechanical ventilation, if we fix the rate at which a given mode of weaning can be reduced, we may inadvertently force a minimum length of stay (LOS) upon the mode. This will confound our ability to interpret the results of the study. This problem is most likely when our outcomes of interest include intermediate or surrogate markers since such markers (e.g., LOS or cost) may be artificially driven by study design and not by the therapy under study *per se*. Nevertheless, by reducing signal-to-noise, attempts to standardize conventional therapy ought to help improve the power of our studies given a similar sample size.

Choosing End-Points

Mortality

Short-term, all-cause mortality has traditionally been used as the end-point in clinical trials of critical illness. The reason to use short-term is because critical illness is thought to be acute, therefore the patient will declare himself as a survivor or non-survivor from this acute process in a relatively short time. The two traditional short-term measures have been hospital discharge status and a fixed time-point (e.g., day 28 or day 30).

Hospital discharge status is relatively easy to collect and represents the end of the acute care time period. Thus, it allows for variation in the length of the acute process between patients. However, the disadvantage of hospital mortality is that it can be biased by differences in practice patterns between different hospitals and regions. For example, in a region where patients are often transferred earlier to a second care facility for chronic ventilator management, a patient may be discharged alive only to die in another facility. Alternatively, in another setting, as long as a patient remains on the ventilator, he may remain at the original hospital. Thus, should that same patient die, his hospital discharge status would be death, hence the same patient would be counted as a survivor or non-survivor depending on the hospital at which he was treated.

To avoid this problem, researchers have increasingly moved to a fixed time point [6, 36–40]. This choice is unbiased by clinical practice but may arbitrarily fail to capture the duration of the episode of illness. For example, a patient with severe sepsis and ARDS may still be critically ill and requiring life support at day 28 yet be called a survivor even though he may die within one or two weeks following the end-point. A recent National Institute of Health – American College of Chest Physicians (NIH-ACCP) Consensus panel stated that, regardless, this remains the best end-point, arguing that prior sepsis studies had shown that most patients dying from sepsis will have died within this time period and that deaths beyond this point are both rare and probably unrelated to the septic process [8].

This position may be a little hard to defend for several reasons. First, Schein et al. [41] recently showed there is a persistent elevated risk of death for several months after the onset of severe sepsis. Failure to capture the associated mortality may confound interpretation of new therapies that only delay death, and stopping follow-up too early increases the likelihood of committing this error. Second, the clinical relevance to the patient is less clear if 28-day mortality does not translate into meaningful differences in survival. The question of whether mortality should be further qualified by the quality of life among the survivors is a further issue discussed below.

Finally, the use of mortality rate as an end-point produces some oddities when attempting to measure other end-points. For example, it is common to explore the extent to which resource use varies between treatments; this might include differences in LOS or hospital costs. Commonly, non-survivors are found to have shorter LOS than survivors in sepsis trials. Interestingly, when calibrating a cost-effectiveness model of sepsis, Chalfin et al. [42] generated LOS data for hospital survivors and non-survivors of sepsis from their own institution and found non-survivors had longer LOS. Why the difference? One possible explanation is the 28-day end-point. Since survival is determined at day 28, the non-survivor group includes only those with LOS < 28 days. This has the potential to distort not only estimates of effect but also estimates of cost-effectiveness as therapies that delay death will result in the miscounting of patients in the wrong outcome cohort and falsely low estimates of mean costs in the non-survivor group.

Ideally, an ICU patient cohort should be followed until their death rate appears to have returned to the norm expected in an age- and co-morbidity-matched population. However, this ideal is complicated since there is still only a paucity of information regarding the duration of the episode of critical illness and also because follow-up for several months beyond enrollment can be expensive and time-consuming. A pragmatic solution is to better delineate the relationship between short-term and long-term mortality in epidemiologic studies, and thus understand better the implications of differences in short-term mortality in future studies. Alternatively, we could attempt limited follow-up in some or all of the patients enrolled.

Another problem with mortality is whether to choose all-cause versus selected cause mortality. While most studies gather information regarding whether the death was related or unrelated to the critical illness, most regulatory bodies approve or disapprove therapies depending on all-cause mortality. While this may seem counter-intuitive, the reason is simple – it is exceedingly difficult to classify a death as related or unrelated. Both death certificates and independent physician reviews of deaths yield poor and inconsistent data whereas the simple recording of death itself remains elegantly simple and accurate. It is unlikely that any solution to increase the objectivity of the cause of death will come soon.

Morbidity

Much of the value of intensive care may be derived from the mitigation of morbidity. Unfortunately, intensive care may save a life only to produce a survivor wracked by terrible infirmity with low quality of life and high reliance on continued, expensive health care. Thus, measures of outcome other than pure survival data are important. Several approaches to evaluate morbidity exist. First, morbidity can be recorded "physiologically" by assessing change in organ function [43, 44]. Second, morbidity can be considered in terms of its effects on resource consumption (e.g., hospital costs, lost wages, cost of home help, or new requirement for chronic dialysis) [45, 46]. Third, the impact of illness on quality of life can serve as a measure of morbidity [45–52]. Of these three, the first is gaining favor in critical care, the second continues to be used confusedly, and the third is gaining favor in other realms of clinical and health service research.

Measuring morbidity by some type of physiologic score has the apparent advantage that it should be relatively easy to quantitate. Unfortunately, problems persist. First, there remains no consensus over which score to use. Indeed, there are a plethora of organ failure scores [19, 27, 43, 44, 53]. Furthermore, there are now the addition of organ failure-free scores [25]. These scores look at the number of days within a defined follow-up period when the patient is free of organ failure or organ failure support. Such scores are tantalizing in that they combine morbidity with mortality (since dying patients do not incur organ failure free days and thus are scored appropriately low). Unfortunately, there is little exploration or validation of these scores and significant concerns remain regarding defining the duration of the period during which days are counted, the sensitivity of the measure to changing that duration, the equality of different organ failure days, and the appropriate way to assess the power of studies based on such calculations.

Another problem of this approach is that it assumes implicit value in avoiding or reducing organ-failure-related morbidity. Unfortunately, such an assumption is not necessarily well founded. For example, while a serum creatinine of 3 mmol/L may score worse than 2 mmol/L in a definition of renal dysfunction, the consequences either in terms of societal or hospital costs or in terms of a patient's quality of life may be difficult to demonstrate. The extent to which inter-organ interactions and differential effects of different organ failures on outcome influence the utility of organ failure scores is also unclear.

Attempting to measure morbidity in dollar terms yet express it as an outcome, though common (e.g., duration of mechanical ventilation), is somewhat problematic. This is because, if measured as an outcome, it becomes an "effect" (denominator) in a cost-effectiveness ratio. Yet resource consumption during the intervention is part of the "cost" (numerator). This creates two problems. First, there is no clear rule determining at what point in time costs would stop being counted as the resources required by the therapy and become the effects of that therapy. Second, the ratio of costs per effects can become distorted by errors of omission.

The solution is to not use resource use as a proxy for morbidity. Rather, all costs are counted in the numerator and all effects in the denominator. For example, if a therapy produced excess renal failure that persisted long after discharge, that therapy would be charged both with the increase in costs associated with ongoing hemodialysis and the decrease in quality of life associated with living with renal failure. To have counted the post-discharge renal failure only as the requirement for hemodialysis, regardless of whether that was expressed in the numerator or denominator, would have failed to attribute the full penalty of excess renal failure to the therapy under study. This approach has recently been endorsed by the NIH Panel on cost-effectiveness in health care [54].

This approach to measuring morbidity has the attraction of capturing the extent to which morbidity detracts from the overall value of survivorship. However, it is barely used currently in clinical trials of critical illness. There are several reasons for this. First, it is expensive to collect. Second, there is as yet little agreement over which quality of life scores should be used. Third, many still debate the entire approach, pointing out that quality is, by its very nature, a subjective opinion not tied to physiology or functional capability. Fourth, determining the extent to which the decrease in quality is due to the critical illness and its sequelae as opposed to other co-morbidities is difficult, especially since pre-illness quality of life is rarely known. Fifth, using this approach alone would not capture any of the negative effects of decreasing morbidity, and therefore delaying death, in those who die from the critical illness.

Nevertheless, quality of life is perhaps the most intuitive patient-oriented outcome since it incorporates survivorship with the perceived value of that survivorship. As such, it is widely adopted as the principal method by which to compare the relative benefits of different therapies in different diseases and has recently been suggested by the NIH panel on cost-effectiveness in health care as the primary endpoint for cost-effectiveness analyses [54].

In summary, end-points from clinical trials in critical illness should probably involve longer follow-up of mortality. Furthermore, the quality of survivors should probably be qualified by some type of health-related quality of life. Alternatively, mortality could be counted with some form of physiology-based morbidity score. Ideally, both approaches should be taken but since morbidity cannot be counted twice, each approach should be calculated separately. In the event that the two approaches yield conflicting data, it is unclear which approach should be considered more valuable. The answer is probably that the approach involving physiology would tell us more about the effect the therapy is having on the body while the latter would yield more information about whether that effect is worth having.

Observational Outcomes Studies as Alternatives to RCTs

As mentioned earlier, the RCT is neither always possible nor always applicable. The principal alternative approach to the RCT involves observation rather than experiment. Prior experience has biased us to favor RCTs but, partly in response to the increasing need to answer questions unanswerable by the RCT, we have become much more sophisticated in our design and execution of observational outcomes studies.

In critiquing such studies, rather than making the knee-jerk response "just a retrospective study", we should consider carefully the different elements most susceptible to bias. First of all, we must consider the data source. Observational outcomes studies are often performed on large data sets wherein the data were collected for purposes other than research. This can lead to error due to either a lack of pertinent information or a bias in the information recorded [55]. It is important to appreciate that the data should be considered separately from the trial design, that a lack of accuracy of the data may or may not be important depending on its pertinence to the question asked, and that it is not inconceivable that an observational outcomes study could be performed on an excellent data source.

Second, we must consider how the authors attempt to control for confounding. The measured effect size of a variable on outcome (e.g., the effect of the pulmonary artery catheter on mortality) can be confounded by the distribution of other known and unknown variables. There are several techniques that attempt to account for known variables, including matching, stratification, and regression modeling. All have advantages and disadvantages and it is incumbent on the investigators to defend the rationale for their choice and present evidence supporting how well their technique performed [56].

Even if the investigators have devised a reliable and valid technique to adjust for known confounders, they still have the problem of controlling for unknown variables. Though there are methods that attempt to measure the extent to which an unmeasured variable may be present in an observational outcome study (e.g., by inserting imaginary variables), there is no well-accepted test for this. The reader must therefore ask the question, "Is there anything unaccounted for in this study that I believe could explain the magnitude and direction of effect otherwise attributable to the intervention?".

It may appear that the alternative to randomization is quite burdensome. However, observational outcomes studies are very powerful tools for addressing many questions that RCTs cannot address, including measuring the effect of harmful substances (e.g., smoking and other carcinogens), organizational structures (e.g., payor status, open versus closed ICUs), or geography (e.g., rural versus urban access to healthcare). Recently investigators have reproduced many of the large cardiology intervention trials in the Duke Cardiovascular Registry using observational outcomes techniques, exploring the effectiveness of therapies previously tested only under efficacious conditions. Investigators have also explored the effects of different therapies that are already accepted, but used variably, in clinical practice [57]. Randomization would be ethically problematic in such situations. Thus, as questions not addressable by RCTs become more important, we must embrace the challenge to adopt and understand observational outcomes studies as part of our methodologic toolset.

Furthermore, we should even be prepared to deal with situations where a well-conducted RCT and a well-conducted observational outcomes study on the same intervention yield opposite results and conclude that both studies are correct. In other words, the RCT demonstrated that a therapy had a significant effect under ideal conditions but the observational outcomes study demonstrated that the effect was lost in the real world. Either study alone would only tell part of the story. The combined information would allow policymakers and clinicians to examine practice patterns and devise strategies to ensure the therapy was used properly in the real world.

Adding Cost to the Equation

The reasons to perform a cost-analysis are to determine whether a new therapy is worth using with respect to existing therapies, and whether existing resources should be allocated to pay for a new therapy [58]. Thus, a cost analysis should estimate the likely costs and effects in the community and express those estimates in units comparable to other cost analyses [54]. Incorporating into an RCT the elements necessary to generate cost-effectiveness estimates is somewhat complicated. Generally, the problems can be considered as related to efficacy versus effectiveness, estimation of costs; and choice of end-points.

Cost-Effectiveness or Cost-Efficacy?

Until we have conducted RCTs that show a positive result, we are likely to focus on efficacy trials. In other words, we will do our best to increase the likelihood of measuring a positive effect. If a cost analysis is part of the trial, and the estimate of effect is generated from the trial, then the cost analysis will be a cost-efficacy ratio, rather than a cost-effectiveness ratio. The differences in such ratios are not trivial [59]. There are two ways to deal with this problem. First, the RCT design can be adapted to measure effectiveness [58, 59]. However, this is likely to be expensive, with the need for either additional study arms or separate trials. Furthermore, study sponsors may simply be unwilling to expose their therapy before approval to the risks of an effectiveness trial where the likelihood of demonstrating effect is reduced.

Alternatively, the costs and effects generated from the RCT can be entered into an economic decision model and exposed to a sensitivity analysis driven by observational data about current practice patterns and assumptions of likely use of the therapy if approved. Such models could determine the impact of loosening the patient eligibility criteria (treating additional patients not likely to benefit), treating patients with alternative therapies, and prescribing the therapy inappropriately. Clinicians are often skeptical of such decision models, in part because the models rely on assumptions, data gathered from multiple sources, and simulated, rather than real, patients. While such skepticism may have been warranted in the past, it is important to appreciate that simulation modeling plays an important role in many other sciences and represents the most practical solution to this problem currently.

Furthermore, recent guidelines from the NIH panel on cost-effectiveness in health care should lead to improved standardization and comparability of such models in healthcare.

Estimating Costs

Cost-effectiveness ratios are the incremental change in costs divided by the incremental change in effects between two study arms. Therefore, only those costs that behave differently between study arms affect the ratio. This is convenient since attempting to measure all costs incurred, including all indirect costs (such as patient and family suffering) would be a gargantuan task. In practice, the costs most likely to differ between therapies are the direct hospital costs (including the estimated "street" price of the therapy) and the costs of managing post-discharge problems that occur at different rates between groups (e.g., if acute renal failure is a more frequent complication in one arm, then the costs of post-discharge hemodialysis must be estimated). The detail with which the cost of a particular element is measured should depend on the sensitivity of the ultimate ratio to that cost. In other words, if the only element that differs is the duration of mechanical ventilation then the ratio will be exquisitely sensitive to the cost of mechanical ventilation and this should therefore be measured very carefully.

There are several methods by which to estimate the costs of health expenditure too numerous to mention here. In general, the methods consist of relying on existing cost-accounting and billing systems (including detailed hospital billing data, summary bills, and patient-specific resource tracking), collecting information prospectively on resources consumed, or measuring the LOS. The number of resources consumed can be converted to costs by multiplying the numbers of each resource by an estimated cost generated from another source (number of units of resource A x estimated cost per unit A), or expressing resource use in a common metric (e.g., the therapeutic intervention scoring system [TISS]) and multiplying that metric by a unit cost (e.g., the number of TISS points x estimated monetary value per TISS point) [60]. LOS can be converted to cost by estimating daily costs such as typical daily ICU costs. Each of these methods represents a different balance of the cost of collecting the information and its accuracy. It should be noted that the more detailed measures may not even be available in certain situations or may require not only patient consent but also hospital or provider cooperation. Consequently, when designing an RCT with a cost component, investigators should be careful to choose wisely which cost elements to measure and how to measure them.

Difficulty with Combined End-Points

The unit of effect, or utility, recommended by the NIH panel for cost effectiveness in health care is quality-adjusted survival [54]. This allows comparison of different cost analyses to each other. Currently we rarely measure quality of life, but we do measure survival which can be adjusted to incorporate quality of life using simulation modeling. Unless there is a belief that the two treatment arms will affect quality of life differently, the error associated with such adjustment will largely be a function of the magnitude of effect. On the other hand, if we do not set mortality as the primary end-point, we run the risk of creating uncertainty not over the magnitude of effect but of whether there is an effect at all.

To illustrate, the recent neonatal inhaled nitric oxide study (NINOS) of inhaled nitric oxide (NO) in the treatment of hypoxic distress of the newborn was powered for the combined end-point of extracorporeal membrane oxygenation (ECMO) or death [61]. The study was terminated when an overwhelming difference in this combined end-point was measured. However, there was no significant difference in mortality. When constructing a cost-effectiveness model, it is unclear how to treat ECMO [62]. Theoretically, ECMO is a resource, and is thus associated with a cost. Therefore, it should be placed in the numerator. Death, on the other hand, is placed in the denominator. In short, the combined end-point is split. Once split, we re-introduce the uncertainty (i.e., no statistical significance) of whether inhaled NO achieved an effect. A cost model can still be constructed and exposed to a sensitivity analysis where the model is tested across the confidence boundaries of the costs and effects [62]. However, although this analysis may be helpful, clinicians and policymakers alike will be left with considerable uncertainty over the value of inhaled NO. The likely result will be that further trials, with different end-points, will be required.

An even more complicated situation may occur with the use of organ failure free days. For example, using ventilator-free days (VFDs) in an ARDS trial, we may create a scenario where we have a significant decrease in VFDs with no significant change in mortality. What would this mean in terms of costs and effects? VFDs are poor proxies for cost since they do not account for potential differences in the LOS of non-survivors (all non-survivors receive a value of zero even though a therapy may well delay the onset of death by temporarily ameliorating the illness). Therefore, VFDs cannot be placed in the numerator. They may also be poor proxies for survival since those alive but ventilated at the end of follow-up are counted as equal to non-survivors, regardless of whether they are subsequently weaned and discharged home alive. Thus, we have a single significant end-point, the meaning of which is unclear with regard to both costs and effects. Again, such data may leave clinicians and policy-makers uncertain over the implications of the trial, with a need for further trials.

Conclusion

The issues facing clinical research in the ICU are quite complex. First, unless we find a better way to identify the correct patients, we probably need to conduct much larger trials than we currently perform. This raises many logistic problems. Second, economic pressures demand that we determine not only efficacy but also effectiveness and cost. Solutions to the first problem largely drive us towards efficacy, decreasing our ability to solve the second problem. Approaches to measure effectiveness require even larger trials and may therefore force us to include observational outcomes studies and simulation models in our current methodology toolset. Though well established in other fields, these new methods have played little role in intensive care to date and will require our time and effort if we are to embrace them and use them optimally.

Perhaps to solve these dilemmas, we might begin with Descartes' lesson that pragmatism and good sense is a fine place to start: "Good sense is the most evenly shared thing in the world, for each of us thinks he is so well endowed with it that even those who are the hardest to please in all other respects are not in the habit of wanting more than they have" [1].

References

1. Descartes R (1979) Discourse on the method of properly conducting one's reason and of seeking the truth in the sciences. In: Sutcliffe FE (ed) Discourse on method and the meditations, Penguin Books Ltd., Harmondsworth, pp 25–92
2. Ware JH, Antman EM (1997) Equivalence trials. N Engl J Med 337:1159–1161
3. Lamas GA, Pfeffer MA, Hamm P, Wertheimer J, Rouleau JL, Braunwald E (1992) Do the results of randomized clinical trials of cardiovascular drugs influence medical practice? The SAVE Investigators. N Engl J Med 327:241–247
4. Lavori PW, Louis TA, Bailar JCI, Polansky M (1986) Designs for experiments – Parallel comparisons of treatments. In: Bailar JI, Mosteller F (eds) Medical uses of statistics. NEJM Books, Waltham, pp 41–66
5. Committee for evaluating medical technologies in clinical use, Division of health sciences policy, Division of health promotion and disease prevention, Institute of Medicine (1985) Assessing medical technologies. National Academy Press, Washington
6. Brun-Buisson C (1994) The HA-1A saga: the scientific and ethical dilemma of innovative and costly therapies. Intensive Care Med 20:314–316
7. Sibbald WJ, Vincent J (1995) Roundtable conference on clinical trials for the treatment of sepsis. Chest 107:522–527
8. Dellinger RP (1997) From the bench to the bedside: The future of sepsis research executive Summary of an American College of Chest Physicians, national institute of allergy and infectious disease, and national heart, lung, and blood institute workshop. Chest 111:744–753
9. Bone RC (1996) Why sepsis trials fail. JAMA 276:565–566
10. Opal SM (1995) Lessons learned from clinical trials of sepsis. J Endotoxin Res 2:221–226
11. Eidelman LA, Sprung CL (1994) Why have new effective therapies for sepsis not been developed. Crit Care Med 22:1330–1334
12. Russell LB, Gold MR, Siegel JE, Daniels N, Weinstein MC (1996) The role of cost-effectiveness analysis in health and medicine. Panel on cost-effectiveness in health and medicine. JAMA 276:1172–1177
13. The global use of strategies to open occluded coronary arteries (GUSTO III) investigators (1997) A comparison of reteplase with alteplase for acute myocardial infarction. N Engl J Med 337:1118–1123
14. The GUSTO investigators (1993) An international randomized trial comparing four thrombolytic strategies for acute myocardial infarction. N Engl J Med 329:673–682
15. Collins R, Peto R, Baigent C, Sleight P (1997) Aspirin, heparin, and fibrinolytic therapy in suspected acute myocardial infarction. N Engl J Med 336:847–860
16. Hornberger J, Wrone E (1997) When to base clinical policies on observational versus randomized trial data. Ann Intern Med 127:697–703
17. Piper RD, Cook DJ, Bone RC, Sibbald WJ (1996) Introducing critical appraisal to studies of animal models investigating novel therapies in sepsis. Crit Care Med 24:2059–2070
18. Galanos C, Freudenberg MA (1993) Mechanisms of endotoxin shock and endotoxin hypersensitivity. Immunobiology 187:346–356
19. Bone RC, Balk RA, Cerra FB, et al (1992) Definitions for sepsis and organ failure and guidelines for the use of innovative therapies in sepsis. Chest 101:1644–1655
20. Angus DC, Kramer DJ (1993) Sepsis: a clinical perspective. In: Pinsky MR, Dhainaut JF (eds) Pathophysiologic foundations of critical care medicine. Williams and Wilkins, Baltimore, pp 96–111

21. Bernard GR, Artigas A, Brigham KL, et al (1994) The American-European consensus conference on ARDS. Definitions, mechanisms, relevant outcomes, and clinical trial coordination Am J Respir Crit Care Med 149:818–824
22. Knaus WA, Sun X, Nystrom O, Wagner DP (1992) Evaluation of definitions for sepsis. Chest 101:1656–1662
23. Rubenfeld GD, Doyle RL, Matthay MA (1995) Evaluation of definitions of ARDS. Am J Respir Crit Care Med 151:1270–1271
24. Knaus WA, Harrell FE Jr, Fisher CJ Jr, et al (1993) The clinical evaluation of new drugs for sepsis. A prospective study design based on survival analysis. JAMA 270:1233–1241
25. Marshall JC, Cook DJ, Christou NV, Bernard GR, Sprung CL, Sibbald WJ (1995) Multiple organ dysfunction score: a reliable descriptor of a complex clinical outcome. Crit Care Med 23:1638–1652
26. Vincent JL, Moreno R, Takala J, et al (1996) The SOFA (sepsis-related organ failure assessment) score to describe organ dysfunction/failure. Intensive Care Med 22:707–710
27. Rangel-Frausto MS, Pittet D, Costigan M, Hwang T, Davis CS, Wenzel RP (1995) The natural history of the systemic inflammatory response syndrome (SIRS). A prospective study. JAMA 273:117–123
28. Salvo J, de Cian W, Musicco M, et al (1995) The Italian SEPSIS study: preliminary results on the incidence and evolution of SIRS, sepsis, severe sepsis and septic shock. Intensive Care Med 21 (suppl 2):S244–S249
29. Sands KE, Bates DW, Lanken PN, et al (1997) Epidemiology of sepsis syndrome in 8 academic medical centers. JAMA 278:234–240
30. Vincent JL (1997) Dear SIRS, I'm sorry to say that I don't like you. Crit Care Med 25:372–374
31. Dougnac A, Hernandez G, Angus DC, et al (1996) Severe SIRS in Chile: Natural history and new organ dysfunction score. Intensive Care Med 22:S321 (Abst)
32. Angus DC, Dougnac A, Hernandez G, et al (1996) Sepsis and SIRS: Are we any nearer to consensus? Intensive Care Med 22:273–280
33. Bone RC, Grodzin CJ, Balk RA (1997) Sepsis: A new hypothesis for pathogenesis of the disease process. Chest 112:235–243
34. Morris AH (1993) Protocol management of adult respiratory distress syndrome. New Horizons 1:593–602
35. Morris AH, Wallace CJ, Menlove RL, et al (1994) Randomized clinical trial of pressure-controlled inverse ratio ventilation and extracorporeal CO_2 removal for adult respiratory distress syndrome. Am J Respir Crit Care Med 149:295–305
36. Greenman RL, Schein RM, Martin MA, et al (1991) A controlled clinical trial of E5 murine monoclonal IgM antibody to endotoxin in the treatment of gram-negative sepsis. JAMA 266:1097–1102
37. Ziegler EJ, Fisher CJ, Jr., Sprung CL, et al (1991) Treatment of gram-negative bacteremia and septic shock with HA-1A human monoclonal antibody against endotoxin. A randomized, double-blind, placebo-controlled trial. N Engl J Med 324:429–436
38. Morris AH, Wallace CJ, Menlove RL (1994) Randomized controlled trial of pressure-controlled inverse ratio ventilation and extracorporeal CO_2 removal for adult respiratory distress syndrome. Am J Respir Crit Care Med 149:295–305
39. Willatts SM, Radford S, Leitermann M (1995) Effect of the antiendotoxic agent, taurolidine, in the treatment of sepsis syndrome: a placebo-controlled, double-blind trial. Crit Care Med 23:1033–1039
40. Reinhart K, Wiegand-Lohnert C, Grimminger F, et al (1996) Assessment of the safety and efficacy of the monoclonal anti-tumor necrosis factor antibody-fragment, MAK 195F, in patients with sepsis and septic shock: A multicenter, randomized, placebo-controlled, dose-ranging study. Crit Care Med 24:733–742
41. Quartin AA, Roland MH, Kett DH, Peduzzi PN, for the Department of Veterans Affairs Systemic Sepsis Cooperative Studies Group (1997) Magnitude and duration of the effect of sepsis on survival. JAMA 277:1058–1063
42. Chalfin DB, Holbein MEB, Fein AM, Carlon GC (1993) Cost-effectiveness of monoclonal antibodies to gram-negative endotoxin in the treatment of gram-negative sepsis in ICU patients. JAMA 269:249–254

43. Knaus WA, Draper EA, Wagner DP, Zimmerman JE (1985) Prognosis in acute organ-system failure. Ann Surg 202:685–693

44. Raffin TA (1989) Intensive care unit survival of patients with systemic illness. Am Rev Respir Dis 140:S28–S35

45. Anonymous (1994) Predicting outcome in ICU patients. 2nd European consensus conference in intensive care medicine. Intensive Care Med 20:390–397

46. Weinstein MC, Stason WB (1977) Foundations of cost-effectiveness analysis for health and medical practices. N Engl J Med 296:716–721

47. Ridley SA, Wallace PG (1990) Quality of life after intensive care. Anaesthesia 45:808–813

48. Tarlov AR, Ware JE Jr, Greenfield S, Nelson EC, Perrin E, Zubkoff M (1989) The Medical Outcomes Study. An application of methods for monitoring the results of medical care. JAMA 262:925–930

49. Visser MC, Fletcher AE, Parr G, Simpson A, Bulpitt CJ (1994) A comparison of three quality of life instruments in subjects with angina pectoris: the Sickness Impact Profile, the Nottingham Health Profile, and the Quality of Well Being Scale. J Clin Epidemiol 47:157–163

50. Kaplan RM, Atkins CJ, Timms R (1984) Validity of a quality of well-being scale as an outcome measure in chronic obstructive pulmonary disease. J Chronic Dis 37:85–95

51. Chelluri L, Grenvik AN, Silverman M (1995) Intensive care for critically ill elderly mortality, costs, and quality of life. Review of the literature. Arch Intern Med 155:1013–1022

52. Slatyer MA, James OF, Moore PG, Leeder SR (1986) Costs, severity of illness and outcome in intensive care. Anaesth Intensive Care 14:381–389

53. Barriere SL, Lowry SF (1995) An overview of mortality risk prediction in sepsis. Crit Care Med 23:376–393

54. Weinstein MC, Siegel JE, Gold MR, Kamlet MS, Russell LB, for the Panel on Cost-Effectiveness in Health and Medicine (1996) Recommendations of the panel on cost-effectiveness in health and medicine. JAMA 276:1253–1258

55. Iezzoni LI, Foley SM, Daley J, Hughes JS, Fisher ES, Heeren T (1992) Comorbidities, complications, and coding bias. Does the number of diagnosis codes matter in predicting in-hospital mortality? JAMA 267:2197–2203

56. Angus DC, Pinsky MR (1997) Risk Prediction – Judging the Judges. Intensive Care Med 23:363–365

57. McClellan M, McNeil BJ, Newhouse JP (1994) Does more intensive treatment of acute myocardial infarction in the elderly reduce mortality? Analysis using instrumental variables. JAMA 272:859–866

58. Freemantle N, Drummond MF (1997) Should clinical trials with concurrent economic analyses be blinded? JAMA 277:63–64

59. Linden PK, Angus DC, Chelluri L, Branch RA (1995) The influence of clinical study design on cost-effectiveness projections for the treatment of gram-negative sepsis with human anti-endotoxin antibody. J Crit Care 10:154–164

60. Cullen DJ (1989) Reassessing critical care: illness, outcome, and cost. Crit Care Med 17:S172–S173

61. The Neonatal inhaled nitric oxide study group (1997) Inhaled nitric oxide in full-term and nearly full-term infants with hypoxic respiratory failure. N Engl J Med 336:597–604

62. Roberts MS, Angus DC, Clermont G, Linde-Zwirble WT, Pinsky MR (1998) From efficacy to effectiveness: problems in translating the results of clinical trials into CE analysis. Med Decis Making (Abst, in press)

Severe Infections

Antimicrobial Therapy for ICU-Acquired Infection: Time for a Reappraisal

J. C. Marshall and D. C. Evans

Introduction

Infections acquired in the intensive care unit (ICU) commonly complicate the course of critical illness. Approximately one fourth to one third of patients admitted to an ICU develop one or more episodes of nosocomial infection [1]; both mortality and morbidity are sharply elevated in this population [2] (Table 1). Yet the extent to which such infections are the cause of excess morbidity and mortality, rather than an additional manifestation of organ dysfunction in a subset of the sickest of critically ill patients, is unclear. Equally, although antibiotics are among the most prescribed pharmaceutical agents in contemporary ICUs, it is not at all established that their widespread use in the management of suspected or proven ICU-acquired infection results in net clinical benefit. Indeed there are reasons to suspect that the opposite may be true. A recent analysis of nosocomial infection following cardiac surgery found that the administration of empiric post-operative antibiotics was an independent risk factor for the development of subsequent nosocomial infection [3].

An informed medical decision involves a careful weighing of the risks and benefits of a planned intervention, and a consideration of the alternate options. The decision to initiate antimicrobial therapy is based on the tacit assumption that antimicrobial therapy will result in sufficient benefit, measured as improved survival or reduced dependence on ICU technology, to warrant the financial costs, and the impact on microbial ecology. Is such an assumption justified by the available data? And do the merits of antimicrobial chemotherapy outweigh those of other, non-pharmacologic strategies for the therapy of nosocomial infection? A review of the

Table 1. Impact of infection with ICU morbidity and mortality. (From [2] with permission)

Infectious status	Length of ICU stay (days)	p value	Per cent mortality	p value
No infection (N = 123)	3.7 ± 0.1	...	3.3	...
Primary infection (N = 56)	7.1 ± 1.0	< 0.001	19.6	0.03
ICU-acquired infection (N = 51)	11.2 ± 1.2	< 0.001	23.5	0.002

published literature suggests that the answer to both these questions is "no", and that current practice merits a critical re-evaluation.

The Costs of Antimicrobial Therapy

Economic Costs

The provision of intensive care is enormously expensive. It has been estimated that the costs of intensive care in Canada in 1986 exceeded $ 1 billion, 8% of all inpatient costs and 0.2% of the gross national product. In the United States, the costs were even higher, 20% of inpatient costs and 0.8% of the gross national product [4]. Estimates of the contribution of pharmaceutical costs to these totals are not readily available. In our own unit, a 20-bed mixed medical/surgical ICU in a tertiary care teaching hospital, anti-infective agents were the most costly item in the budget for patient-specific medications, accounting for 36% of the total drug budget during the most recent fiscal year, and consuming 3% of the entire ICU operating budget.

Antimicrobial Resistance

Resistance to specific antimicrobial agents is encoded in the genetic structure of a microorganism. Resistance may arise spontaneously, or it may be acquired through plasmid or transposon-mediated gene transfection. For a given organism, the probability of acquisition of resistance in the ICU is influenced by the baseline genetic resistance of the organism, the extent of exposure to exogenous antibiotics, the degree of patient to patient contact, and the CD50, or dose of antibiotic at which 50% of patients become colonized [5]. Exposure to antibiotics selects for resistance by limiting the growth of sensitive strains, and promotes colonization by altering mucosal colonization resistance as a result of its effects on the indigenous flora that normally inhabits these surfaces. Both of these factors influence the microbial ecology of the contemporary ICU.

Intrinsic Microbial Resistance: Microbial isolates obtained from hospitalized patients show a higher degree of antibiotic resistance than isolates of the same organism obtained from outpatients; the highest prevalence of antibiotic resistance is seen in isolates from ICU patients [6] (Table 2). The most common infecting species in the ICU demonstrate a high degree of antibiotic resistance. For example, more than 80% of coagulase-negative staphylococci are methicillin resistant; moreover a number of strains of S. epidermidis are able to transfer resistance to multiple antimicrobial agents to other coagulase-negative staphylococci, and to S. aureus. Enterococci rapidly acquire transposon-mediated aminoglycoside resistance and have recently acquired a readily-transmissible resistance to vancomycin, the last widely available effective agent against these organisms. Vancomycin resistance has spread rapidly amongst enterococci: Its prevalence in American ICU's increased from 0.4% in 1989 to 13.6% in 1993 [7].

Table 2. Resistance patterns in patient and out-patient isolates. (From [6] with permission)

Organism	Resistance	% Resistant		
		Inpatients	Outpatients	p value
Pseudomonas	Imipenem	12.0	6.5	<0.01
	Ceftazidime	7.8	4.0	<0.01
S. aureus	Methicillin	32.7	14.6	<0.01
Enterobacter	Ceftazidime	26.0	11.9	<0.01
S. epidermidis	Methicillin	49.0	35.3	<0.01
Enterococcus	Vancomycin	6.3	1.4	<0.01

Gram-negative organisms commonly isolated from nosocomial infections in the ICU also show rapid acquisition of antibiotic resistance. Third generation cephalosporin use has been linked to the emergence of multi-drug resistance in enterobacter species, and infections with these organisms are associated with a higher mortality [8]. Cephalosporin usage has been associated with the emergence of resistant Gram-negative bacilli [9], suggesting that more conservative use of this class of antimicrobials is warranted [10]. Many common ICU Gram-negative organisms carry chromosomally-mediated inducible β-lactamases and cephalosporinases. Second and third generation cephalosporins and imipenem are known to derepress the genetic sequences encoding this resistance, rendering organisms resistant to β-lactamase stable cephalosporins and monobactams, and perhaps explaining some antibiotic treatment failures seen in the ICU [9].

Colonization Resistance: Most epithelial surfaces of the human body are normally colonized by a complex microbial flora that is acquired shortly following birth, and that persists largely unchanged throughout the life of the individual. The indigenous colonizing flora of the gastrointestinal tract is particularly complex, comprising in excess of 400 separate species, selectively found in discrete ecologic niches [11]. Interactions between carbohydrates on the cell surface of the microorganism and on epithelial cells of the mucosa result in stable colonization. The presence of this indigenous flora prevents the attachment of exogenous pathogens to the mucosal surface, and hence prevents the initial steps in the establishment of invasive infection, a phenomenon that has been termed "colonization resistance" [12].

Colonization resistance is thought to be conferred largely by the anaerobic flora associated with the intestinal mucosa [13]. Antimicrobial agents with activity against this flora can promote pathologic colonization by exposing potential binding sites, although inhibition of colonization resistance is only one of a number of factors that promote gut bacterial overgrowth in critical illness.

The proximal gastrointestinal tract of the critically ill patient becomes colonized with the same microbial species that predominate in ICU-acquired infections, i.e., Candida, spp. enterococci, coagulase-negative staphylococci, and Pseudomonas spp., and gut colonization is highly correlated with the development of invasive infection with the same species [14] (Table 3). Additional support for the concept that altered colonization resistance predisposes to nosocomial infection with resistant orga-

Table 3. Association of proximal GI colonization with invasive infection. (From [14] with permission)

Organism	Patients (%) with invasive infection with same organism[a]		
	GI colonization	No GI colonization	p[b]
Candida	15/19 (79%)	9/22 (41%)	0.03
S. fecalis	8/15 (53%)	17/26 (65%)	N.S.
Pseudomonas	9/10 (90%)	6/31 (19%)	0.0003
S. epidermidis	8/10 (80%)	10/31 (32%)	0.02

[a] Indicates the number of patients developing invasive systemic infection with the particular organism whose upper GI tract was colonized (GI colonization) or not (No GI colonization) with the organism in question
[b] Chi square with Yates' continuity correction

nisms derives from a large body of literature, summarized in several recent meta-analyses, showing that suppression of gut colonization using the technique of selective decontamination of the digestive tract can prevent nosocomial infections following trauma and critical illness [15].

Empiric Versus Directed Antimicrobial Therapy

Ideally, antimicrobial therapy is initiated on the basis of objective data derived from Gram stain and culture documenting the presence of a known pathogen and its antimicrobial sensitivities. To minimize the potential adverse impact of therapy, the agent or agents selected should be microbicidal, should reach high concentrations in the target tissue, and should be limited in spectrum to the organism isolated. Such a rational approach to antimicrobial therapy in the ICU has proven difficult. Culture data are not immediately available, and the gravity of the clinical situation makes the intensivist reluctant to withhold therapy. Accurate microbial diagnosis may be difficult. On the one hand, colonization of invasive devices such as endotracheal tubes, venous catheters, or urinary catheters can be difficult to differentiate from invasive infection [16, 17], particularly when clinical signs of systemic inflammation are so poorly predictive of invasive infection. On the other hand, prior use of systemic antimicrobial agents may mask the presence of infection by inhibiting microbial growth [18, 19].

The net result of diagnostic uncertainty and clinician discomfort with the possibility that the critically ill patient has an untreated infection, is a clinical attitude that favours the empiric use of broad spectrum agents. This approach has certainly had a significant impact in altering microbial ecology and resistance patterns. There is less evidence that it has yielded clinical benefit.

Empiric therapy is founded on three assumptions:
1) That appropriate antimicrobial therapy will alter the clinical course, and hence outcome, of ICU-acquired infections.

2) That early therapy will provide superior results to therapy initiated 24 to 48 hours after the onset of clinical manifestations of infection.
3) That the benefits of liberal antibiotic use in a given patient outweigh the detrimental effects on colonization resistance in that individual, and on the microbial ecology of the local ICU.

Although there are limited data to support some of these assumptions for certain nosocomial infections, the net body of evidence is far from compelling.

Pneumonia

The magnitude of the attributable mortality of ICU-acquired pneumonia is uncertain. The reported attributable mortality increases when more rigorous quantitative diagnostic techniques are used [20], underlining the importance of diagnostic uncertainty as a confounding factor in the evaluation of the role of empiric therapy. The accurate diagnosis of nosocomial pneumonia in the ventilated ICU patient is notoriously difficult, with the result that antimicrobial therapy is usually initiated empirically – in 100% of cases in a primary care centre, and in 78% of cases in a referral centre according to a recent report [21]. However, the use of empiric therapy has been evaluated better for ICU-acquired pneumonia than for any other ICU-acquired infection.

Conclusions regarding the impact of the adequacy of antimicrobial therapy on outcome from ICU-acquired pneumonia derive largely from retrospective analyses of descriptive cohort studies. For example, both Torres et al. [22] and Celis et al. [23] found that inappropriate antibiotic therapy was an independent risk factor for mortality from nosocomial pneumonia. Similarly, Luna and co-workers [24] reported that for patients with bacteriologically-proven pneumonia by broncho-alveolar lavage, appropriate antimicrobial therapy at the time of diagnosis resulted in a mortality of 38% compared to 91% for patients in whom antibiotic therapy was inappropriate; interestingly, patients who received no antibiotics had an intermediate risk of death, 60%, that was not significantly different from that of patients receiving appropriate antibiotics. When antibiotics were changed following bronchoscopy, the mortality figures were comparable to those of patients who continued to receive inappropriate antibiotics [24].

These analyses support the contention that early empiric therapy is associated with clinical benefit, although they must be interpreted with caution, for it is unknown to what extent unmeasured confounding variables may explain the different outcomes. Increased mortality may, for example, reflect a greater prevalence of infection with resistant strains, in turn a reflection of more advanced physiologic derangement and previous antibiotic therapy. Several authors have reported the predominance of resistant species such as *Pseudomonas* and *Acinetobacter* in patients who have received prior antibiotic therapy [25, 26], and it has been found that previous antibiotic therapy is a risk factor for mortality [27].

In summary, there are suggestive, but imperfect data to suggest that empiric therapy of ICU-acquired pneumonia may improve outcome. Conversely, similar retrospective analyses raise the possibility that treatment of one episode of pneumonia may jeopardize recovery from a subsequent episode.

Intravenous Catheter Infections

Bacteremia in the ICU patient may arise as a consequence of systemic dissemination of organisms from a local focus of infection, or from the colonization of an indwelling intravascular device. The majority of episodes of bacteremia that occur following admission to the ICU appear to arise from devices, rather than as systemic spread from a remote focus, and involve the characteristic spectrum of ICU-acquired pathogens: S. epidermidis (28%), S. aureus (16%), enterococci (8%), Candida spp. (5–10%), and Gram-negative bacilli [28].

In contrast to the descriptive data on the importance of appropriate antimicrobial therapy in the prognosis of ICU-acquired pneumonia, the adequacy of antibiotic coverage does not exert a significant impact on the outcome of ICU-acquired bacteremias [29–32]. Rather, prognosis is most strongly determined by the severity of the accompanying physiologic derangements. Consistent with this conclusion, Mainous and colleagues [33] reported that although vancomycin resistance has become more common in bacteremic isolates of enterococcus in the ICU, vancomycin resistance does not portend a worse clinical outlook. Independent of therapy, however, Gram-negative or fungal isolates are associated with a worse prognosis than the more common Gram-positive isolates [29].

Pittet and coworkers [30] evaluated 176 bacteremic patients in a cohort of 5,457 ICU admissions, and found that prior antibiotic therapy (odds ratio 2.40, 95% CI 1.59–3.62) predicted a higher mortality for bacteremic patients.

Urinary Tract Infection

Urinary tract infections in patients in the ICU usually arise as a consequence of retrograde colonization of in-dwelling urinary catheters. The duration of catheterization is an important risk factor for the development of bacteriuria. Although urinary tract infections are second only to pneumonia as the most common ICU-acquired infection, there are few studies evaluating their impact on outcome, or the merits of antimicrobial therapy. It has been a consistent observation that the crude mortality associated with ICU-acquired urinary tract infection is lower than that seen with other infections [31].

Tertiary Peritonitis

Recurrent, persistent, or tertiary peritonitis occurs in up to three fourths of patients admitted to the ICU with peritonitis, and involves not the characteristic enteric mixed flora of secondary peritonitis, but the same spectrum of organisms isolated from other sites during nosocomial ICU-acquired infections: Coagulase-negative staphylococci, Candida spp., enterococci, Enterobacter, and Pseudomonas [34]. The principles of empiric therapy for secondary peritonitis are well-established [35], but the role of antibiotics in tertiary peritonitis is unclear. Descriptive studies have failed to demonstrate any impact on outcome with the use of appropriate systemic antibiotics [34, 36].

The Impact of Antibiotic Therapy on ICU Outcome

In the absence of well-designed clinical trials with an appropriate placebo arm, conclusions regarding the impact of ICU-acquired infection on ICU morbidity and mortality must be derived from analyses of descriptive data, and are subject to the inherent biases of this approach. As discussed above, such analyses suggest benefit of appropriate therapy for nosocomial pneumonia, however alternate conclusions can be drawn.

To assess the impact of antimicrobial therapy on ICU mortality and the development of the multiple organ dysfunction syndrome (MODS), we analyzed a prospectively-collected database of 477 patients admitted to the ICU of a tertiary care center for at least 24 hours. Organ dysfunction was quantified using the multiple organ dysfunction (MOD) score [37]. Microbiologically-proven ICU-acquired infection developed in 74 patients (15.5%). Antimicrobial agents were started at least two days following ICU admission in 133 patients (27.9%). Overall, patients receiving antibiotics that were started at least 48 hours after admission had a worse ICU outcome as evidenced by an increased length of ICU stay (12.8 ± 10.5 vs 3.4 ± 2.2 days, $p < 0.0001$), a higher mean MOD score (8.9 ± 4.7 vs 3.3 ± 4.2, $p < 0.0001$), and a higher ICU mortality, 21.1% vs 4.4% (odds ratio 5.8; 95% CI 3.0–11.4). Patients without proven ICU-acquired infection had a worse outcome if they received antibiotics (Table 4), and even for those patients with ICU-acquired infections, the use of antibiotics was associate with worsening organ dysfunction without evidence of benefit measured as ICU mortality or length of stay (Table 5).

Table 4. The impact of antibiotic therapy started at least 48 hours after admission on outcome of patients without ICU-acquired infection

	Antibiotics	No antibiotics	Odds ratio/p value
Number of patients	76	327	
Admission APACHE II score	14.8 ± 7.3	12.5 ± 6.5	0.07
MOD score	7.5 ± 3.9	4.0 ± 3.1	< 0.0001
ICU mortality	11.8%	3.4%	3.9 (1.5–9.7)

Table 5. The impact of antibiotic therapy started at least 48 hours after admission on outcome of patients with ICU-acquired infection

	Antibiotics	No antibiotics	Odds ratio/p value
Number of patients	57	17	
Admission APACHE II score	15.7 ± 6.6	16.2 ± 7.4	0.26
MOD score	10.9 ± 5.0	7.9 ± 4.7	0.03
ICU mortality	33.3%	23.5%	1.6 (0.5–5.7)

Conclusion

Despite the fact that antibiotics are one of the most prescribed classes of drug in the contemporary ICU, and despite the increasing awareness that injudicious antibiotic use has created a crisis in antimicrobial resistance, data supporting a beneficial role for antibiotics in common nosocomial ICU-acquired infections are sparse and of sub-optimal quality. Intensivists, on the other hand, are naturally reluctant to adopt a more restrictive practice towards the prescribing of antibiotics because of concerns that patient safety might be jeopardized through the deliberate withholding of antimicrobial therapy.

There are solid grounds for believing that the benefits of antibiotics in ICU-acquired infection are less impressive than commonly believed, and, conversely, that the adverse effects on both the individual patient and the ICU microbial ecology are greater. There is an urgent need for rigorous randomized, blinded, and controlled studies to define the roles of antibiotics in both empiric therapy, and the treatment of common discrete infections such as catheter-related bacteremias and urinary tract infections.

References

1. Nathens AB, Chu PTY, Marshall JC (1992) Nosocomial infection in the surgical intensive care unit. Infect Dis Clin North Am 6:657–675
2. Marshall JC, Sweeney D (1990) Microbial infection and the septic response in critical surgical illness. Sepsis, not infection, determines outcome. Arch Surg 125:17–23
3. Kollef MH, Sharpless L, Vlasnik J, Pasque C, Murphy D, Fraser VJ (1997) The impact of nosocomial infections on patient outcomes following cardiac surgery. Chest 112:666–675
4. Jacobs P, Noseworthy TW (1990) National estimates of intensive care utilization and costs: Canada and the United States. Crit Care Med 18:1282–1286
5. Barza M (1996) Transmission of antibiotic-resistant bacteria in the ICU. New Horizons 4:333–337
6. Archibald L, Phillips L, Monnet D, McGowan JE, Tenover F, Gaynes R (1997) Antimicrobial resistance in isolates from inpatients and outpatients in the United States: Increasing importance of the intensive care unit. Clin Infect Dis 24:211–215
7. Centers for Disease Control (1993) Nosocomial enterococci resistant to vancomycin – United States – 1989–1993. MMWR 42:597–599
8. Chow JW, Fine MJ, Shlaes DM, et al (1991) Enterobacter bacteremia: clinical features and emergence of antibiotic resistance during therapy. Ann Intern Med 115:585–590
9. Sanders CC, Sanders Jr WE (1985) Microbial resistance to newer generation B-lactam antibiotics: Clinical and laboratory implications. J Infect Dis 151:399–406
10. Berkelman RL, Hughs JM (1993) The conquest of infectious diseases: who are we kidding? Ann Intern Med 119:426–428
11. Lee A (1985) Neglected niches. The microbial ecology of the gastrointestinal tract. Adv Microbial Ecol 8:115–162
12. Van Der Waaij D, Berghuis De Vries JM, Lekkerkerk Van Der Wees JEC (1971) Colonization resistance of the digestive tract in conventional and antibiotic treated mice. J Hyg Camb 69:405–411
13. Van Der Waaij D (1989) The ecology of the human intestine and its consequences for overgrowth by pathogens such as *Clostridium difficile*. Annu Rev Microbiol 43:69–87
14. Marshall JC, Christou NV, Meakins JL (1993) The gastrointestinal tract. The "undrained abscess" of multiple organ failure. Ann Surg 218:111–119
15. Heyland DK, Cook DJ, Jaeschke R, Griffith L, Lee HN, Guyatt GH (1994) Selective decontamination of the digestive tract. An overview. Chest 105:1221–1229

16. Fagon J, Chastre J, Hance AJ, Domart Y, Trouillet J, Gibert C (1993) Evaluation of clinical judgment in the identification and treatment of nosocomial pneumonia in ventilated patients. Chest 103:547–553

17. Sterling TR, Ho EJ, Brehm WT, Kirkpatrick MB (1996) Diagnosis and treatment of ventilator-associated pneumonia – impact on survival. Chest 110:1025–1034

18. Timsit JF, Misset B, Renaud B, Goldstein FW, Carlet J (1997) Effect of previous antimicrobial therapy on the accuracy of the main procedures used to diagnose nosocomial pneumonia in patients who are using mechanical ventilation. Chest 108:1036–1040

19. Montravers P, Fagon JY, Chastre J, et al (1993) Follow-up protected specimen brushes to assess treatment in nosocomial pneumonia. Am Rev Respir Dis 147:38–44

20. Wunderink RG (1998) Attributable mortality of ventilator-associated pneumonia. Sepsis (In Press)

21. Thomas M, Govil S, Moses BV, Joseph A (1996) Monitoring of antibiotic use in a primary and tertiarry care hospital. J Clin Epidemiol 49:251–254

22. Torres A, Aznar R, Gatell JM, et al (1990) Incidence, risk and prognosis factors of nosocomial pneumonia in mechanically ventilated patients. Am Rev Respir Dis 142:523–528

23. Celis R, Torres A, Gatell JM, Almela M, Rodriguez-Roisin R, Agusti-Vidal A (1988) Nosocomial pneumonia. A multivariate analysis of risk and prognosis. Chest 93:318–324

24. Luna C, Vujacich P, Niederman MS, et al (1997) Impact of BAL data on the therapy and outcome of ventilator-associated pneumonia. Chest 111:676–685

25. Rello J, Ausina V, Ricart M, et al (1994) Risk factors for infection by Pseudomonas aeruginosa in patients with ventilator-associated pneumonia. Intensive Care Med 20:193–198

26. Kollef MH, Silver P, Murphy DM, Trovillion E (1995) The effect of late-onset ventilator-associated pneumonia in determining patient mortality. Chest 108:1655–1662

27. Rello J, Ausina V, Ricart M, Castella J, Prats G (1993) Impact of previous antimicrobial therapy on the etiology and outcome of ventilator associated pneumonia. Chest 104:1230–1235

28. Banerjee SN, Emori TG, Culver DH, et al (1997) Secular trends in nosocomial primary bloodstream infection in the United States, 1980–1989. National Nosocomial Infections Surveillance System. Am J Med 91 (suppl 3B):86S–89S

29. Valles J, Leon C, Alvarez-Lerma F (1997) Nosocomial bacteremia in critically ill patients: a multicenter study evaluating epidemiology and prognosis. Clin Infect Dis 24:387–395

30. Pittet D, Thievent B, Wenzel RP, Li N, Auckenthaler R, Suter PM (1996) Bedside prediction of mortality from bacteremic sepsis. A dynamic analysis of ICU patients. Am J Respir Crit Care Med 153:684–693

31. Fagon JY, Novara A, Stephan F, Girou E, Safar M (1994) Mortality attributable to nosocomial infections in the ICU. Infect Control Hosp Epidemiol 15:428–434

32. Rello J, Ricart M, Mirelis B, et al (1994) Nosocomial bacteremia in a medical-surgical intensive care unit: epidemiologic characteristics and factors influencing mortality in 111 episodes. Intensive Care Med 20:94–98

33. Mainous MR, Lipsett PA, O'Brien M (1997) Enterococcal bacteremia in the surgical intensive care unit. Does vancomycin resistance affect mortality? Arch Surg 132:76–81

34. Nathens AB, Rotstein OD, Marshall JC (1998) Tertiary peritonitis: Clinical features of a complex nosocomial infection. World J Surg (In Press)

35. Bohnen JMA, Solomkin JS, Dellinger EP, Bjornson HS, Page CP (1992) Guidelines for clinical care: Anti-infective agents for intra-abdominal infection. A Surgical Infection Society policy statement. Arch Surg 127:83–89

36. Rotstein OD, Pruett TL, Simmons RL (1986) Microbiologic features and treatment of persistent peritonitis in patients in the intensive care unit. Can J Surg 29:247–250

37. Marshall JC, Cook DJ, Christou NV, Bernard GR, Sprung CL, Sibbald WJ (1995) Multiple organ dysfunction score: A reliable descriptor of a complex clinical outcome. Crit Care Med 23:1638–1652

Nosocomial Sinusitis:
A Critical Appraisal of the Evidence

T. Sinuff and D. J. Cook

Introduction

Nosocomial sinusitis has long been established as a complication of endotracheal intubation, predominantly the nasotracheal route, in critically ill patients. Prolonged intubation causes direct irritation of the nasal mucosa, resulting in sufficient edema to occlude the maxillary sinus ostium. With the advent of low pressure cuffs, prolonged nasotracheal intubation occurs regularly. The combination of these two factors predisposes to the development of paranasal sinusitis. The diagnosis of nosocomial sinusitis is difficult, and often unrecognized, because of its subtle presentation. In contrast to outpatient acute sinusitis, which commonly presents with overt clinical symptoms, paranasal sinusitis in the critically ill is often clinically silent, and the presenting manifestation may be fever or sepsis. Symptoms of headache, facial pain, localized swelling and complaints of purulent nasal discharge are either absent or difficult to elicit in a critically ill intubated patient. Moreover, the sequelae can be catastrophic [1]. There is often a further dilemma in diagnosis since on clinical grounds we do not do routine computerized tomography (CT) scans of the sinuses or sinus aspiration for definitive diagnosis of sinusitis. Consequently, it has been difficult to elucidate the true incidence of nosocomial sinusitis, and the best method of diagnosis. In recent intensive care literature, there has been a resurgence of interest in paranasal sinusitis as an important factor in the etiology of infections in the intensive care unit (ICU), because of new evidence indicating that it is a major risk factor in nosocomial pneumonia [2, 3, 4].

Epidemiology

Dating back to the early 1970s, paranasal sinusitis in mechanically ventilated patients was recognized increasingly as an important nosocomial infection and a source of sepsis in the ICU patient. Initially, there were several case reports of paranasal sinusitis associated with nasotracheal intubation first reported only in the anesthesia literature [5, 6], and soon followed by reports in the medical literature [7, 8]. Since these case reports, there have been numerous studies characterizing paranasal sinusitis in the ICU population. These have been varied for two main reasons: First the patient population studied has been fairly heterogeneous; and second, patients were thought predominantly to be from high risk groups, such as head injury, trauma, and burn patients admitted to a critical care setting. Many critically ill partients with sinusitis often have other concurrent infections and, as such, the exact role of sinusitis as the primary or only source of occult, unexplained, or ongoing fever has not been well characterized and is rather controversial. However, the early work by Caplan and Hoyt [1], O'Reilly et al. [9], Grindlinger et al. [10], and Deutschman et al. [11], studied nosocomial sinusitis associated with naso-pharyngeal intubation. These studies elucidated a closer association of paranasal sinusitis (predominantly maxillary) with unexplained fever in certain ICU popula-tions. Maxillary sinusitis accounts for 85% of the paranasal sinusitis in ICU patients [12]. These prospective cohort studies used either plain roentgenograms [1] or CT [9, 10, 11] of the paranasal sinuses as part of their diagnostic protocol. In most cases, the portable plain roentgenogram method was used because of the hemodynamic and respiratory instability of the population studied. Plain radiographs taken at the bedside were performed with Water's view technique and were sufficient for exami-nation of the maxillary sinuses. Sinusitis was consistently judged to be present if roentgenograms showed either an air-fluid level or complete opacification of one or more sinuses. Diagnosis was made only when roentgenographic findings consistent with acute sinusitis were confirmed with purulent material aspirated from the in-volved sinus, or purulent nasal discharge was present. This is a fundamental point as radiologic signs of sinusitis alone, such as mucosal thickening, opacification of spa-ces or air-fluid levels in the sinus cavity, are a non-specific and common finding in mechanically ventilated patients regardless of the mode of intubation [13, 14].

The radiologic signs described above do not imply a bacterial infection, as the differential diagnosis is broad. However, radiographic signs may be precursors of infection in this particular setting. Therefore, radiologic suspicion of sinusitis should be distinguished from infectious maxillary sinusitis, the latter being defined by positive cultures from sinus aspirate. These studies, as well as subsequent investi-gations of nosocomial sinusitis have used sinus aspiration for culture to correlate clinical and radiologic suspicion of sinusitis. Sinusitis aspiration must be performed aseptically to prevent contamination by nosocomial bacteria that have colonized the nasopharynx in ICU patients, but are not pathologic.

Since these early clinical studies, more recent investigations from 1987 to 1992 have utilized CT scans to a greater degree to aid in the radiographic diagnosis of sinusitis. The value of conventional sinus radiography has been demonstrated to be limited in both the outpatient and ICU settings [15]. CT scans have associated sensi-tivities of approximately 66–80%, although the specificity remains low [15]. CT scans are better than radiographs for the evaluation of the sphenoid, ethmoid, and frontal sinuses, together with the maxillary sinuses [15]. The drawback, however, is that an unstable patient must be taken to the radiology department, at some increas-ed risk from the transport. Therefore, if maxillary sinusitis has been demonstrated to account for approxinately 85% of cases of paranasal sinusitis, and portable plain radiographic analysis is sufficient, is the added risk to the patient warranted? There have been no studies, to date, directly comparing the utility of CT scan versus plain radiograph in the ICU patient and any resulting differences in diagnostic efficacy, treatment, morbidity, or mortality.

In 1987, Humphrey et al. [16], prospectively investigated paranasal sinusitis as an important source of sepsis and morbidity in head injured patients. This was a methodologically sound, prospective cohort study in which 208 consecutive head-injured patients were followed for 36 months. A diagnosis of nosocomial sinusitis was made in 24, an incidence of 11%. In these patients, sinusitis was suspected when opacification or an air fluid level persisted on CT scan and the patient remained febrile despite culture-specific antibiotic treatment of concurrent infections. In every patient, the diagnosis was confirmed only when purulent material was aspirated from an involved sinus. Air fluid levels were present on the initial CT scan in 17 (8%) patients. All patients were persistently febrile (T > 38.5 °C) and had a leukocytosis (WBC count > 10 500/mm³), which were not part of the initial inclusion criteria.

In 1988, a group of investigators from France [17] prospectively studied 35 critically ill patients intubated by the nasotracheal route for at least eight days. All patients had a CT scan of their paranasal sinuses with radiologic presence of opacity or an air fluid level within the sinuses. A sinus aspirate was performed to confirm the diagnosis of sinusitis. CT scan revealed sinusitis in 23 (66%) patients and pathological bacteria were isolated in 31 patients. In addition, all patients had persistent fever.

When analyzing any body of research for possible implementation into practice, it is useful to critically appraise it to determine its validity and to understand the results, then whether, and if so, how, the results of the research can be applied in practice. Well established guides for determining the validity of diagnostic tests [21] can be applied to the above four studies.

Is there an Independent, Blind Comparison with a Reference Standard?

The first critical appraisal guide for a diagnosis article is to determine whether there is an independent, blind comparison with a reference standard. In these studies, the reference standard for the diagnosis of paranasal sinusitis is sinus aspiration, while the initial screening test is radiographic evaluation. Here, verification bias [21] is avoided because all patients in the cohort identified by the inclusion criteria received both radiographic evaluation and confirmatory sinus aspiration. This was rigorously met by all the studies. One limitation, however, is that within Grindlinger and colleagues' analysis [10], a combination of plain sinus films and CT scans was used. It then becomes difficult to determine which investigation can be utilized with a high enough sensitivity relative to the reference standard.

Did the Patient Sample Include an Appropriate Spectrum of Patients to Whom the Diagnostic Test will be Applied in Clinical Practice?

This critical appraisal guide is to evaluate whether the patient sample includes an appropriate spectrum of patients to whom the diagnostic test will be applied in clinical practice. The individual studies examined a specific group of ICU patients at high risk of developing nosocomial sinusitis, within their individual ICUs. Therefore, the spectrum of patients studied may not delineate the patients at risk in any given ICU. This becomes more relevant to the issue of generalizability, and less crucial to the issue of validity because the studies, in combination, cover a rather broad spectrum of high risk patients, provided they meet independently the criteria for validity.

Did the Results of the Test being Evaluated Influence the Decision to Perform the Reference Standard?

This guide helps determine whether the results of the test being evaluated influence the decision to perform the reference standard. All studies rigorously adhered to the issue of performing the reference standard on all patients that had the initial radiographic evaluation.

Were the Methods for Performing the Test Described in Sufficient Detail to Permit Replication?

The final guide asks whether the methods for performing the test are described in sufficient detail to permit replication. While the radiographic evaluation was described in sufficient detail by all investigators, only one study [16] described the method of sinus aspiration. This is an important consideration, as improper technique can result in contamination of the aspirate and, potentially, incorrect diagnosis.

In summary, overall the studies were well performed, valid, and have offered much insight into the nature of paranasal sinusitis in the ICU patient. Furthermore, they defined important diagnostic parameters for the foundation of subsequent randomized trials.

Recent randomized controlled trials (RCTs), are more powerful designs to evaluate the relationship between nasotracheal (NT) intubation and orotracheal (OT) intubation. There have been five prospective RCTs on NT versus OT intubation evaluating the outcome of nosocomial sinusitis [2, 3, 18–20] (Table 1).

Bach et al. [18] conducted an RCT enrolling 68 post-operative patients requiring mechanical ventilation for more than four days. After an initial radiograph demonstrating no pathologic findings in the paranasal sinuses, patients were assigned randomly to one of two groups. In one group, OT intubation was continued, and in the other group, the original method of endotracheal intubation was changed to the NT route. All patients had a nasogastric tube in place for enteral feeding. Patients were screened for sinusitis with bedside AP plain radiograph of the skull on the fourth, seventh, and tenth post-operative days, and at weekly intervals thereafter. Patients who developed signs of infection with no apparent source were subjected to CT scan of the head, amongst other investigations, to rule out all other possible sources of infection. Sinusitis was suspected if radiologic examination showed opacification of sinuses or air fluid levels. Diagnosis was made if there were positive radiographic signs associated with fever ($T > 38.5\,^{\circ}C$), leukocytosis (WBC count $> 15 \times 10^{-9}$), and confirmed with needle aspirate and culture positive of at least one pathologic microorganism. Of the 68 patients, 15 (22%) patients in the OT group and 25 (37%) patients in the NT group developed radiologic signs of sinus infection. A suspected diagnosis was confirmed by sinus needle aspirate and culture in 2 of the

Table 1. Randomized controlled trials of oral versus nasal intubation in nosocomial sinusitis

Author (year)	Population	Sinusitis definition	Patients with NTI (%)	Patients with OTI (%)	p value
Bach et al. (1992) [18]	SICU MV > 4 days	– bedside sinus x-ray – sinus puncture	RS: 25/36 (69.4) IS: 29/36 (41.7)	RS: 15/32 (46.8) IS: 2/32 (6.2)	not specified <0.01
Salord et al. (1990) [19]	ICU MV > 2 days	– bedside sinus x-ray	RS: 25/58 (43.1)	RS: 1/52 (1.8)	< 0.001
Michelson et al. (1992) [20]	SICU MV duration not specified	– bedside sinus US – sinus puncture in some positive US	RS: 19/20 (95) IS: 7/13 (53.8)	RS: 5/24 (62.5) IS: 2/9 (22.2	<0.03 <0.3
Holzapfel et al. (1993) [2]	ICU MV > 7 days	– CI scan sinuses – sinus puncture	RS: 45/149 (30.2) IS: 25/149 (19.4)	RS: 33/151 (28.3) IS: 25/151 (16.5)	0.08 0.75
Rouby et al. (1994) [3]	SICU MV > 7 days	– CT scan sinuses – sinus puncture	RS: 21/22 (95.5) IS: not specified	RS: 4/18 (22.5) IS: not specified	<0.001

SICU: surgical intensive care unit; ICU: intensive care unit; MV: mechanical ventilation; NTI: nasotracheal intubation; OTI: orotracheal intubation; RS: radiographic sinusitis; IS: infectious sinusitis; US: ultrasound

15 (6%) patients in the OT group and 15 of the 25 (42%) in the NT group (p<0.01). Both patients in the OT group developed culture confirmed sinusitis on the side of insertion of the nasogastric tube.

This study further substantiated the increase in incidence of sinusitis associated with NT intubation. Bach et al. [18] suggested that the incidence of sinusitis in oro-tracheally intubated patients may actually be attributed to the placement of naso-gastric tubes. Moreover, this work further substantiates that the diagnosis can only be made by a combination of radiologic examination, microbial culture, and clinical parameters of infection, such as fever and leukocytosis in a clinical situation where no other infection can be isolated. This also confirms previous work done by Salord et al. [19].

Michelson and colleagues [20] randomized 44 patients to OT intubation (N = 24) versus NT intubation (N = 20) post-operatively. Daily ultrasound scans of the maxil-lary sinuses were performed. Patients with positive sinus ultrasounds had a diagno-stic sinus aspiration for confirmation of the radiographic findings. Initially, 15 of the 24 (63%) patients with OT intubation compared to 19 of the 20 (95%) patients with NT inhibation demonstrated radiographic sinusitis (p < 0.03). Diagnostic aspiration was performed in only 22 (13 nasally and 9 orally intubated) of the 34 patients with positive radiographic findings. Of this group, sinus aspirates confirmed the presence of pathologic organisms in 7/13 nasotracheally intubated patients and 2/9 patients with oral tubes (p < 0.3). This study, therefore, although suggestive that NT intubation increases the risk of nosocomial sinusitis compared to OT intubation, was under powered to substantiate previously established differences.

Holzapfel et al. [2] and Rouby et al. [3] utilized CT scans in their trials and sinus aspiration consistently in all patients as per a protocol outlined in their studies. Holzapfel and colleagues [2] randomized 300 patients in the setting of a general adult ICU, with a foreseeable need for mechanical ventilation for more than 7 days. The study population was heterogeneous with reasons for admission including coma, pneumonia, infection, surgery, and trauma. Patients received daily chest radiographs and CT scans of their sinuses every 7 days routinely, or earlier if the temperature was greater than 38 °C or purulent nasal discharge was noted. Patients with signs on CT of air fluid level or opacification within a maxillary sinus along with a temperature > 38 °C all had sinus aspiration for culture and quantification, with drain insertion. Nosocomial sinusitis was diagnosed only when all of the following criteria were met: sinus CT scan findings consistent with sinusitis (air-fluid level and/or opacification); mechanical ventilation for at least 48 hours; purulent sinus aspiration; and quantitative culture of the aspirated material with > 10^3 colony-forming units/mL.

Radiographic sinusitis was observed in 78 patients: 45 (30%) in the NT intubated group and 33 (22%) in the OT intubated group (p = 0.08). Following sinus aspiration, however, 54 patients met the criteria outlined above for a diagnosis of infectious sinusitis, with 29 (19%) in the NT intubated group and 25 (17%) in the OT intubated group. This difference was not statistically significant (p = 0.75). In this RCT, radiographic sinusitis occurred more frequently than infectious sinusitis, confirming Michelson's data [20], but with a higher powered study with more stringent diagnostic criteria.

Finally, Rouby and colleagues [3] studied 162 consecutive surgical ICU patients who were mechanically ventilated for a period of more than 7 days. All patients had CT scans of their sinuses within 48 hours of admission to the ICU. These patients were subsequently divided into 3 groups according to radiographic findings of their sinuses: Group 1 – normal maxillary sinuses (40 patients), group 2 – maxillary mucosal thickening (26 patients), group 3 – radiologic maxillary sinusitis (96 patients). Patients with normal maxillary sinuses were randomized to either NT or OT intubation. This group was subsequently followed with CT scan at day 7 and had sinus aspiration if radiographic changes were present. Patients from group 2 were followed prospectively in their original group. All patients from group 3 underwent sinus aspiration. A management protocol of nasal disinfection was followed with a drain left in the sinus cavity. Sinus aspirates were cultured and quantified. Diagnostic criteria for infectious maxillary sinusitis included sinus aspirate containing > 5 polymorphonuclear cells per high powered field and a positive culture. A separate group of non-intubated patients served as control.

In the randomized group, the incidence of radiographic maxillary sinusitis was 21/22 (95.5%) in patients with NT intubation compared to 4/18 (22.5%) in patients with OT intubation (p < 0.001). After sinus aspiration, however, fewer patients actually had infectious maxillary sinusitis. However, the exact number of patients in the randomized group with infectious sinusitis is not specified. These data were grouped and reported in terms of all 3 groups, without specification of the route of intubation. Thus, although a well designed study, in the final analysis, the exact extent of the correlation between infectious sinusitis in NT intubated patients compared to OT intubated patients is unknown.

The three last studies described above demonstrated a non-significant trend in favor of OT with respect to lower rates of infectious sinusitis, compared to the findings of Salord et al. [19] and Bach et al. [18]. This is an important issue and because of variations in study design, it is difficult to compare these studies. However, the differences in study results between these two groups of studies may reflect the fact that higher powered multicentered RCTs with standardized design protocols are required to confirm whether there is a true difference in sinusitis due to the two different methods of intubation.

With previous suggestions that nosocomial sinusitis is a risk factor for the development of nosocomial pneumonia, both Holzapfel et al. [2] and Rouby et al. [3] sought to evaluate the incidence of pneumonia associated with sinusitis in their study populations. Holzapfel and colleagues [2] demonstrated, with multivariate analysis, that sinusitis increased the risk of nosocomial pneumonia by a factor of 3.8. Rouby et al. [3] showed that nosocomial pneumonia occurred more frequently in patients with infectious sinusitis than in those with radiographic sinusitis (67% versus 43%, $p < 0.02$).

As with the previous non-randomized trials, it is important to apply guides for determining the validity of these RCT's. Here, we can consider the following guides [22]:
1) was the assignment of patients to treatments randomized?
2) were all patients who entered the trial properly accounted for and attributed at its conclusion? Was follow up complete? Were patients analyzed in the groups to which they were randomized?
3) were patients, health workers, and study personnel "blind" to treatment?
4) were the groups similar at the start of the trial?
5) aside from the experimental intervention, were the groups treated equally?

Working through these guidelines, most of the above RCTs fulfill the criteria for validity. Double blinding in this situation is difficult since the physicans treating these patients must be aware of the results of all the tests. Therefore, in these studies, the radiologists reading the sinus radiographs or CT scans were blinded to any information on the patients. These RCTs were rigorously performed in a setting in which it is often difficult to perform methodologically sound clinical trials, owing to the complexity of these patients and the vast potential for bias and confounders.

Conclusion

Nosocomial sinusitis will continue to be an important infection to diagnose among ICU patients, given the frequency of nasotracheal intubation and the use of nasogastric enteral feeding tubes. Nosocomial sinusitis is a cause of unrecognized fever in some critically ill patients, and a high index of suspicion is warranted for its diagnosis. Current diagnostic approaches vary, and surveillance testing is not standardized, nor recommended. The relation between radiographic sinusitis and clinical sinusitis is, moreover, unclear. The precise contribution of sinusitis to the development of nosocomial pneumonia warrants further investigation.

References

1. Caplan ES, Hoyt NS (1982) Nosocomial sinusitis. JAMA 247:639–641
2. Holzapfel L, Chevret S, Madinier G, et al (1993) Incidence of long term oro-or nasotracheal intubation on nosocomial maxillary sinusitis and pneumonia. Results of a randomized clinical trial. Crit Care Med 21:1132–1138
3. Rouby JJ, Laurent P, Gasnach M, et al (1994) Risk factors and clinical relevance of nosocomial maxillary sinusitis in the critically ill. Am J Respir Crit Care Med 150:776–783
4. Bert F, Lambert-Zechovsky N (1995) Pneumonia associated with nosocomial sinusitis: a different risk according to the pathogen involved. Am J Respir Crit Care Med 152:1422–1423
5. Arens FT, LeJeune FE, Webre DR (1974) Maxillary sinusitis, a complication of nasotracheal intubation. Anaesthesiology 4:415–416
6. Gallagher T, Civetta J (1976) Acute maxillary sinusitis complicating nasotracheal intubation: a case report. Anesth Anal 55:885–886
7. Pope TE Jr, Stelling CB, Leitnem YB (1981) Maxillary sinusitis after nasotracheal intubation. South Med J 74:610–612
8. Knodel AR, Beekman JF (1982) Unexplained fevers in patients with nasotracheal intubation. JAMA 248:868–870
9. O'Reilly MJ, Reddick EJ, Black W, et al (1984) Sepsis from sinusitis in nasotracheally intubated patients. Am J Surg 147:601–604
10. Grindlinger GA, Niehoff J, Hughes SL, Humphrey MA, Simpson G (1987) Acute paranasal sinusitis related to nasotracheal intubation of head injured patients. Crit Care Med 5:214–217
11. Deutschman CS, Wilton P, Sinow J, Thienprasit P, Konstantinides FN, Cerra FB (1985) Paranasal sinusitis: a common complication of nasotracheal intubation in neurosurgical patients. Neurosurgery 17:296–299
12. Michelson A, Schuster B, Kamp HD (1992) Paranasal sinusitis associated with nasotracheal and orotracheal long term intubation. Arch Otolaryngol Head Neck Surg 118:937–939
13. Chideckel N, Jensen C, Axelsson A, Gregelins N (1970) Diagnosis of fluid in the maxillary sinus. Acta Radiologica Diag 10:433–440
14. Illum P, Jeppesen F, Langebaek E (1972) X-ray examination and sinoscopy in maxillary sinus disease. Acta Otolaryngol 75:287–292
15. Bilaniuk LT, Zimmerman RA (1982) Computed tomography in evaluation of the paranasal sinuses. Radiol Clin North Am 20:51–66
16. Humphrey MA, Simpson GT, Grindlinger GA (1987) Clinical characteristics of nosocomial sinusitis. Ann Otol Rhinol Laryngol 96:687–690
17. Guerin JM, Meyer P, Habib Y, Levy C (April 1993) Purulent rhinosinusitis is also a cause of sepsis in critically ill patients. Chest 93:893–898
18. Bach A, Boehrer H, Schmidt H, Geiss HK (1992) Nosocomial sinusitis in ventilated patients nasotracheal versus orotracheal intubation. Anaesthesia 47:335–339
19. Salord F, Gaussorgues P, Marti-Flich J, et al (1990) Nosocomial maxillary sinusitis during mechanical ventilation: a prospective comparison of orotracheal versus the nasotracheal route for intubation. Intensive Care Med 16:390–393
20. Michelson A, Kamp HD, Schuster B (1991) Sinusitis in long term intubated, intensive care patients: nasal versus oral intubation. Anaesthesist 40:100–104
21. Jaeschke R, Guyatt G, Sackett DL, for the evidence-based medicine working group (1994) Users' guides to the medical literature. III. How to use an article about a diagnostic test. A. Are the results of the study valid? JAMA 271 (5):389–391
22. Guyatt G, Sackett DL, Cook DJ, for the evidence-based working group (1993) Users' guides to the medical literature. II. How to use an article about therapy or prevention. A. Are the results of the study valid? JAMA 270 (21):2598–2601

The Importance of Initial Empiric Antibiotic Selection in Ventilator-Associated Pneumonia

M. H. Kollef

Introduction

Nosocomial pneumonia is the leading cause of death from hospital-acquired infections [1,2]. The estimated prevalence of nosocomial pneumonia within the intensive care unit (ICU) setting ranges from 10 to 65%, with case fatality rates greater than 25% in most studies [3–6]. Ventilator-associated pneumonia (VAP) specifically refers to pneumonia developing in mechanically ventilated patients later than 48 hours after intubation (i.e., late-onset VAP with no clinical evidence suggesting the presence or likely development of pneumonia at the time of intubation) [7]. VAP occurring within 48 hours of intubation is frequently due to aspiration, and is usually associated with a better prognosis compared to late-onset VAP which is more often due to antibiotic-resistant bacteria [7–9]. The clinical importance of VAP is demonstrated by several investigations suggesting that its occurrence is an independent determinant of mortality for critically ill patients requiring mechanical ventilation [10, 11].

Recently, a consensus appears to be emerging regarding the variability present among the different etiologic bacterial agents of VAP and their propensity to cause patient deaths [8–18]. In general, these reports suggest that specific bacterial pathogens which are associated with high levels of antibiotic resistance, [e.g., *Pseudomonas aeruginosa*, *Acinetobacter* species, and methicillin-resistant *Staphylococcus aureus* (MRSA)] are associated with greater mortality rates compared to more antibiotic sensitive pathogens [e.g., *Haemophilus influenza* and methicillin-sensitive *Staphylococcus aureus* (MSSA)]. Even within the same bacterial species, those bacteria possessing antibiotic-resistance are frequently associated with greater mortality rates in patients with VAP, as well as in patients with other nosocomial infections, compared to antibiotic-sensitive strains of the same bacteria [16, 19, 20]. Recently, several groups of investigators have demonstrated that patients with VAP receiving inadequate antibiotic therapy, based on the findings of lower airway cultures obtained by either bronchoalveolar lavage (BAL), a protected specimen brush (PSB), or tracheal aspirates, have a greater mortality rate compared to patients receiving antibiotics to which the isolated bacteria were sensitive [21–24]. More importantly, these studies also suggest that the increased risk of mortality persists despite changing antibiotic therapy based on the findings of the lower airway cultures. The various authors of these studies independently concluded that the microbiologic etiology of VAP, and the antimicrobial resistance patterns of the isolated pathogens, represent important determinants of patient outcomes.

The purpose of this chapter is to review the four recent clinical studies which highlight the importance of the initial empiric antibiotic selection for the treatment of VAP [21–24]. The findings of these outcome investigations are remarkably similar, despite their wide geographic representation, and their results are probably applicable to most ICU settings caring for patients with VAP. The overall additive importance of these studies is that they may suggest new strategies for the administration of antibiotics in patients with suspected VAP in order to improve their outcome.

Literature Review

South American Perspective

Luna and colleagues [21] examined 132 patients requiring mechanical ventilation with clinically suspected VAP in a medical-surgical ICU. All 132 patients underwent bronchoscopy with BAL. Sixty-five (49.2%) patients had a microbiologically positive BAL culture. The BAL-positive patients had no difference in hospital mortality, prior antibiotic use, and demographic characteristics compared to the patients with no identified pathogens from their BAL cultures (i.e., BAL-negative patients). A total of 50 BAL-positive patients received empiric antibiotic therapy prior to bronchoscopy. However, within this group, patients receiving adequate antibiotic therapy (n = 16), based on the culture results of the BAL fluid, had a significantly lower mortality rate compared to patients receiving inadequate antibiotic therapy (n = 34, 37.5% versus 91.2%; p < 0.001, (Fig. 1). The mortality rate of the patients receiving inadequate antibiotic therapy was also greater than the mortality rate of patients receiving no empiric antibiotic therapy prior to BAL (n = 15), however this difference was not statistically significant (p = 0.372).

Subsequent changes in antibiotic therapy, following the results of the bronchoscopically obtained BAL cultures, did not appear to alter the outcomes of the BAL-positive patients. More of these patients received adequate antibiotic therapy following the results of the BAL cultures (42 of 65 patients), however their mortality rate was similar to the mortality rate of patients continuing to receive inadequate antibiotic therapy following the BAL culture results (71.4% versus 69.6%, p = 0.899).

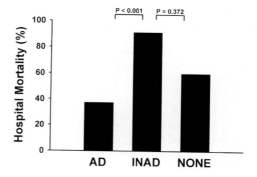

Fig. 1. Hospital mortality rates according to whether patients received adequate (AD) empiric antibiotic treatment prior to obtaining lower airway culture results, inadequate (INAD) antibiotic treatment, or no empiric antibiotics (none). (From [21] with permission)

Overall, it appeared that the identification of Gram-negative bacteria with resistance to broad-spectrum cephalosporin antibiotics and the presence of MRSA in the BAL cultures accounted for the majority of the inadequate antibiotic regimens. Finally, these authors [21] also found that there was no difference in the pathogens recovered from the BAL cultures among patients receiving prior antibiotic therapy compared to patients not having received prior antibiotics (p > 0.05).

European Perspective

Two studies from Spain have examined the influence of the adequacy of initial empiric antibiotic therapy on the outcomes of patients with VAP. The first study by Alvarez-Lerma and coworkers [22] followed 530 patients who developed 565 episodes of pneumonia (91.9% during mechanical ventilation) in the ICU setting. Empiric antibiotics were administered during 490 (86.7%) of the 565 episodes of suspected nosocomial pneumonia. The appropriateness of the empiric antibiotic treatment was assessed using the results of cultures obtained from tracheal aspirates or expectorated sputum, blood or pleural fluid specimens, and from BAL fluid or PSB samples. Among the 565 episodes of nosocomial pneumonia acquired in the ICU, 430 (76.1%) cases were evaluated for the appropriateness of the prescribed empiric antibiotic regimen. The remaining patients were excluded due to the lack of a definitive diagnosis in 116 cases and no prescribed antibiotic treatment in the remaining 19 cases. Inadequate antibiotic treatment was assessed to be present in 146 (34.0%) of the 430 evaluated cases. Table 1 provides the outcome data for these patients according to the appropriateness of their initial empiric antibiotic therapy.

In 214 episodes of ICU-acquired pneumonia treated initially with empiric antibiotic therapy, a change in the subsequent antibiotic regimen occurred. The indications for changing antibiotics in these patients included the following: The isolation of uncovered microorganisms from the available cultures (62.1%); poor clinical response suggesting the possibility of a treatment failure (36.0%); detection of a resistant bacterial strain during treatment (6.5%); and a miscellaneous category

Table 1. Outcomes of patients with nosocomial pneumonia according to the adequacy of the initial empiric antibiotic regimen. (From [22] with permission)

Outcome	Adequate initial empiric antibiotic therapy (n = 284)	Inadequate initial emipiric antibiotic therapy (n = 146)	p value
Attributable mortality, n (%)	46 (16.2)	36 (24.7)	0.039
Crude mortality, n (%)	92 (32.4)	51 (34.9)	NS
Shock, n (%)	49 (17.3)	42 (28.8)	<0.005
Empyema, n (%)	10 (3.5)	6 (4.1)	NS
No. of complications per patient	1.73 ± 1.82	2.25 ± 1.98	<0.001
Gastrointestinal bleeding, n (%)	30 (10.6)	31 (21.2)	0.003
Multiple organ failure, n (%)	36 (12.7)	31 (21.2)	NS

(11.7%). In 35 cases, more than one indication for an antibiotic change was identified. Multivariate analysis found that the presence of microorganisms in clinical cultures uncovered by the initial empiric antibiotic regimen, the administration of more than one antibiotic, and the previous use of antibiotics were independently associated with modification of the initial empiric antibiotic regimen.

Rello et al. [23] described 113 ventilated patients judged to have VAP on the basis of clinical criteria. In 100 (88.5%) of these patients an etiologic agent for VAP was established using cultures from either blood, pleural fluid, or lower airway secretions obtained bronchoscopically using BAL or a PSB. Antibiotic therapy was changed on the basis of the culture results in 51 (51.0%) microbiologically-positive patients. Among the patients undergoing a change in their antibiotic regimens, 27 (52.9%) were changed due to the presence of inadequate antibiotic therapy based on the isolated pathogens. The most common reason for inadequate initial empiric antibiotic therapy was the isolation of *Pseudomonas aeruginosa* resistant to at least one of the prescribed antibiotics in 20 (74.1%) cases. The crude and related mortality rates of the patients with inadequate therapy was found to be significantly greater than the respective mortality rates of patients receiving adequate initial empiric antibiotics (Fig. 2).

North American Experience

Kollef and Ward [24] investigated 130 mechanically ventilated patients with clinically identified VAP in a medical ICU. Mini-BAL was performed in all patients at the time that VAP was suspected using a previously described technique [25]. Sixty (46.2%) patients had a positive mini-BAL culture yielding at least one potential pathogen accounting for the episode of VAP. Among these 60 patients with microbiologically-positive mini-BAL cultures, 44 (73.3%) were classified as receiving inadequate antibiotic therapy (i.e., identification of a microorganism resistant to the empiric antibiotic regimen). Seven additional patients not prescribed initial empiric antibiotic treatment were also found to have pathogens in their mini-BAL cultures. The hospital mortality rate of these 51 patients, requiring a change or start of antibiotic therapy, was significantly greater than the mortality rate of patients having no

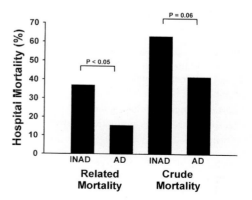

Fig. 2. Related and crude hospital mortality rates plotted according to the adequacy of the initially prescribed empiric antibiotic regimen in patients with microbiologically positive ventilator-associated pneumonia. INAD = inadequate antibiotic treatment. AD = adequate antibiotic treatment

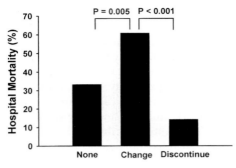

Fig. 3. Mortality rates are plotted in relation to antibiotic management changes made following the results of mini-BAL cultures. "None" indicates that no changes occurred; "Change" indicates that antibiotic therapy was started or changed; and "Discontinue" indicates that antibiotic therapy was stopped altogether following the mini-BAL culture results. BAL = bronchoalveolar lavage. (From [24] with permission)

change in their antibiotic management (n = 51) and patients having their antibiotics discontinued altogether (n = 28) (Fig. 3). In the latter two groups, mini-BAL cultures revealed either no growth or pathogens (n = 70), or pathogens appropriately treated by the initial empiric antibiotic regimen (n = 9). Multiple logistic regression analysis demonstrated that being immunocompromised and receiving inadequate antibiotic therapy (i.e., the presence of a microorganism in the mini-BAL culture resistant to the initially prescribed empiric antibiotic regimen) were variables independently related to the likelihood of hospital mortality (Table 2).

Discussion

In summary, these investigations have demonstrated that an inadequate antibiotic regimen, initiated before obtaining the results of cultures from respiratory secretions, blood, and pleural fluid, was associated with a greater hospital mortality rate

Table 2. Variables independently associated with hospital mortality by logistic regression analysis. (From [24] with permission)

Variable	Adjusted odds ratio	95% CI	p value
Age (1-year increments)	1.01	1.00 to 1.03	0.381
Immunocompromised	2.45	1.56 to 3.85	0.047
Premorbid lifestyle score (1-point increments)	1.18	0.91 to 1.54	0.526
Cancer	2.56	1.51 to 4.36	0.076
Start or change of antibiotic therapy[a]	1.27	0.96 to 1.69	0.394
Receiving inadequate antibiotic therapy[b]	3.28	2.12 to 5.06	0.006
Constant	0.098	0.043 to 0.220	–

[a] Following mini-bronchoalveolar lavage (BAL)
[b] Defined as patients having a microorganism isolated from their mini-BAL cultures resistant to the prescribed antibiotic regiment

compared to an antibiotic regimen which provided adequate antimicrobial coverage of all identified pathogens from the obtained cultures. More importantly, the study by Luna et al. [21] found that subsequent changes in antibiotic therapy, based on the results of BAL cultures, did not reduce the risk of hospital mortality in patients initially prescribed inadequate antibiotic therapy. Although Alvarez-Lerma et al. [22] did not find a significant difference in crude hospital mortality between patients receiving adequate versus inadequate antibiotic therapy, a statistically significant difference in attributable mortality was identified between these two groups (Table 1). The findings from Rello et al. [23] and Kollef et al. [24, 25] confirm the presence of a statistically greater attributable mortality related to VAP in patients with inadequate initial antibiotic therapy compared to patients receiving adequate initial antibiotic treatment. These three studies emphasize the importance of analyzing patient outcomes according to appropriately defined end points (e.g., attributable mortality) in order to determine the actual impact of an intervention on patient outcome. Additionally, these investigations suggest that inadequate antibiotic therapy is most frequently due to the omission of treatment for MRSA or the presence of Gram-negative bacteria with resistance to previously prescribed antibiotics.

The data summarized in these reports support the hypothesis that bacteriologic data obtained from respiratory secretions may not be clinically useful for improving the outcomes of patients with VAP [26]. The absence of a beneficial impact from such bacteriologic data is most likely due to the delay in the availability of the culture results and the antibiotic sensitivities of the identified pathogens (usually available greater than 24 to 48 hours following the cultures). These data also suggest that there is a need to develop a comprehensive clinical approach to the assessment of patients with suspected VAP which is not primarily dependent on the results of cultures obtained from respiratory secretions. Such a clinical approach appears to be necessary in order to optimally determine a patient's requirement for starting antibiotic therapy when VAP is initially suspected, as well as selecting the most appropriate antibiotic regimen. Therefore, based on the experiences of these investigators [21–24], the following recommendations for the empiric treatment of VAP seem reasonable. These recommendations are also consistent with a recent consensus statement on the treatment of VAP published by the American Thoracic Society [27].

First, early use of adequate antibiotic therapy, prior to obtaining culture results appears to have the greatest likelihood of improving patient outcome. Delaying the administration of adequate antibiotic therapy to patients with microbiologically documented VAP is associated with a greater risk of hospital mortality [21–24]. Broad spectrum antibiotic therapy should be started in most patients immediately following a clinical diagnosis of VAP. Cultures of lower airway secretions should primarily be used to confirm the diagnosis of VAP and to allow narrowing of the antimicrobial regimen. Such an approach, based on the initial empiric administration of antibiotics, seems reasonable unless the risks of administering antibiotics are judged to be extreme [28]. Second, the initial selection of empiric antibiotic therapy should be broad enough to insure that adequate coverage of all likely bacterial pathogens is provided. Initial treatment of both Gram-negative bacteria and Gram-positive bacteria, including MRSA, should be provided unless infection due to these organisms is excluded. Given the high yield of Gram's stain examination for Gram-positive cocci in the tracheal aspirates and BAL fluid of patients with VAP due to

Staphylococcus aureus, initial administration of vancomycin should be considered in all patients with Gram-positive cocci identified in their respiratory secretions [29]. Third, the prior use of antibiotics is common among critically ill patients presenting with a clinical picture suggestive of VAP. Therefore, bacterial resistance to a previously prescribed class of antibiotics should be suspected when selecting an empiric antibiotic regimen until culture results become available. The importance of this last point is highlighted by Alvarez-Lerma et al. [22] who found that the previous use of antibiotics was an independent risk factor for the modification of empiric antibiotic treatment in their patients with VAP.

Several groups of clinical investigators have demonstrated a strong association between prior antibiotic administration and the emergence of VAP, as well as other nosocomial infections, due to antibiotic-resistant bacteria [8–11, 14, 16, 19, 20, 30, 31]. More importantly, infection due to antibiotic-resistant bacteria has been associated with an increased risk of hospital mortality [10–12]. Rello and coworkers [11], using a multivariable analysis, demonstrated that prior antibiotic use was the only variable significantly influencing the risk of death from VAP. Prior antibiotic exposure appears to accelerate the development of antibiotic-resistant infection by selecting bacteria with constitutive and inducible β-lactamases, aminoglycoside modifying enzymes, altered penicillin binding proteins, and membrane porin proteins that confer antibiotic resistance [32]. Many of these properties can be transferred between organisms by plasmids or transposons facilitating the spread of antibiotic resistance within hospitals. Patients in intensive care units are at increased risk of developing antibiotic-resistant bacterial infections [12, 16, 19, 20]. This is in large part due to the frequent administration of antibiotics to this group of patients and the geographic localization of the critically ill within confined areas of the hospital [32].

It is important to note the limitations of the investigations reviewed above, which suggest an association between the presence of inadequate initial empiric antibiotic therapy and increased hospital mortality. First, they represent observational studies and therefore do not prove a causal relationship between these two variables. A randomized clinical trial of patients receiving adequate initial antibiotic therapy compared to standard medical therapy (including the use of inadequate antibiotic therapy) would be a more appropriate design to test this hypothesis. Second, the results of these investigations may not be applicable to other institutions without similar antibiotic practices and bacterial resistance patterns. Finally, various methods were used to establish the diagnosis of VAP, and uniform mortality outcomes (i.e., crude versus attributable) were not examined in these studies. Although these variations may identify different sets of patients with VAP, recent investigations suggest that patient outcomes are similarly predicted by the presence of VAP regardless of the methods used to make the diagnosis [33, 34].

Conclusion

In summary, our present understanding of the treatment of VAP suggests the presence of an association between inadequate initial empiric antibiotic therapy and an increased risk of hospital mortality (Table 3). These data also support the hypothesis

Table 3. Summary of outcome investigations linking inadequate initial empiric antibiotic therapy with increased patient mortality

Authors	Crude mortality rates of patients receiving inadequate antibiotic treatment	Crude mortality rates of patients receiving adequate antibiotic treatment	p value
Luna et al. [21]	92.2% (n = 34)	37.5% (n = 16)	<0.001
Alvarez-Lerma et al. [22]	34.9% (n = 146)	32.4% (n = 284)	0.597
Rello et al. [23]	63.0% (n = 27)	41.5% (n = 58)	0.06
Kollef et al [24]	60.8% (n = 51)	26.6% (n = 79)	0.001
Cumulative results	50.4% (n = 258)	32.7% (n = 437)	0.001

that the method used to establish the diagnosis of VAP may not be important in altering patient outcomes [26]. It appears that the initial selection of empiric antibiotics may be one of the most important determinants of outcome for patients with VAP. However, patient microbiologic surveillance, using lower respiratory tract cultures obtained bronchoscopically or non-bronchoscopically, may be useful to identify early development of resistance to empirically prescribed antibiotics [30]. Clinicians should be aware of these findings when assessing their patient's need for empiric antibiotic therapy as well as the selection of the antibiotic regimen. Future studies are necessary to determine if the early use of adequate empiric antibiotics will result in improved patient outcomes. Until such studies are performed, clinicians should consider the early use of broad-spectrum antibiotic therapy in their patients with clinically suspected late-onset VAP. The initial selection of antibiotics should be based on patient characteristics, institutional resistance patterns, and the patient's prior exposure to specific classes of antibiotics [27]. Figure 4 offers a treatment strategy for patients with suspected VAP based on the data presented in this chapter. Finally, the clinical use of respiratory specimens appears to be most helpful in narrowing the spectrum of antibiotic therapy and should not be routinely used as a means of broadening initially inadequate antibiotic therapy.

References

1. Craven DE, Steger KA, Barber TW (1991) Preventing nosocomial pneumonia: state of the art and perspectives for the 1990s. Am J Med 91:44S–53S
2. Niederman MS, Craven DE, Fein AM, et al (1990) Pneumonia in the critically ill hospitalized patient. Chest 97:170–181
3. Kollef MH (1993) Ventilator-associated pneumonia: a multivariate analysis. JAMA 270: 1965–1970
4. Torres A, Aznar R, Gatell JM, et al (1990) Incidence, risk, and prognosis factors of nosocomial pneumonia in mechanically ventilated patients. Am Rev Respir Dis 142:523–528
5. Craven DE, Kunches LM, Lichtenberg DA, et al (1988) Nosocomial infection and fatality in medical and surgical intensive care unit patients. Arch Intern Med 148:1161–1168
6. Leu HS, Kaiser DL, Mori M, et al (1989) Hospital-acquired pneumonia. Attributable mortality and morbidity. Am J Epidemiol 129:1258–1267

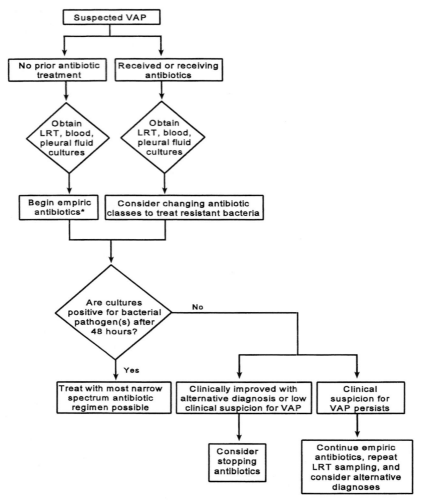

Fig. 4. Strategy for the evaluation and treatment of patients with suspected ventilator-associated pneumonia (VAP). *Initial empiric antibiotic therapy should be based on patient characteristics, the results of Gram's stain examination of respiratory secretions, and the antibiotic susceptibility patterns for pathogenic bacteria at a given institution. LRT = lower respiratory tract

7. Pingleton SK, Fagon JY, Leeper KV Jr (1992) Patient selection for clinical investigation of ventilator-associated pneumonia. Criteria for evaluating diagnostic techniques. Chest 102: 553S–556S
8. Kollef MH, Silver P, Murphy DM, et al (1995) The effect of late-onset ventilator-associated pneumonia in determining patient mortality. Chest 108:1655–1662
9. Rello J, Ausina V, Ricart M, et al (1994) Risk factors for infection by Pseudomonas aeruginosa in patients with ventilator-associated pneumonia. Intensive Care Med 20:193–198
10. Fagon JY, Chastre J, Hance AJ, Montravers P, Novara A, Gilbert C (1993) Nosocomial pneumonia in ventilated patients: a cohort study evaluating attributable mortality and hospital stay. Am J Med 94:281–288

11. Rello J, Ausina V, Ricart M, Castella I, Prats G (1993) Impact of previous antimicrobial therapy on the etiology and outcome of ventilator-associated pneumonia. Chest 104:1230–1235
12. Fagon JY, Chastre J, Domart Y, et al (1996) Mortality due to ventilator-associated pneumonia or colonization with Pseudomonas or Acinetobacter species: assessment by quantitative culture of samples obtained by a protected specimen brush. Clin Infect Dis 23:538–542
13. Stevens RM, Teres D, Skillman JJ, et al (1974) Pneumonia in an intensive care unit. Arch Intern Med 134:106–111
14. Fagon JY, Chastre J, Domart Y, et al (1989) Nosocomial pneumonia in patients receiving continuous mechanical ventilation. Prospective analysis of 52 episodes with use of a protected specimen brush and quantitative culture technique. Am Rev Respir Dis 139:877–884
15. Tillotson JR, Lerner AM (1968) Characteristics of nonbacteremic Pseudomonas pneumonia. Ann Intern Med 68:295–307
16. Rello J, Torres A, Ricart M, et al (1994) Ventilator-associated pneumonia by Staphylococcus aureus. Comparison of methicillin-resistant and methicillin-sensitive episodes. Am J Respir Crit Care Med 150:1545–1549
17. Celis R, Torres A, Gatell JM, Almela M, Rodriguez-Roisin R, Agusti-Vidal A (1988) Nosocomial pneumonia. A multivariate analysis of risk and prognosis. Chest 93:318–324
18. Rello J, Ricart M, Ausina V, et al (1992) Pneumonia due to Haemophilus influenzae among mechanically ventilated patients. Incidence, outcome, and risk factors. Chest 102:1562–1565
19. Chow JW, Fine MJ, Shlaes DM, et al (1991) Enterobacter bacteremia: clinical features and emergence of antibiotic resistance during therapy. Ann Intern Med 115:585–590
20. Meyer KS, Urban C, Eagan JA, et al (1993) Nosocomial outbreak of Klebsiella infection resistant to late-generation cephalosporins. Ann Intern Med 119:353–358,
21. Luna CM, Vujacich P, Niederman MS, et al (1997) Impact of BAL data on the therapy and outcome of ventilator-associated pneumonia. Chest 111:676–685
22. Alvarez-Lerma F (1996) Modification of empiric antibiotic treatment in patients with pneumonia acquired in the intensive care unit. ICU-acquired pneumonia Study Group. Intensive Care Med 22:387–394
23. Rello J, Gallego M, Mariscal D, et al (1997) The value of routine microbial investigation in ventilator-associated pneumonia. Am J Respir Crit Care Med 156:196–200
24. Kollef MH, Ward S (1998) The influence of mini-BAL cultures on patient outcomes: Implications for the antibiotic management of ventilator-associated pneumonia. Chest (In press)
25. Kollef MH, Bock KR, Richards RD, et al (1995) The safety and diagnostic accuracy of minibronchoalveolar lavage in patients with suspected ventilator-associated pneumonia. Ann Intern Med 122:743–748
26. Niederman MS, Torres A, Summer W (1994) Invasive diagnostic testing is not needed routinely to manage suspected ventilator-associated pneumonia. Am J Respir Crit Care Med 150:565–569
27. American Thoracic Society (1995) Hospital-acquired pneumonia in adults: diagnosis, assessment of severity, initial antimicrobial therapy, and preventive strategies. A consensus statement. Am J Respir Crit Care Med 153:1711–1725
28. Baker AM, Bowton DL, Haponik EF (1995) Decision making in nosocomial pneumonia. An analytic approach to the interpretation of quantitative bronchoscopic cultures. Chest 107:85–95
29. Marquette CH, Copin MC, Wallet F, et al (1995) Diagnostic tests for pneumonia in ventilated patients: prospective evaluation of diagnostic accuracy using histology as a diagnostic gold standard. Am J Respir Crit Care Med 151:1878–1888
30. Montravers P, Fagon JY, Chastre J, et al (1993) Follow-up protected specimen brushes to assess treatment in nosocomial pneumonia. Am Rev Respir Dis 147:38–44
31. Petit D, Thievent B, Wenzel RP, et al (1996) Bedside prediction of mortality from bacteremic sepsis. A dynamic analysis of ICU patients. Am J Respir Crit Care Med 153:684–693
32. Jenkins SG (1996) Mechanisms of bacterial antibiotic resistance. New Horizons 4:321–332
33. Timsit JF, Chevret S, Valeke J, et al (1996) Mortality of nosocomial pneumonia in ventilated patients: influence of diagnostic tools. Am J Respir Crit Care Med 154:116–123
34. Bregeon F, Papazian L, Visconti A, et al (1997) Relationship of microbiologic diagnostic criteria to morbidity and mortality in patients with ventilator-associated pneumonia. JAMA 277:655–662

Why, When, and How to Prescribe a Combination of Antibiotics

X. Viviand, S. Arnaud, and C. Martin

Introduction

The aim of antibiotic treatment is to cure infection, documented or not, while fulfilling, if possible, certain conditions: The lowest risk of toxicity; the lowest cost; and the least impact on bacterial ecology in order to limit the emergence of resistant strains.

The decision to use or not to use a combination of antibiotics depends on numerous factors: The bacteria responsible for the infection (some of which are considered as "difficult to treat", e.g., *Pseudomonas aeruginosa*, *Staphylococcus aureus*, *Serratia*, *Enterobacter*); the antibiotics (some can easily induce the emergence of resistant mutants, e.g., fosfomycin, rifampin, fusidic acid and fluoroquinolones); and finally, the patients (sites of infection that are difficult to reach e.g., bone infections, meningitis; foreign body; immunodepression; underlying pathology) [1–5]. The debate over the use of monotherapy (single-drug therapy) or combination therapy would seem to be merely academic when analysis of the patient, site of infection, and bacterial agent(s) potentially responsible is properly performed. Obviously, the first episode of pyelonephritis (very probably caused by *Escherichia coli*) in a 20-year-old immunocompetent woman will be treated and cured without problem by monotherapy using a recent cephalosporin or a fluoroquinolone. Equally evident, a case of septic shock or a severe nosocomial infection, whatever the site, will require, at least at first, a combination of antibiotics.

The aim of this paper is to provide information in order to know why, when and how to prescribe a combination of antibiotics [1–7]. The special problems that are encountered with tuberculosis and brucellosis will not be described here.

Arguments in Favor of the Use of Monotherapy (Single-Drug Therapy)

Obviously, the choice of a monotherapy has undeniable advantages: Reduced cost; absence of interaction between antibiotics; no competition at the elimination site; reduced side effects; and efficacy in numerous situations.

Outside the hospital, the use of monotherapy is almost always the rule. For more severe infections that require hospitalization, monotherapy using a third-generation cephalosporin or a fluoroquinolone can be a very good solution [1, 8, 9] (Table 1). However, in many situations (Tables 2 and 3), monotherpy may not be sufficient:

Table 1. Clinical situations in which serious infections may be treated with a single antibiotic

Background
- No septic shock
- No organ dysfunction
- No immunodepression (?)

Infections
- Meningitis (>2 months and <60 years)
  3rd generation cephalosporin
- Pyelonephritis (1st episode)
  3rd generation cephalosporin or fluoroquinolone
- Typhoid
  fluoroquinolone
- Lower urinary tract infection
  3rd generation cephalosporin or fluoroquinolone

Table 2. Indications for antibiotic combinations (to broaden the spectrum of activity)

- Fever in neutropenic patients
  recent beta-lactam + aminoglycoside or fluoroquinolone + vancomycin
- Septic shock
  recent beta-lactam + aminoglycoside or fluoroquinolone + vancomycin
- Severe infections in neonates
  ampicillin + aminoglycoside + cefotaxime
- Reccurent pyelonephritis
  3rd generation cephalosporin + aminoglycoside or fluoroquinolone
- Severe community acquired pneumonia
  Co amoclav + macrolide
- Bacterial meningitis (>60 years)
  3rd generation cephalosporin + ampicillin
- Peritonitis
  aminoglycoside + imidazole derivative
- Failure of prior monotherapy
- Multifocal infection

- immunodeficiency;
- numerous bacteria responsible for the infection;
- bacteria with reduced sensitivity;
- bacterial inoculum at a very high concentration ($>10^5$ bacteria/ml);
- sites of infection that are difficult to reach;
- difficult to treat bacteria (such as *P. aeruginosa*, *Staphylococcus*, *Enterobacter*).

In such situations, the use of combined antibiotic therapy is considered as providing the following advantages [1, 7]:
- broadening of the spectrum of activity (Table 2);
- a synergistic antibacterial effect with an increase in the rate of bacterial killing (Tables 3, 4, 5);
- prevention or limitation of the risk of selection or the emergence of resistant or mutant strains (Table 4) [10, 11].

Table 3. Indications for antibiotic combinations (synergistic effect)

- *Enterococcus* endocarditis
  penicillin G + aminoglycoside
- Streptococcus prosthesis endocarditis
  penicillin G + aminoglycoside
- Listeriosis
  ampicillin + aminoglycoside
- *Pseudomonas* infection
  beta-lactam + aminoglycoside
- Methicillin resistant Staphylococcus infection
  vancomycin + rifampin

Table 4. Synergistic effects of antibiotic combinations

Combination	Mechanism	Bacteria
beta-lactam + aminoglycoside	increased penetration of aminoglycoside	– Gram + cocci – Gram − bacteria – *Listeria*
vancomycin + aminoglycoside	idem	Gram + cocci
beta-lactam + fosfomycin	inhibition of PBP 2a synthesis	methicillin-resistant Staphylococcus penicillin-resistant Pneumococcus
2 beta-lactams	– inhibition of beta-lactamases – simultaneous effect on several PBP	Gram − bacteria
trimethoprim + sulfamethoxazole	Blockade at two levels of the same metabolic pathway	Gram + bacteria Gram − bacteria
vancomycin + rifampin	?	Staphylococcus
beta-lactam + fluoroquinolone	?	Gram − bacteria

PBP: penicillin binding proteins

Table 5. Possible antagonistic effects of antibiotic combinations

Combinations	Bacteria
aminoglycoside + chloramphenicol	*Proteus mirabilis* *Klebsiella pneumoniae*
ampicillin + chloramphenicol	Pneumococcus *Listeria monocytogenes*, Streptcococcus B
rifampin + beta-lactam vancomycin + rifampin pefloxacin + rifampin	*Staphylococcus aureus*[a]

[a] *In vitro* antagonism, but frequent clinical efficacy

While all of these elements have been proposed, one must not forget that they have all been criticized, that a large number of nuances have clouded interpretation, and that there is no shortage of contradictions between studies [1–7]. Clinically, studies that bring indisputable arguments for the use of a bitherapy are not very numerous and Tables 2 and 3 list some of the accepted indications.

Combinations of Antibiotics and Broadening the Spectrum of Activity [1, 7]

Broadening the spectrum of activity is the most usual justification for combination antibiotic therapy in intensive care and surgical units, as well as hematology and oncology departments. It is also the reason for the great amount of misuse. The use of a combination requires a documented plurimicrobial infection or a severe infection that is potentially plurimicrobial for which treatment must be administered immediately in a life-threatening situation (Table 2). Indications for combination therapy include the following:

1) In neutropenic patients, several studies have shown that monotherapy can be effective e.g., a third-generation cephalosporin, (mainly ceftazidime) or impipenem [1, 12]. However, numerous authors consider that it is better to combine a beta-lactam treatment with a glycopeptide (generally vancomycin) in order to better act on *Staphylococcus* and *Enterococcus*. Moreover, the use of a beta-lactam alone can favor the emergence of resistant strains [13].
2) In septic shock patients, the importance of an antibiotic therapy with a very broad spectrum of activity is evident, justifying a beta-lactam-aminoglycoside (or fluoroquinolone) combination. A glycopeptide can be added as a third partner if a methicillin-resistant staphylococcus is suspected.
3) Severe neonatal infections are often polymicrobial, multiresistant and almost always require urgent empiric therapy. The triple combination of a third-generation cephalosporin-aminoglycoside-ampicillin is efficient on *E. coli*, group B streptococcus and *Listeria monocytogenes.*
4.) After multiple treatments, recurring pyelonephritis requires the use of a combination of antibiotics, e.g., third-generation cephalosporin or fluoroquinolone plus aminoglycoside.
5) In cases of severe and hypoxemic community-acquired pneumonia, the combined responsibility of *Haemophilus influenzae, Streptococcus pneumoniae, Staphylococcus aureus* and intracellular germs, justify the use of the combination amoxicillin-clavulanic acid with a macrolide [14, 15]. Nosocomial pulmonary infections are due to enterobacteria (*E. coli, Klebsiella, Enterobacter, Serratia*), *Pseudomonas* and *Staphylococcus* which is sometimes methicillin-resistant. An anaerobic germ of buccopharyngeal origin is often associated. It is often recommended to add a third-generation cephalosporin, an aminoglycoside (or a fluoroquinolone), an imidazole derivative, or even a glycopeptide [16].
6) In patients over 60 years of age, meningitis is often due to *Listeria monocytogenes* and Gram-negative bacilli. *H. influenzae, S. pneumoniae* and *N. meningitidis* represent less than half the cases. In addition to the usual treatment by a third-generation cephalosporin, an aminopenicillin is systematically used in order to cover *L. monocytogenes.* In nosocomial meningitis, *Klebsiella, E. coli, P. aerugi-*

nosa as well as *S. aureus* (often methicillin-resistant) are the cause. In addition to a third-generation cephalosporin, one can use an aminoglycoside, fosfomycin or a fluoroquinolone. Fosfomycin and/or vancomycin are used in case of *Staphylococcus* infection.

7) For peritoneal infections, the combination usually recommended (aminoglycoside-imidazole or clindamycin) is efficient on aerobic and anaerobic bacteria. The addition of a beta-lactam inhibitor to an aminopenicillin makes it possible to avoid these combinations [17]. Similarly, single-drug therapy could be considered using agents that are active against anaerobic bacteria e.g., cephamycins (cefoxitin, cefotetan, moxalactam) [17], ureidopenicillins, imipenem [18], meropenem [18,19] and piperacillin-tazobactam. In gynecopelvic infections, monotherapy can only be employed if the infection is bacterially documented. However, it may not be considered with empiric treatments that include the combination of a beta-lactam and a cycline or a fluoroquinolone.

8) It is strongly advisable to re-evaluate continuing with a bitherapy for prolonged periods. From day 3 to 5, the physician must re-evaluate his therapeutic strategy based on microbiologic results and clinical evolution. It is then often possible to change to one antibiotic (under the following conditions):
   – bacteria responsible for the infection identified or highly suspected,
   – urinary, abdominal, pulmonary infections,
   – clinical improvement.
   Continuing an antibiotic combination essentially depends on the site (endocarditis, prosthetic infection, brain abscess) and the bacteria (*Pseudomonas*). Even so, the use of aminoglycosides should not be prolonged beyond day 7. Knowing when to reasonably stop therapy is certainly preferable to the "don't change a winning team" attitude in terms of bacterial ecology and in order to conserve the current efficacy of antibiotics.

9) Can new antibiotics with favorable microbiologic properties be used in monotherapy? There are some strong arguments in favor of this attitude [20–26]. Imipenem and other carbapenems have a very broad spectrum of bacterial activity that covers aerobic-anaerobic Gram-negative bacilli (*Enterobacter, Haemophilus*), strictly aerobic bacteria (*Pseudomonas, Acinetobacter*), Gram-positive cocci (*Staphylococcus, Streptococcus, E. faecalis*), strictly anaerobic Gram-positive and Gram-negative bacteria. However, there are several gaps: *X. maltophilia, P. cepacia, E. faecium* and especially methicillin-resistant staphylococci. The hydrolysis stability to beta-lactamases is excellent. Only the beta-lactamases of *X. maltophilia, P. cepacia*, a beta-lactamase of *B. fragilis* and one of *Aeromonas hydrophilia* can hydrolyze these antibiotics. Bacterial killing is powerful, rapid, concentration-dependent (except for *P. aeruginosa*) approaching that of aminoglycosides and fluoroquinolones. Carbapenems have very little sensitivity to the inoculum effect and maintain an activity on quiescent bacteria (that do not multiply) while the other beta-lactams are inactive in these conditions. Intracellular bactericidal activity is powerful and the post-antibiotic effect exists for Gram-negative bacilli, contrary to other beta-lactams. All these microbiologic properties underline the use of monotherapy [18-21, 24–26] with these newer antibiotics but the gaps in their spectrum of activity must not be ignored. Moreover, the therapeutic coefficients of imipenem (its bacteriologic strength determined

by the "antibiotic concentration minimal inhibitory concentration (MIC) of the pathogenic strains" ratio) on some enterobacter (*Enterobacter, Citrobacter, Serratia, Proteus*) are inferior to those of third-generation cephalosporins [27]. Clinically, the resistance acquired during the treatment of *Pseudomonas* infections is high (up to 40% of the strains). This resistance which is not crossed with that of other beta-lactams, is linked to the modification of a membrane porine. The use of imipenem in combination should therefore be considered in some patients and the general rules for combination therapy must not be modified for this antibiotic or those in the same family [20, 21].

Antibacterial Synergy [1, 2, 4, 5, 7]

Antibacterial synergy is often sought after but less often reached as such a synergy is difficult to document *in vivo* [28].

The Mechanism of a Synergistic Effect [29]

Synergism can be obtained by blocking two different metabolic pathways such as that of the synthesis of the bacterial wall by the beta-lactams combined with that of the synthesis of DNA by the fluoroquinolones. A synergistic effect is also obtained by blocking two different levels of the same metabolic pathway as in the combination sulfamethoxazole-trimethoprim. One antibiotic can also act on the bacterial wall, modifying its permeability (beta-lactams) and thus facilitating the penetration of the other antibiotic toward its site of intracellular action (ribosome for aminoglycosides on Gram-positive cocci). The synergistic effect is defined by the fact that the bactericidal effect is more pronounced than the sum of the effects of each antibiotic alone [29]. The fact that a combination is more effective than each antibiotic alone is not necessarily synonymous with synergy, but could reflect a mere additive effect. Numerous factors can influence the accomplishment of a synergistic effect (Table 4). Pharmacokinetic factors are essential as it is necessary to obtain sufficient levels for both antibiotics, both in serum and in the tissue implicated in the infectious process. Doses, rate and speed of administration, and tissue penetration of the antibiotics will strongly influence the results and vary from one patient to another. Immunosuppression, the pre-existing conditions, type of infection, size of the bacterial inoculum, and the time between the onset of infection and treatment will also have an influence on efficacy.

The Risks of Antibiotic Antagonism [29]

This is the opposite of the desired effect and while antibiotic antagonism is rare (at least it does not seem to worry practitioners ... !), it can have negative clinical consequences. The principal combinations with a risk of antibiotic antagonism are presented in Table 5. Curiously enough, certain *in vitro* antagonist combinations provide excellent results *in vivo*, particularly for *Staphylococcus* bone infections

[30–32]. A possible explanation is that the limitation on bacterial killing is greatly compensated *in vivo* by excellent tissue penetration. This is the case for rifampin when it is combined with vancomycin or a fluoroquinolone [30, 33]. For the same reasons, the combination ampicillin-chloramphenicol is used in the treatment of cerebral infections [34].

The Experimental Basis of Antibacterial Synergy [28]

Despite all the difficulties of interpretation, certain antibiotic combinations have proven their superiority over single-drug therapy both in animal experiments and in man [2, 28, 35, 36]. Rapid sterilization of infectious lesions, the possibility of shortening treatment tine, increase in the rate of cure, and reduction in the number of relapses when treatment is stopped are the principal criteria that strongly suggest the superiority of a combination of antibiotics over monotherapy (Tables 2 and 3). In general, a synergistic effect will provide better therapeutic results in severe infections with virulent bacteria poorly eliminated by monotherapy, and lowered patient defenses. One can therefore understand why the most obvious examples of an *in vivo* benefit following *in vitro* synergy are endocarditis, infections in neutropenic patients, *Listeria monocytogenes* meningitis, and *Enterococcus* and *P. aeruginosa* infections.

Streptococcus infections [28]: In an experimental model of *Streptococcus sanguis* endocarditis, 9 days of penicillin are required to sterilize the vegetations versus 3 to 4 days if gentamicin or streptomycin are included [38]. In penicillin-resistant strains combination with one of the aminoglycosides will provide better efficacy [39]. In man, the clinical data are less apparent. Penicillin alone provides a relapse rate of 0.6% after 4 weeks of treatment, while the rate is 1% if streptomycin is combined with penicillin. On the other hand, the penicillin-streptomycin combination for a shorter period (only two weeks) is also effective [39].

Enterococcus infections: The penicillin-aminoglycoside combination is synergistic *in vitro* on enterococci with a marked bactericidal effect [40]. The efficacy and superiority of the combination have been clearly demonstrated in experimental models [40]. The clinical data are equivalent and the very high failure rate observed when only beta-lactams are used supports the choice of a combination. Gentamicin is substituted for streptomycin in cases of major resistance ($>1,000$ mg/l). In *Enterococcus faecium* endocarditis with a low level of resistance to vancomycin, the combination with gentamicin is very synergistic [28]. In high-level resistance, the triple combination of penicillin-vancomycin-gentamicin provides a synergistic bactericidal effect *in vitro* [35].

Staphylococcus infections [28]: In methicillin-sensitive *Staphylococcus* endocarditis or osteomyelitis, the addition of an aminoglycoside will sterilize infected lesions more rapidly in experimental models [38]. However, clinical data have not confirmed these findings [41] although treatment of endocarditis by aminoglycosides in drug addicts reduces the duration of the bacteremia period [42]. Therefore, the use of a combination is recommended during the first 3 to 5 days of treatment. In experimental methicillin-sensitive *Staphylococcus* endocarditis, the combination vancomycin-rifampin is significantly more effective than monotherapy in terms of sterilization of the vegetations and cure [32]. A beneficial effect has also been found in cases of experimental osteomyelitis [33]. In drug addicts, the clinical results obtained with vancomycin alone are identical to combinations with rifampin or an aminoglycoside [43].

Gram-negative bacilli infections: The combination beta-lactam-aminoglycoside has generally had a marked synergistic effect in numerous experimental infection models [28]. This has been found for enterobacteriaceae and *P. aeruginosa*. Clinically, the use of a combination is strongly recommended for *P. aeruginosa* [1, 44, 45] but is much less clear for enterobacteriaceae.

Prevention of Resistant Mutants [1–7]

Prevention of resistance is demonstrated in the treatment of tuberculosis. However, the ability of combinations to avoid the selection of resistant variants is less obvious for other bacteria. Since the beginning of the 1980s there have been many observations of therapeutic failure after the use of third-generation cephalosporins or monobactams due to the emergence of resistant mutants, particularly with *P. aeruginosa*, *E. cloacae*, *Serratia*, *Citrobacter* and *Acinetobacter* [13]. In any bacterial population there are resistant strains to a given antibiotic for which the number depends on the rate of mutation (which in turn depends on the bacterial species and the antibiotic) and other environmental factors (Table 6). If the rate of mutation ($f(A)$) is 10^{-7} for a beta-lactam and 10^{-5} for an aminoglycoside ($f(B)$), the predicted mutation rate in combination therapy is dramatically lower and equal to:

$$f(AB) = 10^{-7} \times 10^{-5} = 10^{-12}$$

(the probability of a double mutation is equal to the product of the probability of each mutation). This principle is the basis for the treatment of tuberculosis by triple or quadritherapy (with the probability being even lower) and the association of two

Table 6. Factors favoring the emergence of resistant bacterial strains

Antibiotics
fusidic acid, fosfomycin, rifampin, fluoroquinolones, novibocin
Bacteria
Pseudomonas, Stenostrophomonas, Enterobacter, Serratia, Proteus indole +, Acinetobacter, Staphylococcus
Other factors
- low antibiotic tissue level: MIC of pathogenic bacteria ratio (< 10)
- high bacterial inoculum ($> 10^5$ to 10^7/ml)
- foreign body
- deep infection (endocarditis, meningitis …)
- combination of two beta-lactams

antibiotics for the treatment of other bacterial infections. However, the combination does not act on all the factors responsible for the emergence of resistant strains (Table 6). For example, a very high inoculum increases the risk of mutation for a given combination. It is then essential that the two antibiotics be present simultaneously and at a sufficient dose ("antibiotic tissue level/MIC of pathogenic bacteria" ratio ≥ 10) at the site of infection. If diffusion problems or physicochemical conditions (acid medium for aminoglycosides) affect the activity of one of the two drugs in the combination, one is confronted with monotherapy at the site of infection which can cause a mutation that one was attempting to avoid. Such failures are frequent in cases of mediastinitis, bronchopulmonary suppurations, or peritonitis. In practice, severe infections with elevated inoculum caused by above-mentioned species, particularly P. aeruginosa, justify the use of a combination of a beta-lactam and aminoglycoside, or fluoroquinolone antibiotic [1, 7].

Experimental Model for the Prevention of the Emergence of Resistant Mutants [5, 10, 28]

In an experimental model of peritonitis in the mouse, the use of quinolones in monotherapy is accompanied by the frequent emergence of resistant strains for K. Pneumoniae, S. marcescens, E. cloacae and especially for P. aeruginosa (Table 7). On the other hand, no emergence of resistance has been found for E. coli and S. aureus strains [10, 11]. When quinolones are combined with a beta-lactam or an aminoglycoside, the emergence of resistance is reduced but not totally prevented (Table 7). Beta-lactams seem to be more effective than amikacin for the prevention of resistance to pefloxacin. Ceftazidime has a very marked effect which is probably due to elevated intraperitoneal concentrations. In this experimental model, the observed reduction in the emergence of resistance with the use of a combination has not always been accompanied by a synergistic bactericidal effect when compared with the use of monotherapy [10, 11].

P. aeruginosa Infections: In the above experimental model, the protective effect of a quinolone-beta-lactam combination is superior to that of a quinolone-amikacin combination [10, 11]. As for the association beta-lactam-aminoglycoside, the emergence of resistance can easily occur in cases of P. aeruginosa infection, all the more because there is an elevated inoculum and the presence of foreign bodies [45]. All the evidence points to the fact that with this bacteria, the risk of emergence of resistance in vitro, in vivo, and clinically, is high [21]. Using the method of successive antibiotic exposure in experimental models mimicking repeated injections of antibiotics, resistance is encountered after the second or third exposure. It occurs as rapidly for penicillins and recent cephalosporins, as for aminoglycosides. On the other hand, the use of combinations makes it possible to slow down or inhibit this phenomenon. While there has been no clinical confirmation that the use of a combination of antibiotics will prevent the emergence of resistant mutants, experimental results and clinical experience support this hypothesis [1, 20, 44, 46, 47].

Staphylococcus Infections [48]: The treatment of reference for methicillin-resistant staphylococci infections is still vancomycin in monotherapy and no study has demonstrated the superiority of a combination [43, 48]. The beneficial effect of a combination on the emergence of resistant mutants, however, has a solid experimental basis when antibiotics other than vancomycin are used. In an endocarditis model, fosfomycin and pefloxacin were respectively responsible for the emergence of resistance in 36% and 4% of the animals. A combination of both drugs totally suppressed this phenomenon [28]. In an infection model on a foreign body caused by methicillin-resistant staphylococcus, the combination of rifampin-pefloxacin (two antibiotics with good tissue diffusion) prevented the emergence of resistance whereas vancomycin (with lower tissue diffusion) combined with rifampcin did not prevent the emergence of resistance [28]. The explanation is probably that resistance to rifampicin is more likely to be prevented if the combination includes a partner with good tissue and intracellular penetration [28]. In man, the combination vancomycin-fosfomycin has proven to be very effective for prevention of the emergence of resistance to fosfomycin in the treatment of endocarditis with the risk of mutation appearing to be close to zero.

Indications for Combinations Linked to the Use of Certain Antibiotics

Fosfomycin [49]: The association of another antibiotic with fosfomycin has effectively prevented the emergence of resistant mutants in experimental models of *Staphylococcus* and Gram-negative meningitis and endocarditis. These results have been clinically confirmed and its use in combination is imperative.

Rifampin: *In vitro* results have confirmed *in vivo* studies and studies in man [31, 32] that bitherapy reduces the frequency of the emergence of resistant germs. The combination partners are usually fluoroquinolones, fusidic acid, vancomycin and oxacillin. There have, however, been failures and only tritherapy (with vancomycin and an aminoglycoside) effectively prevents this risk. Proof of the efficacy of a combination of antibiotics in the prevention of the emergence of resistant mutants is no longer needed in the treatment of tuberculosis.

Fusidic Acid: Its use in combination reduces the risk of the selection of resistant mutants. Its usual partners are rifampin, the aminoglycosides and the beta-lactams. Its use as monotherapy is not foreseeable.

Fluoroquinolones: Animal models and clinical studies have confirmed the data obtained *in vitro* concerning the relatively high frequency of the selection of resistant bacteria during monotherapy with fluoroquinolones. The antibiotic tissue level/MIC of the pathogenic bacteria ratio at the site of the infection is the most important favorable factor for such a selection. The association of another antibiotic that is active against the bacteria in question reduced this risk in experimental *P. aeruginosa* peritonitis but did not cancel it, and certain combinations are no more effective than a monotherapy (Table 7) [10, 11].

Table 7. Emergence of resistant strains in an experimental peritonitis model [10–11]

Emergence of resistance after treatment of *Pseudomonas infection* (10^8 CFU) with a single antibiotic

Antibiotics	Prevalence of resistance (%)
ceftazidime	25 (p<0.01)
cefepime	<10
imipenem	<5
ciprofloxacin	>60 (p<0.01)
amikacin	<5

Effect of an antibiotic combination on the emergence of resistance

Antibiotics	Efficacy
ciprofloxacin + ceftazidime	+++
cirprofloxacin + amikacin	+++
ciprofloxacin + penicillin	++
pefloxacin + piperacillin	–
pefloxacin + amikacin	+/–

Critical Analysis

Reduction or suppression of the emergence of resistant strains is a difficult goal to acheive during antibiotic treatment and the use of a combination does not solve all problems – far from it. For example, in the treatment of *Enterobacter* septicemia, the association of aminoglycoside with third generation cephalosporin did not have a favorable effect on the emergence of resistance [50]. In the treatment of nosocomial pneumonia, the rate of superinfection by resistant bacteria increased with the use of a combination with gentamicin when compared with a third generation cephalosporin alone [22]. Of course, this study suffered from a lack of randomization but it confirmed just the same that a combination was not the always the answer. In ICU patients, the addition of netilmicin to imipenem did not modify the frequency of the emergence of resistant mutants nor the rate of superinfection [20]. Patients in that study presented with elevated inoculum infections but their disease severity was minor (APACHE II: 9) which explains the low rate of treatment failure and therefore resistant bacteria superinfections. Only one study has shown the benefit of the association of an aminoglycoside with a carboxypenicillin for the prevention of the emergence of resistance in the treatment of severe infections [51]. The small number of studies and their methodological limitations therefore do not make it possible to draw definite conclusions [18, 19, 23–26].

The risks of monotherapy at the infected site have already been mentioned highlighting the importance of choosing products with sufficient tissue diffusion at the infection site. This is not always possible: Certain antibiotics possess variable tissue diffusion (glycopeptides, aminoglycosides); some sites are always difficult to reach (endocarditis, osteomyelitis, meningitis). It is therefore important to act on the factors that the clinician can easily control, i.e., doses and rate of drug injection. For the fluoroquinolones and in particular for ciprofloxacin, the use of a unit dose of 400 mg instead of 200 mg and a rate of 3 injections per day makes it possible to limit the emergence of resistant strains [51]. As for beta-lactams, obtaining antibiotic serum levels superior to the MIC of the treated germs for more than 50% of the time between two injections is a major factor for limiting or even suppressing the emergence of resistant strains. In clinical practice, single-drug treatment of severe pneumonias by ciprofloxacin or imipenem is accompanied by an excessively high level of resistance during treatment [51]. For imipenem, this level reaches nearly 40% for *P. aeruginosa* [53]. This supports an analysis of the literature reporting that the emergence of resistance ranges from 8% to 32% for monotherapy versus 0% to 12% for combinations [4].

From Theory to Practice

Beta-Lactam-Aminoglycoside Combinations

Such combinations are synergistic *in vivo* in Gram-negative bacilli and *P. aeruginosa* infection models [28]. Clinically, while some studies have not demonstrated significant differences between monotherapy and the beta-lactam-aminoglycoside combination, others, on the contrary, have confirmed the superiority of the combination, subject to the requirement that the bacteria are sensitive to both antibiotics [2]. The penicillin-streptomycin combination is synergistic *in vivo* and clinically for *Streptococcus* and penicillin-sensitive *Enterococcus* endocarditis. In the same manner, the methicillin-aminoglycoside combination is synergistic for methicillin-sensitive *Staphylococcus* endocarditis. Finally, the ampicillin-aminoglycoside combination is synergistic for severe neonatal *Listeria* and streptococcus B infections.

Combinations with a Fluoroquinolone [2, 3]

In severe documented infections, quinolones must be used in combination with other antibiotics if the infection is due to *Staphylococcus* or *P. aeruginosa*. These species develop resistance very rapidly and the aim of combinations is to limit the emergence of resistant variants. Moreover, the fluoroquinolone MIC for these species are very close to critical concentrations and a mutation at any stage can transform sensitivity to resistance. In cases of *Enterobacter* infections where the MIC is much lower, monotherapy is possible since tissue penetration is excellent, except in certain sites with difficult access such as meningitis and neurological locations. For infections treated empirically, it is the gap in the spectrum of activity that justifies the use of a combination [2, 3].

On a bacteriologic level, the argument against beta-lactam-aminoglycoside combinations is that the resistance with two antibiotic families is often genetically cross-linked because the genetic determinants are carried by the same plasmid. However, due to a resistance that is strictly chromosomic, there is no crossed resistance between quinolones and the other antibiotic families. On a practical level, a quinolone-aminoglycoside or quinolone-third-generation cephalosporin combination can be envisaged. For reasons of lower toxicity, the latter association is perhaps preferable but there are not as yet definitive results to confirm this. Elsewhere, for bone or meningeal locations, or if the medium is without oxygen or at a low pH, aminoglycosides could be inactivated.

The Special Case of a Combination of Two-Beta-Lactams [4]

The combination of two beta-lactams can be, depending on the agents and the bacteria, synergistic or antagonistic. The synergy is the result of several different mechanisms:
1) synergy by action on the different penicillin binding proteins (PBP) for each of the agents in the combination (meticillnam PBP_2 cephalexin PBP_3);
2) synergy by enzyme inhibition; one of the beta-lactams neutralizes the beta-lactamases produced by the bacteria. The other beta-lactam which is normally inactivated by the beta-lactamases can then become active.

Antagonism can be the result of different mechanisms:
1) antagonism by competition between the beta-lactams at the level of the porins (allowing the passage of the antibiotics to the periplasmic space) or at the level of the PBP.
2) antagonism by depression of beta-lactamase synthesis is by far the most frequent mechanism. Synthesis of these enzymes of chromosomic origin is either permanent (a chromosomic mutation triggers a constant beta-lactamase secretion) or temporary (beta-lactamase secretion occurs only when the bactericia is in contact with an inductor agent (such as a beta-lactam). *Enterobacter, Serratia* and *Pseudomonas aeruginosa* are the most frequently involved. The inductor agents can be the beta-lactams themselves which include cefoxitin, imipenen, cefamandol, cefaloridine, cefotaxime, ceftizoxime and moxalactam. The beta-lactamases will hydrolyze certain beta-lactams (penicillins and first and second-generation cephalosporins) or fix onto the beta-lactams that are resistant to hydrolysis (sponge effect or barrier phenomenon).

In practice, the combination of two beta-lactams is employed for the empiric treatment of infectious syndromes in neutropenic patients. According to the literature, however, there are major risks of resistant mutant selection, especially for *Enterobacter, Serratia,* and *Pseudomonas aeruginosa.* Apart from the empiric treatment of infectious syndromes in neutropenic patients, combinations of two beta-lactams cannot reasonably be recommended given the number of side effects of such an association as well as the major risks of the selection of resistant bacteria [4].

Pseudomonas aeruginosa Infections [26]

Reinforced bacterial killing is the reason given by clinicians to justify the use of a combination of *in vitro* synergistic antibiotics on *Pseudomonas* [1, 36, 45, 47]. The benefit of such an association has been found *in vivo* in peritoneal, septicemia and pulmonary infection models with associations of imipenem-amikacin (versus imipenem alone), ceftazidime-tobramycin (versus tobramycin alone and amikacin alone), or ciprofloxacin-azlocillin (versus ciprofloxacin alone) [45]. Clinically, the superiority of an association over monotherapy has not been definitely demonstrated [45]. In a study of 200 patients with a *P. aeruginosa* infection with bacteremia, Hilf et al. [54] noted a reduction in mortality in 143 patients treated with the combination beta-lactamine-aminoside compared with 43 patients treated by monotherapy (respective mortality: 27% and 47%). This reduction was significant in certain subgroups (neutropenic patients, cancers, patients treated by immunosuppressors) but while the overall reduction in mortality existed, it was no longer significant. The main drawback of this study is that it was not randomized.

In conclusion, while current clinical studies do not permit us to definitively close the debate "combination of antibiotics or monotherapy?", the association of two synergistic antibiotics *in vitro* is strongly recommended for *P. aeruginosa* infections [1–7, 36, 47, 54].

Staphylococcus Infections

In methicillin-sensitive *Staphylococcus* infections, the use of an isoxazolylpenicillin is imperative. For the best renal tolerance, oxacillin (Bristopen®) replaces methicillin. The use of a combination with an aminoglycoside is often recommended in order to obtain a synergistic effect and/or to prevent an evolution towards resistance [41, 42, 48]. However, this type of treatment has not proven its superiority. In the treatment of right heart endocarditis, only the period of bacteremia was reduced (by one day) in patients treated by bitherapy, whereas mortality was not affected [42].

In methicillin-resistant *Staphylococcus* infections, the value of combination therapy with glycopeptides remains to be demonstrated [43, 48]. The use of glycopeptides in monotherapy can in fact be theoretically justified with rare exceptions because staphylococci are always sensitive to glycopeptides and they do not develop resistance to this antibiotic, even in monotherapy. Thus, an association is not justified to prevent the emergence of resistant mutants. However, the slow bacterial killing of the glycopeptide can be a disadvantage in severe or life-threatening infections. For the same reason, given their low therapeutic margin and their poor diffusion, antibiotic tissue levels can be inferior to the MIC. Clinically, infections with methicillin-resistant *Staphylococcus* bacteremias have been treated by vancomycin in monotherapy with an efficacy equal to that of oxacillin in methicillin-susceptible *Staphylococcus* septicemias, with mortality at approximately 30% [43]. However, *in vitro* results have demonstrated that an association can improve the rate of glycopeptide bacterial killing. These results have been confirmed in animal models and in clinical observations [32, 30]. They make it possible to recommend a combination for the treatment of severe methicillin-resistant *Staphylococcus* infections. This is particularly the case not only for endocarditis of the left heart which requires rapid sterilization of the valves, but also for meningo-encephalitis and bone infections. Finally, the combination therapy would seem to be necessary in cases of infection with secondary organ dysfunction, and in treatment failure (persistence of fever and/or positive blood cultures after 72 hours). Five antibiotics can be combined with glycopeptides: Rifampin; fosfomycin; fusidic acid; cotrimoxazole; and the synergistines. Association with rifampin is the best documented. However, this combination does not always prevent the emergence of mutants resistant to rifampin [31], particularly in tissues where the glycopeptides have insufficient diffusion (bone, meninges, peritoneum) [48]. Finally, a perfect *in vitro* sensitivity to rifampin must be ensured. As with rifampin, the utilization of fusidic acid in monotherapy is accompanied by the emergence of resistant mutants by chromosomic mutation. Good results have been obtained particularly in combination with vancomycin in severe infections, although clinical experience remains limited. The same is true for fosfomycin [49], a bactericidal antibiotic for staphylococci. This activity is relatively slow and time-dependent. Combination with vancomycin yields either indifferent, additive, or synergistic effects.

Conclusion

The use of a single antibiotic presents indisputable advantages: Reduced cost, lack of interference between antibiotics; reduction of undesirable side effects, frequent clinical efficacy. A combination of antibiotics is considered in certain situations: Immunodeficiency; bacterial inoculum at a high concentration; bacteria with reduced sensitivity; sites of infection that are difficult to reach (bone, endocardium, meninges); or bacteria that are "difficult to treat" (*P. aeruginosa*, *Staphylococcus*, *Enterobacter*). The combination of two antibiotics can provide the following advantages: A broadening of the antibacterial spectrum; increased bacterial killing; a limitation of the emergence of resistant strains. All of these arguments in favor of the use of a combination of antibiotics have been examined critically and none has been indisputably proven. The need to continue a combination of antibiotics must be re-evaluated after 3–5 days according to the clinical data.

References

1. Moellering RC (1985) Can the third-generation cephalosporins eliminate the need for antimicrobial combinations? Am J Med (suppl 2A): 104–109
2. Eliopoulos GM, Moellering BC (1991) Antimicrobial combinations. In: Lorian V (ed) Antibiotics in laboratory medicine. Williams and Wilkins Co, Baltimore, pp 432–492
3. Denis JP, Gouin (1992) Association d'antibiotiques In: Martin C, Gouin F (eds) Antibiothérapie en réanimation et en chirurgie. Arnette, Paris, pp 351–362
4. Dejace P, Klatersky J (1986) Comparative review of combination therapy: two beta-lactams versus beta-lactam plus aminoglycoside. Am J Med 80 (suppl. 6B): 29–37
5. Barriere SL (1991) Monotherapy versus combination antimicrobial therapy. A review. Pharmacotherapy 11: 645–654
6. Joly-Guillou ML, Bergogne-Berezin E (1986) Synergies ou antagonismes des associations d'antibiotiques. Presse Med 15: 1037–1040
7. Regnier B (1987) Utilisation des associations d'antibiotiques. Presse Med 16: 2186–2191
8. Martin C, Perrin G, Lambert D (1992) Les quinolones. In: Martin C, Gouin F (eds) Antibiothérapie en réanimation et en chirurgie. Arnette, Paris, pp 109–112
9. Martin C, Gouin F, Fourrier F, Juninger W, Prieur BL (1988) Pefloxacin in the treatment of nosocomial lower respiratory tract infections in intensive care patients. J Antimicrob Chemother 21: 795–799

10. Pechere JC, Marchou B, Michea-Hamlehpour M, Aukenthaler A (1986) Emergence of resistance after therapy with antibiotics used alone or combined in a murine model. J Antimicrob Chemother 17 (suppl A) 11–18
11. Michea-Hamzehpour M, Pechere JC, Marchou B, Auckenthaler RC (1986) Combination therapy: a way to limit the emergence of resistance. Am J Med 80 (suppl 6B):138–142
12. Boogaerts MA (1995) Anti-infective strategies in neutropenia. J Antimicrob Chemother 36 (suppl A):167–178
13. Perronne C, Regnier B, Legrand P, et al (1986) Echec des nouvelles béta-lactamines dans le traitement d'infections sévères *Enterobacter cloacae*. Presse Med 15:1813–1818
14. Anonymous (1991): Respiratory infections of the lower respiratory airway. 4th Consensus Conference of the French Society of Infectious Diseases. Med Mal Inf 21 (suppl 1):1–8
15. Niederman MS, Bass JB, Campbell GD, et al (1993) Guidelines for the initial management of adults with community-acquired pneumonia: diagnosis, assessment of severity, and initial antimicrobial therapy. Am Rev Respir Dis 142:1418–1426
16. American Thoracic Society (1995) Hospital-acquired pneumonia in adults: diagnosis, assessment of severity, initial antimicrobial therapy, and preventive strategies. Am J Respir Crit Care Med 143:1711–1725
17. Bohnen JMA, Solomkin JS, Dellinger EP, Bjornson S, Page CP (1992) Guidelines for clinical care: anti-infective agents for intra-abdominal infections. Arch Surg 127:83-89
18. Geroulanos SJ and the Meropenem Study Group (1995) Meropenem versus imipenem/cilastatin in intra-abdominal infections requiring surgery. J Antimicrob Chemother 36 (suppl A):191–205
19. Huizinga WKJ, Warren BL, Baker LW, et al (1995) Antibiotic monotherapy with meropenem in the surgical management of intra-abdominal infections. J Antimicrob Chemother 36 (suppl A): 79–89
20. Cometta A, Baumgartner JD, Lew D, et al (1994) Prospective randomized comparison of imipenem monotherapy with imipenem plus netilmicin for the treatment of severe infections in non-neutropenic patients. Antimicrob Agents Chemother 38:1309–1313
21. Winston DJ, Mc Grattan MA, Busuttil RW (1984) Imipenem therapy of *Pseudomonas aeruginosa* and other serious bacterial infections. Antimicrob Agents Chemother 26:673–677
22. Croce MA, Fabian TC, Stewart RM, et al (1993) Empiric monotherapy versus combination therapy of nosocomial pneumonia in trauma patients. J Trauma 35: 303–309
23. Solberg CO, Sjursen H (1995) Safety and efficacy of meropenem in patients with septicemia: a randomised comparison with ceftazidime, alone or combined with amikacin. J Antimicrob Chemother 36 (suppl A):157–166
24. Norrby SR, Finch RG, Glauser M, et al (1993) Monotherapy of serious hospital-acquired infections: a clinical trial of ceftazidime versus imipenem/cilastatin. J Antimicrob Chemother 31: 927–937
25. Cometta A, Calandra T, Gaya H, et al (1996) Monotherapy with ceftazidime plus amikacin as empiric therapy for fever in granulocytopenic patients with cancer. Antimicrob Agents Chemother 40:1108–1115
26. Leibovici L, Paul M, Poznanski O, et al (1997) Monotherapy versus β-lactam-aminoglycoside combination treatment for Gram-negative bacteremia: a prospective, observational study. Antimicrob Agents Chemother 41:1127–1133
27. Martin C (1992) Rapports thérapeutiques (taux tissulaires/CMI 90). In: Martin C, Gouin F (eds) Antibiothérapie en réanimation et en chirurgie. Arnette, Paris, pp 717–741
28. Fantin B, Carbon C (1992) *In vivo* antibiotic synergism: contribution of animal models. Antimicrob Agents Chemother 36:907–912
29. Mallet MN (1992) Bactériostase, bactéricidie, étude des associations d'antibiotiques. In: Martin C, Gouin F (eds) Antibiothérapie en réanimation et en chirurgie. Arnette, Paris, pp 281–304
30. Kaatz GW, Seo SM, Barriere SL, Albrecht LM, Rybak MJ (1989) Ciprofloxacin and rifampin, alone and in combination, for therapy of experimental *Staphylococcus aureus* endocarditis. Antimicrob Agents Chemother 33:1184–1187
31. Acar JF, Goldstein FW, Duval J (1983) Use of rifampin for the treatment of serious staphylococcal and gram-negative bacillary infections. Rev Infect Dis 5 (suppl 3):502–506
32. Bayer AS, Lam KJ (1985) Efficacy of vancomycin plus rifampicin in experimental aortic valve – endocarditis due to methicillin-resistant *Staph aureus: in vitro – in vivo* correlations. J Infect Dis 151:157–165

33. Norden CW, Shaffer M (1983) Treatment of experimental chronic osteomyelitis due to *Staphylococcus aureus* with vancomycin and rifampin. J Infect Dis 147:352–357

34. Wispelwey B, Scheld WM (1990) Brain abcess. In: Mandell GL, Douglas RG, Bennett JE (eds) Principles and practice of infectious diseases. Churchill Livingstone, New York, pp 777–787

35. Caron F, Carbon C, Gutmann L (1991) Evaluation of the triple combination penicillin-vancomycin-gentamicin in an experimental endocarditis caused by moderately penicillin and a highly glycopeptide-resistant strain of *Enterococcus faecium*. J Infect Dis 164:888–893

36. Klatersky J, Zinners SH (1982) Synergistic combinations of antibiotics in Gram-negative bacillary infections. Rev Infect Dis 4:294–301

37. Sande MA, Irvin RG (1975) Penicillin-aminoglycoside synergism in experimental *Streptococcus vidans* endocarditis. J Infect Dis 136:327–335

38. Sande MA, Courtney KB (1976) Nafcillin-gentamicin synergism in experimental staphylococcal endocarditis. J Lab Clin Med 88:118–124

39. Wilson WR (1987) Antimicrobial therapy of streptococcal endocarditis. J Antimicrob Chemother 20 (suppl A):147–159

40. Henry NK, Wilson WR, Geraci JE (1986) Treatment of streptomycin-susceptible enterococcal experimental endocarditis with combinations of penicillin and low- or high-dose streptomycin. Antimicrob Agents Chemother 30:725–728

41. Levine DP, Cushing RD, Jui J, Brown WJ (1982) Community-acquired methicillin-resistant *Staphylococcus aureus* endocarditis in the Detroit Medical Center. Ann Intern Med 97:330–338

42. Korzeniowski O, Sande MA and the NCESG (1982) Combination antimicrobial therapy for *Staphylococcus aureus* endocarditis in patients addicted to parenteral drugs and in non addicts. Ann Inter Med 97: 496–504

43. Rahal JJ (1986) Treatment of methicillin-resistant staphylococcal infection. In: Peterson PK, Verhoef J (eds) The antimicrobial agents annual I. Elsevier, Amsterdam, pp 489–514

44. Reyes MP, Lerner AM (1983) Current problems in the treatment of infective endocarditis due to *Pseudomonas aeruginosa*. Rev Infect Dis 5:314–321

45. Martin C, Saux P, Perrin G (1992) Choix d'une antibiothérapie pour le traitement d'une infection à *Pseudomonas*. In: Martin C, Gouin F (eds) Antibiothérapie en réanimation et en chirurgie. Arnette, Paris, pp 389–406

46. Quinn JP, Dubek EJ, Divincenzo CA, Lucks DA, Lerner SA (1986) Emergence of resistance to imipenem during therapy for *Pseudomonas infection*. J Infect Dis 16:289–294

47. Nichols L, Maki DG (1985) The emergence of resistance to beta-lactam antibiotics during treatment of *Pseudomonas aeruginosa* lower respiratory tract infections: is combination therapy the solution? Chemotherapia 4:102–109

48. Martin C, Albanèse J, Thomachot L, Quinio B (1993) Choix d'une antibiothérapie pour le traitement d'une infection staphylocoques. In: Confèrences d'actualisation 35e Congrés National d'Anesthésie et Réanimation. Masson, Paris, pp 601–620

49. Saux P, Martin C, Perrin G (1992) La fosfomycine. In: Martin C, Gouin F (eds) Antibiothérapie en réanimation et en chinurgie. Arnette, Paris, pp 189–194

50. Chow JW, Fine MJ, Shlaes DM (1991) *Enterobacter* bacteremia: clinical features and emergence of antibiotic resistance during therapy. Ann Intern Med 115:585–590

51. Gribble MJ, Chow AW, Naiman SC, et al (1983) Prospective randomized trial of piperacillin monotherapy versus carboxypenicillin-aminoglycoside combination regimens in the empirical treatment of serious bacterial infections. Antimicrob Agents Chemother 24:388–393

52. Fink MP, Snydman DR, Niederman MS (1994) Treatment of severe pneumonia in hospitalized patients: results of a multicenter, randomized, double blind trial comparing intravenous ciprofloxacin with imipenem-cilastin. Antimicrob Agents Chemother 38:547–557

53. Thabaut A (1992) Impénème: Monotherapie ou associations? Arguments microbiologiques. Lettre Infect 7:151–153

54. Hilf M, Yu VL, Sharp J, et al (1989) Antibiotic therapy for *Pseudomonas aeruginosa* bacteremia: outcome correlation in a prospective study of 200 patients. Am J Med 87:540–546

Prevention of Infections Associated with Vascular Catheters

R. O. Darouiche and I. I. Raad

Introduction

Intravascular devices have become indispensable tools in the care of seriously and/or chronically ill patients. However, the benefits derived from these devices may be offset by the morbidity and mortality resulting from catheter-related infection and the high cost of managing such a complication. Catheter-related bloodstream infection (CRBSI) represents the most frequent life threatening complication of intravascular catheters [1, 2]. Moreover, most nosocomial bloodstream infections are related to the use of intravascular devices. For instance, an intensive care units (ICU) surveillance by the National Nosocomial Infection Surveillance (NNIS) system hospitals during the years 1986–1990 showed that patients with intravascular devices had substantially higher rates of bloodstream infection than those without such devices [3].

The reported rates of CRBSI have ranged from 4–14% with non-cuffed central venous catheters (CVC) [4–7], to 8–43% in association with the use of long term cuffed silastic catheters [8]. More than 5 million CVC [9], including half a million cuffed silastic catheters [10], are inserted annually in the United States. Using an average conservative estimate of a CRBSI rate of 8%, one would expect at least 400 000 cases of CVC-related bloodstream infections per year [11]. Such cases of CRBSI can be associated with major morbidity and mortality. For instance, the case-fatality rate associated with CRBSI in ICU patients is reportedly 35% [5]. By prolonging hospitalization and incurring excess cost, the occurrence of CRBSI has substantial financial implications. A recent report estimated the extra hospital and surgical ICU length of stay of patients who survived nosocomial blood infection to be 24 and 8 days, respectively, with an extra cost of treating one episode of CRBSI of $ 40 000 per patient [12]. Based on these figures, the annual economic burden resulting from the infectious complications of CVC amounts to billions of dollars in the United States alone.

Several protective measures have been suggested to guard against catheter-related infection. A review of the pathogenesis, microbiology, routes of acquiring the infecting organisms, and risk factors is essential for understanding the scientific reasoning for the efficacy, or lack thereof, of various measures aimed at preventing catheter related infection.

Pathogenesis and Microbiology

Bacterial adherence to the vascular catheter is a prelude to catheter-related infection. The ability of various microorganisms to adhere to and colonize the catheter is dependent on a number of factors, including:
1) microbial factors, such as the fibroglycocalyyx, also known as extracellular slime, which constitutes the microbial component of the biofilm produced by coagulase-negative staphylococci;
2) the host reaction which is initially manifested by the formation around the catheter of a thrombin sleeve that is rich in fibronectin, fibrinogen, fibrin and other host factors that may selectively enhance the adherence of certain microorganisms; and
3) the type of catheter material as, for instance, *Staphylococcus aureus* and *Candida* organisms tend to adhere better to polyvinylchloride catheters than to Teflon catheters [7].

The organisms responsible for vascular catheter colonization and infection originate from four potential sources, including the skin insertion site, the catheter hub, hematogenous seeding of the catheter, and infusate contamination. Of these four potential sources, the skin insertion site and the catheter hub are by far the two most important and will be further discussed in this chapter.

The skin insertion site is the most common source for colonization and infection of short-term catheters [4]. When studying short-term CVC and arterial catheters, a strong correlation between high-level bacterial colonization of the skin insertion site, external catheter colonization, and catheter-related sepsis was established [13]. Skin flora can migrate from the insertion site along the external surface of the catheter, causing colonization of the intracutaneous segment, then the distal intravascular segment (tip) of the catheter, ultimately resulting in CRBSI. The major contribution of the skin to the pathogenesis of catheter-related infection is reflected by the predominance of staphylococci (coagulase-negative organisms and *S. aureus*) as causative agents for catheter-related infection. The relationship between skin contamination and catheter infection was best demonstrated by documenting the efficacy of practices that either decrease the colonization of the insertion site, such as the application of topical antibiotics and disinfectants [14, 15], or interrupt the intercutaneous migration of organisms, such as the use of subcutaneous silver-impregnated cuffs [4]. On the other hand, practices that tend to enhance the multiplication of organisms at the skin insertion site (by applying an occlusive transparent plastic dressing) [16], or lead to site contamination (by using heavily contaminated disinfectants) [17], may increase the risk of developing catheter-related infection.

The pathogenesis of catheter-related infection that is initiated by contamination of the catheter hub differs from that related to skin insertion site in that organisms are usually introduced into the hub from the hands of medical personnel, then migrate along the internal surface of the catheter. However, both these sources of catheter-related infection are predominantly caused by skin organisms, although the organisms are transmitted from a different skin source (the skin of the medical personnel in the case of hub contamination vs the skin of the patient in the case of microbial migration from the skin insertion site). The contribution of hub contamination to catheter-related infection helps explains why CRBSI can occur without inflammation at the skin entry site and despite the use of aseptic techniques during catheter insertion and why catheter tunneling may not necessarily protect from catheter-related infection [18]. Although Maki and co-workers [4] found the hub to be the second most common source of catheter-related infections. Sitges-Serra et al. [18, 19], Salzman et al. [20], and other investigators highlighted the hub as the most common source for CRBSI. This discrepancy in findings could be explained by the fact that the former group of investigators studied short-term catheters with a mean duration of placement of 7.2–9.1 days, whereas the latter group of investigators studied longer term CVCs with a mean duration of placement of 23.4 to 26.5 days. The validity of such an explanation for those seemingly discrepant reports was confirmed by a recent evaluation of the ultrastructural colonization on the internal and external surfaces of CVSs using semiquantitative scanning electron microscopy [21]. For CVCs with a relatively short placement duration (mean 10 days) colonization of the external catheter surface predominated, whereas the prolonged use of the hub in CVCs that remained in place for longer periods (>30 days) resulted in a high degree of internal surface colonization that exceeded the external surface colonization originating from the skin insertion site [21]. Therefore, it is reasonable to conclude that the catheter insertion site is the major source of organisms causing infection of catheters in place for a short time, but that entry of organisms via the catheter hub may become more important in infection of long-term catheters [22].

The microbiology of vascular catheter-related infection is a direct reflection of the various sources of infection. The fact that most episodes of catheter-related infection are caused by skin organisms (originating from the skin of the patient at the catheter insertion site or the hands of medical personnel), explains why staphylococci (coagulase-negative staphylococci and *S. aureus*) account for about two-thirds of these episodes [7]. *Candida* species (most commonly *C. albicans* followed by *C. parapsilosis*) are becoming increasingly important as a cause of catheter-related infection and are thought to originate either from the hands of medical personnel or from hematogenous seeding of the catheter from the gastrointestinal tract. *Corynebacterium*, especially JK strains, and *Bacillus* species can cause catheter-related infection and are usually introduced from the skin or the hub. The contribution of Gram-negative bacilli to catheter-related infection is mostly due to bacteria acquired from the hospital environment (such as *Acinetobacter* species, *Pseudomonas* species, and *Stenotrophomonas maltophilia*) rather than enteric organisms (such as *Escherichia coli* and *Klebsiella pneumoniae*).

Risk Factors

A clear understanding of the various risk factors implicated in catheter-related infection is essential to planning an effective strategy for prevention. A risk factor applicable to infection of CVCs [23], peripheral arterial catheters [24], and pulmonary arterial Swan-Ganz catheters [25] is the prolonged duration of catheterization. The location of the catheter can also affect the predisposition to infection. A review of 30 prospective clinical studies showed that the risk of catheter infection per day of catheterization was 1.3% for peripheral plastic venous catheters, 1.9% for peripheral arterial catheters, and 3.3% for CVCs [26]. It has also been suggested that internal jugular CVCs are more likely to become infected than subclavian catheters [25], probably owing to higher bacterial concentrations in areas that are more likely to be covered by hair, such as the neck; however, this suggestion could not be confirmed by others [27]. CVCs inserted into the femoral veins, an area that is easily accessible to a large number of enteric flora, are generally thought to be associated with the highest rates of infection. However, this association is not necessarily causal since femoral cannulation is likely to be preceded by failed attempts at cannulation of the subclavian or jugular veins, a practice that, in and by itself, is expected to reduce sterile precautions.

Frequent manipulation of the catheter as with pulmonary artery Swan-Ganz catheters can predispose to catheter-related infection [26]. A similar predisposition to infection was also thought to apply when comparing frequently-manipulated triple-lumen CVCs vs less-manipulated single-lumen CVCs. However, although several non-randomized, and most retrospective studies have suggested that triple-lumen CVCs are associated with a higher risk of infection than single-lumen CVCs [28, 29], some recent prospective randomized trials have failed to demonstrate any significant difference in infection rates [30, 31]; it is possible that patients who require triple-lumen catheters generally have more serious underlying illnesses than those in whom a single-lumen catheter is inserted and, therefore, are more likely to develop catheter-related infection.

The catheter material may be an important factor in promoting thrombogenesis and adherence of organisms. For instance, flexible silicone and polyurethane catheters are less thrombogenic than polyvinylchloride catheters, which may explain why, as previously mentioned, staphylococci and fungi adhere better to polyvinylchloride catheters than to Teflon catheters [7].

Another risk factor is the direct application of occlusive transparent plastic dressings to the CVC insertion site. This type of dressing leads to a warm, moist insertion site with a high microbial burden, thereby increasing the risk of catheter colonization and septicemia [16]. The findings of a meta-analysis of all pertinent randomized controlled trials demonstrated a higher risk for catheter tip infection in patients with either central or peripheral venous catheters who received occlusive transparent polyurethane film compared with gauze dressings [32]. It is important to note, however, that the largest prospective randomized studies reviewed in that meta-analysis [32] failed to show significant differences in catheter-related septicemia between the two groups of patients. Moreover, the results of studies done with occlusive transparent dressings might not be applicable to the more recently marketed non-occlusive transparent dressings.

Other risk factors for vascular catheter-related infection include violation of aseptic techniques for insertion and maintenance of catheters by inexperienced medical personnel [33], and using cutdowns for the insertion of catheters [34].

Prevention

A number of protective measures have been reported to possibly reduce the rate of catheter-related infection. In this chapter, only those measures that have been reported in clinical trials to be protective against catheter-related infection will be discussed, and potentially controversial issues will be addressed. These protective measures can be divided into two general categories depending on whether or not they utilize some form of antimicrobial agent(s) (Table 1).

Measures that Utilize Antimicrobials

Sterilization of the Insertion Site: The most commonly used antimicrobial-utilizing measure consists of the application of topical antibiotics or disinfectants in an attempt to lower the microbial burden at the skin insertion site. For instance, the use of a topical polyantibiotic regimen (polymyxin-neomycin-bacitracin) was associated with a significantly lower rate of catheter related infection [14], at the expense, though, of a higher risk of acquiring fungal (*Candida*) colonization and infection. In a randomized controlled trial, the application of mupirocin (a topical antibiotic with high anti-staphylococcal activity) was shown to decrease by five-fold the risk of significant colonization of CVCs inserted in the internal jugular vein [35]. In a three-arm trial that compared the efficacy of topical application of 70% alcohol vs. 10% povidone iodine vs. 2% chlorhexidine gluconate, the rate of catheter-related bacteremia was almost four-fold lower in the group of patients who received chlorhexidine vs the other two groups [15].

Silver-Impregnated Subcutaneous Cuff: This measure is intended to provide both an antimicrobial deterrent (due to the silver) and a mechanical barrier (due to the subcutaneously placed collagen cuff) to the migration of bacteria. Although the use of the silver-impregnated subcutaneous cuff has been reported in two prospective, randomized clinical trials to reduce the incidence of infection of short-term CVCs [4, 36], a recent prospective non-randomized study failed to demonstrate any protective effect [37]. Moreover, the use of silver-impregnated subcutaneous cuffs failed to protect against infection of the longer-term CVCs (mean duration 20 days) [unpublished observations] or of the long-term, tunneled Hickman catheters [38]. Given

Table 1. Measures reported to protect against catheter-related infection in human subjects

---

Measures that utilize antimicrobials
- Sterilization of insertion site
- Silver-impregnated cuff
- Flushing catheters with antimicrobial/antithrombotic agents
- Antimicrobial coating of catheters with effective antimicrobials
- Antiseptic catheter hub

Measures that do not utilize antimicrobials
- Maximal sterile barriers
- Skilled infusion therapy team

---

the biodegradable nature of the collagen to which the silver ions are chelated, it is quite understandable why the potential anti-infective activity of this silver-impregnated collagen cuff is short-lived and does not apply to long-term CVCs.

Flushing Catheter with Antimicrobial/Antithrombotic Agents: Since some coagulase-positive organisms, such as *S. aureus* and *Candida* species, adhere tightly to fibronectin and fibrin present in the thrombin sleeve around the catheter, it is conceivable that flushing the CVC lumen with a combination of antimicrobial and antithrombotic agents could potentially protect against catheter-related infection. Because of the extremely small amounts of antimicrobial agents present in the catheter flush solution, the use of this approach is not expected to produce any systemic antimicrobial activity. When compared to flushing with heparin alone, daily flushing of tunneled CVCs with a solution containing heparin plus vancomycin was reported to significantly decrease the frequency of catheter-related bacteremia due to vancomycin-susceptible Gram-positive organisms colonizing the lumen [39]. Although seemingly efficacious, the impact of this approach on the overall incidence of catheter-related bacteremia due to both vancomycin-susceptible and vancomycin-resistant organisms was not examined. The use of vancomycin/heparin solutions for flushing the catheter raises some potential concerns, including the possibility of developing superinfection with Gram-negative bacilli and *Candida* species. Moreover, the use of this catheter flush solution may theoretically predispose to the emergence of vancomycin-resistant Gram-positive cocci, a potentially serious event given the fact that vancomycin is the only therapeutic drug of choice for treatment of established infections due to methicillin-resistant staphylococci and penicillin-resistant enterococci.

Another antimicrobial/anticoagulant alternative for flushing catheters consists of the combination of minocycline and ethylenediaminetetraacetate (EDTA). Neither minocycline nor EDTA are used for the treatment of bloodstream infections and, hence, the emergence of organisms resistant to this combination, if it ever occurs, should not cause a therapeutic dilemma. This antimicrobial/antithrombotic combination possesses a broad spectrum, and often synergistic, *in vitro* activity against methicillin-resistant staphylococci, Gram-negative bacilli, and *C. albicans* [40]. Although the minocycline/EDTA flush solution has not been evaluated yet in a prospective controlled study, it has been reported to successfully prevent the recurrence of catheter infection in several high risk patients [40].

The major limitation of the general approach of flushing the lumen of catheters is that organisms adherent to the external surface of the catheter are not directly exposed to the antimicrobial/antithrombotic flush solution, which would theoretically limit the potential clinical efficacy of this approach for preventing infections of short-term CVCs. It is yet to be determined whether this approach is clinically successful in preventing infection of long-term vascular catheters where colonization of the internal surface of the catheter predominates.

Antimiocrobial Coating of Catheters: Coating catheters with antimicrobial agents (antibiotics or antiseptics) may prove to be the most protective antimicrobial-utilizing approach for the prevention of vascular catheter-related infection. This approach can be particularly effective if both the external and internal surfaces of the catheter are coated with antimicrobial agent(s) that provide strong, durable and broad spectrum antimicrobial activity against the vast majority of organisms that can cause catheter-related infection

The potential clinical efficacy of this approach was initially demonstrated in a prospective randomized study that showed that the immersion of CVCs that had been pre-treated with a positively charged cationic surfactant (tridodecyl methylammonium chloride; TDMAC), in a solution of cefazolin (a negatively charged antibiotic) just prior to catheter insertion significantly reduced the rate of catheter colonization, when compared to untreated catheters [41]. Although seemingly effective, the immersion of the catheter in an antimicrobial solution by the bed-side prior to insertion in patients is rather impractical and time-consuming. Therefore, the utility of the approach of antimicrobial coating of catheters is best addressed by examining the anti-infective efficacy of CVCs that are pre-coated with antimicrobial agent(s).

In that regard, a prospective, randomized, multi-center study demonstrated that CVCs coated with the combination of chlorhexidine and silver sulfadiazine were two-fold less likely to become colonized, and were at least four-fold less likely to be associated with bacteremia, when compared to uncoated catheters [42]. However, the protective efficacy of CVCs coated with chlorhexidine and silver sulfadiazine could not be demonstrated in three recently reported, randomized, single-center studies [43–45].

The novel approach of coating catheters with the unique combination of minocycline and rifampin provides a broad spectrum inhibitory activity *in vitro* against Gram-positive bacteria, Gram-negative bacteria and *C. albicans* [46, 47]. The clinical efficacy of short-term CVCs coated with minocycline/rifampin was demonstrated, in a recently reported, prospective, randomized, multi-center study, to produce at least a three-fold reduction in the rate of catheter colonization and to prevent the occurrence of catheter-related septicemia when compared to uncoated catheters [48]. The potential concern of developing antibiotic resistance was addressed in this study which found no evidence for the emergence of antibiotic resistance among bacteria recovered from the patients who had received catheters coated with minocycline/rifampin; the presence of one coating antibiotic may serve to prevent emergence of bacterial resistance to the other coating antibiotic in the clinical scenario of catheter infection where the concentration of infecting bacteria is relatively low.

The use of catheters coated with either chlorhexidine/silver sulfadiazine or minocycline/rifampin was reported to be very cost-beneficial [42, 48]. Moreover, by decreasing the likelihood of administering drugs (such as vancomycin) for the treatment of suspected or documented catheter-related infection, the use of catheters coated with effective antimicrobials (antiseptics or antibiotics) may, in fact, help reduce the development of antibiotic resistance. The antimicrobial activity of catheters coated with minocycline/rifampin was reportedly significantly superior both *in vitro* and in a rabbit model of *S. aureus* infection to that of catheters coated with chlorhexidine/silver sulfadiazine [46, 47]. Moreover, both the external and internal surfaces of the former catheter are coated with minocycline/rifampin, whereas only the external surface of the latter catheter is coated with chlorhexidine/silversulfadiazine. Therefore, it is anticipated that catheters coated with minocycline/rifampin will prove clinically superior to catheters coated with chlorhexidine/silver sulfa-diazine.

The novel method of ion beam-assisted deposition of silver ions on the catheter surface has been used to construct silver-coated catheters. *In vitro* adherence experiments and *in vivo* rat studies have demonstrated that such silver-coated catheters are less prone to bacterial colonization than uncoated catheters [49]. However, there have been no randomized prospective clinical trials that evaluate the efficacy of these silver-coated catheters in reducing catheter-related bloodstream infection. In that regard, it is important to note that the silver ions are not released from the surface of these catheters in sufficient enough magnitude to affect the bacteria that are embedded in the layer of biofilm around the catheter that contains host tissue ligands (such as fibronectin, fibrin, fibrinogen, etc.,) to which organisms are likely to adhere, and, therefore, produce no detectable zones of inhibition.

Antiseptic Catheter Hub: A novel hub model that allows passage of the needle through an antiseptic chamber that contains iodinated alcohol has been shown both *in vitro* [50] and in an animal model [51] to protect against hub colonization. When tested in patients with a mean duration of CVC placement of two weeks, this new hub model was shown to decrease catheter-related sepsis by four-fold [52]. The major limitation of this approach, particularly in patients with short-term CVCs, is that it only protects against organisms migrating through the hub along the internal surface of the catheter and offers no antimicrobial activity against skin organisms that migrate along the external surface of the catheter.

Measures that do not Utilize Antimicrobials

Aseptic Insertion: The practice of using maximal sterile barriers (i.e., wearing sterile gloves, a mask, a gown, and a cap, and using a large drape) during the insertion of a CVC may help protect against catheter-related infections, when compared to the routine aseptic procedure of wearing gloves and using a small drape. In addition to producing a more than six-fold decrease in the rate of CVC-related sepsis [53] and a four-fold decrease in the rate of pulmonary artery catheter-related bacteremia [25], the use of maximal sterile barriers was found to be highly cost-effective. The efficacy of maximal sterile barriers in preventing field contamination during insertion of CVCs is highlighted by the finding that all cases of catheter infection in the maximal sterile barrier group occurred more than two months following catheter insertion, whereas two-thirds of cases of catheter infections in the control group occurred during the first week post-insertion of the catheter [53].

Skilled Infusion Therapy Team: The use of an experienced infusion therapy team has been demonstrated to decrease the rates of catheter infection by five- to eight-fold [8, 54]. Establishing such a skilled team for the insertion and maintenance of vascular catheters can be cost-effective, particularly in medical centers with high rates of catheter-related infection or with large numbers of immunocompromised patients.

Although some other practices have been suggested to have preventive potential, clinical trials have failed to demonstrate any protection against catheter-related infection. For instance, changing the dressing at the insertion site, and the infusate tubing every 24 hours is no more protective than changing them every 72 hours [55, 56]. Although the use of in-line filters can reduce the rate of phlebitis, it does not decrease the frequency of catheter infections [57]. The protective role of routine exchange of CVC over a guide wire remains most controversial. Although earlier uncontrolled trials that did not entail performing quantitative catheter cultures suggested that routine exchange of CVCs can reduce the risk of CVC-related infections [58, 59], more recent prospective, randomized clinical trials failed to demonstrate any protection from regularly scheduled CVC exchange every three days over a guidewire versus replacing the CVC only when clinically indicated [60, 61]. On the contrary, one of these studies showed that routine exchange of CVC over a guidewire may actually increase the risk of bloodstream infection, though it may be protective against mechanical complications of catheter insertion such as pneumothorax [61]. A reasonable approach to adopt might be to routinely culture the removed catheter whenever a new CVC is inserted over a guide wire. If the removed catheter is colonized (which is the case with only a minority of catheters), the newly exchanged catheter may then be removed and another CVC inserted via a fresh venous stick, preferably on the contralateral side.

Conclusion

Catheter-related bloodstream infection represents the most common life threatening complication of intravascular catheters and is very expensive to manage. By reducing the adherence to the catheter of organisms originating from either the skin or the catheter hub, a number of measures have been reported in clinical trials to successfully reduce the rate of vascular catheter-related infection. These include measures such as application of topical disinfectants (particularly chlorhexidine), use of silver-impregnated subcutaneous cuffs (for short-term central venous catheters), flushing catheters with the combination of antimicrobial and antithrombotic agents, antimicrobial coating of catheters with either antiseptic (chlorhexidine plus silver sulfadiazine) or antibiotic combinations (minocycline plus rifampin), use of an antiseptic catheter hub, institution of maximal sterile barriers, and placement and maintenance of vascular catheters by a skilled infusion therapy team. Fortunately, the majority of cases of catheter-related infection appear to be preventable, particularly those associated with the short-term use of catheters. More work is needed on the prevention of infection of long-term vascular devices, including catheters used for hemodialysis, parenteral nutrition and chemotherapy.

References

1. Maki DG (1992) Infections due to infusion therapy. In: Bennett JV, Brachman PS (eds) Hospital infections . Little, Brown and Co, Boston, pp 849–898
2. Farr BM (1994) Prevention and management of vascular catheter infections. Crit Care Med 6:29–42
3. Jarvis WR, Edwards JR, Culver DH, et al (1991) Nosocomial infection rates in adult and pediatric intensive care units in the United States. Am J Med 91 (suppl 3B):185S–191S

4. Maki DG, Cobb L, Garman JK, Shapiro JM, Ringer M, Helgerson RB (1988) An attachable silver-impregnated cuff for prevention of infection with central venous catheters: a prospective randomized multicenter trial. Am J Med 85:307–314
5. Powell C, Kudsk KA, Kulich PA, Mandelbaum JA, Fabri PJ (1988) Effect of frequent guidewire changes on triple-lumen catheter sepsis. J Parenter Enteral Nutr 12:464–465
6. Gill RT, Kruse JA, Thill-Baharozian MC, Carlson RW (1989) Triple vs single-lumen central venous catheters. Arch Intern Med 149:1139–1141
7. Raad II, Bodey GP (1992) Infectious complications of indwelling vascular catheters. Clin Infect Dis 15:197–210
8. Groeger JS, Lucas AB, Thaler HT, et al (1993) Infectious morbidity associated with long-term use of venous access devices in patients with cancer. Ann Intern Med 229:168–174
9. Maki DG (1991) Infection caused by intravascular devices: pathogenesis, strategies for prevention. Royal Society of Medicine Sevices Limited, London
10. Groeger JS, Lucas AB, Coit D (1991) Venous Access in the cancer patient. In: DeVita VT Jr, Hellman S, Rosenbert SA (eds) Cancer: Principles and Practice of Oncology. JB Lippincott, Philadelphia, 3rd ed, pp 1–14
11. Darouiche RO, Raad II (1997) Prevention of catheter-related infections: the skin. Nutrition 13 (suppl. 4):26S–29S
12. Pittet D, Tarara D, Wenzel RP (1994) Nosocomial bloodstream infection in critically ill patients: excess length of stay, extra costs, and attributable mortality. JAMA 271:1598–1601
13. Bjornson HS, Colley R, Bower RH, Duty VP, Schwartz-Fulton JT, Fisher JE (1982) Association between microorganism growth at the catheter insertion site and colonization of the catheter in patients receiving total parenteral nutrition. Surgery 192:720–726
14. Maki DG, Band JD (1981) A comparative study of polyantibiotic and iodophor ointments in prevention of vascular catheter-related infection. Am J Med 70:739–744
15. Maki DG, Ringer M, Alvarado CJ (1991) Prospective randomized trial of povidone-iodine, alcohol, and chlorhexidine for prevention of infection associated with central venous and arterial catheters. Lancet 338:339–343
16. Conly JM, Grieves K, Peters B (1989) A prospective, randomized study comparing transparent and dry gauze dressings for central venous catheters. J Infect Dis 159:310–318
17. Frank MJ, Schaffner W (1976) Contaminated aqueous benzalkonium chloride. An unnecessary hospital infection hazard. JAMA 236:2418–2419
18. Sitges-Serra A, Hernandez R, Maestro S, Pi-Suner T, Garces JM, Segura M (1997) Prevention of catheter sepsis: the hub. Nutrition 13 (suppl 4):30S–35S
19. Sitges-Serra A, Puig P, Linares J, et al (1984) Hub colonization as the initial step in an outbreak of catheter-related sepsis due to coagulase negative staphylococci during parenteral nutrition. J Parenter Enter Nutr 8:668–672
20. Salzman MB, Isenberg HD, Shapiro JF, Lipsitz PJ, Rubin LG (1993) A prospective study of the catheter hub as the portal of entry for microorganisms causing catheter-related sepsis in neonates. J Infect Dis 167:487–490
21. Raad I, Costerton JW, Sabharwal U, Sacilowski M, Anaissie E, Bodey GP (1993) Ultrastructural analysis of indwelling vascular catheters: a quantitative relationship between luminal colonization and duration of placement. J Infect Dis 168:400–407
22. Salzman MB, Rubin LG (1997) Relevance of the catheter hub as a portal for microorganisms causing catheter-related bloodstream infections. Nutrition 13 (suppl 4):15S–17S
23. Norwood SH, Jenkins G (1990) An evaluation of triple-lumen catheter infections using a guidewire exchange technique. J Trauma 30:706–712
24. Shinozaki T, Deane RS, Mazuzan JE Jr, Hamel AJ, Hazelton D (1983) Bacterial contamination of arterial lines. JAMA 249:223–225
25. Mermel LA, McCormick RD, Springman SR, Maki DG (1991) The pathogenesis and epidemiology of catheter-related infection with pulmonary artery Swan-Ganz catheters: a prospective study utilizing molecular subtyping. Am J Med 91 (suppl 3B):197S–205S
26. Hampton M, Sherertz RJ (1988) Vascular-access infections in hospitalized patients. Surg Clin North Am 68:57–71
27. Senagore A, Waller JD, Bonell BW, Bursch LR, Scholten DJ (1987) Pulmonary artery catheterization: a prospective study of internal jugular and subclavian approaches. Crit Care Med 15:35–37

28. Pemberton LB, Lyman B, Lander V, et al (1986) Sepsis from triple vs. single-lumen catheters during total parenteral nutrition in surgical or critically ill patients. Arch Surg 121:591–594

29. Hilton E, Haslett TM, Borenstein MT, et al (1988) Central catheter infections: single vs triple-lumen catheters influence of guidelines on infection rates when used for replacement of catheters. Am J Med 84:667–672

30. MacCarthy MC, Shives JK, Robison RJ, Broadie TA (1987) Prospective evaluation of single and triple lumen catheters in total parenteral nutrition. J Parenter Enteral Nutr 11:259–262

31. Farkas JC, Liu N, Bleriot JP, Chevret S, Goldstein FW, Carlet J (1992) Single- versus triple-lumen central catheter-related sepsis: a prospective randomized study in a critically ill population. Am J Med 93:277–282

32. Hoffmann KK, Weber DJ, Samsa GP, Rutala WA (1992) Transparent polyurethane film as an intravenous catheter dressing. A meta-analysis of the infection rates. JAMA 167:2072–2076

33. Armstrong CW, Mayhall CG, Miller KB, et al (1986) Prospective study of catheter replacement and other risk factors for infection of hyperalimentation catheters. J Infect Dis 154:808–816

34. Moran JM, Atwood RP, Rowe MI (1965) A clinical and bacteriologic study of infections associated with venous cutdowns. N Engl J Med 272:554–558

35. Hill RLR, Fisher AP, Ware RJ, Wilson S, Casewell MW (1990) Mupirocin for the reduction of colonization of internal jugular cannulae: a randomized controlled trial. J Hosp Infect 15:311–321

36. Flowers RH III, Schwenzer KJ, Kopel RF, Fisch MJ, Tucker SI, Farr BM (1989) Efficacy of an attachable subcutaneous cuff for the prevention of intravascular catheter-related infection. A randomized, controlled trial. JAMA 261:878–883

37. Hasaniya NW, Angelis M, Brown MR, Yu M (1996) Efficacy of subcutaneous silver-impregnated cuffs in preventing central venous catheter infections. Chest 109:1030–1032

38. Groeger JS, Lucas AB, Coit D, et al (1993) A prospective randomized evaluation of silver-impregnated subcutaneous cuffs for preventing tunneled chronic venous access catheter infections in cancer patients. Ann Surg 218:206–210

39. Schwartz C, Henrickson KJ, Roghmann K, Powell K (1990) Prevention of bacteremia attributed to luminal colonization of tunneled central venous catheters with vancomycin-susceptible organisms. J Clin Oncol 8:591–597

40. Raad I, Buzaid A, Rhyne J, et al (1997) Minocycline and ethylenediaminetetraacetate for the prevention of recurrent vascular catheter infections. Clin Infect Dis 25:149–151

41. Kamal GD, Pfaller MA, Rempe LE, Jebson PJR (1991) Reduced intravascular catheter infection by antibiotic bonding. JAMA 265:2364–2368

42. Maki DG, Stolz SM, Wheeler S, Mermel LA (1997) Prevention of central venous catheter-related bloodstream infection by use of an antiseptic-impregnated catheter: a randomized, controlled study. Ann Intern Med 127:257–266

43. Ciresi D, Albrecht RM, Volkers PA, Scholten DJ (1996) Failure of an antiseptic bonding to prevent central venous catheter-related infection and sepsis. Am Surg 62:641–646

44. Pemberton LB, Ross V, Cuddy P, Kremer H, Fessler T, McGurk E (1996) No difference in catheter sepsis between standard and antiseptic central venous catheters. A prospective randomized trial. Arch Surg 131:986–989

45. Heard SO, Wagle M, Vijayakumar E, et al (1998) The influence of triple-lumen central venous catheters coated with chlorhexidine/silversulfadiazine on the incidence of catheter-related bacteremia: a randomized, controlled clinical trial. Arch Intern Med 158:81–87

46. Raad I, Darouiche R, Hachem R, Sacilowski M, Bodey GP (1995) Antibiotics and prevention of microbial colonization of catheters. Antimicrob Agents Chemother 39:2397–2400

47. Raad I, Darouiche R, Hachem R, Mansouri M, Bodey GP (1996) The broad spectrum activity and efficacy of catheters coated with minocycline and rifampin. J Infect Dis 173:418–424

48. Raad I, Darouiche R, Dupuis J, et al (1997) Central venous catheters coated with minocycline and rifampin for the prevention of catheter-related colonization and bloodstream infections: a randomized, double-blind trial. Ann Intern Med 127:267–274

49. Bambauer R, Mestres P, Schiel R, Klinkman J, Sioshansi P (1997) Surface-treated catheters with ion beam-deposition process evaluation in rats. Artif Organs 21:1039–1041

50. Segura M, Alia C, Oms L, Sancho JJ, Torres-Rodriguez JM, Sitges-Serra A (1989) *In vitro* bacteriological study of a new hub model for intravascular catheters and infusion equipment. J Clin Microbiol 27:2656–2659

51. Segura M, Alia C, Valverde J, Franch G, Torres-Rodriguez JM, Sitges-Serra A (1990) Assessment of a new hub design and the semiquantitative catheter culture method using an *in vivo* experimental model of catheter sepsis. J Clin Microbiol 28 :2551–2554
52. Segura M, Alvarez-Lerma F, Tellado JM, et al (1996) Advances in surgical technique: a clinical trial on the prevention of catheter-related sepsis using a new hub model. Ann Surg 223:363–369
53. Raad II, Hohn DC, Gilbreath BJ, et al (1994) Prevention of central venous catheter-related infections by using maximal sterile barrier precautions during insertion. Infect Control Hosp Epidemiol 15:231–238
54. Nelson DB, Kien CL, Mohr B, et al (1986) Dressing changes by specialized personnel reduce infection rates in patients receiving central venous parenteral nutrition. J Parenter Enteral Nutr 10:220–222
55. Maki DG, Ringer M (1987) Evaluation of dressing regimens for prevention of infection with peripheral intravenous catheters. JAMA 258:2396–2403
56. Josephson A, Gombert ME, Sierra MF, et al (1985) The relationship between intravenous fluid contamination and the frequency of tubing replacement. Infect Control 6:367–370
57. Rusho WJ, Bair JN (1979) Effect of filtration complications of postoperative intravenous therapy. Am J Hosp Pharm 36:1355–1356
58. Gregory JA, Schiller WR (1985) Subclavian catheter changes every third day in high risk patients. Am Surg 51:534–536
59. Bozetti F, Terno G, Bonfanti G, et al (1983) Prevention and treatment of central venous catheter sepsis by exchange via guidewire: a prospective controlled trial. Ann Surg 198:48–52
60. Eyer S, Brummitt C, Crossley K, Siegel R, Cerra F (1990) Catheter-related sepsis: prospective, randomized study of three methods of long-term catheter maintenance. Crit Care Med 18:1073–1079
61. Cobb DK, High KP, Sawyer RG, et al (1992) A controlled trial of scheduled replacement of central venous and pulmonary-artery catheters. N Engl J Med 327:1062–1068

Management of Fever in Cancer Patients with Acquired Neutropenia

P. Eggimann

Introduction

During the past few decades, substantial progress in multidrug immunosuppressive and cytotoxic chemotherapeutic treatments have greatly improved the prognosis of most cancer patients. However, infectious complications due to acquired neutropenia have become a major medical issue, often requiring intensive care management. The infections may be lethal if empiric broad-spectrum treatment is not instituted at the first sign of infection. Although this is now considered standard practice, the selection and evaluation of the efficacy of antibiotic agents has generated considerable controversy for nearly 25 years. After reviewing some particularities of infection in neutropenic patients, this paper will discuss the options and suggest a comprehensive algorithm for the non-infectious diseases specialist.

Particularities of Infection in Neutropenic Patients

Evaluation of the Infectious Risk

Among all the factors involved in the development of an infection in a patient with cancer, the most important is dysfunction of the immune system [1]. This immunosuppression may be subdivided into three types which predispose to the acquisition of distinct pathogens: These are granulocytopenia or neutropenia, defects of immune function related to the diminished capacity to opsonise microorganisms, and defects of cellular immunity related to T-cell functions (Table 1).

Neutropenic cancer patients are a heterogeneous group of patients, but the risk of infection is proportional to the granulocyte count and to the duration of immunosuppression. Although this risk substantially increases with granulocyte counts below 500/mm^3, many authorities consider that it becomes clinically relevant below 1 000/mm^3, and that severe infections and almost all bacteremias are observed below 100/mm^3 [2]. The presence of comorbidity, deep tissue infections, and the patient's underlying neoplastic disease are the other major factors. While the risk appears to be low for ambulatory patients with solid tumors, as many as 60% of leukemic patients will develop an infection during the aplastic phase of their treatment [3, 4].

Table 1. Common pathogens in immune dysfunction

Dysfunction of neutrophils (granulocytopenia)

Bacteria:	Staphylococcus epidermidis	Fungi:	Candida spp
	Staphylococcus aureus		Aspergillus spp
	Viridans streptococci		Mucorales
	Escherichia coli		
	Pseudomonas aeruginosa		

Dysfunction of immune function (hypogammaglobulinemia)

Bacteria:	Streptococcus pneumoniae
	Haemophilus influenzae

Dysfunction of cellular immunity

Bacteria:	Listeria monocytogenes	Viruses:	Cytomegalovirus
	Salmonella spp		Herpes simplex
	Mycobacterium spp		Varicella zoster
	Legionella spp	Protozoa:	Pneumocystis carinii
Fungi:	Cryptococcus neoformans		Toxoplasma gondii
	Histoplama capsulatum		Cryptosporidium
	Coccidioides immitis	Helminths:	Strongyloides stercoralis

Significance of Fever

The lack of cells able to carry out the inflammatory response explains why paramount signs and symptoms of infection are often absent in neutropenic patients. Of these, fever, that may be related to the tumor, to some drugs or to transfusion products, is often the mainstay of an infection [5, 6]. Although not specific, the development of fever in such patients should be considered to be the first sign of a potentially life-threatening infection and requires prompt empiric initiation of broad-spectrum antibiotic treatment [2, 4, 7]. Until the validation of this concept late in the 1960s, almost all neutropenic cancer patients died before the results of blood cultures were available, but since then, continuous progress has been made in the management of these patients [3, 8].

Definition of Fever: Generally, a single temperature measurement of $\geq 38.3\,°C$ orally, or $\geq 38.0\,°C$ over at least 1 hour in the absence of obvious other causes is considered as

Table 2. Initial diagnostic work-up of neutropenic patients with fever

Complete comprehensive history

Detailed physical examination, without rectal examination

Complementary diagnostic work-up
- Blood culture (2 sets)
- Complete blood count
- Blood chemistry (electrolytes, creatinine, BUN, liver function test)
- Urine analysis and urine culture
- Chest roentgenogram
- Throat and sputum culture
- Other microbiological studies based on physical findings

fever [2]. Febrile neutropenic cancer patients require a complete diagnostic work-up (Table 2), and microbiological studies must be obtained before the start of any antimicrobial agents.

Etiology of Fever: According to the classification of the International Immunocompromised Host Society (ICHS), febrile episodes in neutropenic cancer patients are microbiologically documented in 30 to 40% of cases, including an episode of bacteremia in two thirds of them. The infection is clinically documented in 25 to 30% of episodes. The oral cavity, the oropharynx, the lungs, the digestive tract, the skin, particularly the anal region and the sites of catheter insertion are the most commonly infected sites. In 30 to 40% the origin of the fever remains, unknown. However, until formal demonstration of another origin (in only about 5 to 10% of cases), infection remains the most probable etiology of these episodes, known as unexplained fever [2].

Etiologic Agents

During the 1950s, *Staphylococcus aureus* was the primary documented pathogen. A shift occurred in the 1960s, and for more than two decades, Gram-negative microorganisms (*Escherichia coli, Klebsiella* spp and *Pseudomonas aeruginosa*) were responsible for more than two-thirds of microbiologically documented infections in febrile neutropenic cancer patients. Most empiric antibiotic regimens were specifically directed against these organisms and this strategy allowed a significant reduction of their related mortality [9, 10]. Within the past decade, Gram-positive microorganisms have emerged as increasingly important pathogens [7, 11]. Presently, coagulase-negative staphylococci, alpha-hemolytic streptococci, methicillin-sensitive and methicillin-resistant *Staphylococcus aureus* (MSSA/MRSA) are responsible for the majority of episodes in most centers [12–15].

The factors responsible for this evolution are not completely understood, and the clinical data to establish them are scarce. The increasing use of venous access over long periods and indwelling catheters, which seem to promote bacteremia with microorganisms of the skin flora, is one factor [11,16]. Viridans streptococci are common in blood cultures of patients with extensive ulceration of the oral cavity, such as those treated with aggressive chemotherapy, and in those developing herpes gingivostomatitis [17, 18]. In leukemic patients receiving high dose cytarabine the course of streptococcal infections may be particularly fulminant with the development of acute respiratory distress syndrome (ARDS) [17, 19]. Finally, it is possible that the increasing use of oral quinolones as prophylaxis in neutropenic patients may have promoted the emergence of streptococci which are naturally resistant to them [20–23].

Fungal infections may occasionally be responsible for an initial febrile episode in a neutropenic host, but they present more commonly as superinfections occurring later in the course of a prolonged neutropenia. The risk appears to be particularly high if corticosteroids are associated, and their incidence has been reported to be as high as 15 to 30% [24–26]. The persistence of fever for more than 5 to 7 days, despite adequate broad-spectrum antibacterial coverage with a negative diagnostic work-up, is their usual mode of presentation. When a fungal infection is suspected, the incubation time of blood cultures must be prolonged to detect the presence of *Candida* spp, and chest and sinus X-rays obtained in order to detect early signs of aspergillosis [27]. Outside endemic areas, *Histoplasma* spp, *Coccidioides* spp and other deep-sited mycoses are uncommon. Their treatment is mostly empirical and essentially based on amphotericin B since the advent of potent prophylaxis with tri-azole agents such as fluconazole or itraconazole [28–30].

Reactivation of the *Herpes simplex* virus group is very common in neutropenic cancer patients, and their morbidity justifies systematic prophylaxis by acyclovir for all seropositive patients [31]. This approach limits the development of *Herpes zoster* group infections, which may disseminate in these patients. *Cytomegalovirus* infections are characterized by multiorgan involvement and their severity is directly related to the degree of T-cell dysfunction. They occur in transplant recipients and in human immundeficiency virus (HIV) positive patients. Bone marrow transplant patients cumulate all risks, but the prognosis of these infections has improved dramatically with the advent of potent antiviral agents such as gancyclovir and forcarnet [32, 33].

Empiric Antimicrobial Therapy

It is difficult to provide precise guidelines for initial empiric antibiotic therapy for fever occurring during neutropenia, because the choice of a specific regimen must be adapted to local and institutional patterns in microorganism ecology, as well as to individual characteristics of the infected patients. However, some concepts are well-established. Initial empiric agent(s) must be characterized by
1) bactericidal serum levels rapidly reached after administration
2) broad-spectrum activity against most Gram-negative and some Gram-positive bacteria
3) a good tolerance for potential administration during a long period of time.

For 30 years, numerous authors have reported on the efficacy of empiric treatment [2, 34]. Presently, although data support the use of combination regimens, the advent of advanced-generation cephalosporins and the data from recent carbapenem studies may strongly argue in favor of monotherapy.

Combination Therapy

The combination of antibiotic agents as initial empiric therapy has been widely accepted as standard clinical practice. A rapid bactericidal effect, an enhanced killing of microorganisms afforded by synergism, and a reduction in the emergence of resistance were until recently the rationale for using such regimens [4, 35].

Combination of Two β-Lactam Agents: These combinations present the advantage of a low toxicity potential, but their coverage is less effective than that of a β-lactam plus an aminoglycoside, so that they are practically no longer used. The combination of more recent agents would be very costly, without broadening the coverage, and would probably increase the selection of resistant microorganisms [2, 7].

Anti-pseudomonal β-Lactam plus Aminoglycosides: The combination of an anti-pseudo-monal β-lactam (anti-pseudomonal penicillin or third-generation cephalosporin) plus an aminoglycoside is the well established empiric initial treatment of fever in neutropenic cancer patients. A series of studies from the international antimicrobial therapy cooperative group (IATCG) of the European organization for research on treatment of cancer (EORTC) which each includes several hundreds of patients from 30 to 40 centers provided the essential data supporting this strategy [14, 15, 35–39]. The fourth study from this group [35] demonstrated the superiority of a long course (9 days) versus a short course (3 days) of the combination of an aminoglycoside (amikacin) with a third-generation cephalosporin (ceftazidime) in 872 febrile gra-nulocytopenic cancer patients [39]. The eighth study showed, early in the 1990s, a similar efficacy for single daily doses of ceftriaxone plus amikacin as compared with ceftazidime plus amikacin three times a day, suggesting that aminoglycosides admi-nistered once daily are as effective and no more toxic than multiple daily doses. In order to adapt the β-lactam agent to the evolution of the spectrum of infecting agents to Gram-positive cocci, the ninth study [14] showed that a combination of piperacillin-tazobactam (an extended spectrum penicillin combined with a potent β-lactamase inhibitor) plus amikacin was more effective than ceftazidime plus ami-kacin [14].

Antipseudomonal β-Lactam plus Aminoglycoside plus Glycopeptide: In order to extend the coverage to Gram-positive cocci, including those resistant to methicillin, several authors reported that the addition of a glycopeptide (vancomycin/teicoplanin) to the combined regimens previously described enhanced their efficacy [40, 41]. Two large studies suggested however, that this addition may be safely delayed until there is strong clinical or microbiological evidence for it [38, 42]. In addition, the recent emergence of staphylococci and enterococci resistant to glycopeptides strongly ar-gues against their widespread use [43, 44].

Monotherapy

The very broad spectrum of some third-generation cephalosporins (ceftazidime, cefepime), quinolones, and carbapenems (imipenem-cilastatin, more recently mero-penem) incited many groups to study their efficacy in monotherapy as empiric in-itial treatment for fever in neutropenic cancer patients. The arguments favoring this approach are
1) a decrease in costs
2) reduced equipment for intra-venous administration
3) less frequent monitoring of drug levels
4) the absence of aminoglycoside, allowing a better safety profile when the admini-stration of nephrotoxic drugs such as amphotericin or chemotherapy are needed [7, 12].

Third-Generation Cephalosporins: After an early trial conducted at the National Cancer institute, a meta-analysis indicated that except for profound neutropenia and Gram-positive bacteremia (< 50% failure), ceftazidime monotherapy could be considered as an alternative to the traditional combined regimens [4, 45]. Preliminary results with extended spectrum cephalosporins, considered by some authors as fourth generation (cefepime) are promising, and large trials are in progress [46, 47].

Quinolones: The lack of activity aqainst streptococci of the old quinolones (ciprofloxacin, ofloxacin, pefloxacin) may explain why the fifth study of the IACTG of the EORTC [37] did not support sufficient efficacy of ciprofloxacin monotherapy. Newer generation quinolones (sparfloxacin, levofloxacin) with an extended spectrum against Gram-positive cocci should probably be reserved for some subgroups of low-risk patients for which recent preliminary data suggest that they may be managed ambulatory with oral therapy [48–51].

Carbapenems: The coverage of carbapenems extends to almost all Gram-negative and Gram-positive aerobic bacteria. They are the most potent agents against anaerobes, and their stability is preserved against most beta-lactamase producing species. This very broad spectrum and their low toxicity profile have contributed to their position as first line agents in many severe nosocomial infections, including those due to *Pseudomonas aeruginosa* or *Enterobacter cloacae*, as well as for intra-abdominal infections [9, 52]. Several studies demonstrated that carbapenem monotherapy is a valuable and realistic alternative for the empiric treatment of fever in cancer patients, and the eleventh study of the IACTG of the EORTC confirmed that this option is also applicable for patients with profound and prolonged neutropenia [12, 15, 53].

Of the 958 patients included, whose main duration of neutropenia was 16–17 days, 483 received meropenem (1 g every 8 hours) and 475 the combination (ceftazidime 2 g every 8 h plus amikacin 20 mg/kg once daily). Stringent ICHS consensus criteria were used, with success defined as the resolution of fever and clinical signs of infection and eradication of the infecting organism without modification of the initial empiric regimen [34]. The success rates were 270/483 (56%) for monotherapy and 245/475 (52%) for combination, and were comparable (p = 0.20). They were similar for all types of infection (single Gram-negative bacteremia, single Gram-positive bacteremia, clinically documented infections and possible infections), as were the modification rates of the allocated regimen (glycopeptide in 33% versus 37%; empirical antifungal therapy in 23% versus 25%) and further infection rates (12%). At 30 days, the overall mortality rate was 5% in both groups, and the mortality attributed to the presenting infection or to further infection was very low (1.7% versus 2.7%) [15].

Indeed, this study pointed out that the three main traditional arguments in favor of combined therapy are probably obsolete. The time to defervescence was similar in the group treated with meropenem monotherapy and in the group treated with a combination of ceftazime plus amikacin, suggesting that the aminoglycoside did not enhance the bactericidal effect. In the same way, the comparable efficacy in two subgroups in which synergism was previously demonstrated as important (patients with streptococcal bacteremia and those with profound neutropenia) suggests that enhancing the killing of bacteria by synergy is no longer necessary with carbapenems. Colonization with resistant organisms was not studied in this trial, but it was recently demonstrated that a combination of imipenem-cilastatin plus netilmicin for the treatment of severe ICU infections did not prevent colonization or superinfections with resistant microorganisms [52].

Duration of Treatment

The duration of antimicrobial therapy must be determined by the type of infection, and by the evolution of the patient's clinical condition. Unfortunately, there is no consensus in the literature. Short term treatments are associated with a high level of relapse, and prolonged antibiotic therapy is associated with an increased risk of superinfections [4]. For microbiologically documented infections, for those with a severe clinical course or if profound neutropenia persists, the treatment has to be prolonged for more than the traditional 14 days, and some authors prolong it until the time of recovery from neutropenia. For each episode of fever, the initial empiric regimen has to be re-evaluated after 72 hours, and eventually adapted or restricted to the identified causative agent. When the origin of the fever is not attributed to a documented infection (fever of unknown origin), the treatment can be stopped after 5–7 days without fever [2, 4, 7, 54].

Adjunctive Therapy

Numerous approaches aimed at enhancing the immune function of neutropenic patients have been studied.

White Blood Cell Transfusion: Despite positive results, complications including alloimmunization and transmission of infection have led us to abandon the transfusion of heterologous white blood cells which was one of the earliest approaches studied [55, 56].

Immunotherapy: After a long history and vigorous debate in septic shock patients, passive immunization with either polyclonal or monoclonal antibodies has no defined role in the treatment of neutropenic patients [57–59]. Patients in whom neutropenia is anticipated should to be actively immunized against numerous potentially infecting agents including pneumococci [60, 61].

Hematopoietic Growth Factors: Colony-stimulating factors (G-CSF and GM-CSF) produce a dose-dependent increase in neutrophil counts and some side effects such as bone pain and fever in almost all acquired and congenital granulocytopenias. They induce secondary cytokine production and there are theoretical concerns about the acceleration of disease in patients with myeloid disorders, but there is at present no evidence that these may be clinically relevant. Hence, they are presently widely used as adjuvant therapy for aggressive chemotherapy [62, 63]. This contributes to an intensification of many chemotherapeutic regimens, and will probably result in increased neutropenic episodes. However, despite impressive preliminary clinical data suggesting that, when combined with antibiotics in neutropenic febrile cancer patients, they may reduce the duration of neutropenia, hospital stay, and antibiotic therapy, there is presently no consensus about hematopoietic growth factor use in this indication [10, 64].

Prophylaxis of Infection in Neuropenic Cancer Patients

Physical measures, including rigorous respect of hospital hygiene rules are important. Systematic hand washing and disinfection, special clothes for patient handling, and systematically cooked meals are of paramount importance to limit colonization with potentially pathogenic microorganisms. A consensus on the efficacy of special isolation wards ventilated in positive pressure with filtered air has not been reached, and must be restricted to patients with an anticipated long and profound neutropenia such as bone marrow transplant recipients and acute leukemic patients [2, 65].

For two decades, oral chemoprophylaxis with either non-resorbable agents (neomycin/garamycin/polymixine/vancomycin) or antibiotics (trimethoprim-sulfamethoxazole) was shown to reduce the number of febrile episodes [66]. However, the rapid emergence of resistant species has motivated the use of more effective agents of which oral fluoroquinolones are the most studied. Their efficacy against most potentially pathogenic Gram-negative enterobacteria is excellent. Their complete absorption by the digestive tract is responsible for limitation of the lymphatic spread of microorganisms, and preservation of the anaerobic flora contributes, by competition for substrates, to limit the proliferation of potentially resistant species [22, 67]. The combination of quinolones with agents effective against streptococci (penicillin/rifampin) reduces the incidence of Gram-positive infections, but may be ineffective in reducing the overall incidence of febrile neutropenic episodes [21, 23]. Here again, the emergence of resistant species of *Escherichia coli* and viridans streptococci may limit their utilization [17, 68]. In summary, chemoprophylaxis remains very controversial and is actually not systematically recommended [65].

Practical Guidelines

The management of fever occurring in a neutropenic cancer patient requires prompt extensive evaluation in order to initiate early empiric broad-spectrum antimicrobial therapy. Several particularities must be taken into account to implement this strategy. The infectious risk is proportional to the degree and the duration of the immunosuppression. All infectious signs or symptoms other than fever may be absent. The choice of antibiotic agent(s) must be determined by the degree of immunosuppression, by clinical findings and by local epidemiologic data. The empiric regimen should be re-evaluated after 72 h. An algorithm is proposed as a practical guide for the clinician in Fig. 1, but the patient's clinical condition remains determinant and consulting with an infectious disease specialist may be required in difficult cases.

Conclusion

Severe infectious complications among cancer patients with acquired neutropenia remain a major medical issue, and as they may present with fever only, early empiric broad-spectrum antibiotic therapy is the cornerstone of their management. To adapt to the evolving spectrum of the infecting organisms to Gram-positive cocci and taking into account the most recent data from large clinical studies, empiric

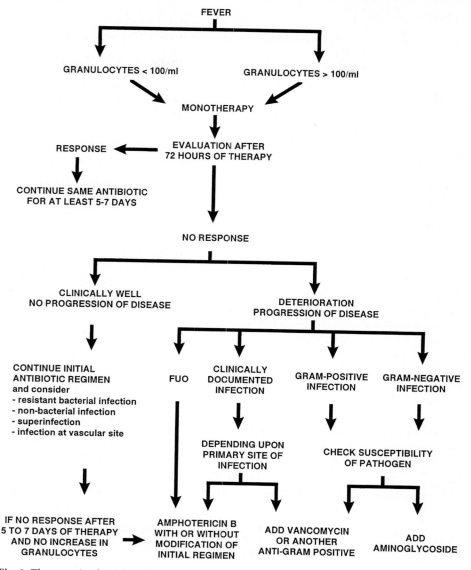

Fig. 1. Therapeutic algorithm for fever in neutropenic cancer patients. FUO: fewer of unknown origin

monotherapy with carbapenems may be chosen as first line treatment of fever in all neutropenic cancer patients including those high-risk patients with profound and persistent neutropenia. The combination of an anti-pseudomonal β-lactam with an aminoglycoside remains a well established alternative. For some particular sub-groups of low-risk patients, preliminary data suggests that ambulatory management with oral therapy may be feasible.

References

1. Mcgeer A, Feld R (1994) Epidemiology of infection in immunocompromised oncological patients. In: Balliere's Clinical Infectious Diseases 1, pp 415–438
2. Hughes WT, Armstrong D, Bodey GP, et al (1990) Guidelines for the use of antimicrobial agents in neutropenic patients with unexplained fever. J Infect Dis 161:381–396
3. Bodey GP, Buckley M, Sathe YS, Freireich EJ (1966) Quantitative relationships between circulating leukocytes and infection in patients with acute leukemia. Ann Intern Med 64:328–340
4. Schimpff SC (1995) Infections in cancer patients – diagnosis, prevention and treatment. In: Mandell GL, Douglas RG, Bennett JE (eds) Principles and practice of infectious diseases, 4th ed. Churchill Livingstone, New York, pp 2266–2275
5. Talcott GP, Siegel RD, Finberg R, et al (1992) Risk assessment in patients with cancer with fever and neutropenia: A prospective two-center validation of a prediction rule. J Clin Oncol 10:316–322
6. Talcott GP, Finberg R, Mayer RJ, et al (1988) The medical course of patients with cancer with fever and neutropenia. Arch Intern Med 148:2561–2568
7. Pizzo PA (1993) Management of fever in patients with cancer and treatment-induced neutropenia. N Engl J Med 328:1323–1332
8. Bodey GP (1986) Infection in patients with cancer: A continuing association. Am J Med 81 (suppl 1A):11–26
9. Calandra T, Cometta A (1991) Antibiotic therapy for Gram-negative bacteremia. Infect Dis Clin North Am 5:817–834
10. Hathorn JW, Lyke K (1997) Empirical treatment of febrile neutropenia: Evolution of current therapeutic approaches. Clin Infect Dis 24 (suppl 2):S256–S265
11. The EORTC International Antimicrobial Therapy Cooperative Group (1990) Gram-positive bacteraemia in granulocytopenic cancer patients. Eur J Cancer 26:569–574
12. Rolston KVI, Berkey P, Bodey GP, et al (1992) A comparison of imipenem to ceftazidime with or without amikacin as empiric therapy in febrile neutropenic patients. Arch Intern Med 152:283–291
13. Coullioud D, Van der Auwera P, Viot M, Lasset C (1993) Prospective multicentric study of the etiology of 1051 bacteremic episodes in 782 cancer patients. Cemic (french-belgian study club of infectious diseases in cancer). Support Care Cancer 1:34–46
14. Cometta A, Zinner SH, De Bock R, et al (1995) Piperacillin-tazobactam plus amikacin versus ceftazidime plus amikacin as empiric therapy for fever in granulocytopenic patients with cancer. Antimicrob Agents Chemother 39:445–452
15. Cometta A, Calandra T, Gaya H, et al (1996) Monotherapy with meropenem versus combination therapy with ceftazidime plus amikacin as empiric therapy for fever in granulocytopenic patients with cancer. Antimicrob Agents Chemother 40:1108–1115
16 Winston DJ, Dudnick DV, Chapin M, Ho WG, Gale RP, Martin WJ (1983) Coagulase-negative staphylococcal bacteremia in patients receiving immunosuppressive therapy. Arch Intern Med 143:32–36
17. Bochud PY, Eggimann P, Calandra T, Van Melle G, Saghafi L, Francioli P (1994) Viridans streptococcal bacteremias in neutropenic cancer patients: clinical spectrum and risk factors. Clin Infect Dis 18:25–31
18. Bochud PY, Calandra T, Francioli P (1994) Bacteremia due to viridans streptococci in neutropenic patients: a review. Am J Med 97:256–264
19. Dybedal I, Lamvik J (1989) Respiratory insufficiency in acute leukemia following treatment with cytosine arabinoside and septicemia with streptococcus viridans. Eur J Haematol 42:405–406
20. Karp JE, Merz WG, Hendricksen C, et al (1987) Oral norfloxacin for the prevention of gram-negative bacterial infections in patients with acute leukemia and granulocytopenia. Ann Intern Med 106:1–7
21. International Antimicrobial Therapy Cooperative Group of the European Organization for Research and Treatment of Cancer (1994) Reduction of fever and streptococcal bacteremia in granulocytopenic patients with cancer. JAMA 272:1183–1189
22. GIMEMA Infection Program (1991) Prevention of bacterial infection in neutropenic patients with hematologic malignancies: a randomized, multicenter trial comparing norfloxacin with ciprofloxacin. Ann Intern Med 117:7–12

23. Bow EJ, Mandell LA, Louie TJ, et al (1996) Quinolone-based antibacterial chemoprophylaxis in neutropenic patients: Effect of augmented gram-positive activity on infectious morbidity. Ann Intern Med 125:183–190

24. Anaissie E (1992) Opportunistic mycoses in the immunocompromised host: experience at a cancer center and review. Clin Infect Dis 14 (suppl 1):S43–S53

25. EORTC International Antimicrobial Therapy Cooperative Group (1989) Empiric antifungal therapy in febrile granulocytopenic patients. Am J Med 86:668–672

26. Bodey G, Bueltmann B, Duguid W, et al (1992) Fungal infections in cancer patients: an international autopsy survey. Eur J Clin Microbiol Infect Dis 11:99–109

27. Schaffner A (1994) Prophylaxis and treatment of fungal infections in cancer patients. In: Balliere's Clinical Infectious Diseases 1, pp 499–522

28. Winston DJ, Chandrasekar PH, Lazarus HM, et al (1993) Fluconazole prophylaxis of fungal infections in patients with acute leukemia. Results of a randomized placebo-controlled, double-blind, multicenter trial. Ann Intern Med 118:495–503

29. Menichetti F, Del Favero A, Martino P, et al (1994) Preventing fungal infection in neutropenic patients with acute leukemia: fluconazole compared with oral amphotericin B. Ann Intern Med 120:913–918

30. Powderly WG, Finkelstein D, Feinberg J, et al (1995) A randomized trial comparing fluconazole with clotrimazole troches for the prevention of fungal infections in patients with advanced human immunodeficiency virus infection. N Engl J Med 332:700–705

31. Novakova I, Donnelly JP, De Pauw B (1991) Ceftazidime as monotherapy or combined with teicoplanin for initial empiric treatment of presumed bacteremia in febrile granulocytopenic patients. Antimicrob Agents Chemother 35:672–678

32. Gold D, Corey (1987) Acyclovir prophylaxis for herpes simplex virus infection. Antimicrob Agents Chemother 31:361–367

33. Reusser P (1994) Prophylaxis and treatment of herpes virus infections in immunocompromised cancer patients. In: Balliere's Clinical Infectious Diseases 1, pp 523–544

34. Jones RN, Thornsberry C, Barry AL (1984) In vitro evaluation of HR810, a new wide-spectrum aminothiazol α-methoxyimino cephalosporin. Antimicrob Agents Chemother 25:710–718

35. EORTC International Antimicrobial Therapy Cooperative Group (1987) Ceftazidime combined with a short or long course of amikacin for empirical therapy of Gram-negative bacteremia in cancer patients with granulocytopenia. N Engl J Med 317:1692–1698

36. Klastersky J, Zinner SH, Calandra T, et al (1988) Empirical antimicrobial therapy for febrile granulocytopenic cancer patients: lessons from four EORTC trials. Eur J Cancer Clin Oncol 24:535–545

37. Meunier F, Zinner SH, Gaya H, et al (1991) Prospective randomized evaluation of ciprofloxacin versus piperacillin plus amikacin for empiric antibiotic therapy of febrile granulocytopenic cancer patients with lymphomas and solid tumors. Antimicrob Agents Chemother 35:873–878

38. The EORTC International Antimicrobial Therapy Cooperative Group (1991) Vancomycin added to empirical combination antibiotic therapy for fever in granulocytopenic cancer patients. J Infect Dis 163:951–958

39. EORTC International Antimicrobial Therapy Cooperative Group (1993) The efficacy and toxicity of single daily dose of amikacin and ceftriaxone versus multiple daily doses of amikacin and ceftazidime for infection in patients with cancer and granulocytopenia. Ann Intern Med 119:584–593

40. Karp JE, Hick JD, Angelopulos C, et al (1986) Empiric use of vancomycin during prolonged treatment induced granulocytopenia. Am J Med 81:237–242

41. Rubin M, Hathorn JW, Marshall D, Gress J, Steinberg SM, Pizzo PA (1988) Gram-positive infections and the use of vancomycin in 550 episodes of fever and neutropenia. Ann Intern Med 108:30–35

42. Ramphal R, Bolger M, Oblon DJ, et al (1992) Vancomycin is not an essential component of the initial empiric treatment regimen for febrile neutropenic patients receiving ceftazidime: a randomized prospective study. Antimicrob Agents Chemother 36:1062–1067

43. Edmond MB, Wenzel RP, Pasculle AW (1996) Vancomycin-resistant staphylococcus aureus: perspectives on measures needed for control. Ann Intern Med 124:329–334

44. Coque TM, Tomayko JF, Ricke SC, Okhyusen PC, Murray BE (1996) Vancomycin-resistant enterococci from nosocomial, community, and animal sources in the united states. Antimicrob Agents Chemother 40:2605–2609

45. Sanders JW, Powe NR, Moore RD, et al (1991) Ceftazidime monotherapy for empiric treatment of febrile neutropenic patients: a metaanalysis. J Infect Dis 164:907–916
46. Eggimann P, Glauser MP, Aoun M, Meunier F, Calandra T (1993) Cefepime monotherapy for the empirical treatment of fever in granulocytopenic cancer patients. J Antimicrob Chemother 32 (Suppl B):151–163
47. Ramphal R, Gucalp R, Rotstein C, Cimino M, Oblon D (1996) Clinical experience with single agent and combination regimens in the management of infection in the febrile neutropenic patient. Am J Med 100:83S–89S
48. Malik IA, Khan WA, Karim M, Aziz Z, Khan MA (1995) Feasibility of outpatient management of fever in cancer patients with low-risk neutropenia: Results of a prospective randomized trial. Am J Med 98:224–231
49. Freifeld AG, Pizzo PA (1996) The outpatient management of febrile neutropenia in cancer patients. Oncology 10:599–612
50. Escalante CP, Rubenstein EB, Rolston KV (1997) Outpatient antibiotic therapy for febrile episodes in low-risk neutropenic patients with cancer. Cancer Invest 15:237–242
51. Freifeld A, Pizzo P (1997) Use of fluoroquinolones for empirical management of febrile neutropenia in pediatric cancer patients. Pediatr Infect Dis J 16:140–146
52. Cometta A, Baumgartner JD, Lew D, et al (1994) Prospective randomized comparison of imipenem monotherapy with imipenem plus netilmicin for treatment of severe infections in non-neutropenic patients. Antimicrob Agents Chemother 38:1309–1313
53. The meropenem study group of Leuven (1995) Equivalent efficacies of meropenem and ceftazidime as empirical monotherapy of febrile neutropenic patients. J Antimicrob Chemother 36:185–200
54. Santolaya ME, Villarroel M, Avendano LF, Cofre J (1997) Discontinuation of antimicrobial therapy for febrile, neutropenic children with cancer: a prospective study. Clin Infect Dis 25:92–97
55. Clift RA, Sanders JE, Thomas ED, Buckner CD (1978) Granulocyte transfusions for the prevention of infection in patients receiving bone-marrow transplant. N Engl J Med 298:1052–1057
56. Strauss RG, Conett JE, Gale RP, et al (1981) A controlled trial of prophylactic granulocyte transfusions during initial induction chemotherapy for acute myelogenous leukemia. N Engl J Med 305:597–638
57. Cohen J, Heumann D, Glauser MP (1995) Do monoclonal antibodies and anticytokines still have a future in infectious diseases? Am J Med 99:45S–52S
58. Cohen J, Carlet J (1996) Intersept: an international, multicenter, placebo-controlled trial of monoclonal antibody to human tumor necrosis factor-alpha in patients with sepsis. International sepsis trial study group. Crit Care Med 24:1431–1440
59. Fisher CJ Jr, Agosti JM, Opal SM, et al (1996) Treatment of septic shock with the tumor necrosis factor receptor:fc fusion protein. The soluble tnf receptor sepsis study group. N Engl J Med 334:1697–1702
60. Gardner P, Schaffner W (1993) Immunization of adults. N Engl J Med 328:1252–1258
61. Fedson DS (1994) Adult immunization. Summary of the national vaccine advisory committee report. JAMA 272:1133–1137
62. American society of clinical oncology (1994) Recommendations for the use of hematopoietic colony-stimulating factors: evidence-based, clinical practice guidelines. J Clin Oncol 12:2471–2508
63. Boogaerts M, Cavalli F, Cortes-Funes H, et al (1995) Granulocyte growth factors: achieving a consensus. Ann Oncol 6:237–244
64. Freifeld A, Pizzo P (1995) Colony-stimulating factors and neutropenia: intersection of data and clinical relevance. J Natl Cancer Inst 87:781–782
65. Pizzo PA (1995) Empiric therapy and prevention of infection in the immunocompromised host. In: Mandell GL, Bennett JE, Dolin R (eds) Principles and practice of infectious diseases. 4th ed. Churchill Livingstone, New York, pp 2686–2696
66. EORTC International Antimicrobial Therapy Cooperative Group (1984) Trimethoprim-sulfamethoxazole in the prevention of infection in neutropenic patients. J Infect Dis 150:372–379
67. Maschmeyer G (1993) Use of the quinolones for the prophylaxis and therapy of infections in immunocompromised hosts. Drugs 45 (Suppl 3):73–80
68. Cometta A, Calandra T, Bille J, Glauser MP (1994) Escherichia coli resistant to fluoroquinolones in patients with cancer and neutropenia. N Engl J Med 330:1240–1241

Measuring Lung Mechanics

Determination of Lung Volume in the ICU

H. Burchardi, H. Wrigge, and M. Sydow

Introduction

Acute lung injury (ALI) and early acute respiratory distress syndrome (ARDS) are characterized by increased pulmonary membrane permeability leading to interstitial and intraalveolar edema. Under gravitational influence alveoli are compressed particularly in the dependent parts, whereas aerated alveoli are found in the non-dependent areas. In severe cases, no more than one third of the alveoli may remain patent ("baby lung"). By this mechanism, venous admixture and intrapulmonary shunt perfusion is increased and oxygenation is severely impaired.

In the non-dependent aerated and ventilated areas of the lungs, gas exchange may be unaltered and maintained if any additional impairment, like alveolar hyperinflation, can be avoided. Alveolar hyperinflation by mechanical ventilation, however, may severely damage these lungs. The mechanisms of this ventilator-induced lung injury [1] are various, e.g., regional alveolar overdistension by high airway inflation pressures [2, 3] and large tidal volumes [4, 5], as well as shear forces generated by local alveolar overdistension in inhomogeneous lungs [6]. Alveolar overdistension may cause increased microvascular permeability ("stress failure") which *per se* may induce lung edema [4, 5]. Alveolar overdistension also increases the risk of barotrauma which is still an often deleterious complication of mechanical ventilation [7, 8].

Thus, in an ARDS patients with "baby lungs" the clinical action must be to reduce tidal volume considerably in order to avoid high inflation pressures and alveolar overdistension [9]. Indeed, the high tidal volumes (12 to 15 ml/kg), formerly proposed, will certainly overdistend the ventilated alveoli. It is completely misleading to recommend a tidal volume by ml per kg body weight as tidal volume depends on the actual lung volume accessible for ventilation. Thus, it would be much more reasonable to relate tidal volume to functional residual capacity (FRC). At least airway pressure will give us more useful information than body weight. Restriction of the ventilatory excursion may be even more important in inhomogeneous lungs in order to reduce local tissue stress forces [6]. Moreover, the end-expiratory lung volume may be a valuable parameter to titrate positive end-expiratory pressure (PEEP) in ARDS because it is more strongly correlated to PEEP than to compliance or gas exchange [10].

Considering that the key phenomenon in the ARDS lung is the reduced lung volume ("baby lungs"), it is difficult to understand why lung volume is rarely measured in these critically ill patients. One of the reasons may be that determination of lung volume is considered to be complicated and elaborate.

Lung Volume Measurement

In principle, lung volume can be determined by two different procedures: Body plethysmography (a routine technique in lung function laboratories); and indicator gas washout techniques (either by a gas mixing technique in a closed circuit or by multiple breath washout in an open circuit). However, the resulting lung volume is different according to the measurement technique. Washout techniques can only perceive lung volumes which are available to ventilation, closed or trapped volumes will not be included in the resulting lung volume. On the other hand, by body-plethysmographic determination, total gas volume is measured which includes non-ventilated alveolar areas, and even (if present) non-thoracic gas spaces, like gastric air spaces.

For lung volume measurement and monitoring in the intensive care the body-plethysmographic methods are not applicable, thus, only the indicator gas mixing procedures have been used. As indicator gas, inert, poorly soluble gases like helium, argon, sulfur hexafluoride (SF6), or nitrogen are used. For bedside use in the ICU closed circuit indicator gas mixing systems are impractical and awkward. Thus, the multiple breath indicator gas washout technique is the most useful and applicable technique for this purpose.

In the multiple breath indicator gas washout procedure the subject inspires a certain concentration of the indicator gas until it is homogeneously distributed over the lungs. Then, after switching back to ventilation with the previous inspiratory gas mix, the indicator gas is withdrawn from the respiratory system. During this, flow and indicator gas-concentrations are continuously measured. The quotient of the amount of indicator gas washed out and the difference of indicator gas concentrations between the beginning and the end of the washout procedure is equal to the lung volume. Multiple breath washout procedures using SF6 [11, 12] or argon [13] as the indicator gas have been described. However, the nitrogen washout technique has the advantage of not using a special indicator gas, it only requires a modification of the nitrogen concentration by changing the oxygen concentration. Thus, it is the most frequently used technique.

FRC Measurement by Multibreath Nitrogen Washout

Since the open-circuit multibreath nitrogen-washout method (MBNW) was first established by Darling et al. in 1940 [14], several investigators have used washout techniques to measure FRC in ventilated patients [e.g. 13, 15, 16, 17, 18]. Although MBNW can easily be performed, a significant problem of this method is the considerable changes in gas viscosity during the washout maneuver. Variations in viscosity not only affect the accuracy of the gas flow measurement by pneumotachography [19, 20], moreover, they affect the gas signal since the gas flow through the sampling capillary is viscosity dependent [21]. Thus, sidestream analysis of gas fractions (e.g. by mass-spectrometry) via a capillary and mainstream gas flow measurement, result in a substantial time delay (T_D) between both signals, caused by the transport time of the sampled gas. For determination of the lung volume by the MB-NW technique these signals must be synchronized.

To improve the accuracy of nitrogen volume calculation during MBNW a continuous off-line correction of gas flow and T_D for changes in dynamic gas-viscosity has been proposed by Brunner et al. [21]. Below we describe a procedure for determining FRC by a multibreath nitrogen washout maneuver with automated compensation of gas viscosity variations. The accuracy and repeatability of the method and the influence of the dynamic adjustment of T_D were evaluated in a lung model and in mechanically ventilated patients.

Measurement Equipment

Gas flow was measured with a heated pneumotachograph (Fleisch no. 2, Fleisch, Lausanne, Switzerland) (Fig. 1). Inspiratory and expiratory gases were continuously sampled via a capillary connected to the Y-piece of the breathing circuit. Concentrations of nitrogen (N_2), oxygen (O_2) and carbon dioxide (CO_2) were measured with a mass spectrometer (MGA 1100, Perkin-Elmer, Pomona CA, USA). All data were sampled on-line by an analog/digital converter (DT 2801-A, Data Translation, Marlboro MA, USA) at a rate of 40 Hz and processed by an IBM AT compatible personal computer. The data acquisition and processing software were programmed with a commercially available software program (Asyst® 4.0, Keithley Asyst, Taunton, MA, USA).

The flow measuring system was calibrated with a gas mixture of known gas concentrations (65% N_2, 30% O_2 and 5% CO_2) and viscosity using a precision calibration pump with sinusoidal flow pattern. The instantaneous gas viscosity was determined from the analyzed gas fractions to correct the measured flow signal [20]. Volume was then obtained from the corrected flow signal during off-line analysis. To minimize a drift of the volume signal by an off-set of the flow signal the pressure transducer was adjusted meticulously during zero flow conditions before each measurement. Furthermore, for every minute, the inspiratory and expiratory volume was corrected as the arithmetic mean of both.

Determination of FRC

The N_2-washout maneuver was started by changing the inspired oxygen fraction (FiO_2) from baseline to 1.0. The N_2-fraction (F_{N_2}) at baseline was determined as the average N_2 concentration before the start of washout. As the first breath usually still contains a certain amount of nitrogen this inspired N_2-volume was subtracted from the cumulative N_2-volume calculated from the washout procedure. The measurement was finished at 3% ot the baseline F_{N_2} and then extrapolated. FRC was determined by the equation:

$$FRC = \frac{\int_{t_B}^{t_E} -\dot{V}(t) \cdot F_{N_2}(t) dt}{F_{N_2}(t_B) - F_{N_1}(t_E)}$$

where $\dot{V}$ is gas flow, t_B is the time at the beginning of the washout and t_E the time at the end of the calculation. $F_{N_2}(t_E)$ was defined as 3% of $F_{N_2}(t_B)$. Note that expiratory flow is negative by definition. Additionally, a correction tor tissue N_2 by Cournand et al. [22] was used in all patient measurements.

Delay Time and Viscosity Corrections

The entire T_D between gas sampling and data output of the mass spectrometer consists of a viscosity dependent part and a viscosity independent part ("internal delay time") which refers to the time between gas analysis and data output. The viscosity dependent part depends on the vacuum pressure of the gas analyzer as well as on the diameter and length of the capillary. During the washout procedure the momentary delay time $T_D(t_i)$ of the gas signal was calculated from the momentary gas viscosity $\eta(t_i)$ in the sampling line, according to Brunner et al. [21].

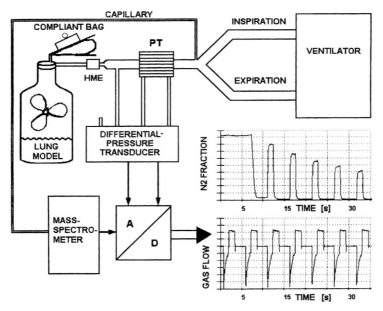

Fig. 1. General schematic diagram of the open circuit multiple breath nitrogen washout system for evaluating accuracy: a custom made lung model consisting of a 10 l glass bottle and a 1.5 l rubber bag (representing the compliant part of the lung). The bag was placed between two perspex plates with a weight on top of the upper plate to provide complete emptying of the bag during expiration. The compliance of the lung model was 40 ml/mbar. Different end-expiratory lung model volumes were achieved by different water fillings of the bottle. The end-expiratory volumes were measured by volume replacement (water filling) at the beginning and the end of each measurement series. PT: pneumotachograph, ASD: analog/digital converter; HME: heat and moisture exchanger. An original tracing of nitrogen fraction and gas flow is shown as an example of the output of the personal computer

Lung Model Measurements

In order to evaluate accuracy, experimental measurements were performed with a custom made lung model (Fig. 1). The end-expiratory volumes were measured by volume replacement (water filling) at the beginning and the end of each measurement series. Different end-expiratory lung model volumes were achieved by different amounts of water filling of the bottle. Three different end-expiratory volumes of the test lung were chosen: 2600 ml, 5100 ml and 7600 ml. FRC was determined 5 times in each.

To test the accuracy of the nitrogen washout method during ventilation with different FiO$_2$ five determinations of test lung volume were performed at FiO$_2$ of 0.21, 0.3, 0.4, 0.5, 0.6, 0.7, and 0.8 at an end-expiratory volume of 2580 ml. Using the automatic delay time and dynamic viscosity correction, the mean deviation of volume (measured vs. real: 2600 ml, 5100 ml, 7600 ml,) was 0.2% (=9 ml) with a doubled standard deviation (2 SD) of 2.4% (=123 ml) (Fig. 2). Washout maneuvers at different FiO$_2$ (0.21 up to 0.8) in the lung model revealed no obvious differences in accuracy of FRC determination. In contrast, FRC determination without viscosity correction by off-line analysis of the same MBNW curves resulted in systematic differences compared with the real model volume: Relative deviation of measured FRC and real model volume was 8% during measurements with FiO$_2$ of 0.21 increasing to 12% with FiO$_2$ of 0.8.

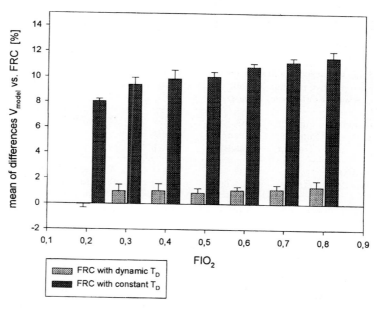

Fig. 2. Mean of differences of model volume (2600 ml) versus 5 FRC determinations depending on the different baseline FiO$_2$ MBNW was started at. The light boxes represent FRC determinations with continuous correction of mass spectrometer delay time (dynamic T$_D$) for changes in dynamic viscosity; the dark boxes represent FRC determinations from the same data without viscosity correction of delay time (constant T$_D$)

Patient Measurements

To test the *in vivo* reproducibility of the method we performed duplicated MBNW measurements in 30 mechanically ventilated adult intensive care patients (Table 1). 16 postoperative adults (NORM) without history or evidence of lung pathology were studied in the first 4 hours after major extrathoracic surgery. 14 critically ill patients with either acute lung injury (ALI, n = 8) or acute decompensation of chronic obstructive pulmonary disease (COPD, n = 6) were included. All patients were mechanically ventilated with continuous positive pressure ventilation (CPPV), 10–20 breaths/min., constant inspiratory flow, V_T 6–12 ml/kg, and FiO_2 0.3–0.7 depending on the individual pulmonary status and needs. After each measurement a nitrogen washout lasting 15–20 min. was performed to regain baseline conditions. To investigate the influence of different baseline FiO_2 on the reproducibility of FRC measurement MBNW was started from 4 different baseline FiO_2 levels (0.3, 0.6, 0.7, 0.8) in 6 NORM patients.

In patients the relative coefficient of repeatability (2 SD of differences between repeated measures) for 30 double FRC measurements was 3.8% (NORM), 5.2% (ARI) and 7.3% (COPD) (Fig. 3). Over all the repeatability was 6.0%. On the other hand, FRC determined without the dynamic viscosity correction was 10.9 ± 4.2% (mean ± 1 SD!) smaller than that using dynamic adjustment of T_D for viscosity changes. These deviations varied in the different patient groups: NORM 6.4 ± 1.0%; ALI 13.7 ± 3.0%, COPD 14.5 ± 2.5% (mean ± 1 SD!).

Table 1. Demographic characteristics, FiO_2 and PEEP of the 30 patients enrolled in the study. NORM: Postoperative patients without significant lung pathology, ALI: Acute lung injury; COPD: Chronic obstructive pulmonary disease

Group	Age mean (range)	FiO_2 mean (range)	PEEP mean (range)	Diagnosis	Number of patients
NORM (n = 12)	43.1 (18–68)	0.31 (0.3–0.4)	3.8 (0–6)	Abdominal surgery	9
				Bone surgery	2
				ENT surgery	1
ALI (n = 6)	58.0 (32–75)	0.45 (0.4–0.6)	6.8 (5–8)	Sepsis	4
				Pneumonia	1
				Near drowning	1
COPD (n = 6)	68.6 (57–85)	0.40 (0.3–0.6)	5.4 (5–8)	Respiratory failure due to:	
				– bronchopulmonary infection	4
				– respiratory muscle fatigue	2
Total (n = 24)	52.9 (18–85)	0.36 (0.3–0.6)	4.9 (0–8)		

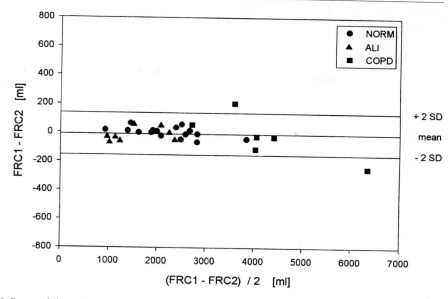

Fig. 3. Repeatability of duplicate FRC measurements in 30 patients with different pulmonary status. Absolute differences of FRC values against their means are plotted according to Bland and Altman [23]. NORM: post-operative patients, ALI: patients with acute lung injury, COPD: patients with chronic obstructive pulmonary disease.

Conclusion

Determination of end-expiratory lung volume by multibreath nitrogen washout is only accurate if the varying delay time of the side-stream sampled gas analysis is continuously corrected for gas viscosity changes. In experimental measurements with a lung model this continuous correction for gas viscosity improves accuracy to an average of $< 1.5\%$ (2 SD). The absence of systematic differences during ventilation with different FiO_2 (range 0.21–0.8), indicates a very precise compensation for viscosity changes influencing the gas flow measurement and T_D.

In patients these high levels of accuracy cannot be obtained, which may mainly be due to real variations in FRC as well as actual influences on gas exchange by variation of FiO_2. The results, however, still remain within a very acceptable mean range of 6% for doubled SD. On the other hand, FRC determined without automatic compensation for viscosity encompasses large errors (up to 24%!) due to incorrect synchronization of flow and gas concentration signals depending on the flow pattern for the individual ventilatory setting. The method can be easily performed at the bedside, only requiring a switch to 100% oxygen for 10 to 15 min. The only drawback for using this method in clinical practice is the need for a high-performance gas analyzer (e.g., mass spectrometer or fast nitrogen meter).

In view of the accurate and easy determination of lung volume now possible, this important parameter merits more attention in intensive care medicine.

References

1. Parker JC, Hernandez LA, Peevy KJ (1993) Mechanisms of ventilator-induced lung injury. Crit Care Med 21:131–143
2. Dreyfuss D, Basset G, Soler P, Saumon G (1985) Intermittent positive-pressure hyperventilation with high inflation pressures produces pulmonary microvascular injury in rats. Am Rev Respir Dis 132:880–884
3. Parker JC, Hernandez LA, Longnecker GL, Peevy K, Johnson W (1990) Lung edema caused by high peak inspiratory pressures in dogs. – Role of increased microvascular filtration pressure and permeability. Am Rev Respir Dis 142:321–328
4. Dreyfuss D, Soler P, Basset G, Saumon G (1988) High inflation pressure pulmonary edema. Respective effects of high airway pressure, high tidal volume, and positive end-expiratory pressure. Am Rev Respir Dis 137:1159–1164
5. Fu Z, Costello ML, Tsukimoto K, et al (1992) High lung volume increases stress failure in pulmonary capillaries. J Appl Physiol 73:123–133
6. Mead J, Takishima T, Leith D (1970) Stress distribution in lungs: a model of pulmonary elasticity. J Appl Physiol 28:596–608
7. Haake R, Schlichtig R, Ulstad DR, Henschen RR (1987) Barotrauma: Pathophysiology, risk factors, and prevention. Chest 91:608–613
8. Marcy TW (1993) Barotrauma: detection, recognition and management. Chest 104:578–584
9. Bernard GR, Artigas A, Brigham KL, et al and the Consensus Committee (1994) The American-European consensus conference on ARDS. Definitions, mechanisms, relevant outcomes, and clinical trial coordination. Am J Respir Crit Care Med 149:818–824
10. East TD, in't Veen JCC, Pace NL, McJames S (1988) Functional residual capacity as a noninvasive indicator of optimal positive end-expiratory pressure. J Clin Monit 4:91–98
11. East TD, Andriano KP, Pace NL (1987) Automated measurement of functional residual capacity by sulfur hexafluoride washout. J Clin Monit 3:14–21
12. Jonmarker C, Jansson L, Jonson B, Larsson A, Werner O (1985) Measurement of functional residual capacity by sulfur hexafluoride washout. Anesthesiology 63:89–95
13. Huygen PE, Feenstra BW, Holland WP, Ince C, Stam H, Bruining HA (1990) Design and validation of an indicator gas injector for multiple gas washout tests in mechanically ventilated patients. Crit Care Med 18:754–759
14. Darling RC, Richards DW, Cournant A (1940) Studies on intrapulmonary mixture of gases. Open circuit method for measuring residual air. J Clin Invest 19:609–618
15. Saidel GM, Salmon RB, Chester EH (1975) Moment analysis of multibreath lung washout. J Appl Physiol 38:328–334
16. Hylkema BS, Barkmeyer-Degenhart P, van der Mark TW, Peset R, Sluiter HJ (1982) Measurement of functional residual capacity during mechanical ventilation for acute respiratory failure. Chest 81:27–30
17. Brunner JX, Wolff G (1988) Pulmonary function indices in critical care patients. Springer-Verlag, Berlin, Heidelberg, New York
18. Fretschner R, Deusch H, Weitnauer A, Brunner JX (1993) A simple method to estimate functional residual capacity in mechanically ventilated patients. Intensive Care Med 19:372–376
19. Sullivan WJ, Peters GM, Enright PL (1984) Pneumotachographs: Theory and clinical application. Respir Care 29:736–749
20. Brunner JX, Langenstein H, Wolff G (1983) Direct accurate gas flow measurement in the patient: compensation for unavoidable error. Med Prog Technol 9:233–238
21. Brunner JX, Wolff G, Cumming G, Langenstein H (1985) Accurate measurement of N_2 volumes during N_2 washout requires dynamic adjustment of delay time. J Appl Physiol 59:1008–1012
22. Cournand A, Yarmouth IG, Riley RL (1941) Influence of body size on gaseous nitrogen elimination during high oxygen breathing. Proc Soc Exp Biol. 48:280–286
23. Bland JM, Altman DG (1986) Statistical methods for assessing agreement between two methods of clinical measurement. Lancet 1:307–310

Chest Wall Mechanics: Methods of Measurement and Physiopathologic Insights

P. Pelosi, A. Aliverti, and R. Dellaca

Introduction

There is a common belief that respiratory mechanics are representative of the lung status and unaffected by the chest wall behaviour. In reality, altered mechanical properties of the chest wall may limit ventilation, influence the work of breathing [1], affect the interaction between the respiratory muscles [2], hasten the development of respiratory failure and interfere with gas exchange [3]. Despite this central role of the chest wall in respiratory function, the understanding of its behavior has evolved slowly due to difficulties in making direct measurements in humans. However, recently several methods have been developed to evaluate chest wall mechanics, allowing better definition of the role of the chest wall in different clinical situations.

In this chapter we will discuss:
1) the methods available to evaluate the chest wall;
2) the mechanical behaviour of the chest wall during spontaneous breathing and during mechanical ventilation, both in normal subjects and in critically ill patients; and
3) some clinical consequences of these findings.

General Concepts

The respiratory system is composed of the lung and chest wall components, and the individual mechanical properties of each of them determine the behaviour of the respiratory system as a whole. We define the chest wall as those parts of the body that surround the lung and that move with ventilation, passive or active.

The airway pressure (P_{ao}) required to inflate the respiratory system is the sum of the pressure required to inflate the lung (P_L) plus the pressure required to inflate the chest wall (P_w):

$$P_{ao} = P_L + P_w \tag{1}$$

P_{ao} is easily obtained directly by measuring the pressure at the airway opening from a side tap in the mouthpiece, face mask, or tracheal cannula. P_w is more difficult to measure, since it would require the direct measurement of the pressure in the pleural space with needles, trocars, catheters, balloons, etc. [4]. This is possible in animals but, obviously not in humans. In humans it is usually measured indirectly from the esophagus (P_{es}) [5]. Furthermore, the P_w results from the different components of the chest wall (rib cage, the diaphragm and the abdomen). To assess the mechanical properties of these different components, it is necessary to additionally measure their volume variations and the intra-abdominal pressure (P_{ab}) [6].

Measurement of Esophageal and Intra-Abdominal Pressure

Esophageal Pressure: The most widely used method for recording P_{es} in the study of respiratory mechanics employs air-containing latex balloons (10 cm long, perimeter 3.5 to 4.8 cm, wall thickness 0.1 mm, minimum unstretched volume 0.2 ml, and pressure 0 to 0.5 cmH_2O within the balloon when it contains 0.5 ml of air) which in turn transmit balloon pressures to manometers [7]. Although the esophageal balloon technique is widely used in the measurements of lung and chest wall mechanics, its validity has been questioned by several authors due to the influence of the balloon volume, position and body posture on the measurement itself [8].

1) Influence of balloon volume: For accurate transmission of pressure, gas must be introduced into the balloon taking care to stay within the range of volume over which the rubber is unstretched. The changes in P_{es} resulting from changes in balloon volume vary at different lung volumes.
2) Influence of balloon position: The best place to measure P_{es} seems to be the lower part of the esophagus. In this position, P_{es} accurately reflects changes in pleural pressure.
3) Influence of body posture: P_{es} is relatively more positive in the supine position than in other postures. This is thought to result from the weight of structures anterior to the esophagus. However, it should be remembered that what is important is not the absolute value of P_{es} but its modifications with gas movements in the respiratory system.

The most widely used method to validate the esophageal balloon technique as a measure of the pleural surface pressure consists of having subjects perform static voluntary or involuntary efforts (glottis open) against a closed airway, and comparing the changes in P_{es} (DP_{es}) with the corresponding changes in airway pressure (DP_{ao}). An agreement between DP_{es} and DP_{ao} is taken to indicate that P_{es} provides a valid measure of changes in pleural surface pressure [9, 10].

Intra-Abdominal Pressure: Two methods are currently available to estimate P_{ab}: One is the direct measurement of gastric pressure (P_{ga}) [6], while the other is the measurement of bladder pressure [11]. P_{ga} is easily obtained using a gastric balloon similar to the esophageal one, positioned in the gastric cavity. The bladder pressure is measured by means of the bladder catheter, after the infusion of 50–250 ml of saline in the bladder. The bladder pressure is considered representative of the P_{ab} and correlates well with P_{ga} [12].

In conclusion, the esophageal balloon technique is the only method applicable in humans to separate the individual contribution of the chest wall, as a whole, on the respiratory system. Measurement of intra-abdominal pressure is needed to have more detailed information regarding the rib cage, diaphragm and abdomen.

How to Evaluate Chest Wall Mechanics

The mechanics of the chest wall may be investigated according to its static, dynamic and kinematic characteristics.

"Statics" describes the elastic ("static elastance") properties in equilibrium conditions, i.e., in the absence of flow, at different volumes. It is assessed in relaxed situations, both induced by drugs (i.e., paralyzing agents) or intentionally (i.e., relaxation maneuvers).

"Dynamics" describes the relationships between forces (pressures) and movements (volume derivatives) both in passive (i.e., during active inflation of gas into the airways) and active (i.e., during active breathing movements) conditions. These relationships are usually described in terms of viscoelastic properties (resistance, "dynamic elastance", and inertance).

"Kinematics" describes the shape and the movements considered as pure motion without reference to the masses or forces involved.

Different methods have been developed to evaluate the static, dynamic and kinematic behavior of the chest wall during passive and active breathing.

Statics and Dynamics: Measurement of Elastic and Resistive Properties

Rapid Airway Occlusion Method: The rapid airway occlusion method is one of the most commonly used methods to evaluate static and dynamic characteristics of the chest wall both during passive and active breathing [13 14]. Briefly, this method necessitates the recording of the P_{es}, the flow and the volume. It consists of a rapid occlusion of the airways at the end of an inspiration (Fig. 1). After the occlusion, it is evident that there is a decay of P_{es} tracings from a maximum value (P_{max}) to a plateau value (P_2). The ratio of the difference between P_{es} at end-inspiration (P_2) and at end-expiration and the inflation volume gives the elastance of the chest wall at that volume (Est_w). Similarly, the ratio of the difference between P_{max} and P_2 and the inspiratory flow at the moment of the occlusion, gives the resistance of the chest wall (R_w) at that volume and flow. The change in P_{es} after the interruption may follow two characteristic behaviors: 1) a rapid initial decay from P_{max} to P_1 (immediately after the occlusion) and then a slow decay from P_{max} to P_2; 2) no rapid initial decay and only a slow decay to plateau. In the first case, the resistance of the chest wall may be further partitioned into two components; the interrupter resistance ($Rint_w$); and the "viscoelastic resistance" (DR_w).

The "interrupter resistance" may be computed as

$$(P_{max} - P_1)/\text{flow} \tag{2}$$

while the "viscoelastic resistance" as

$$(P_1 - P_2)/\text{flow} \tag{3}$$

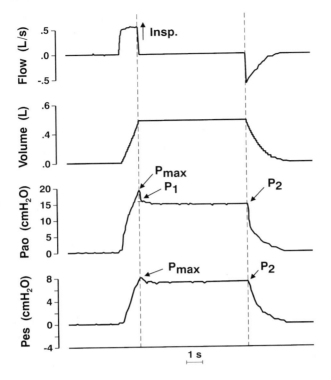

Fig. 1. Rapid airway occlusion method. Tracings (*top to bottom*) of flow, volume, airway pressure (Pao) and esophageal pressure (Pes). After an end-inspiratory occlusion, there is an immediate drop in Pao from a maximum pressure (Pmax) to a lower value (P_1), followed by a slow decay to a plateau (P_2) that represents the end-inspiratory recoil pressure of the respiratory system (Pst_{rs}). The end-inspiratory recoil pressure of the lung (Pst_L) is obtained as the difference between Pst_{rs} and Pst_w.

When P_1 is not identifiable, the resistance of the chest wall is represented by the viscoelastic resistance alone. The occlusion maneuver may also be performed during spontaneous breathing or during assisted ventilation [14]. In general, P_1 of P_{es} has been identified only in animals [15] and not in humans [13]. However, a recent study suggested the possible presence of an interrupter resistance of the chest wall in normal anesthetized subjecs using a valve with a short occlusion time [16].

Forced Oscillations Technique: In 1956, Dubois et al. [17] introduced a simple, minimally invasive forced oscillation approach to measure the mechanical impedance of the respiratory system. There are two common methods for applying forced oscillations to measure a mechanical impedance. With input impedance (Z_{in}), forced pressure oscillations are imposed at the airway opening and the complex ratio between airway opening pressure (P_{ao}) and flow (F_{ao}) is measured, i.e., ($Z_{in} = P_{ao}/F_{ao}$). With transfer impedance (Z_{tr}), forced oscillations are imposed around the chest wall (P_{cw}) and the ratio P_{cw}/F_{ao} is measured [18]. Starting from the assessment of Z_{in} and Z_{tr} it is possible to estimate the resistance and the elastance of the respiratory system, basing on different element models [19]. All of these models consider the respiratory system as a series combination of airways, lung tissues and chest wall, with an additional shunt alveolar gas compression capacitor. In any case, without the measurement of P_{es}, it is impossible to separate all these different components.

This technique does not require patient co-operation and for this reason it is an attractive potential pulmonary function test, particularly for infants and ventilator dependent patients. The disadvantages are that the measurements are influenced by all respiratory structures, and their physiological and clinical interpretation are dependent on the model used and the considered frequency range [20].

Kinematics: Measurement of Shape and Motion

Respiratory-Inductive Plethysmography (RIP): The RIP, originally described by Milledge et al. [21], has become the most widely accepted non-invasive method of measuring ventilation. The plethysmograph [22] comprises two separate coils of Teflon-insulated wire sewn in a zigzag pattern onto elastic-fabricated bands measuring approximately 10 cm in height, normally placed just under the axilla and at the umbilical line. The self-inductance of the coil, and so the frequencies of the oscillator which is connected to it, is proportional to the cross-sectional area enclosed by the coil. The signals from the oscillator are sent to a demodulator unit which provides output voltage signals (AC or DC). The device measures the average of an infinite number of cross-sectional areas over its complete height rather than the circumference of the enclosed part.

To obtain accurate results, an appropriate calibration for rib cage and abdomen cross-sectional area changes should be applied and, in the past, different methods have been developed [23, 24]. Possible limitations of RIP calibration are the need for co-operative and trained subjects, difficulty in performing the particular respiratory maneuvers (isovolume maneuvers), and the dependency on body posture and lung volume. In addition, all these calibration methods are based on the assumption, not always verified [25], that the respiratory system possesses only two degrees of freedom, rib cage and abdominal motion.

Optoelectronic Method: In recent years, a new method for kinematic analysis of chest movements during respiration has been implemented and validated [26, 27] (Fig. 2).

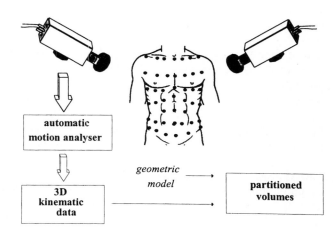

Fig. 2. Schematic diagram of the optoelectronic method for the analysis of the chest wall shape, volume changes and movements

It is based on an automatic motion analyzer [28] which measures the 3D co-ordinates of several markers applied to body landmarks. The markers are small (6–10 mm of diameter) and light plastic hemispheres coated with retroreflective paper. The co-ordinates of the landmarks are measured with a system configuration with four TV-cameras at a sampling rate up to 100 Hz. Different experimental set-up and marker positioning have been considered, for sitting, standing and supine positions. In the sitting and standing positions the subject wears the markers on the front and on the back, while in the supine position the markers are put only on the anterior chest wall surface as the back is considered to be fixed by lying on the bed.

The anterior markers are usually positioned at different horizontal levels (typically second rib, nipple, xiphoid process, costal margin, abdominal transverse line, pubic line) and vertical rows from the anterior axillary line, symmetric with respect to the parasternal line: On the back, the different levels of markers correspond to those on the front.

Starting from these co-ordinates the volume variations inside the whole thoraco-abdominal surface or inside a part of it can be computed by using different mathematical methods [26, 27, 28]. The positioning of the markers allows the computation of the volume changes of the different compartments of the rib cage (pulmonary rib cage (RC_p) and diaphragmatic rib cage (RC_a)) and of the abdomen (AB); the contribution of the left and right part of each of these compartments can also be computed.

The optoelectronic method, compared to other devices, has several advantages:
1) it is highly accurate in the quantification of total chest wall absolute volume and its changes with time;
2) it provides a measurement of the volume changes of the different compartments (two-compartment rib cage and abdomen);
3) it provides information on the relative contribution of the right and left chest wall compartments to volume changes;
4) it is completely non-invasive;
5) calibration is independent of the subject;
6) it can analyze the subject in different body postures (upright, sitting, supine, prone and lateral decubitus).

The main limitation of this method, up to now, is the complexity of data analysis which requires trained staff.

Other Devices: In the past many other devices have been developed for the measurement of linear dimensions, such as magnetometers [29], bellows pneumographs [30], mercury-in-silastic strain gauges [31], impedance pneumographs [32], Jerkin plethysmographs [33], and linear differential transducers [34]. Their clinical applications were very limited, because of numerous problems: Low accuracy, non-linearity; dependence on lung volumes and body postures, sizes and dimensions limiting the naturality of the respiratory movements; invasivity. The chest wall and its motion can be visualized using different techniques that rely on light [35], X-rays [36] or ultrasound [37]. In particular, the use of three-dimensional X-ray computed tomography using the dynamic spatial reconstructor [38, 39] has increased the possibilities of investigation, but it is still too slow, not suitable for long analyses, limited to the supine position and ionising.

Normal Subjects

The Chest Wall during Spontaneous Breathing

In order to describe chest wall mechanics during spontaneous breathing in normal subjects, several models have been proposed. The simplest was developed by Konno and Mead [34], who showed that chest wall motion is influenced by the rib cage and the abdomen, which are highly independent of each other. The limitations of this approach, however, have long been recognized. In fact different authors [40, 41] have demonstrated that the rib cage cannot be considered as a single compartment with a single degree of freedom. Available evidence suggests that its behaviour is the result of the highly co-ordinated action of the inspiratory muscles rather than inherent rigidity of the rib cage.

Ward et al. [42] proposed a model that incorporates a two-compartment rib cage, separated into the part apposed on its inner surface to the lung (RC_p) and the part apposed to the diaphragm (RC_{ab}). Recently, a modified version of this model has been proposed [43, 44] (Fig. 3). Briefly, the total chest wall is divided into RC_p (pulmonary rib cage), RC_a (abdominal rib cage) and AB (abdomen) components. RC_p is apposed to the lung, while RC_a is the part of the rib cage apposed to the diaphragm. Inspiratory and expiratory rib cage muscles (RCM_i and RCM_e, respectively) act on RC_p. The diaphragm is considered as being composed of two muscles [45]: the costal diaphragm (COS), which acts on the abdominal rib cage, and the crural diaphragm (CRU). The abdominal muscles are divided into their insertional (ABM_{ins}) and non-insertional (ABM_{nins}) components on the rib cage. The spring represents the mechanical linkage between RC_p and RC_a and describes the restoring force developed by distortions between the two compartments away from the relaxation configuration.

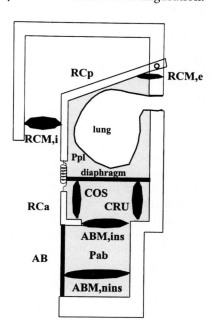

Fig. 3. Simplified mechanical model of the chest wall incorporating a two-compartment rib cage, i.e.,pulmonary (RC_p) and abdominal (RC_a) rib cage, and the abdomen (AB). The respiratory muscles are grouped into: inspiratory and expiratory rib cage muscles (RCM_i and RCM_e), costal and crural diaphragm (COS and CRU), insertional and non insertional abdominal muscles (ABM_{ins} and ABM_{nins}). P_{pl} and P_{ab} represent the pleural and intra-abdominal pressures, respectively

During spontaneous breathing, only the inspiratory muscles are active, while the expiratory muscle activity is negligible [43, 44]. The diaphragm's contraction plays the major role of the inspiratory muscles.

In conclusion, the partitioning of the pressure differences across different parts of the respiratory system, and the methodology to describe the volume displacements of the rib cage and abdomen have been major advances in our knowledge of the act of breathing in normal conditions. This is important to better understand the behaviour of the chest wall in different "pathologic" conditions.

The Chest Wall During Anesthesia and Paralysis

It has been well recognized that the induction of general anesthesia reduces oxygenation and functional residual capacity [46], while it increases respiratory elastance and resistance [47, 48]. These abnormalities are rapid, do not change with time and are unaffected by administration of neuromuscular blockade. A loss of tonic activity in the chest wall muscles, both rib cage and diaphragm, is one of the possible factors explaining these physiologic changes induced by anesthesia.

The primary source of the increased static respiratory system elastance appears to be the lung, since the static chest wall elastance appears to be little influenced over most lung volumes [47, 48]. Respiratory resistance increases after induction of anesthesia, but does not significantly affect chest wall resistance [47, 48]. Data relative to changes in chest wall shape with the induction of anesthesia are scanty and involve very small samples of subjects. Anesthesia and paralysis, in fact, decrease the external antero-posterior diameter and increase the lateral diameter of the thorax and abdomen. Froese and Bryan [49] examined the diaphragmatic shape and found that the induction of anesthesia caused a cephalad shift of the end-expiratory position of the dependent part of the diaphragm, with no further modification after paralysis. Shifts in the non-dependent part were inconsistent. In contrast, Krayer et al. [50] found no consistent net cephalad shift in end-expiratory diaphragmatic position with induction of anesthesia, concluding that the contribution of the diaphragm to the reduction in lung volume caused by anesthesia may be generally smaller than originally thought. Moreover, they found that an inward displacement of the rib cage accounts for most of the decrease in lung volume.

Another interesting aspect is related to the pattern of the diaphragmatic movement during mechanical ventilation. Several authors [49, 50] found in the supine position, a prevalent motion of the non-dependent regions of the diaphragm and a more uniform motion during large tidal volumes. Moreover, during anesthesia the relative movement of the rib cage and the abdomen is reversed. While during spontaneous breathing the prevalent movement is in the abdomen, during anesthesia and paralysis rib cage movement is prevalent. The antero-posterior diameters of both the rib cage and abdomen increase during a tidal breath, while the lateral diameters decrease [51].

In conclusion, it seems that:
1) anesthesia changes the shape and and pattern of motion of the chest wall, but not its elastic and resistive properties;

2) the reduction in lung volume seems more related to changes in the rib cage than in the diaphragm;

3) distribution of inspired gases during mechanical ventilation is prevalent in the rib cage and the movement of the diaphragm is prevalent in the non-dependent lung regions; and

4) the added paralysis has no effect.

All these changes in chest wall mechanics may be implicated in the abnormalities in respiratory function after induction of anesthesia.

Acute Respiratory Distress Syndrome Patients

The Chest Wall During Sedation and Paralysis

The mechanical properties of the respiratory system are severely affected in the acute respiratory distress syndrome (ARDS) and are supposed to mainly reflect alterations in lung, rather than chest wall mechanics. However, only a few studies have reported chest wall mechanical data in patients with ARDS during sedation and paralysis [52, 53, 54, 55]. On average the mean value of the chest wall elastance was 10.2 ± 2.5 cmH$_2$O/L, markedly lower than that reported in normal subjects [13]. However, all these studies had some limitations since they were performed in a limited number of inhomogenous patients, often not including a control group, and using different methods of measurement. More recently, we reported [56], in a selected group of patients with different degrees of acute lung injury (ALI), a substantial increase in chest wall elastance (i.e., decrease in compliance) compared to normal subjects (Fig. 4). The increase in elastance of the chest wall was attributed to dif-

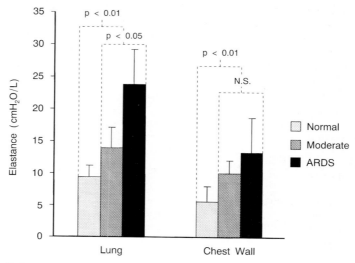

Fig. 4. Lung and chest wall elastance in normal subjects and in patients with moderate and severe acute lung injury, PEEP at 0 cmH$_2$O. Data are expressed as mean $\pm$ SD. (Modified from [56] with permission)

ferent factors: A decrease in lung volume, which could produce a decrease in the volume of the rib cage-abdominal compartment, moving it to a less compliant portion of its pressure-volume curve; and true alterations of the chest wall due to abdominal distension, edema, pleural effusion and so forth. The first hypothesis was ruled out since a direct relationship between lung and thoracic volume does not apply in ARDS, a significant portion of the thoracic volume being occupied by blood, exudate, edema and pleural fluid [57]. Consequently, these results were ascribed to alterations of the intrinsic properties of the chest wall. Although in that study [56] the authors were unable to identify the specific factors affecting chest wall elastance, some hypotheses were proposed. Common causes of increased chest wall elastance are summarized in Table 1. Among them the most attractive is an increase in the intra-abdominal pressure. It is well known that both in animals [58] and in normal subjects [59] that the increase in intra-abdominal pressure may significantly affect chest wall mechanics. Both surgical procedures on the abdomen, the continuous use of sedatives and the fluid overload treatment commonly used in these patients, may impair abdominal function producing a possible increase in the intra-abdominal pressure [60].

Moreover, the mechanical properties of the chest wall may be influenced by the etiology of ARDS. We studied two groups of patients with ARDS: one group with ARDS due to a "direct" insult to the lung (e.g., bacterial, viral or fungal pneumonia, etc.), the other group had ARDS due to an "indirect" insult to the lung (e.g., surgical abdominal problems) [61]. We found that the first group was characterized by severe alterations in lung mechanics with the chest wall substantially unaffected, while the second group was characterized by severe alterations in the chest wall with minimal alterations in the lung. Interestingly, the increase in chest wall elastance was paralleled by an increase in the intra-abdominal pressure. It was thus evident that the alteration of the chest wall is not a hallmark of all kinds of ARDS, but specific of indirect lung injury, at least in the first days of the disease. However, it is possible that other factors, such as the duration of mechanical ventilation, sedation, and nutrition

Table 1. Common causes of decreased chest wall compliance in critically ill patients

Rib cage
- anatomic deformities
- edema
- obesity
- supine positioning

Abdomen
- obesity
- supine positioning
- ascites
- abdominal distension

Pleural space
- pleural effusion
- pneumothorax
- hemothorax
- empyema

may lead to an increase in the intra-abdominal pressure, and thus to abnormalities in chest wall mechanics. Finally, the chest wall behavior may influence the distribution of ventilation and gas-exchange [62]. There is evidence that the characteristics of chest wall elastance in the supine position may be useful in predicting the oxygenation response in the prone position in patients with ALI, i.e., the higher the chest wall elastance, the lower the oxygenation response, and the lower the elastance, the higher is the oxygenation response. Moreover, the improvement in oxygenation, while prone, is directly related to the increase in elastance while prone.

In conclusion, contrary to common belief, the mechanics of the chest wall may be altered in patients with ARDS, and influence the respiratory function during mechanical ventilation.

Chronic Obstructive Pulmonary Disease Patients

The Chest Wall During Sedation and Paralysis

Chronic obstructive pulmonary disease (COPD) with acute exacerbation of acute respiratory failure is characterized by an increase in airway resistance and a loss of lung elastic recoil with a normal contribution of the chest wall [63]. As a result, airflow limitation develops, leading to the presence of dynamic hyperinflation and intrinsic positive end-expiratory pressure (PEEPi) [64]. These alterations lead to increased work of breathing, but the role of the chest wall is usually considered as negligible [65]. However, recent data suggest that the chest wall contribution to the elastic properties of the respiratory system may be substantial [66, 67]. We systematically investigated the chest wall mechanics in a group of mechanically ventilated COPD patients with acute respiratory failure compared to normal subjects of similar age [68]. We found an increased chest wall elastance compared to normal subjects, despite a substantially normal lung elastance. The chest wall resistance was also increased compared to normal.

As for ARDS patients, we may hypothesize that several factors contributed to our finding. Altered intestinal motility, eventually leading to colonic pseudo-obstruction, has been shown to occur with an unexpectedly high frequency in mechanically ventilated COPD patients with acute respiratory failure [69]. Narcotic sedation, which is frequently used in critically ill patients may further aggravate this condition. The resulting abdominal distension might increase the intra-abdominal pressure and thus the chest wall elastance.

In conclusion, COPD patients with acute respiratory failure are characterized not only by an abnormal increase in airway resistance but also by severe alterations in the mechanical properties of the chest wall, elastance and resistance.

Physiopathologic and Clinical Implications

The findings outlined above indicate that the evaluation of chest wall behavior is not only important from a speculative point of view, but also from a clinical one. It may have "important" physiopathologic and clinical consequences on:

Interpretation of Respiratory Mechanics: We now have evidence that chest wall mechanics may be abnormal in critically ill patients. Consequently, the data relative to the whole respiratory system may not always be considered representative of the lung. For example, two patients may have the same respiratory system elastance but, if the chest wall contribution is different, lung elastance will be different. Thus, if a physician measures the respiratory system elastance alone to have an idea of the lung elastance, he may be misled.

Current Recommendations on Ventilatory Treatment: The recommendations of the consensus group regarding high airway pressure during the ventilatory management of ARDS emphasized that a respiratory system plateau pressure higher or equal to 35 cmH_2O is of concern and that reductions in tidal volume may be necessary [70]. They went on to point out that if a clinical situation is associated with decreased chest wall compliance then a plateau pressure higher than 35 cmH_2O may be acceptable. This is an issue that has not been addressed by more recent trials. Lung distension is directly related to transpulmonary pressure. A normal lung will reach its maximum distension when the transpulmonary pressure reaches 30–35 cmH_2O. Lung overdistension can usually be avoided by preventing transpulmonary pressures exceeding 30–35 cmH_2O. A treatment strategy which uses the plateau pressure of the respiratory system as a surrogate for transpulmonary pressure may overestimate the true transpulmonary pressure.

Interpretation of Hemodynamics: The different mechanical characteristics of the chest wall influence the transmission of the airway pressure in the pleural space. In fact, for the same airway pressure, patients with lower chest wall elastance will have a lower increase in pleural pressure. On the contrary, patients with higher chest wall elastance will have a greater increase in pleural pressure. This means that the venous return to the heart is less affected, for the same airway pressure, in patients with low chest wall elastance compared to those with a high chest wall elastance. This will influence the interpretation of intravascular pressures and the effects of application of different airway pressures on hemodynamics.

Evaluation of the Work of Breathing: The work of breathing is frequently measured both for research and clinical purposes. However, what is generally called "work of breathing" is really the work of breathing done by the respiratory muscles on the lung alone. But the patient's work of breathing results from the action of the respiratory muscles to inflate not only the lung but also to expand the chest wall (rib cage, diaphragm and abdomen). Thus in the presence of alterations of the chest wall, measurement of the work of breathing on the lung may markedly underestimate the total respiratory work of breathing. This should be remembered in the evaluation and interpretation of this kind of measurement.

Conclusion

The role of the chest wall on respiratory function during passive and active ventilation has not been widely investigated. This is due to difficulties in measuring chest wall behavior, both as a whole and divided into its components, separate from the total respiratory system. Nevertheless, the chest wall appears to substantially influence the mechanics of breathing, distribution of ventilation and gas-exchange. Moreover, the knowledge of chest wall behaviour may have important clinical implications both in normal and pathologic conditions. In the future, the development of new technologies and their applications in the clinical setting will allow us to understand in more detail the importance of the chest wall during spontaneous breathing, anesthetic procedures and mechanical ventilation.

Acknowledgements. The authors wish to thank Prof. L. Gattinoni and Prof. A. Pedotti for their thoughtful contributions.

References

1. Agostoni E (1964) Action of respiratory muscle. In: Fenn WO, Rahn H (eds) Handbook of physiology, 2nd edn. American Physiological Society, Washington, pp 377–386
2. Zocchi L, Garzaniki N, Newman S, Macklem PT (1987) Effect of hyperventilation and equalization of abdominal pressure on diaphragmatic action. J Appl Physiol 62:1655–1664
3. Liu S, Margulies SS, Wilson TA (1990) Deformation of the dog lung in the chest wall. J Appl Physiol 68:1979–1987
4. Lai-Fook SJ, Rodarte JR (1991) Pleural pressure distribution and its relationship to lung volume and interstitial pressure. J Appl Physiol 70:967–978
5. Milic-Emili J, Mead J, Turner JM (1964) Improved technique for estimating pressure from esophageal balloons. J Appl Physiol 19:207–211
6. Agostoni E, Rhan H (1960) Abdominal and thoracic pressures at different lung volumes. J Appl Physiol 15:1087–1092
7. Maxted KJ, Shaw A, Macdonald TH (1977) Choosing a catheter system for measuring intraesophageal pressure. Med Biol Eng Comput 15:398–401
8. Knowles JH, Hong SK, Rhan H (1959) Possible errors using esophageal balloon in determination of pressure-volume characteristics of the lung and thoracic cage. J Appl Physiol 14:525–530
9. Baydur A, Behrakis PK, Zin WA, Jaeger M, Milic-Emili J (1982) A Simple method for assessing the validity of the esophageal balloon technique. Am Rev Respir Dis 126:788–791
10. Higgs BD, Bherakis PK, Bevan DR, Milic-Emili J (1983) Measurement of pleural pressure with esophageal balloon in anesthetized humans. Anesthesiology 59:349–343
11. Iberti TJ, Kelly KM, Gentili DR, Hirsch S (1987) A simple technique to accurately determine intra-abdominal pressure. Crit Care Med 15:1140–1142
12. Collee GG, Lomax DM, Ferguson C, Hanson GC (1993) Bedside measurement of intraabdominal pressure (IAP) via an indwelling nasogastric tube: clinical validation of the technique. Intensive Care Med 19:478–480
13. D'Angelo E, Robatto FM, Calderini E, Tavola M, Bono D, Milic-Emili J (1991) Pulmonary and chest wall mechanics in anesthetized and paralyzed humans. J Appl Physiol 70:2602–2610
14. Pesenti A, Pelosi P, Foti G, D'Andera L, Rossi N (1992) An interrupter technique for measuring respiratory mechanics and the pressure generated by respiratory muscles during partial ventilatory support. Chest 102:918–923
15. Bates JHT, Ludwig M, Sly PD, Brown K, Martin JG, Fredberg JJ (1988) Interrupter resistance elucidated by alveolar pressure measurement in open-chested normal dogs. J Appl Physiol 65:408–414

16. D'Angelo E, Prandi E, Tavola M, Calderini E, Milic-Emili J (1994) Chest wall interrupter resistance in anesthetized paralyzed humans. J Appl Physiol 77:883–887
17. DuBois AB, Brody AW, Lewis DH, Burgess BF (1956) Oscillation mechanics of lung and chest in man. J Appl Physiol 8:587–594
18. Michaelson ED, Grassman ED, Peters WR (1975) Pulmonary mechanics by spectral analysis of forced random noise. J Clin Invest 56:1210–1230
19. Peslin R, Papon J, Duvivier C, Richalet J (1975) Frequency response of the chest: modeling and parameter estimation. J Appl Physiol 39:523–534
20. Lutchen KR, Everett JR, Jackson AC (1993) Influence of frequency range and input impedance on interpreting the airways tissue separation implied from transfer impedance. J Appl Physiol 73:1089–1099
21. Milledge JS, Stott FD (1977) Inductive plethysmography – a new respiratory transducer. J Physiol 267:4–5
22. Cohn MA, Rao AS, Broudy M, et al (1982) The respiratory inductive plethysmograph: a new non-invasive monitor of respiration. Bull Eur Physiopathol Respir 18:643–658
23. Stagg D, Goldman M, Davis JN (1978) Computer aided measurement of breath volume and time components using magnetometers. J Appl Physiol 44:623–633
24. Stadling JR, Chadwick GA, Quirk C, Phillips T (1985) Respiratory inductance plethysmography: calibration techniques, their validation and the effects of posture. Bull Eur Physiopathol Respir 21:317–324
25. Smith JC, Mead J (1986) Three degree of freedom description of movement of the human chest wall. J Appl Physiol 60:928–934
26. Ferrigno G, Carnevali P, Aliverti A, Molteni F, Beulke G, Pedotti A (1994) Three-dimensional optical analysis of chest wall motion. J Appl Physiol 77:1224–1231
27. Cala SJ, Kenyon C, Ferrigno G, et al (1996) Chest wall and lung volume estimation by optical reflectance motion analysis. J Appl Physiol 81:2680–2689
28. Ferrigno G, Pedotti A (1985) ELITE: a digital dedicated hardware system for movement analysis via real time TV signal processing. IEEE Trans Biomed Eng BME 32:943–950
29. Mead J, Peterson N, Grimby G, et al (1967) Pulmonary ventilation measured from body surface movements. Science 156:1383–1384
30. Morel DR, Forster A, Suter PM (1983) Noninvasive ventilatory monitoring with bellows pneumographs in supine subjects. J Appl Physiol 55:598–606
31. Wade OL (1954) Movements of the thoracic cage and diaphragm in respiration. J Physiol 124:193–197
32. Grenvik A, Ballou S, McGinley E, et al (1972) Impedance pneumography: comparison between chest impedance changes and respiratory volumes in 11 healthy volunteers. Chest 62:439–443
33. Spier S, England S (1983) The respiratory inductive plethysmograph: bands vs jenkins. Am Rev Respir Dis 127:784–785
34. Konno K, Mead J (1967) Measurement of the separate volume changes of rib cage and abdomen during breathing. J Appl Physiol 22:407–422
35. Peacock AJ, Morgan MDL, Gourlay S, Tourton C, Denison DM (1984) Optical mapping of the thoraco-abdominal wall. Thorax 39:93–100
36. Krayer S, Rehder K, Beck KC, Cameron PD, Didier EP, Hoffman EA (1987) Quantification of thoracic volumes by three-dimensional imaging. J Appl Physiol 62:591–598
37. McCool FD, Hoppin FG (1995) Ultrasonography of the diaphragm. In: Roussos C (ed) The thorax, 2nd edn., Marcel Dekker Inc, New York, pp 1295–1311
38. Warner DO, Krayer S, Rehder K, Ritman EL (1989) Chest wall motion during spontaneous breathing and mechanical ventilation in dogs. J Appl Physiol 66:1179–1189,
39. Warner DO, Warner MA, Ritman EL (1995) Human chest wall function while awake and during halothane anesthesia. Anesthesiology 82:6–19
40. McCool FD, Liu S, Mead J (1985) Rib cage distortion during voluntary and involuntary breathing acts. J Appl Physiol 58:1703–1712
41. Jiang TX, Demedts M, Decramer M (1988) Mechanical coupling of upper and lower canine rib cages and its functional significance. J Appl Physiol 64:620–626
42. Ward ME, Ward JW, Macklem PT (1992) Analysis of human chest wall motion using a two-compartment rib cage model. J Appl Physiol 72:1338–1347

43. Aliverti A, Kenyon CM, Yan S, et al (1997) Human respiratory muscle actions and control during exercise. J Appl Physiol 83:1256–1269
44. Kenyon CM, Cala SJ, Aliverti A, et al (1998) Rib cage mechanics during quiet breathing and exercise in humans. J Appl Physiol (in press)
45. De Troyer A, Sampson M, Sigrist S, et al (1981) The diaphragm: two muscles. Science 213: 237–241
46. Tokics L, Hedenstierna G, Strandberg A, Brismar B, Lunquist H, Hedenstierna G (1987) Lung collapse and gas exchange during general anesthesia: effects of spontaneous breathing, muscle paralysis, and positive end-expiratory pressure. Anesthesiology 66:157–167
47. Rehder K, Mallow JE, Fibuch EE, Krabill DR, Sessler AD (1974) Effects of isoflurane anesthesia and muscle paralysis on respiratory mechanics in normal man. Anesthesiology 41: 477–485
48. Westbrook PR, Stubbs SE, Sessler AD, Rheder K, Hyatt RE (1973) Effects of anesthesia and muscle paralysis on respiratory mechanics in normal man. J Appl Physiol 44:114–123
49. Froese AB, Bryan AC (1974) Effects of anesthesia and paralysis on diaphragmatic mechanics in man. Anesthesiology 41:242–255
50. Krayer S, Rehder K, Vettermann J, Didier EP, Ritman EL (1989) Position and motion of the human diaphragm during anesthesia and paralysis. Anesthesiology 70:891–898
51. Hedenstierna G, Lofstrom B, Lundh R (1981) Thoracic gas volume and chest-abdomen dimensions during anesthesia and muscle paralysis. Anesthesiology 55:499–506
52. Suter PM, Fairley HB, Isenberg MD (1978) Effect of tidal volume and positive end-expiratory pressure on compliance during mechanical ventilation. Chest 73:158–162
53. Katz JA, Zinn SE, Ozanne GM, Fairley HB (1982) Pulmonary, chest wall and lung-thorax elastances in acute respiratory failure. Chest 80:304–311
54. Jardin F, Genevray B, Brun-ney D, Bourdarias JP (1985) Influence of lung and chest wall compliances on transmission of airway pressure to the pleural space in critically ill patients. Chest 88:653–658
55. Polese G, Rossi A, Appendini L, Brandi G, Bates JHT, Brandolese R (1991) Partitioning of respiratory mechanics in mechanically ventilated patients. J Appl Physiol 71:2425–2433
56. Pelosi P, Cereda M, Foti G, Giacomini M, Pesenti A (1995) Alterations in lung and chest wall mechanics in patients with acute lung injury: effects of positive end-expiratory pressure. Am J Respir Crit Care Med 152:531–537
57. Pelosi P, D'Andrea L, Vitale G, Pesenti A, Gattinoni L (1994) Vertical gradient of regional lung inflation in adult respiratory distress syndrome. Am J Respir Crit Care Med 149:8–13
58. Mutoh T, Lamm WJE, Hildebrandt J, Albert RK (1991) Abdominal distension alters regional pleural pressures and chest wall mechanics in pigs in vivo. J Appl Physiol 70:2611–2618
59. Pelosi P, Foti G, Cereda M, Vicardi P, Gattinoni L (1996) Effects of carbon dioxide insufflation for laparoscopic cholecystectomy on the respiratory system. Anaesthesia 51:744–749
60. Schein M, Rucinski J, Wise L (1996) The abdominal compartment syndrome in the critically ill patients. Curr Opinion Crit Care 2:287–294
61. Pelosi P, Croci M, Chiumello D, Pedoto A, Gattinoni L (1996) Direct or indirect lung injury differently affects respiratory mechanics during acute respiratory failure. Intensive Care Med 22:105
62. Pelosi P, Tubiolo D, Mascheroni D, et al (1998) The effects of prone position on respiratory mechanics and gas exchange during acute lung injury. Am J Respir Crit Care Med (in press)
63. Guerin C, Coussa ML, Eissa NT, et al (1993) Lung and chest wall mechanics in mechanically ventilated COPD patients. J Appl Physiol 74:1570–1580
64. Pepe PE, Marini JJ (1982) Occult positive end-expiratory pressure in mechanically ventilated patients with airflow obstruction: the auto-PEEP effect. Am Rev Respir Dis 126:166–170
65. Coussa ML, Guerin C, Eissa NT, et al (1993) Partitioning of work of breathing in mechanically ventilated COPD patients. J Appl Physiol 75:1711–1719
66. Ranieri VM, Giuliani R, Mascia L, et al (1996) Chest wall and lung contribution to the elastic properties of the respiratory system in patients with chronic obstructive pulmonary disease. Eur Respir J 9:1232–1239
67. Ranieri VM, Giuliani R, Cinnella G, et al (1993) Physiologic effects of positive end-expiratory pressure in patients with chronic obstructive pulmonary disease during acute ventilatory failure and controlled mechanical ventilation. Am Rev Respir Dis 147:5–13

68. Musch G, Foti G, Cereda M, Pelosi P, Poppi D, Pesenti A (1998) Lung and chest wall mechanics in normal anesthetized subjects and in patients with COPD at different PEEP levels. Eur Respir J (in press)
69. Bonmarchand G, Denis P, Weber J, Lerebours-Pigonierre G, Massari P, Leroy J (1989) Motor abnormalities of digestive and urinary tracts in patients on ventilator for acute exacerbation of chronic obstructive pulmonary disease. Digest Dis Sciences 34:1231–1237
70. Slutsky AS (1993) Mechanical ventilation. Chest 104:1833–1859

Modes of Mechanical Ventilation

Emergency Intubation: The Difficult Airway

J. Kofler, B. Stoiser, and M. Frass

Introduction

One of the fundamental responsibilities of anesthesiologists, intensive care and emergency physicians is to maintain adequate gas exchange. In order to perform this goal, the airway must be managed in such a way that it is almost continuously patent. Inadequate lung ventilation results in irreversible brain damage or cardiac arrest within a few minutes.

Adverse outcomes associated with respiratory events constitute the single largest class of injury in the American Society of Anesthesiology (ASA) closed claims study [1]. Death or brain damage occurred in 85% of these cases. Three mechanisms of injury accounted for three-fourths of the adverse respiratory events: Inadequate ventilation (38%); esophageal intubation (18%); and difficult tracheal intubation (17%). Eighty-five (4%) of the first 2000 incidents during anesthesia reported to the Australian incident monitoring study indicated difficulties with intubation; in one fifth of these cases endotracheal intubation was not possible [2].

In contrast to tracheal intubation carried out for routine surgical procedures, airway management of the critically ill patient often requires emergency intubation in an individual suffering from respiratory failure, shock, or cardiopulmonary arrest. Several studies demonstrate that emergency intubations are rather frequently associated with complications such as difficult intubation, esophageal intubation, mainstem intubation, aspiration or death [3, 4]. However, patients do not succumb from failure to be intubated, but from failure to be ventilated. Therefore it is important to become familiar with alternative techniques for emergency airway management. Practice guidelines for the management of the difficult airway as well as indications, advantages, disadvantages and contraindications of various methods for adequate lung ventilation are described in this chapter.

Practice Guidelines for Management of the Difficult Airway

In 1992 the ASA algorithm on the management of the difficult airway was developed by the Task Force on guidelines for management of the difficult airway [5]. The purpose of this algorithm is to facilitate the management of the difficult airway and to reduce the likelihood of adverse outcomes. The algorithm is divided into three main steps:

1) Assess the Likelihood and Clinical Impact of Basic Management Problems

- Difficult intubation
- Difficult ventilation
- Difficulty with patient cooperation or consent

The following tests are recommended for routine evaluation of a patient's airway [6]:
1) Mallampati airway classification, modified by Samsoon and Young [7, 8]
2) Thyromental distance and horizontal length of the mandible [9]
3) Evaluation of atlanto-occipital extension [10]
4) Lateral view of the patient to recognize a maxillary overbite
5) Evaluation of any history of previous difficulties with managing the patient's airway
6) Evaluation of any obvious pathologic condition

If it is recognized that intubation or mask ventilation is going to be difficult because of the presence of a pathologic factor or a combination of anatomic factors (large tongue, small mandibular space, or restricted atlanto-occipital extension), airway patency should be secured and guaranteed (usually by intubation) while the patient remains awake [11].

2) Consider the Relative Merits and Feasibility of Basic Management Choices

- Non-surgical versus surgical techniques for initial approach to intubation
- Awake intubation versus intubation after induction of general anesthesia
- Preservation or ablation of spontaneous ventilation

3) Develop Primary and Alternative Strategies

- Awake intubation; may be useful during routine surgery, but not in emergency situations
- Intubation attempts after induction of general anesthesia
- Non-emergency pathway: Patient is anesthetized, intubation attempts are unsuccessful, but mask ventilation is adequate. In this situation, alternative approaches should be considered (e.g. use of different laryngoscopic blades, laryngeal masks, Combitube, blind oral or nasal intubation, fiberoptic intubation, intubating stylet, light wand, retrograde intubation). In cases of multiple failure of these methods, the patient should be either woken, surgery performed under mask anaesthesia or a surgical airway management considered.
- Emergency pathway: Patient is anesthetized, intubation attempts are unsuccessful and mask ventilation is inadequate. In this case non-surgical (laryngeal mask, esophageal-tracheal Combitube, transtracheal jet ventilation) or emergency surgical airway management (cricothyroidotomy, tracheostomy) must be considered [11].

Situations as described in the emergency pathway of the ASA algorithm occur not infrequently in critically ill patients. Therefore simple and effective devices for managing such "can't ventilate, can't intubate" situations should be immediately available. All emergency and intensive care physicians should be familiar with techniques to improve mask ventilation and with at least one of the methods described in the following sections.

Mask Ventilation

The correct use of a face mask depends on obtaining a good seal between the mask and the patient's face; successfully doing this is fundamental for administration of adequate ventilation. The mask should comfortably fit both the hand of the user and the face of the patient. Difficulties with mask ventilation can range from zero to infinite [6, 11, 12]. In cases of inadequate ventilation different techniques can be tried such as two-person mask ventilation. Far better mask seal, jaw thrust, and therefore tidal volume can be achieved with two persons than with one. The first person stands at the head of the patient with the left hand effecting jaw thrust at the angle of the left mandible and left-sided mask seal, while the right hand compresses the bag. The second person should stand at the patient's side facing the first person. The right hand should cover the left hand of the first person, thus contributing to left-sided jaw thrust and mask seal, while the left hand should effect right-sided jaw thrust and mask seal. Furthermore, mask ventilation can be improved by the use of oropharyngeal and/or nasopharyngeal airways.

Mask ventilation is relatively contraindicated in situations requiring general anesthesia but also where these is a large likelihood of gastric contents soiling the trachea (such as a full stomach, hiatus hernia, esophageal motility disorders and pharyngeal diverticula). In addition, whenever there is a likelihood of gas inflating the stomach, a need for high airway pressures (e.g., decreased compliance of lungs or chest wall, obesity, marked kyphoscoliosis, or marked bronchospasm) or an adverse position (headdown or prone), use of a mask for positive pressure ventilation must be done cautiously. Mask ventilation is also relatively contraindicated whenever there is a need to avoid head and neck manipulation (head tilt) or an inability to seal the mask (e.g., facial trauma, edentulous mouths with alveolar recession).

The effectiveness of ventilation should be judged by the exhaled tidal volume, movement of the chest, good bilateral breath sounds, vital signs and available monitors of oxygenation and ventilation. It is important to limit positive airway pressure to 25 cmH_2O to avoid inflating the stomach, which will in turn restrict diaphragmatic movement and increase the chance of regurgitation through the esophageal sphincters. If the patient cannot be ventilated with 25 cmH_2O positive pressure, either the airway is obstructed at the pharynx by the tongue or at the larynx by cord spasm, the patient has sufficient muscle tone to prevent chest expansion, or there is a decrease in pulmonary compliance or an increase in airway resistance. The oral airway corrects the first, a small dose of succinylcholine decreases laryngeal spasm and muscle tone, and definite treatment of the compliance and resistance issues depends on the etiologic factors.

Laryngeal Mask Airway (LMA)

The LMA was designed to allow an end-to-end connection between the anatomical airway and the breathing circuit [13, 14, 15]. The LMA achieves this by surrounding the opening of the larynx as it enters into the hypopharynx (Fig. 1). It consists of an obliquely cut tube mounted into the concave central part of an inflatable oval mask. Because the cuff is soft, it can conform to the contours of the larynx, thereby forming a relatively good seal. Before insertion the cuff must be deflated and the rear surface lubricated. After induction of anesthesia, the LMA is placed in the mouth and pressed back against the hard palate so that the LMA is seen to flatten. From this point, the LMA is slid behind the tongue and into the pharynx. A definite resistance is felt when the LMA reaches its final location (LMA is at the esophageal sphincter). Now the cuff is inflated, thus leading to a slight protrusion of the LMA [16].

The advantages of this method are:
1) The LMA can be placed easily in the majority of patients
2) No need for muscle-relaxant drugs
3) In contrast to a face mask, the use of the LMA allows the physician to perform other tasks
4) Hemodynamic responses following the placement of the LMA are reduced compared to laryngoscopy and endotracheal intubation
5) The LMA is well tolerated in the postoperative period and can be left *in situ* to provide an unobstructed airway and adequate oxygenation until return of consciousness ensures a clear airway
6) The incidence of sore throat is lower than following endotracheal intubation
7) The LMA can serve as a conduit for fiberoptic bronchoscopy

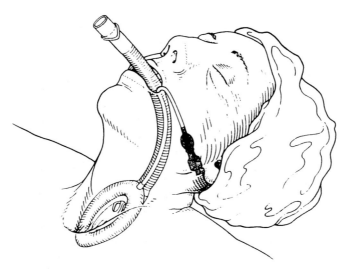

Fig. 1. Correct insertion of the laryngeal mask airway with the tip of the mask reaching the hypopharynx

8) The LMA can serve as a conduit for endotracheal intubation using either a 6 mm ID endotracheal tube, a gum-elastic bougie serving as a guide for the tube after removal of the LMA, or a fiberoptic bronchoscope with premounted endotracheal tube. The latest type of LMA is the intubating LMA or FastTrach, which is inserted without head or neck manipulation and can be used for blind intubation using an 8 mm cuffed tube.

9) The resistance and work of breathing through the LMA is lower than that through an endotracheal tube.

10) The LMA can be re-used 40 to 100 times.

The disadvantages are:

1) The LMA does not guarantee a perfect seal against pulmonary aspiration of gastric contents

2) Application of positive pressure ventilation is limited since the seal between the LMA and the larynx will leak at pressures of 15 to 20 cmH_2O; because the opening of the esophagus often lies within the bowl of the LMA, gastric distension might occur during positive pressure ventilation

3) The LMA cuff is permeable to nitrous oxide and carbon dioxide, which results in significant increases in cuff pressures and volume during its use

4) Edema of the epiglottis resulting from its entrapment in the bars at the distal aperture of the LMA may lead to airway obstruction

5) Laryngospasm is possible

Contraindications are:

1) Risk of regurgitation

2) Low pulmonary compliance

3) High pulmonary resistance

4) Pharyngeal or laryngeal pathology

Esophageal-Tracheal Combitube

The Combitube™ (Kendall-Sheridan Arayl, New York, USA) is a new device for emergency intubation which combines the functions of an esophageal obturator airway (EOA) and a conventional endotracheal airway [17]. The Combitube can be positioned into either the esophagus or the trachea. It is a double-lumen tube: The "esophageal" lumen has an open upper end and a blocked distal end, with perforations at the pharyngeal level; the "tracheal" lumen has a distal open end. The lumens are separated by a partition wall. Each lumen is linked via a short tube with a connector. Proximal to the pharyngeal perforations an oropharyngeal balloon is positioned. This balloon seals the oral and nasal cavity after inflation. At the lower end, a conventional cuff seals either the esophagus or the trachea (Fig. 2).

The lower jaw and tongue are lifted by one hand and the tube is inserted in a curved downward movement until the printed ringmarks lie between the teeth or alveolar ridges. First, the oropharyngeal balloon is inflated via the port with the blue pilot balloon, with 100 ml of air with the large syringe. Then, the distal balloon is inflated via the port with the white pilot balloon with 10 to 15 ml of air with the

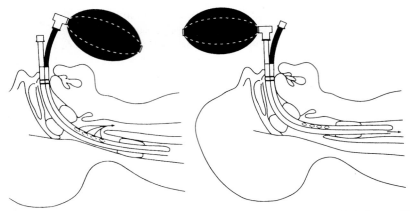

Fig. 2. *Left:* Combitube in esophageal position: Ventilation is performed via longer filled tube. Air flows through holes into pharynx and from there into trachea. *Right:* Combitube in tracheal position: Ventilation is performed via shorter clear tube. Air flows directly into trachea

small syringe. With blind insertion, there is a high probability that the tube will be placed in the esophagus. Air passes through the longer connector, leading to the esophageal lumen, into the pharynx and from there over the epiglottis into the trachea since the mouth, nose and esophagus are blocked by the balloons. The auscultation of breath sounds and the abscence of gastric insufflation confirm adequate ventilation when the Combitube is in the esophagus. Ventilation is continued through this lumen. When no breath sounds are heard over the lungs in the presence of gastric insufflation, the Combitube has been placed in the trachea. Ventilation is changed to the shorter connector, leading to the tracheal lumen, and the position is again controlled by auscultation. Now, air flows directly into the trachea. In a few cases, ventilation does not work via either lumen because the Combitube, and with it the oropharyngeal balloon, may have been placed too deep; move the Combitube about 3 cm out of the patient's mouth and try ventilation again via the esophageal lumen.

Experimental and Clinical Studies

Function and effectiveness of the Combitube were first tested in animal experiments [18] and subsequently in humans [19]. The effectiveness of ventilation with the Combitube was compared to ventilation with conventional endotracheal airways during routine surgery in a cross-over study [20]. In all cases, patients were ventilated with the Combitube without problems. It was demonstrated that ventilation via the Combitube was comparable to an endotracheal airway. In addition, arterial oxygen pressure was higher during ventilation with the Combitube.

The application of the Combitube during cardiopulmonary resuscitation (CPR) was investigated in several studies [21, 22]. Blood gas analysis again showed higher arterial oxygen pressures and a slightly decreased pH during ventilation with the Combitube. Carbon dioxide pressure was not significantly different. Intubation time was shorter with the Combitube, which might improve success rates of CPR.

To investigate the reasons for increased oxygen tension during ventilation with the Combitube, a thin catheter was placed with its tip 10 cm below the vocal cords [23]. Pressures were recorded in the trachea as well as at the airway opening and compared to ventilation via an endotracheal tube. The following differences in intratracheal pressures were found during ventilation with the Combitube: A smaller pressure rise during inspiration; a prolonged expiratory flow time; and the formation of a small positive end-expiratory pressure (PEEP). While pressures at the airway openings may be high due to the resistance of the double-lumen airway, intratracheal pressures were comparable between the two tubes.

The Combitube has shown its value especially in the pre-hospital setting [24, 25] and is the only device recommended by the European Resuscitation Council [26], American Heart Association [27] and American Society of Anesthesiologists [5].

Indications

1) Use in cases of difficult or unexpected intubation in and out of hospital [24, 25]
2) Upper airway bleeding or continued vomiting
3) Face abnormalities (congenital, trauma, lockjaw)
4) Cervical spine abnormalities (rheumatoid arthritis with subluxation of the atlantooccipital joint, fractures, luxations, Bechterew's disease, Klippel-Feil syndrome)
5) Routine surgery in singers and actors
6) Accidental extubation in patients undergoing surgery in prone or sitting position

Advantages

1) Insertion without the need of a laryngoscope; therefore establishment of a patent airway is not hampered by either adverse enviromental factors (difficult access to the patient's head, e.g. patient trapped in a car) or staff unskilled in the use of laryngoscopes.
2) Minimized risk of aspiration
3) Gastric fluids can be suctioned through the tracheal lumen when the tube is in the esophagus
4) No preparations necessary, tube and syringes are ready to use
5) Neck flexion unnecessary
6) Use of controlled mechanical ventilation possible at higher ventilation pressures
7) Simultaneous fixation after inflation of oropharyngeal balloon
8) Independent of power supply
9) Well suited for obese patients

Contraindications

1) Patients with intact gag reflexes, irrespective of their level of consciousness
2) The Combitube 41 F cannot be used in patients smaller than five feet (1.5 m), while the Combitube SA (=small adult, 37 F) may be used in patients between four feet (1.4 m) and five feet six inches (1.68 m) (there is some overlap between the two types)
3) Ingestion of caustic substances
4) Obstruction of the upper airway (foreign bodies, tumors)
5) Esophageal pathology

A new version of the Combitube allows fiberoptic inspection of the tachea, suctioning of tracheal secretions and replacement using a guidewire [28].

Transtracheal Jet Ventilation

For percutaneous transtracheal jet ventilation (TTJV) a large intravenous catheter placed through the cricothyroid membrane is used for immediate restoration of an adequate airway (Fig 3).

Insertion

The cricothyroid membrane is palpated with the neck of the patient extended. Then a 12- to 16-gauge intravenous catheter with the needle pointed 30 degrees off the perpendicular is used to puncture the cricothyroid membrane (the needle stylet/catheter should be pre-angled or pre-curved and/or non-kinkable). The needle should then be connected to either a completely empty 20 ml syringe or a partly clear fluid-

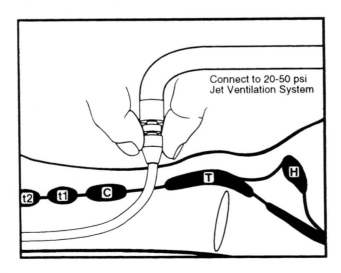

Connect to 20-50 psi Jet Ventilation System

Fig. 3. Transtracheal jet-ventilation catheter is inserted through cricothyroid membrane and connected to jet ventilator. H: hyoid bone; T: thyroid cartilage; C: cricoid cartilage; t1: first tracheal cartilage; t2: second tracheal cartilage; psi: pounds per square inch

filled 20 ml syringe. The syringe will easily fill with air, or air bubbles are seen in the case of fluid-filled syringes, if the tip of the needle is in the trachea. If the tip of the needle is not in the trachea but in some tissue, resistance to pulling the plunger back will be felt because of the development of negative pressure in the syringe. Once entry into the trachea has been identified, the catheter can be threaded over the needle stylet into the trachea, and should be held exactly in place until a definite airway is established. Then the catheter is connected to a jet injector (powered by wall- or tank-oxygen) via a non-compliant tubing. Depending on the size of the catheter, flow rates between 400 and 1600 ml/sec can be achieved using a driving pressure of 50 psi (pounds per square inch) [29]. Numerous animal and human studies have shown that these flow rates are adequate to provide good ventilation and oxygenation (30–35).

During TTJV the natural airway must be maintained as much as possible, so that the expiratory gas can escape through as large a channel as possible under a relatively low driving pressure to avoid air trapping and hyperinflation of the lungs. This means that oropharyngeal and nasopharyngeal airways should be used and maximal jaw thrust maintained.

Indications

1) "Cannot ventilate, cannot intubate" situations
2) Upper airway obstruction (foreign bodies, trauma, infection, neoplasms, laryngeal edema)
3) Lack of equipment and/or trained personnel for conventional airway management
3) Elective diagnostic and surgical procedures of the upper airways to avoid tracheostomy
5) In situations in which an increased risk of developing a "cannot ventilate, cannot intubate" situation can be identified, elective institution of TTJV may prevent the development of a life-threatening gas exchange problem while a more secure permanent airway is established.

Complications

The frequency of complications ranges from about 2 to 29% according to the literature [35, 36, 37]
1) Subcutaneous emphysema
2) Mediastinal emphysema
3) Exhalation difficulty
4) Arterial perforation
5) Barotrauma with resultant pneumothorax; the risk is increased in cases of total airway obstruction because gas cannot escape from the lungs in a normal manner
6) Esophageal puncture
7) Hematoma
8) Hemoptysis

9) Bleeding
10) Damage to tracheal mucosa; the risk is increased in prolonged TTJV without hu-
    midification

Surgical Airway

Emergency Tracheostomy

In a true emergency tracheostomy, where the patient's airway is completely obstructed, a single incision is made though the skin. This is always a vertical incision
and should extend from the cricoid cartilage to the sternal notch. The physician palpates the trachea and with the second cut of the knife incises into the trachea. Then,
using a finger, the endotracheal tube is guided into the trachea. The balloon is inflated and the neck incision is packed with gauze to tamponade bleeding. In contrast to
tracheostomy tubes, endotracheal tubes allow re-inspection of the wound and are
therefore preferred in such situations [38].

Indications

Acute upper airway obstructions:
1) Hypopharyngeal or laryngeal tumours
2) Trauma to the maxilla, mandible or larynx
3) Infection (submental or peritonsillar abscess, epiglottitis)
4) Failed intubation

Emergency Cricothyroidotomy

If a patient cannot be intubated and no intrinsic laryngeal obstruction is seen, entrance into the subglottic airway through the cricothyroid membrane is technically
easier to accomplish and is the technique of choice for those not skilled in neck
surgery. To perform a cricothyroidotomy, one palpates the thyroid cartilage, the
cricoid cartilage, and then identifies the cricothyroid membrane. A scalpel is then
inserted through the skin and through the cricothyroid membrane, and with a single
cut a 1 to 1.5 cm horizontal incision is made. The space is opened and an appropiate
diameter tube is inserted, thereby establishing an airway. Tracheostomy tubes cannot be used because their angles are incorrect [38].

Complications

1) Hemorrhage
2) Complete transection of the trachea
3) Misidentification of the thyrohyoid membrane as the cricothyroid space, surgery
   there is difficult and often unsuccessful

Conclusion

Since "cannot ventilate, cannot intubate" situations occur not infrequently and are often unexpecteod, physicians should be familiar with alternative airway management techniques. In particular, anesthesiologists, emergency and intensive care physicians should be trained in the use of the Combitube and/or laryngeal mask. Since TTJV has a number of serious complications, this procedure should only be undertaken in desperate situations. Both Combitube and LMA are not applicable in patients with laryngeal or pharyngeal pathology. Therefore, in cases of severe upper airway obstruction, emergency cricothyroidotomy or tracheostomy might be the method of choice.

References

1. Caplan RA, Posner KL, Richard JW, Cheney FW (1990) Adverse respiratory events in anesthesia: A closed claims analysis. Anesthesiology 72:828–833
2. Williamson JA, Webb RK, Szekely S, Gillies ERN, Dreosti AV (1993) Difficult intubation: An analysis of 2000 incident reports. Anaesth Intensive Care 21:602–607
3. Schwartz DE, Matthay MA, Cohen NH (1995) Death and other complications of emergency airway management in critically ill adults. Anesthesiology 82:367–376
4. Taryle DA, Chandler JE, Good JT, Potts DE, Sahn SA (1979) Emergency room intubations – complications and survival. Chest 75:541–543
5. American Society of Anesthesiologists Task Force on management of the difficult airway (1993) Practice guidelines for mangement of the difficult airway: a report. Anesthesiology 78:597–602
6. Mallampati SR (1995) Recognition of the difficult airway. In: Benumof JL (ed) Airway management: Principles and practice. Mosby, New York, pp 126–142
7. Mallampati SR, Gatt SP, Gugino LD, et al (1985) A clinical sign to predict difficult tracheal intubation: a prospective study. Can J Anaesth 32:429–434
8. Samsoon GLT, Young JRB (1987) Difficult tracheal intubation: a retrospective study. Anaesthesia 42:487–490
9. Mathew M, Hanna LS, Aldretre JA (1989) Preoperative indices to anticipate a difficult tracheal intubation. Anesth Analg 68:S187
10. Bellhouse CP, Dore C (1988) Criteria for estimating likelihood of difficulty of endotracheal intubation with Macintosh laryngoscope. Anaesth Intensive Care 16:329–337
11. Benumof JL (1995) The American Society of Anesthesiologists' management of the difficult airway algorithm and explanation-analysis of the algorithm. In: Benumof JL (ed) Airway management: Principles and practice. Mosby, New York, pp 143–156
12. McGee II JP, Vender JS (1995) Nonintubation management of the airway: Mask ventilation. In: Benumof JL (ed) Airway management: Principles and practice. Mosby, New York, pp 228–254
13. Joshi GP, Smith I, White PF (1995) Laryngeal mask airway. In: Benumof JL (ed). Airway management: Principles and practice. Mosby, New York, pp 353–373
14. Brain AIJ (1983) The laryngeal mask: a new concept in airway management. Br J Anaesthesia 55:801–805
15. Brain AIJ (1991) The development of the laryngeal mask: a brief history of the invention, early clinical studies and experimental work from which the laryngeal mask evolved. Eur J Anaesthesiol 4:5–17
16. Brain AIJ (1992) The Intravent laryngeal mask instruction manual, 2nd edn., Brain Medical, Berkshire
17. Frass (1995) The Combitube: Esophageal/tracheal double-lumen airway. In: Benumof JL (ed) Airway management: Principles and practice. Mosby, New York, pp 444–454
18. Frass M, Frenzer R, Ilias W, Lackner F, Hoflehner G, Losert U (1987) Tierexperimentelle Ergebnisse mit einem neuen Notfalltubus. Anästh, Intensivther, Notfallmed 22:142–144

19. Frass M, Frenzer R, Zahler J, Ilias W, Lackner F (1987) Ergebnisse erster experimenteller Studien mit einem neuen Notfalltubus (ETC). Intensivmed, Notfallmed 24:390–392
20. Frass M, Frenzer R, Zdrahal F, Hoflehner G, Porges P, Lackner F (1987) The esophageal tracheal combitube: Preliminary results with a new airway for CPR. Ann Emerg Med 16:768–772
21. Frass M, Frenzer R, Rauscha F, Weber H, Pacher R, Leithner C (1987) Evaluation of esophageal tracheal combitube in cardiopulmonary resuscitation. Crit Care Med 15:609–611
22. Frass M, Frenzer R, Rauscha F, Schuster E, Glogar D (1988) Ventilation with the esophageal tracheal combitube in cardiopulmonary resuscitation. Promptness and effectiveness. Chest 93:781–784
23. Frass M, Rödler S, Frenzer R, Ilias W, Leithner C, Lackner F (1989) Esophageal tracheal combitube, endotracheal airway and mask: Comparison of ventilatory pressure curves. J Trauma 29:1476–1479
24. Rumball CJ, MacDonald D (1997) PTL, Combitube, laryngeal mask, and oral airway: A randomized prehospital comparative study of ventilatory device effectiveness and cost-effectiveness in 470 cases of cardiorespiratory arrest. Prehosp Emerg Care 1:1–10
25. Liao D, Shalit M (1996) Successful intubation with the Combitube in acute asthmatic distress by a paramedic. J Emerg Med 14:561–563
26. Baskett PJF, Bossaert L, Carli P, et al (1996) Guidelines for the advanced management of the airway and ventilation during resuscitation. Resuscitation 31:201–230
27. Emergency Cardiac Care Committee and Subcommittees, American Heart Association (1992) Guidelines for cardiopulmonary resuscitation and emergency cardiac care. JAMA 268: 2199–2241
28. Krafft P, Röggla M, Fridrich P, Locker GJ, Frass M, Benumof JL (1997) Bronchoscopy via a re-designed Combitube™ in the esophageal position. A clinical evaluation. Anesthesiology 86: 1041–1045
29. Benumof JL (1995) Transtracheal jet ventilation via percutaneous catheter and high-pressure source. In: Benumof JL (ed) Airway management: Principles and practice. Mosby, New York, pp 455–474
30. Zornow M, Thoma T, Scheller MS (1989) The efficacy of three different methods of transtracheal ventilation. Can J Anaesth 36:624–628
31. Klain M, Smith RB (1988) High frequency percutaneous trantracheal jet ventilation. Crit Care Med 5:280–287
32. Cote CJ, Eavey RD, Todres ID, Jones DE (1988) Cricothyroid membrane puncture: oxygenation and ventilation in a dog using an intravenous catheter. Crit Care Med 16:615–619
33. Weymuller EA, Paugh D, Pavlin EG, Cummings CW (1987) Management of difficult airway problems with percutaneous transtracheal ventilation. Ann Otol Rhinol Laryngol 96:34–37
34. Jacobs HB (1974) Transtracheal catheter ventilation: clinical experience in 36 patients. Chest 65:36–40
35. Monnier PH, Ravussin P, Savary M, Freeman J (1988) Percutaneous transtracheal ventilation for laser endoscopic treatment of laryngeal and subglottic lesions. Clin Otolaryngol 13:209–217
36. Smith BR, Babinski M, Klain M, Pfaeffle H (1976) Percutaneous transtracheal ventilation. J Am Colleg Emerg Physicians 5:765–770
37. Benumof JI, Scheller MS (1989) The importance of transtracheal jet ventilation in the management of the difficult airway. Anesthesiology 71:769–778
38. Davidson TM, Magit AE (1995) Surgical airway. In: Benumof JL (ed) Airway management: Principles and practice. Mosby, New York, pp 513–530

Control of Breathing During Assisted Mechanical Ventilation

D. Georgopoulos

Introduction

The respiratory control system consists of a motor arm which executes the act of breathing, a contol center located in the medulla and a number of mechanisms that convey information to the control center [1, 2]. Based on the information received, the control center activates spinal motor neurons subserving respiratory muscles, with an intensity and rate that varies substantially between breaths. The activity of the spinal motor neurons is conveyed, via peripheral nerves, to respiratory muscles, which contract and generate pressure (P_{mus}). P_{mus} is dissipated to overcome the resistance and elastance of the respiratory system (inertia is assumed to be negligible) and this combination determines volume-time profile and, thus, ventilation. Volume-time profile affects P_{mus} via force-length and force-velocity relationships of the respiratory muscles (mechanical feedback), whereas it modifies the activity of spinal motor neurons and the control center via afferents from various receptors located in the airways, chest wall or respiratory muscles (reflex feedback). Input generated from other sources (e.g., behavioral, temperature, postural) may also modify the function of the control center. On the other hand, ventilation and gas exchange properties of the lung determine arterial blood gases (PaO_2, $PaCO_2$), which, in turn, affect the activity of the control center, via peripheral and central chemoreceptors (chemical feedback). This briefly described complex system may be influenced at any level by various disease states as well as by therapeutic interventions.

During mechanical ventilation another variable, the pressure provided by the ventilator (P_{aw}), is incorporated into the system [3]. Therefore, in mechanically ventilated patients the driving pressure for inspiratory flow (P_{TOT}) is the sum of P_{mus} and P_{aw} [4]. P_{TOT} is dissipated to overcome resistance and elastance of the respiratory system, determining the volume time profile (Fig. 1). The volume time profile, via mechanical, chemical, reflex and behavioral feedback systems, affects the P_{mus} waveform, which, depending on several factors (see below), may alter the P_{aw} waveform. It follows that there is a significant interaction between P_{aw} and P_{mus}. This interaction may alter either the system itself or its expression (i.e., ventilatory output), leading to serious consequences as far as the management of the mechanically ventilated patient is concerned [3].

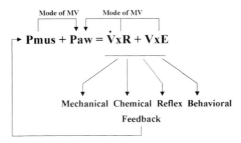

Fig. 1. Schematic representation of the interactions between patient respiratory effort and pressure delivered by the ventilator. P_{mus}: pressure generated by respiratory muscles (inspiratory muscles generate positive pressure and expiratory muscles negative); P_{aw}: pressure generated by the ventilator; $\dot{V}$, V: instantaneous volume above passive FRC and instantaneous flow, respectively (inspiratory flow is positive); R, E: resistance and elastance of respiratory system, respectively, at the relevant flow and volume; MV: mechanical ventilation. Mechanical, chemical, reflex and behavioral feedback systems are the main determinants of P_{mus}. P_{aw} is determined by the mode of ventilatory support, patient's respiratory effort (Pmus) and mechanical properties of the respiratory system (R and E). See text for further details

Determinants of P_{aw} During Assisted Mechanical Ventilation

The waveform of P_{aw} depends on three factors:
1) the mode of mechanical ventilation;
2) the mechanics of the respiratory system; and
3) the characteristics of the P_{mus} waveform (Fig. 1).

Mode of Mechanical Ventilation

I will only discuss assisted modes of ventilatory support. In patients ventilated on controlled modes the P_{aw} waveform is pre-set by the mode of support, the ventilator settings and the mechanics of the respiratory system [4]. In these patients the control center is inactive and the respiratory system represents a passive distensible structure [4]. It follows that during controlled mechanical ventilation the issue of control of breathing is related exclusively to ventilator function.

There are several modes of assisted mechanical ventilation [4, 5]. For teaching purposes these can be classified in three categories [6]:
1) assist volume control (AVC) where the ventilator, once triggered, delivers a pre-set tidal volume (V_T) with a pre-set flow-time profile
2) pressure-support (PSV), where the ventilator delivers a pre-set pressure
3) proportional assist ventilation (PAV), where the ventilator delivers pressure which is proportional (the proportionality is pre-set) to instantaneous flow and volume and, thus, to P_{mus}.

With AVC, mechanical inflation time is determined, theoretically, by the ventilator, whereas with PSV it is influenced both by the patient and the ventilator [4]. On the other hand, with PAV, mechanical inflation time is controlled mainly by the patient [5]. The modern ventilators are able to combine various modes and ventilate the patient simultaneously with more than one mode. Currently, PAV mode is under intense investigation and is not available for general use. In this article, however, the peculiar relationship between P_{aw} and P_{mus} in PAV mode will be used as a tool to clarify some important aspects of control of breathing relevant to mechanical ventilation.

The P_{aw} is greatly influenced by the mode of support. Figures 2 to 4 show the response of the ventilator (i.e., P_{aw}) to respiratory effort in one representative patient ventilated on different modes of support. A carbon dioxide (CO_2) challenge was used to alter the patient effort. With AVC (Fig. 2) the ventilator decreases the P_{aw} to almost zero in order to compensate for the greater patient inspiratory effort due to high $PaCO_2$ and, thus, to maintain the pre-set V_T. It follows that with this mode the ventilator antagonizes the patient effort. With PSV, V_T and inspiratory flows are increased with increasing CO_2, while P_{aw} remains relatively constant (Fig. 3). Therefore, with PSV there is no relationship between patient effort and P_{mus}. Finally, with PAV, CO_2 stimulation causes an increase both in patient effort and pressure provided by the ventilator (Fig. 4). With this mode there is a positive relationship (the gain is pre-set) between P_{mus} and P_{aw}. It is obvious from Figures 2–4 that in mechanically ventilated patients the ventilatory output can not be interpreted properly if the

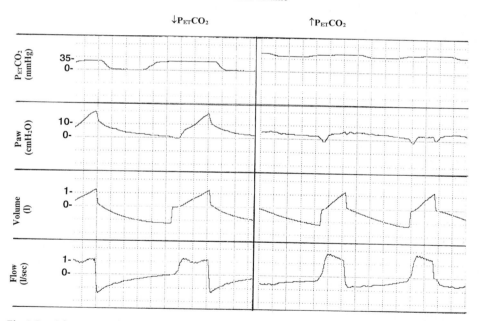

Assist-volume

Fig. 2. Partial pressure of end-tidal CO_2 ($P_{ET}CO_2$), airway pressure (P_{aw}), volume and flow in a patient ventilated on assist volume control mode (AVC). Note the decrease in P_{aw} when the patient's respiratory effort was stimulated by CO_2. Observe also that due to high inspiratory effort the patient was able to increase inspiratory flow above the pre-set level and, thus to achieve the pre-set tidal volume sooner. This was due to the fact that the ventilator was not able to decrease P_{aw} during inflation below a minimum value

Pressure-support

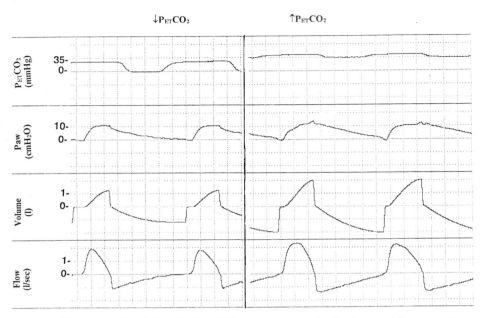

Fig. 3. Partial pressure of end-tidal CO_2 ($P_{ET}CO_2$), airway pressure (P_{aw}) volume and flow in a patient (same patient as Fig. 2) ventilated on pressure-support mode (PSV). Note that P_{aw} remained constant and independent of the patient's respiratory effort

mode of support is not taken into account. During assisted ventilation, changes in ventilatory output may not reflect corresponding changes in patient effort.

Mechanics of Respiratory System

The mechanical properties of the respiratory system and ventilator tubings are important determinants of P_{aw}. These properties may influence P_{aw} independent of P_{mus}, leading to patient-ventilator asynchrony. Asynchrony between P_{mus} and P_{aw} waveforms is mainly due to the phenomenon of dynamic hyperinflation and can be observed with all modes of support [7–12]. Dynamic hyperinflation is a common finding in patients with obstructive lung disease [7]. It is caused by several factors such as low elastic recoil, high ventilatory demands, increased expiratory resistance and short expiratory time [7]. When dynamic hyperinflation is present, end-expiratory lung volume is above passive functional residual capacity (FRC) or the volume determined by external positive end-expiratory pressure (PEEPe) and, therefore, elastic recoil pressure at end-expiration is positive. This positive elastic recoil pressure, referred to as intrinsic PEEP (PEEPi), represents an elastic threshold load for the patient. Indeed, in order to decrease alveolar pressure below PEEPe and trigger the ventilator, the patient must first counterbalance PEEPi. Therefore, a portion of

PAV

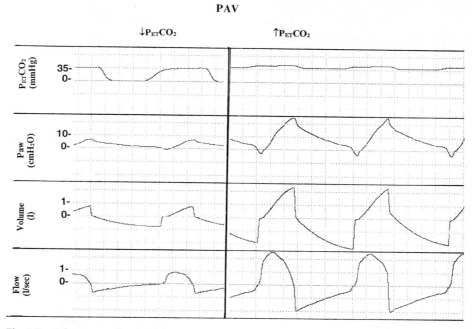

Fig. 4. Partial pressure of end-tidal CO_2 ($P_{ET}CO_2$), airway pressure (P_{aw}) volume and flow in a patient (same patient as Fig. 2) ventilated on proportional assist ventilation (PAV). Note that CO_2 stimulation caused an increase in P_{aw}

the P_{mus} waveform is dissipated to counteract PEEPi (elastic threshold load) and as a consequence there is a delay between the beginning of inspiratory effort and the triggering. At times triggering is so delayed that the ventilator cycles almost completely out of phase with the patient, totally defeating the purpose of assisted ventilators support (Fig. 5). In some circumstances (high PEEPi and or low P_{mus}) the patient can not decrease the P_{aw} below PEEP and his/her inspiratory effort is ineffective. We should note that when asynchrony is present the relation between a patient's spontaneous breathing frequency and the machine rate becomes quite sensitive to changes in ventilator settings or in the patient's respiratory output (Fig. 5).

Ineffective efforts have also been observed with PSV [10, 12], particularly when the PSV level and therefore V_T are relatively high. In mechanically ventilated patients with obstructive lung disease increasing the PSV level usually causes a decrease in the ventilator rate, despite the fact that the patient's spontaneous rate has not been changed. This decrease is the result of the increased number of ineffective efforts due to a higher V_T, which further augments the dynamic hyperinflation. It is thus obvious that this decrease in the ventilator rate can not be interpreted as suggesting a decrease in the patient's respiratory work or an increase in patient comfort. Titration of the PSV level using the ventilator rate as an index should be abandoned; the ventilator rate may not reflect the patient's spontaneous breathing frequency.

With PAV the likelihood of ineffective efforts is considerably reduced [8, 9]. This is mainly due to the fact that with PAV the end of mechanical inflation time occurs

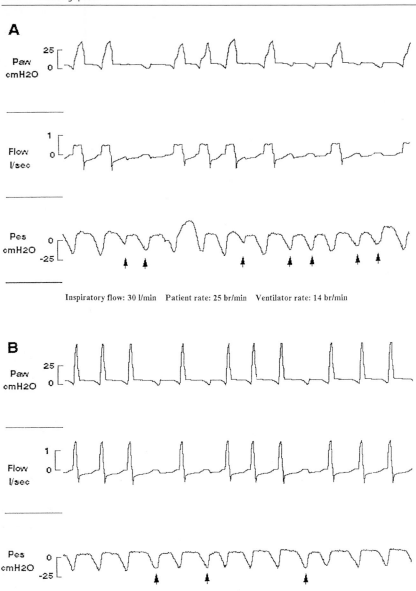

A

Inspiratory flow: 30 l/min   Patient rate: 25 br/min   Ventilator rate: 14 br/min

B

Inspiratory flow: 90 l/min   Patient rate: 22 br/min   Ventilator rate: 18 br/min

Fig. 5. Airway pressure (P_{aw}), flow and esophageal pressure (P_{es}) in a patient with chronic obstructive lung disease ventilated on assist volume-control (AVC) mode with two different inspiratory flow rate (V_I), 30 l/min (**A**) and 90 l/min (**B**). Tidal volume was kept constant (0.55 l). Ineffective efforts are indicated by arrows. Observe the time delay between the onset of inspiratory effort (abrupt decrease in P_{es}) and the ventilator triggering. By increasing the time available for expiration (increase in inspiratory flow at constant V_T, **B**), the number of ineffective efforts reduced and as a result the rate of the ventilator increased at the end of neural inspiration because, by design, the P_{aw} is linked to P_{mus}. Therefore, the mechanical inflation time can not be extended to the neural expiratory time, which is available for lung deflation. Furthermore, a large V_T, an important cause of ineffective efforts, occurs with strong inspiratory efforts. Strong inspiratory efforts, however, may be able to trigger the ventilator, thus reducing the number of ineffective efforts. On the other hand with AVC and PSV a large V_T is usually the result of the ventilator settings and may not be associated with strong inspiratory efforts.

It follows that the phenomenon of ineffective efforts influences considerably the interpretation of ventilatory output in relation to the control of breathing during assisted mechanical ventilation. Furthermore, with ineffective efforts, significant alteration in P_{mus} may occur due to changes in the feedback loop. For example in the patient shown in Fig. 5 breathing frequency decreased with increasing inspiratory flow, most likely because chemical feedback was altered. Indeed, at high inspiratory flow rates minute ventilation increased from 6.2 l/min to 9.4 l/min. This caused a decrease in $PaCO_2$ (not shown), which might be associated with a drop in the patient's spontaneous breathing frequency.

Characteristics of P_{mus} Waveform

The characteristics of the P_{mus} waveform influence the P_{aw} in a complex way, depending on several factors related to both patient and ventilator. Although an extensive review of these factors is beyond the scope of this article, some examples may be helpful for the reader to understand how the characteristics of P_{mus} may affect ventilator function.

The initial rate of P_{mus} increase interacts with the triggering function of the ventilator. A low rate of initial increase in P_{mus}, as occurs with a concave upwards shape of P_{mus} or low respiratory drive (e.g., low $PaCO_2$, sedation, sleep), increases the time delay between the onset of a patient's inspiratory effort and ventilator triggering and promotes asynchrony (see above). In the presence of dynamic hyperinflation this increased triggering time, particularly when it is associated with a relatively short neural inspiratory time and low peak P_{mus}, may result in ineffective efforts with all the consequences described above (Fig. 5). Alternatively, an increase in intensity of inspiratory effort, as occurs, for example, with an increase in metabolic rate, high $PaCO_2$ or decrease in the level of sedation, is manifest in the rate of rise of P_{mus} as well as in the peak P_{mus}. This may cause a decrease in the time delay, thus promoting patient-ventilator synchrony. On the other hand if the patient inspiratory effort is vigorous and longer than the mechanical inflation time, the ventilator may be triggered more than once (double triggering) during the same inspiratory effort (Fig. 6). This may occur when at the end of mechanical inspiration P_{mus} continues to increase and, because inspiratory flow is zero or is reversed, it is dissipated to overcome only the elastic recoil. Thus, during mechanical expiration there might be a situation where the P_{mus} is greater than the elastic recoil, causing the airway pressure to decrease below PEEP and this triggers the ventilator. Short mechanical inflation time (Fig. 6) and low elastic recoil at end-inspiration may promote re-triggering. It follows that changes in the characteristics of the P_{mus} waveform may influence

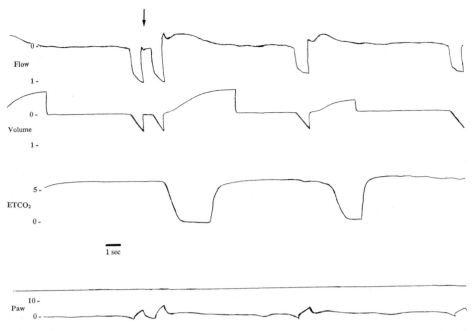

Fig. 6. Flow (l/sec, inspiration down), volume (l, inspiration down)), end-tidal CO_2 (ETCO$_2$, %) and airway pressure (P_{aw}, cm H_2O) in a normal subject ventilated on assist volume-control mode. Note double-triggering (arrow) when inspiratory flow was 60 l/min. This occurred because mechanical inspiratory time, which was pre-set by ventilatory settings, was considerably shorter than neural inspiratory time. In this case, immediately after inflation, P_{mus} decreased P_{aw} below the threshold for triggering and caused the ventilator to re-cycle. The actual tidal volume (V_T) delivered to the subject and the ventilator rate were double the pre-determined V_T (note the expired V_T) and spontaneous subject breathing frequency, respectively. Changing inspiratory flow from 60 to 50 l/min (V_T was kept constant) increased mechanical inflation time from 0.6 to 0.8 sec and double triggering did not occur

the ventilator rate and ventilatory output even in the absence of a change in the patient's breathing frequency. Alteration in ventilatory output may secondarily modify patient effort through various changes in feedback loops [3].

Determinants of P$_{mus}$ During Assisted Mechanical Ventilation

The waveform of P_{mus} during assisted mechanical ventilation is determined mainly by four feedback systems: mechanical; chemical, reflex; and behavioral.

Mechanical Feedback

Mechanical feedback describes the effects of length (i.e. volume) and velocity of respiratory muscle contraction (i.e., flow) on P_{mus} [14]. For a given neural output to inspiratory muscles, P_{mus} decreases with increasing lung volume and flow [141. The-refore, for a similar level of muscle activation, P_{mus} should be smaller during mecha-nical ventilation than during spontaneous breathing if the pressure provided by the ventilator results in greater flow and volume. The influences and consequences of mechanical feedback dunng mechanical ventilation have not been studied. It is like-ly that the effects of mechanical feedback on P_{mus} in mechanically ventilated pa-tients are relatively small, due to low values of operating volume and flow. However, the mechanical feedback should be taken into account when pressure measurements (i.e., transdiaphragmatic pressure) are used to infer changes in respiratory muscle activation. Particularly at high ventilatory demands P_{mus} may considerably under-estimate the neural output to respiratory muscles, leading to erroneous conclusions. Indeed, we have found recently [13] that during hypercapnic hyperventilation mechanical feedback may decrease peak P_{mus} and peak transdiaphragmatic pres-sure by as much as 15%.

Chemical Feedback

Chemical feedback refers to the response of the respiratory system to PaO_2, $PaCO_2$ and pH. Chemical feedback minimizes the changes in blood gas tensions that would otherwise occur as a result of changes in metabolic rate or gas exchange properties of the respiratory system [1, 2]. In spontaneously breathing normal subjects chemi-cal feedback is an important determinant of respiratory motor output both during wakefulness and during sleep. Two crucial questions are raised at this point:
1) To which extent does mechanical ventilation alter the contribution of chemical feedback in determining P_{mus}?
2) Is the effectiveness of chemical feedback in compensating for changes in chemi-cal stimuli modified by mechanical ventilation?

Contribution of Chemical Feedback in Determining P_{mus} during Mechanical Ventilation: Me-chanical ventilation is usually used in order to unload the respiratory muscles. Theoretically, the respiratory control system can follow one of three paths in res-ponse to unloading. First, respiratory muscle activation is down-regulated, so that ventilation remains constant to levels obtained before the unloading. Second, res-piratory muscle activation does not respond to unloading and, thus, ventilation increases according to the degree of unloading. Third, there may be an interme-diate response, whereby ventilation is higher at a lower level of respiratory muscle activity (incomplete down-regulation of respiratory muscle activity). It is gener-ally believed that the respiratory system follows the third pathway. Indeed several studies have shown that with unloading ventilation is higher and respiratory motor output is lower [15–17]. These results were interpreted as indicating that non-chemical feedback related to the load *per se* plays a role in determining the level of respiratory muscle activation. Thus, at first glance it seems that the contribu-tion of chemical feedback to P_{mus} is reduced by mechanical ventilation. However, studies dealing with unloading of the respiratory system were performed using an open loop system and as a result chemical feedback was not rigorously con-trolled. The observed down-regulation of respiratory muscle output could have been related to associated reduction of chemical feedback due to higher ventilation.

Several years ago Milic-Emili and Tyler [18] studied in normal subjects the ventilatory response to CO_2 with different resistive loads and observed that, for a given PCO_2, the work output of inspiratory muscles did not change appreciably with the load. Data in patients during constant flow synchronized intermittent mandatory ventilation [SIMV] have shown that, for a given level of assist, inspiratory effort did not differ between spontaneous and mandatory breaths [19–21]. Recently, Leung et al. [22] studied the respiratory effort of patients ventilated on SIMV and on a combination of SIMV and PSV. Compared to SIMV alone, when PS was added to a given level of SIMV, the inspiratory pressure-time product (an index of the inspiratory work of breathing) was decreased both in mandatory and intervening breaths. This additional reduction during mandatory breaths was proportional to the decrease in respiratory drive (estimated using the change in esophageal pressure before triggering, dp/dt) during intervening breaths. All these studies indicate that inspiratory activity was pre-programmed and it was relatively insensitive to breath-by-breath changes in load seen during SIMV or SIMV and PS. Chemical feedback could be a critical factor for this breath programming [3, 6]. This assumption has been supported by a recent study [13] showing that when the chemical stimulus was rigorously controlled, unloading of the respiratory muscles by PAV (50% reduction of the normal load) did not result in down-regulation of respiratory muscle activation. The waveforms of P_{mus} did not differ significantly with and without unloading (Fig. 7), indicating that the neuromuscular output was tightly linked to CO_2 (i.e. to chemical stimulus) and not to load reduction.

Collectively, the above studies suggest that mechanical ventilation does not significantly alter the contribution of chemical feedback to respiratory muscle activity. It follows that chemical feedback remains an important determinant of P_{mus} even in mechanically ventilated patients.

Effectiveness of Chemical Feedback during Mechanical Ventilation: Although mechanical ventilation *per se* is unlikely to significantly alter the contribution of chemical feedback in determining P_{mus}, its effectiveness in compensating for changes in chemical stimuli may be modified [3, 6]. This issue is of fundamental importance to understand the concept of control of breathing during mechanical ventilation. Furthermore, the effectiveness of chemical feedback may differ between wakefulness and sleep (or anesthesia).

1) Wakefulness: Recent studies have examined the ventilatory response to CO_2 in mechanically ventilated normal conscious subjects [23–25]. These studies demonstrated that, as during spontaneous breathing [26–29], changes in $PaCO_2$ resulted in a progressive increase in the intensity of respiratory effort (P_{mus}) with initially no change in respiratory rate. Respiratory rate increased, to a much lesser extent, when $PaCO_2$ approached values well above eucapnia. It is of interest to note that this response pattern was observed both with PSV and with AVC indicating that there is no fundamental difference in the response to CO_2 between various modes of ventilatory support [23, 25].

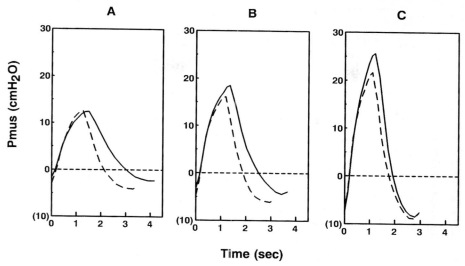

Fig. 7. Average time course of total pressure generated by all respiratory muscles (P_{mus}) at three levels of $P_{ET}CO_2$ with (*dashed lines*) and without (*solid lines*) mechanical ventilatory support. A, B, C: $P_{ET}CO_2$ 50, 55, 59 mmHg, respectively. The traces were aligned at onset of neural inspiration (zero time). Mechanical ventilatory support was achieved using proportional assist ventilation (the assist level was such as to decrease the elastance and resistance of respiratory system by 50%). Observe the similarity of P_{mus} with and without mechanical ventilation particularly at low $P_{ET}CO_2$. At high $P_{ET}CO_2$ P_{mus} at the end of inspiration was slightly lower. This was due to different force-length and force-velocity relationships of respiratory muscles with and without mechanical ventilation; with mechanical ventilation flow and volume were higher and thus, for a given neural output to respiratory muscles P_{mus} must be lower (i.e. mechanical feedback was different) (From [13] with permission)

Although the above studies used CO_2 as a changing chemical stimulus, similar principles should apply if other chemical stimuli (PaO_2, pH) are altered. The steady-state ventilation response to various chemical stimuli is qualitatively similar and mediated mainly by the intensity of the respiratory effort [28, 29]. This ventilatory response pattern has important consequences for the mechanically ventilated patient as far as the effectiveness of chemical feedback is concerned. Figures 8 and 9 demonstrate the basic principles that underly the operation and effectiveness of chemical feedback during assisted modes of mechanical ventilatory support. Fig. 8 shows ventilatory output as a function of $PaCO_2$ in a patient with relatively normal respiratory system mechanics ventilated on different assisted modes of support. On each mode the patient was ventilated with the highest comfortable level of assist, corresponding to an 80% reduction of patient resistance and elastance with PAV, 10 cm H_2O pressure with PSV and 1.2 l V_T with AVC. When the patient was stable on each mode, inspired CO_2 ($FiCO_2$) increased in steps and the response of respiratory system to CO_2 challenge was observed. Several important points are illustrated by Figure 8:

1) The starting PCO_2 point was considerably lower with PSV and AVC than that with PAV; a significant respiratory alkalosis was observed with PSV and AVC but not with PAV;

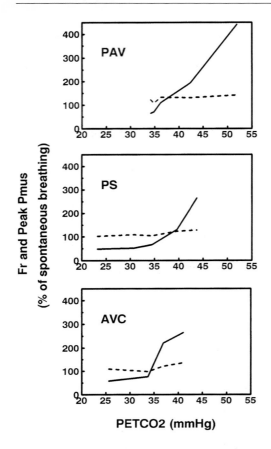

Fig. 8. Breathing, frequency (Fr, *dashed lines*) and peak inspiratory muscle pressure (Peak P_{mus}, *solid lines*) as a function of end-tidal PCO_2 ($P_{ET}CO_2$) in a patient ventilated on three modes of ventilatory support. Fr and peak P_{mus} were expressed as % of the values observed during spontaneous breathing. PAV: proportional assist ventilatione; PS: pressure support; AVC: assist volume control. See text for further details

2) Breathing frequency remained relatively stable at baseline level (spontaneous breathing) over a wide range of PCO_2. Indeed, the patient continued to trigger the ventilator rhythmically despite the severe hypocapnia;

3) At zero $FiCO_2$ and independent of the mode of ventilatory support the intensity of respiratory effort, as expressed by peak P_{mus} (P_{mus} was calculated using esophageal pressure measurements and the Campbell diagram), decreased to approximately 50% of baseline and increased progressively with increasing CO_2 stimulus.

Figure 9 shows in the same patient the relationship between the intensity of patient effort, expressed by peak P_{mus}, and V_T. As expected with AVC, V_T is constant and independent of P_{mus}. With PSV, V_T increased with increasing P_{mus}. However, even when P_{mus} decreased to 50% of baseline, V_T was approximately 40% higher than that during spontaneous breathing. This is because with PSV, in the absence of active termination of inspiration, the V_T has a minimum value which depends on the PS level, mechanical properties of the respiratory system and cycling-off criteria [8, 9]. On the other hand, with PAV the decrease of P_{mus} to 60% of baseline was able to maintain V_T at baseline levels, thus avoiding a significant drop in PCO_2. It follows

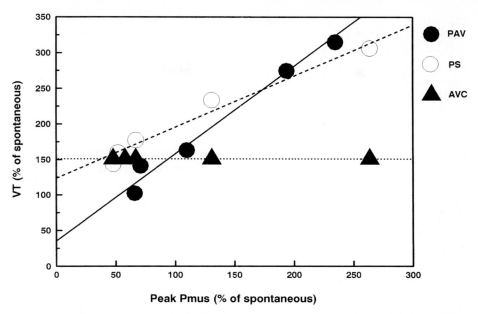

Fig. 9. Same patient as Figure 8. Relationships between V_T and Peak P_{mus} during different modes of support. Regression lines were constructed by the least square method. See Fig. 8 for abbreviations

that modes of ventilatory support that permit the intensity of patient effort to be expressed on the V_T delivered by the ventilator, increase the effectiveness of chemical feedback to regulate $PaCO_2$ and particularly to prevent respiratory alkalosis. Thus, the effectiveness of chemical feedback is increased progressively as we switch from AVC to PSV to PAV. The above considerations are also supported by the recent study of Puntillo et al. [30]. These investigators studied the variability of various ventilatory parameters observed over 12 hours in patients with acute respiratory failure. The patients were studied one day during PSV and the following day during PAV. With PAV arterial blood gases during the 12 hour period of observation were maintained within narrower limits when compared to PSV. This was probably due to the increased ability of patients to change V_T in response to an alteration in ventilatory demands, as suggested by the fact that with PAV the variability of V_T was significantly greater, while that of breathing frequency was significantly less than the values observed during PSV.

The principles described above may be altered by various disease states. This remains an unexplored area and much work needs to be done. A few examples, however, may be useful. We [31, 32] have shown in conscious patients with sleep apnea syndrome that a drop in $PaCO_2$ because of brief (40 sec) hypoxic hyperventilation, resulted, compared to normal controls, in significant hypoventilation and in some cases triggered periodic breathing. Similar results were observed in patients with brain damage [33]. This hypoventilation was interpreted as evidence indicating a defect or reduced effectiveness of short-term post-stimulus potentiation, a brain stem mechanism promoting ventilatory stability. A level of assist that causes a significant decrease in $PaCO_2$ may thus promote unstable breathing, a situation closely resembling that observed during sleep (see below). Ranieri et al. [34] studied the response to added deadspace in patients with abnormal respiratory system mechanics (high resistance and elastance) ventilated either on PSV or PAV. Addition of deadspace (i.e., CO_2 challenge) during PAV resulted in an increase in V_T with no change in breathing frequency. This response pattern was similar to that observed in normal controls. On PSV in the same patients, increased deadspace resulted in an increase in rate with little change in V_T, while they experienced more discomfort. However, because with PSV the ability of patients, particularly in the presence of abnormal respiratory system mechanics, to increase V_T is limited [8, 9], it is likely that the increase in rate is a reflection of greater respiratory distress (i.e., behavioral feedback).

2) Sleep: It is well known that removal of the wakefulness drive to breathe, as occurs during sleep or under anesthesia, increases the dependence of respiratory rhythm on $PaCO_2$ [35–37]. Under these circumstances a drop in $PaCO_2$ by 3–4 mm Hg causes apnea. This has major consequences for the mechanically ventilated patient. An assist level that is associated with a relatively high V_T increases the likelihood of apneas and may trigger periodic breathing [38, 39]. The occurrence of periodic breathing is clearly an indication of over-assist. Periodic breathing may cause significant hypoxemia, an issue that should be seriously considered in critically ill patients. Reducing the assist level to the point where breathing becomes stable may improve oxygenation and sleep quality. Periodic breathing has been observed with PSV and AVC modes of ventilatory support [37–39]. On the other hand, it has been shown that unstable breathing did not occur with PAV despite the fact that the subjects were ventilated at the highest assist level (90% assist) [40]. These results are predictable because, as was discussed already, with PAV the patient is able to maintain V_T constant at different assist levels by appropriate adjustments of P_{mus}. It follows that modes of ventilatory support that decrease the V_T in response to any reduction in P_{mus} promote ventilatory stability. It should be mentioned, however, that in the presence of active lung disease (e.g., pneumonia, ARDS), inputs to respiratory control from other than chemical sources (e.g., reflex feedback) may not permit chemical feedback to prevent respiratory alkalosis during sleep or under anesthesia [41].

In summary the operation of chemical feedback during assisted mechanical ventilation depends on the mode of mechanical ventilatory support; the sleep/awake stage; and the disease state.

Reflex Feedback

Reflex feedback plays an important role in the control of breathing [1, 2]. The characteristics of each breath are influenced by various reflexes, which are related to lung volume or flow and mediated by receptors located in the respiratory tract, lung and chest wall [1, 42, 43]. Mechanical ventilation may stimulate these receptors by changing flow and volume [3]. In addition, changes in ventilatory settings that are inevitably associated with volume and flow changes may also elicit P_{mus} responses

Table 1. Examples of changes in ventilator settings and clinical status, the reflex response of the patient respiratory effort and the possible consequences during assisted mechanical ventilation

Example	Change	Response	Possible consequences during MV
		(Vagal volume related reflexes)	
↑ assist level	↑V_T	↓T_In, ↓ Peak $Pmus_I$	↑ dynamic hyperinflation, ineffective efforts
↓ assist level	↓V_T	↑T_In, ↑ Peak $Pmus_I$	Double triggering
↑ resistance	delayed lung emptying	↑T_En, ↑ $Pmus_E$	↓ dynamic hyperinflation
$T_Im > T_In$	mechanical inflation during T_En	↑T_En, ↑ $Pmus_E$	↓ dynamic hyperinflation
↑ PEEP	sustained increase of lung volume	↑T_En, ↑ $Pmus_E$	↓ PEEP-induced lung volume change
$T_Im < T_In$	withdrawal of lung volume during T_In	↑T_In	Double triggering
		(Chest wall reflexes)	
↑ abdominal pressure	↑E_{CW}	↑ Fr	↑ patient-ventilator asynchrony
		(Flow-related reflexes)	
↓T_Im at constant V_T	↑ inspiratory flow	↓T_In, ↓T_En	↑ dynamic hyperinflation

T_In, T_En: neural inspiratory and expiratory time, respectively; T_Im: ventilator inspiratory time, respectively; E_{CW}: chest wall elastance; Fr: breathing frequency; Pmus, $Pmus_E$: inspiratory and expiratory muscle pressure, respectively; V_T: tidal volume; MV: mechanical ventilation; ↓ decrease; ↑ increase

mediated by various reflexes [3, 6, 8, 9]. Table 1 summarizes the effects of these reflexes on P_{mus} waveform and highlights some possible consequences during mechanical ventilation. Notwithstanding that the final response may be unpredictable depending on the magnitude and type of lung volume change, the level of consciousness and the relative strength of the reflexes involved, reflex feedback should be taken into consideration when ventilatory strategies are planned. However, very few studies have examined specifically the operation of reflex feedback during mechanical ventilation and much work is clearly needed in this field. It is the opinion of the writer that this feedback, under certain circumstances, may be of importance in the management of mechanically ventilated patients. For example, it has been shown that increasing inspiratory flow rate causes tachypnea [44]. This response was also observed during non-rapid eye movement (NREM) sleep, although its magnitude was reduced [45]. This observation confirms that the response is mediated via a reflex pathway (i.e., not a behavioral response) and that its potency is related to the level of vigilance. The response was equally strong in quadriplegic patients, indicating that it was not mediated by rib cage receptors, and was also preserved in patients with double lung transplants [46]. The latter observation does not exclude a vagal mechanoreceptor response, since many of these receptors are located above the resection line, where there is a possibility of regeneration. The excitatory effect of inspiratory flow on breathing frequency has two important clinical implications. First, an increase in flow rate intended to reduce inflation time and provide more time for expiration in order to reduce the dynamic hyperinflation (e.g., in patients with obstructive lung disease) [47] may be detrimental and elicit the opposite response (i.e., decrease in expiratory time). Indeed, in a recent study, Corn et al. [48] increased inspiratory flow rate at a constant V_T in patients ventilated on AVC mode and observed a significant increase in breathing frequency. As a result of the change in breathing frequency, expiratory time showed a variable response to changes in flow rate, with some patients actually demonstrating a reduced expiratory time with higher flow rates (Fig. 10). Second, an increase in inspiratory flow rate may lead to hyperventilation and respiratory alkalosis, important causes of various arrhythmias and weaning difficulty [49].

Behavioral Feedback

The effects of behavioral feedback on the control of breathing in mechanically ventilated patients are unpredictable depending on several factors related to the individual patient and the intensive care unit (ICU) environment. Alterations in ventilator settings, planned to achieve a particular goal (i.e., reduction of dynamic hyperinflation), might be ineffective in awake patients due to behavioral feedback. Manning et al. [50] have shown in normal subjects ventilated on AVC mode that values both higher and lower than the spontaneous inspiratory flow increases breathing discomfort, as estimated using a visual analog scale. This increase in the sense of dyspnea may be manifest by rapid shallow breathing with detrimental effects on patient-ventilator synchrony. Jubran et al. [51] increased the pressure support level in patients with chronic obstructive pulmonary disease (COPD) and observed active expiratory effort. In patients with flow limitation, active expiratory effort causes

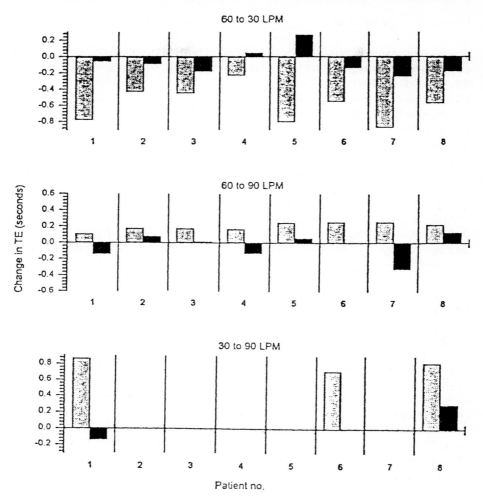

Fig. 10. Individual predicted changes in expiratory time (T_E, gray bars) versus actual change in T_E (black bars) when three inspiratory flow transitions were applied. The patients were ventilated on avssist volume controlled (AVC) mode with square wave flow-time profile. Tidal volume was kept constant. The predicted values of T_E were calculated assuming no change in total breath duration with flow transition. Note that in several patients T_E was actually decreased with increasing inspiratory flow rate. (From [48] with permission)

airway compression downstream to the choke point and breathing discomfort [52]. Thus, increasing the assist level in patients with COPD might force the patient via behavioral feedback to fight with the ventilator. Finally, behavioral feedback may be altered considerably from time to time due to changes in the level of sedation, sleep/awake state, patient status and stimuli of ICU environment. Nevertheless, several factors that are involved in behavioral feedback complicate the study and interpretation of the effects of this feedback on the system that controls breathing in mechanically ventilated patients.

Final Response of P_{mus} to P_{aw}

The above considerations indicate that the final response of P_{mus} to P_{aw} is complex and influenced by several factors. Changes in ventilator settings alter P_{mus} in a way that depends on the:
1) instantaneous flow and volume changes;
2) magnitude of PaO_2, $PaCO_2$ and pH changes;
3) individual sensitivity to chemical stimuli;
4) disease states;
5) level of consciousness; and
6) type and strength of various reflexes involved in the response.

The unpredictable effects of behavioral feedback [53, 54] further complicate the situation. All these determinants of P_{mus} may modify the ventilatory outcome intended from the change in ventilator settings. It follows that when altering ventilatory settings the physician should remember that the respiratory system is not a passive structure but will respond, sometimes vigorously, to the alteration.

Conclusion

In conclusion, the pressure provided by the ventilator considerably alters the effects of the system that controls breathing. On one hand, P_{aw}, by changing the driving pressure for inspiratory flow, modifies the volume-time profile, which via various feedback systems affects the pressure generated by the respiratory muscles of the patient (P_{mus}). On the other hand, P_{aw} is influenced by the mode of mechanical ventilatory support, the mechanics of the respiratory system and the P_{mus} waveform. It follows that during assisted mechanical ventilation a significant interaction between the patient and the function of the ventilator exists. As a result of this interaction various aspects of the control of breathing may be masked and/or modulated.

References

1. Younes M, Remmers J (1981) Control of tidal volume and respiratory frequency. In: Hornbein TF (ed) Lung biology in health and disease, regulation of breathing. Marcel Dekker, New York, pp 621–671
2. Berger AJ (1988) Control of breathing. In: Murray and Nadel (eds) Textbook of respiratory medicine, W.B. Saunders, New York, pp 49–166
3. Georgopoulos D, Roussos C (1996) Control of breathing in mechanically ventilated patients. Eur Respir J 9:2151–2160
4. Slutsky AS (1993) Mechanical ventilation. ACCP consensus conference. Chest 104:1833–1859
5. Younes M (1992) Proportional assist ventilation, a new approach to ventilatory support. Theory. Am Rev Respir Dis 145:114–120
6. Georgopoulos D, Anastasaki M, Katsanoulas K (1997) Effects of mechanical ventilation on control of breathing. Monaldi Arch Chest Dis 52:253–262
7. Rossi A, Polese G, Brandi G, Conti G (1995) Intrinsic positive end-expiratory pressure (PEEPi). Intensive Care Med 21:522–536
8. Younes M (1993) Patient-ventilator interaction with pressure-assisted modalities of ventilatory support. Sem Respir Med 14:299–322

9. Younes M (1995) Interactions between patients and ventilators. In: Roussos C (ed) Thorax, lung biology in health and disease, 2nd edn. Marcel Dekker, New York, pp 2367–2420

10. Fabry B, Guttmann J, Eberhard L, Bauer T, Haberthur C, Wolff G (1995) An analysis of desynchronization between the spontaneous breathing patient and ventilator during inspiratory pressure support. Chest 107:1387–1394

11. Rossi A, Appendini L (1995) Wasted efforts and dyssynchrony: is the patient-ventilator battle back? Intensive Care Med 21:867–870

12. Nava S, Bruschi C, Rubini F, Palo A, Iotti G, Braschi A (1995) Respiratory response and inspiratory effort during pressure support ventilation in COPD patients. Intensive Care Med 21:871–879

13. Georgopoulos D, Mitrouska I, Webster K, Bshouty Z, Younes M (1997) Effects of respiratory muscle unloading on the ventilatory response to CO_2. Am J Respir Crit Care Med 155: 2000–2009

14. Younes M, Riddle W (1984) Relation between respiratory neural output and tidal volume. J Appl Physiol 56:1110–1119

15. Younes M, Puddy A, Roberts D, et al (1992) Proportional assist ventilation. Results of an initial clinical trial. Am Rev Respir Dis 145:121–129

16. DeWeese EL, Sullivan TY, Yu PL (1984) Ventilatory and occlusion pressure responses to helium breathing. J Appl Physiol 54:1525–1531

17. Hussain SNA, Pardy RL, Dempsey JA (1985) Mechanical impedance as determinant of inspiratory neural driving during exercise in humans. J Appl Physiol 59:365–375

18. Milic-Emili J, Tyler JM (1963) Relation between work output of respiratory muscles and end-tidal CO_2 tension. J Appl Physiol 18:497–504

19. Marini JJ, Smith TC, Lamb VJ (1988) External output and force generation during synchronized intermittent mechanical ventilation. Am Rev Respir Dis 138:1169–1179

20. Imsand C, Feihl F, Perret C, Fitting JW (1994) Regulation of inspiratory neuromuscular output during synchronized intermittent mechanical ventilation. Anesthesiology 80:13–22

21. Giuliani R, Mascia L, Recchia F, Caracciolo A, Fiore T, Ranieri VM (1995) Patient-ventilator interaction during synchronized intermittent mandatory ventilation. Am J Respir Crit Care Med 151:1–9

22. Leung P, Jubran A, Tobin MJ (1997) Comparison of assisted ventilator mode on triggering, patient effort, and dyspnea. Am J Respir Crit Care Med 155:1940–1948

23. Patrick W, Webster K, Puddy A, Sanii R, Younes M (1995) Respiratory response to CO_2 in the hypocapnic range in conscious humans. J Appl Physiol 76:2058–2086

24. Scheid P, Lofaso F, Isabey D, Harf A (1994) Respiratory response to inhaled CO_2 during positive inspiratory pressure in humans. J Appl Physiol 77:876–882

25. Georgopoulos D, Mitrouska I, Bshouty Z, Webster K, Patakas D, Younes M (1997) Respiratory response to CO_2 during pressure support ventilation in conscious normal humans. Am J Respir Crit Care Med 156:146–154

26. Rebuck AS, Rigg JRS, Saunders NA (1976) Respiratory frequency response to progressive isocapnic hypoxia. J Physiol 258:19–31

27. Hey EN, Lloyd BB, Cunningham DJC, Juke MGM, Bolton DPG (1966) Effects of various respiratory stimuli on the depth and frequency of breathing in man. Respir Physiol 1:193–205

28. Bechbache RR, Chow HHK, Duffin J, Orsini EC (1979) The effects of hypercapnia, hypoxia, exercise and anxiety on the pattern of breathing in man. J Physiol 293:285–300

29. Gardner WN (1980) The pattern of breathing following step changes of alveolar partial pressures of carbon dioxide and oxygen in man. J Physiol 300:55–73

30. Puntillo F, Grasso S, Fanelli G, et al (1997) Spontaneous variations of ventilatory requirements during mechanical ventilation: Pressure support vs proportional assist ventilation. Intensive Care Med 23 (suppl 1):S6 (Abst)

31. Georgopoulos D, Giannouli E, Tsara V, Argiropoulou P, Patakas D, Anthonisen NR (1992) Respiratory short-term poststimulus potentiation (after-discharge) in patients with obstructive sleep apnea. Am Rev Respir Dis 146:1250–1255

32. Georgopoulos D, Bshouty Z, Younes M, Anthonisen NR (1990) Hypoxic exposure and activation of after-discharge mechanism in conscious humans. J Appl Physiol 69:1159–1164

33. Georgopoulos D, Mitrouska I, Koletsos K, et al (1995) Post-stimulus ventilation in patients with brain damage. Am J Respir Crit Care Med 152:1627–1632

34. Ranieri M, Giuliani R, Mascia L, et al (1996) Patient-ventilator interaction during acute hypercapnia: pressure-support vs. proportional-assist ventilation. J Appl Physiol 81:426–436
35. Younes M (1989) The physiologic basis of central apnea. Cur Pulmonol 10:265–326
36. Fink BR, Hanks EC, Ngai SH, Papper EM (1963) Central regulation of respiration during anesthesia and wakefulness. Ann NY Acad Sci 109:892–899
37. Skatrud JB, Dempsey JA (1983) Interaction of sleep state and chemical stimuli in sustaining rhythmic respiration. J Appl Physiol 55:813–822
38. Morrell MJ, Shea SA, Adams L, Guz A (1993) Effects of inspiratory support uponbreathing during wakefulness and sleep. Respir Physiol 93:57–70
39. Datta AK, Shea SA, Horner RL, Guz A (1991) The influence of induced hypocapnia and sleep on the endogenous respiratory rhythm in humans. J Physiol 440:17–33
40. Meza S, Giannouli E, Younes M (1995) Ventilatore response to inspiratory muscle unloading with PAV during sleep. Am J Respir Crit Care Med 153:A639 (Abst)
41. Rebuck AS, Slutsky AS (1986) Control of breathing in diseases of the respiratory tract and lungs. In: Cherniack NS, Widdicombe JC (eds) Handbook of physiology. The respiratory system, control of breathing, Vol. II, part 2. American Physiological Society, Bethesda, pp 771–791
42. Coleridge HM, Coleridg,e JCG (1986) Reflexes evoked from tracheobronchial tree and lungs. In: Cherniack NS, Widdicombe JC (eds) Handbook of physiology. The respiratory system, vol. 2. American Physiological Society, Bethesda, pp 395–430
43. Shannon R (1986) Reflexes evoked from respiratory muscles and cortovertebral joints. In: Cherniack NS, Widdicombe JG (eds) Handbook of physiology: The respiratory system, vol. 2. American Physiological Society, Bethesda, pp 431–438
44 Georgopoulos D, Mitrouska I, Bshouty Z, Webster K, Anthonisen NR, Younes M (1996) Effects of breathing route, temperature and volume of inspired gas and airway anesthesia on the response of respiratory output to varying inspiratory flow. Am J Respir Crit Care Med 153:168–175
45. Georgopoulos D, Mitrouska I, Bshouty Z, Anthonisen NR, Younes M (1996) Effects of NREM sleep on the response of respiratory output to varying inspiratory flow. Am J Respir Crit Care Med 153:1624–1630
46. Mitrouska I, Georgopoulos D, Younes M, Bshouty Z (1996) Effects of pulmonary and intercostal denervation on the response of respiratory output to varying inspiratory flow. Am Rev Respir Dis 153:A775 (Abst)
47. Georgopoulos, D, Mitrouska I, Markopoulou K, Patakas D, Anthonisen NR (1995) Effects of breathing patterns on mechanically ventilated patients with chronic obstructive pulmonary disease and dynamic hyperinflation. Intensive Care Med 21:880–886
48. Corne S, Gillespie D, Roberts D, Younes M (1997) Effect of inspiratory flow rate on respiratory rate in intubated ventilated patients. Am J Respir Crit Care Med 156:304–308
49. Pierson DJ (1990) Complications of mechanical ventilation. Cur Pulmonol 11:19–46
50. Manning HL, Molinary EJ, Leiter JC (1995) Effect of inspiratory flow rate on respiratory sensation and pattern of breathing. Am J Respir Crit Care Med 151:751–757
51. Jubran A, Van De Graaf WB, Tobin M (1995) Variability of patient-ventilator interaction with pressure support ventilation in patients with chronic obstructive pulmonary disease. Am J Respir Crit Care Med 152:129–136
52. O'Donnell DE (1994) Breathlessness in patients with chronic airflow limitation: mechanisms and management. Chest 106:904–912
53. Killian KJ, Campell EJM (1985) Dyspnea. In: Roussos C, Macklem PT (eds) The thorax. Lung biology in health and disease, vol. 29. Marcel Dekker, New York, pp 787–928
54. Altose MD (1986) Dyspnea. Cur Pulmonol 7:199–226

Proportional Assist Ventilation

J. Mancebo and P. Aslanian

Introduction

Proportional assist ventilation (PAV) is a partial ventilatory support mode in which the ventilator generates pressure (P_{aw}) in proportion to patient effort (P_{mus}). During PAV there is no preset target for flow, volume or airway pressure. Consequently, this mode allows the patient to retain complete control, at least theoretically, over his or her breathing pattern.

Working Principles

PAV has mainly been provided by an experimental, prototype ventilator (Winnipeg ventilator, University of Manitoba, Canada). The gas delivery system consists of a freely moving piston coupled to a motor. The piston moves forward in proportion to the current applied to it. This current, in turn, is proportional to the signals of flow and volume which are continuously measured at the ventilator outlet. The ventilator then generates P_{aw} in proportion to both instantaneous flow and instantaneous volume. The proportionality is given by the respective flow and volume gain signals (the flow assist and the volume assist). The flow assist (FA) determines how much pressure will be generated per unit of flow, and the volume assist (VA) determines how much pressure will be generated per unit of volume [1].

To further understand the working mechanism of PAV it is useful to comment on the equation of motion of the respiratory system. Assuming a linear resistance (R) and elastance (E), the total pressure needed which must be applied to the respiratory system is the sum of the pressure needed to produce flow and the pressure needed to overcome the elastic recoil. Therefore, it follows that:

$$P_{appl} = (E \cdot V) + (R \cdot V'), \tag{1}$$

where V is volume, V′ is flow and P_{appl} is the total pressure which must be applied to the respiratory system to produce V′ and V in accordance with its mechanical properties. P_{appl} may be exclusively generated by the ventilator (P_{aw}), when patients are paralyzed for example (and then P_{mus} equals zero), may be exclusively generated by the patient (P_{mus}), as occurs during spontaneous breathing (and then P_{aw} equals zero) or can be a combination of both, as occurs during PAV and other assisted modes of ventilatory support. In the latter situation $P_{appl} = P_{aw} + P_{mus}$ [1, 2].

According to these principles, the caregiver should set the respective gains for VA and FA. In this way, during PAV, the P_{aw} will follow this equation:

$$P_{aw} = (VA \cdot V) + (FA \cdot V') \qquad (2)$$

and P_{mus} will be

$$P_{mus} = [(E - VA) \cdot V] + [(R - FA) \cdot V'] \qquad (3)$$

For example, if gains for VA and FA are set at 50% of E and 50% of R, respectively, this means that the ventilator (P_{aw}) will deliver 50% of the elastic pressure and 50% of the resistive pressure needed to overcome the E and R of the respiratory system. Consequently, the patient will generate a P_{mus} of the same magnitude as P_{aw}. This 1:1 proportionality implies that patient effort is amplified by a factor of 2, i.e., of a total pressure of 10 units, 5 are provided by the machine (P_{aw}) and 5 by the patient (P_{mus}). In other words, if E is 20 cmH$_2$O/l (compliance 50 ml/cmH$_2$O) and resistance is 10 cmH$_2$O/l/s, and VA is set at 16 and FA is set at 8, then from equation 2, the ventilator will generate a $P_{aw} = (16 \cdot V) + (8 \cdot V')$ and, from equation 3, the patient will develop a $P_{mus} = (4 \cdot V) + (2 \cdot V')$. It then follows that if tidal volume (V_T) is 0.5 l and V' is 0.5 l/s, the ventilator will generate 12 cmH$_2$O P_{aw} (8 cmH$_2$O to overcome elastic recoil and 4 cmH$_2$O to overcome flow resistance) and the patient will generate 3 cmH$_2$O P_{mus}. This represents a proportionality of 4:1 (12 cmH$_2$O P_{aw}: 3 cmH$_2$O P_{mus}) and therefore an amplification factor of 5 because the total pressure applied to the respiratory system is 15 cmH$_2$O of which 3 cmH$_2$O are provided by P_{mus}. Typical tracings of airflow, volume, airway pressure and inspiratory muscle effort during PAV are shown in Fig. 1.

Advantages and Disadvantages

PAV is a mode which, in theory, is very well adapted to follow changes in ventilatory demand provided that there are no concomitant changes in ventilatory mechanics. It has been claimed that for this reason and because there are no preset, physician-selected ventilatory objectives, this mode may be very comfortable [1, 2, 3].

Disadvantages [1, 2] are related to suboptimal assistance in the presence of intrinsic positive end-expiratory pressure (PEEP) because in that case, the pressure developed by the inspiratory muscles before initiating inspiratory flow is not "seen" by the ventilator. Proper adjustment of the FA and VA gains requires estimation of the R and E of the respiratory system, which implies that the patient's muscles be relaxed. Evidently, as in any other assisted ventilatory mode, it is mandatory that patients maintain an adequate central respiratory output.

In the case of inadequate settings, especially when the volume assist gain is greater than the patient's elastance, then the pressure provided by the ventilator at the end of inspiration is higher than the opposing elastic and resistive pressures and then flow and volume delivery continue during neural expiration and the cycle ends either because the machine set limits (airway pressure or tidal volume) are reached, or because the patient fights the ventilator, or even because at high lung volumes the

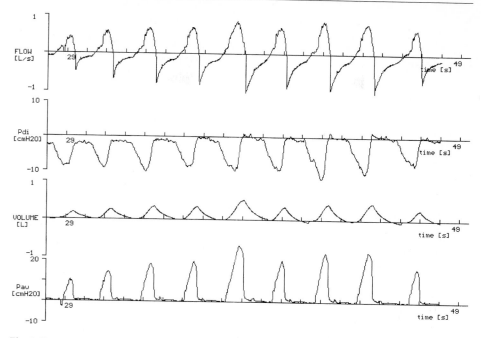

Fig. 1. Representative tracings of (from top to bottom) airflow (flow), transdiaphragmatic pressure (P_{di}), tidal volume (volume) and airway pressure (P_{aw}) in a patient receiving proportional assist ventilation. Note the breath by breath variability in peak P_{aw} and tidal volume in proportion to the different magnitude of inspiratory muscle effort (P_{di})

elastance of the respiratory system increases. This phenomenon of volume overassist is also called "runaway" and is shown in Fig. 2.

Because this mode does not impose any target for flow, volume, time or pressure, variations in the breathing pattern may be difficult to interpret. In fact, in PAV the breathing pattern is often unpredictable. Moreover, PAV is the only mode in which P_{aw} will increase in the presence of leaks because there is an overestimation of the flow and volume received by the patient.

Clinical Studies

Marantz et al. [3], in a group of 11 ventilator-dependent patients, studied the breathing pattern as the level of assist was altered from near maximal to the lowest level that could be tolerated. They observed a high inter-individual variability in breathing pattern at high levels of assist. Respiratory rate, V_T and minute ventilation (V_E) ranged between 18 and 33 breaths/min, 203 and 844 ml, and 5.6 and 18.7 l/min, respectively. The wide ranges in V_T can be explained by normal interindividual variability, by differences in ventilatory demand or respiratory muscle strength or even by different disease-related effects on receptors that modulate breathing pattern. Interestingly, these authors [3] found a high correlation between V_T and V_E at

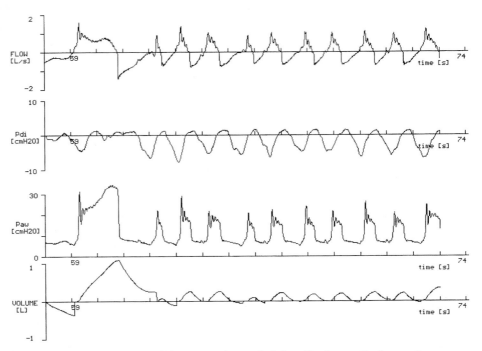

Fig. 2. Representative tracings of (from top to bottom) airflow (flow), transdiaphragmatic pressure (P_{di}), tidal volume (volume) and airway pressure (P_{aw}) in a patient receiving proportional assist ventilation. Note that the first breath from the left shows a typical runaway phenomenon. In this case it probably happened because of a relatively high volume assist and a marked non-linearity of the pressure-volume curve of the respiratory system

high levels of assist, while no changes in breathing pattern or V_E were observed when the level of assist was modified. This means that at high levels of assist, the effort performed by the patient diminishes (there is a down-regulation of P_{mus}) so as to maintain the desired ventilatory target and breathing pattern, or in other words, there exists for each patient's state a level of ventilation and breathing pattern which seems to be independent of the mechanical load.

In another study from the same group [4], non-invasive PAV was rapidly instituted in 11 patients who were deemed to require urgent intubation for acute respiratory failure. Intubation was avoided in 8 patients, and the use of PAV was associated with significant improvements in respiratory rate, accessory muscle use and dyspnea (Borg scale). The lack of a control group in this study makes it difficult to draw firm conclusions. Moreover, PAV was initiated on a rapid basis by a specialized team specifically available for this purpose. Nevertheless, this report suggests that non-invasive PAV may be applied safely and effectively in selected patients.

Ranieri et al. [5], in 12 intubated patients, compared the response to an added deadspace when patients were in PAV and pressure support ventilation (PSV). They found, that after applying the deadspace, there was an increase in respiratory rate during PSV but no change during PAV. However, in these obtunded patients (at PSV levels of 10 cmH$_2$O and at 40% PAV assistance, the patients had an average PaCO$_2$ of 52 and 51 mmHg, respectively, and only an average esophageal pressure-time product (PTP$_{es}$)/min of 110 and 95 cmH$_2$O·s/min, respectively), the response to the same added deadspace, in terms of V$_E$, was much higher in PSV than in PAV. At high levels of assist, V$_E$ changed from 12 to 15 l/min with PAV (80% assist) and from 11 to 19 l/min with PSV (20 cm H$_2$O) when deadspace was added. At low levels of assist, V$_E$ increased from 8 to 13 l/min with PAV (40% assist) and from 9 to 22 l/min with PS (10 cmH$_2$O)). In these circumstances, although the increase in PTP$_{es}$/min during added deadspace was higher in PSV (between 79 and 168%) in comparison with PAV (between 22 and 63%), this increase, when expressed as PTP$_{es}$/l, was only between 8 and 12% during PSV while no change was seen during PAV.

Navalesi et al. [6] studied 8 adult patients whose trachea was intubated because of an episode of acute respiratory failure. The authors found that PAV improved the breathing pattern and reduced inspiratory muscle effort compared with spontaneous breathing. They also observed that at each setting of volume assist, the addition of flow assist significantly reduced the total work of breathing (because of a reduction in its resistive component), thus providing further evidence for the use of both flow and volume assist in the ventilatory management of patients with acute respiratory failure.

More recently, Ranieri et al. [7] studied the effects of continuous positive airways pressure (CPAP) and PAV in 8 intubated patients who had acute decompensation of chronic obstructive pulmonary disease. In these patients, the settings which optimally unloaded the respiratory system and significantly reduced the sense of dyspnea were a combination of flow assist and PEEP. Indeed, the addition of volume assist although further reducing the inspiratory muscle effort, also induced significant patient-ventilator asynchrony.

In a preliminary study performed in 16 intubated patients recovering from acute respiratory failure [8], we observed that at similar levels of assist (both high and low levels), the effects of PAV and PSV were virtually identical in terms of the breathing pattern and respiratory muscle unloading. However, despite a similar breath-by-breath variability in patient's inspiratory efforts (in PAV and in PSV) evaluated in terms of transdiaphragmatic pressure (P$_{di}$) swings, the variability in V$_T$ was significantly higher in PAV than in PSV at both levels of assist. These data suggested that in situations of changing ventilatory demand, and without major changes in respiratory system mechanics, PAV may offer a better adaptation to patient effort in comparison with PSV.

This hypothesis was then tested in another group of ventilator-dependent patients in whom ventilatory demand was suddenly increased by adding carbon dioxide (CO$_2$) to the inspired gas [9]. Once again, we observed a virtually identical breathing pattern and inspiratory muscle effort in PAV and PSV at baseline conditions. However, during CO$_2$ induced hyperventilation, the magnitude of the patient's effort (expressed in PTP$_{es}$/breath and PTP$_{es}$/min) was considerably higher with PSV in comparison to PAV. Moreover, the ratio of patient work to total work (work done by the patient + work done by the ventilator) significantly increased with PSV while it remained unchanged with PAV. These data strongly suggest that PAV allows a better adaptation than PSV to an increase in ventilatory demand. In fact, Bigatello et al. [10] compared the effects of PAV and PSV during variations in tidal volume by using a bellows-in-a-box lung model and they observed that PAV unloaded uniformly the work of breathing (except at low tidal volumes) whereas PSV tended to over-assist low tidal volumes and under-assist high tidal volumes.

Conclusion

PAV represents an interesting and promising approach to partial ventilatory support. Some of its theoretical advantages seem to be borne out by the short-term physiologic studies conducted thus far. Clinical experience with this mode remains limited, however, and further investigation is required to evaluate its potential benefits in terms of comfort and improved patient-ventilator interaction. Most importantly, carefully designed, long-term studies will be essential in assessing the impact of PAV on such outcome measures as ventilator-related complications and duration of weaning.

References

1. Younes M (1998) Proportional assist ventilation (PAV®). In: Brochard L, Mancebo J (eds) Artificial ventilation. Principles and applications. Arnette Blackwell (in press)
2. Younes M (1993) Patient-ventilator interaction with pressure-assisted modalities of ventilatory support. Sem Respir Med 14:299–322
3. Marantz S, Patrick W, Webster K, Roberts D, Oppenheimer L, Younes M (1996) Response of ventilator-dependent patients to different levels of proportional assist. J Appl Physiol 80:397–403
4. Patrick W, Webster K, Ludwig L, Roberts D, Wiebe P, Younes M (1996) Noninvasive positive-pressure ventilation in acute respiratory distress without prior chronic respiratory failure. Am J Respir Crit Care Med 153:1005–1011
5. Ranieri VM, Giuliani R, Mascia L, et al (1996) Patient-ventilator interaction during acute hypercapnia: pressure support vs. proportional-assist ventilation. J Appl Physiol 81:426–436
6. Navalesi P, Hernandez P, Wongsa A, et al (1996) Proportional assist ventilation in acute respiratory failure: effects on breathing pattern and inspiratory effort. Am J Respir Crit Care Med 154:1330–1338
7. Ranieri VM, Grasso S, Mascia L, et al (1997) Effects of proportional assist ventilation on inspiratory muscle effort in patients with chronic obstructive pulmonary disease and acute respiratory failure. Anesthesiology 86:79–91
8. Mancebo J, Aslanian P, Bak E, et al (1997) Effects of pressure-targeted ventilatory support during acute respiratory failure (ARF): PAV vs PSV. Am J Respir Crit Care Med 155:A526 (Abst)
9. Mancebo J, Aslanian P, Straus C, Harf A, Lemaire F, Brochard L (1997) Comparison of the effects of proportional assist ventilation (PAV) and pressure support ventilation (PSV) during variations in ventilatory demand. Am J Respir Crit Care Med 155:A686 (Abst)
10. Bigatello L, Nishimura M, Imanaka H, et al (1997) Unloading of the work of breathing by proportional assist ventilation in a lung model. Crit Care Med 25:267–272

Pressure Controlled Ventilation (PCV): The Ideal Mode of Mechanical Ventilation?

P. Morley

Introduction

Pressure controlled ventilation (PCV) has been used extensively in the ventilation of neonates, but only over the last decade has it taken off as an alternative mode of mechanical ventilation for intensivists in adult intensive care units (ICU). PCV (often linked synonymously with inverse ratio ventilation as PC-IRV) was introduced to many as a mode of last resort when problems were occurring with more traditional forms of ventilation. PCV offers a mode of ventilation suited to the most complex ventilatory challenges, including severe acute respiratory distress syndrome (ARDS), extremes of airflow obstruction and synchrony with a difficult to wean patient.

What is PCV?

PCV is a mode of ventilation available on most mechanical ventilators [1]. During the inspiratory phase, the ventilator delivers a constant pre-set pressure (using whatever flow is necessary) for a chosen inspiratory time.

Volume cycled ventilation (VCV) requires the setting of a tidal volume and respiratory rate (or minute ventilation and respiratory rate) and a flow pattern and inspiratory time (or I/E ratio). Changes in the impedance of the respiratory system (such as increased inspiratory resistance or decreased respiratory system compliance) will result in changes in the inspiratory pressure required (and abnormal cyc-

Table 1. Basic differences between pressure-controlled ventilation and volume-cycled ventilation

	Pressure-controlled ventilation (PCV)	Volume-cycled ventilation (VCV)
Independent variables "What you set"	Pre-set pressure and inspiratory time	Tidal volume and inspiratory flow profile
Dependent variable "What you get"	Tidal volume	Pressure
Common to both	Mode of ventilation (SIMV, Assist-control, etc) FiO_2 and PEEP Triggering (pressure or flow)	

ling if a high pressure limit has been reached). PCV requires setting of a pre-set pressure and an inspiratory time (Table 1).

Just as with VCV, PCV can be used in a control mode, an assist-control mode, or with synchronized intermittent mandatory ventilation (SIMV, with or without pressure support), with flow or pressure triggering of spontaneous breaths, and with various levels of positive end-expiratory pressure (PEEP) and inspired oxygen fraction (FiO$_2$).

Advantages over Alternatives

Limiting the Delivered Pressure

PCV allows the maximum airway pressure delivered by the ventilator to be set at whatever level the operator feels comfortable with. A similar set pressure can be used in volume cycled modes, but this is effectively creating pressure cycling off of the inspiratory phase if this pressure is actually reached. Careful flow and tidal volume (or inspiratory time) settings may allow a PCV-like pressure profile to be approximated, but these settings need to be reviewed whenever changes in respiratory mechanics occur. The use of PCV maximizes the pressure profile for a given peak pressure and inspiratory time [1].

Providing a Decelerating Flow Profile

The provision of a decelerating flow profile may actually be beneficial with regard to gas exchange [1–3]. PCV usually provides such a decelerating flow profile, including a plateau if the inspiratory time is long enough to reach zero flow. PCV also has the advantage that, in situations where the inspiratory resistance is high, the delivered flow rate will be maximized for the given peak pressure (see section on PCV in severe airflow obstruction). When using a decelerating flow profile in VCV, increases in inspiratory resistance will result in higher peak pressures, unless the flow rate is manually adjusted.

Contribution of the Spontaneously Breathing Patient

In VCV (be it SIMV or assist-control) additional spontaneous efforts during the mechanical breaths result in the patient doing more of the work while still achieving the same tidal volume. In PCV, spontaneous efforts are rewarded by increased tidal volumes [as they are in pressure support ventilation (PSV)], because a higher transpulmonary pressure is delivered. In some situations this may be a desired endpoint, especially if tidal volumes had been limited to very low levels (e.g., in situations of high inspiratory resistance).

Traditional Role

PCV-IRV

Early use of PCV with IRV in critically ill patients on very high levels of respiratory support resulted in variable results with regard to improvement in oxygenation and carbon dioxide clearance, and often at the expense of significant gas trapping (autoPEEP) and even barotrauma. The effect of prolonging the inspiratory time to invert the inspiratory/expiratory (I/E) ratio has had variable and inconsistent effects [4]. Prolongation of the inspiratory time seems to have similar effects in PCV and VCV. Many of the potential benefits of PCV probably relate more to its flow profile, opening and maintaining open lung units, than to the duration of inspiration [1–3, 5].

Current Role: Lung Protective Strategies.
Avoiding Iatrogenic Lung Damage and Nosocomial Ventilator Dependency

Over the last decade intensivists have become acutely aware of the potential damage that we are doing to our ventilated patients. This has resulted in three main areas of focus: Keeping the lung open; avoiding overdistension; and encouraging spontaneous breathing while avoiding fatigue.

Open-Lung Strategies

Repetitive collapse and re-opening of some areas of the lung may well contribute to part of the ventilator-induced lung damage that we see. During the opening of collapsed lung units very high shear forces may be generated, despite limiting the overall distending pressure to one considered safe [6]. Animal work has suggested that the use of a minimal level of PEEP may prevent lung damage [7, 8], and the use of moderate levels of PEEP may decrease the release of lung inflammatory mediators [9]. Ventilatory strategies developed on the basis of providing such a minimal level of PEEP actually seem to provide potential benefits for critically ill patients with regard to respiratory function [10, 11] and even mortality [12]. The use of such "open lung" strategies has been recently reviewed [6, 13].

The use of recruitment maneuvers to open the lung in the early phases of ARDS has received more attention recently [6]. Such maneuvers may include the routine use of very high levels of PEEP [14], or the application of a distending pressure for a limited period of time. The immediate effects of such a distending pressure are readily apparent in the open chest with the lung collapsed down for cardiac or thoracic surgery. Anecdotal evidence has suggested that very rapid (and sustained) improvement in oxygenation may result, even in the critically ill patient with acute lung injury. The use of PCV in these circumstances allows the clinician to maximize the tidal volumes delivered while limiting the overall distending pressures (peak and plateau) to a level considered by the clinician to be acceptable.

Pressure-Limiting Strategies

The use of high distending pressures (greater than a plateau pressure of 35–40 cmH$_2$O: "barotrauma") or large tidal volumes (greater than 12–15 ml/kg: "volutrauma") have been associated with ARDS-like damage to even normal lungs. Some clinical evidence has suggested that ventilatory strategies designed to avoid exposing the lung to high pressures or volumes may improve outcome, and have been recommended [15–17], though this is still controversial [18]. Various prospective studies conducted in critically ill patients have been undertaken to confirm this [19–21], but to date only one study [12] (which also used an open-lung strategy) has demonstrated any improvement in survival.

If the goal of the clinician is to maximize the ventilation of the critically ill patient, within limits for applied distending pressures, PCV is the appropriate mode. VCV can be set up to look very much like PCV [2, 3, 22], but if the impedance of the respiratory system changes, for the same pre-set pressure (i.e., high pressure alarm) the delivered tidal volume will be lower in VCV. This is as a result of the peak pressure being reached earlier in the inspiratory cycle, limiting inspiratory time, and preventing the alveolar pressure reaching the desired level. Appropriate titration of PCV ensures that for a given distending pressure, the delivered volume will be maximized, though not constant.

Encouraging Spontaneous Breathing

Prolonged periods of rest of the respiratory muscles, especially when combined with catabolic processes, result in disuse atrophy. PCV may allow spontaneous breathing in patients previously considered too sick to breath spontaneously. (See section on PCV in the spontaneously breathing patient).

"Newer" uses of Pressure Control

PCV in the Spontaneously Breathing Patient

The problem of ICU neuropathy [23] as well as disuse atrophy of the respiratory muscles as a result of prolonged periods of heavy sedation and/or paralysis has encouraged intensivists to let their patients breathe spontaneously while still ventilator dependent. Many components of the delivery of mechanical ventilatory support can be modified to minimize the amount of work needed to be done by the patient to trigger the ventilator, and synchronize with the delivered breath [24–26]. The major components of inspiratory work are those required to overcome 1) triggering the ventilator, 2) the tubing, circuit and connectors, and 3) that due to abnormal resistance or compliance as a result of the patient's disease process.

The best approach seems to be one that allows an appropriate amount of work of breathing to be performed to prevent disuse atrophy, but that the unnecessary impositions of work should be countered by the ventilator [24]. The carefully titrated use of PCV may allow these goals to be more completely achieved [26]. Synchrony of the patient's respiratory efforts and the ventilator, and hence patient comfort, can be improved by decreasing triggering work (e.g., the use of flow cycling), and by better matching of the ventilator's flow delivery with the patient's demands [5]. In general, flow triggering of the ventilator decreases the patient's work of breathing compared with pressure triggering [27]. Flow triggered PCV breaths seem optimal to maximize the synchrony of patient and ventilator [28]. The use of PCV in the spontaneously breathing patient is relatively easy and makes physiologic sense. Adult intensivists in general are not familiar with this technique, and even a recent review of PCV suggested that "the patient should not be assisting the ventilator at the time of the conversion" from VCV to PCV [2].

Synchronized Intermittent Mandatory Ventilation with PCV: SIMV with PCV seems to offer all the potential advantages of SIMV, but with improved patient synchrony with the mandatory breath, and decreased work of breathing [28]. The benefits seem maximized when combined with flow triggering [28]. The use of SIMV as a mode for partial ventilatory support has come under attack more recently. No benefit has been demonstrated for the provision of two different types of breath in the spontaneously breathing patient. The transition from full to partial ventilatory support is not the gradual process that the number of SIMV breaths implies, and SIMV appears inferior to other modes (such as PSV, and intermittent T-tube trials) for the process of weaning from ventilatory support [29, 30].

Assist-Control PCV, Pressure Assist Breaths or Time-Cycled PSV: Rather than the use of the traditional SIMV mode for spontaneous breathing with PCV, it makes sense to use assist-control PCV. By setting a mandatory (control) breath rate below the patient's spontaneous breath rate, all breaths become ventilator assisted breaths, and the control rate becomes a back-up breath rate. All the breaths initiated by the patient are delivered according to the same pre-set pressure and time characteristics, resulting in a patient-triggered, pressure-controlled breath that is time cycled off. Most clinicians are familiar with PSV as a mode for partial ventilatory support (either stand-alone or in conjuction with SIMV). Assist-control PCV can be considered to be the equivalent of pressure support breaths that are time-cycled off. These have also been referred to by MacIntyre as "pressure assist breaths" [26].

Unfulfilled requests (or "desynchronization" [31]), where clinically apparent inspiratory efforts do not result in triggering of the ventilator [25], can occur with this mode as with any other. Examples of clinical scenarios where this can occur include an insufficiently sensitive inspiratory trigger, very weak inspiratory efforts, or the presence of significant autoPEEP. Adjustment of triggering (e.g., change from pressure to flow triggering), minimizing autoPEEP and titration of extrinsic PEEP towards the level of autoPEEP [32] should all be considered. Premature flow cycling off of the pressure support breaths can occur in the setting of weak inspiratory efforts, or high inspiratory flow rates [25, 26]. On the other hand prolonged inspiratory time can occur with pressure support breaths [25] if the patient has airflow obstruction with autoPEEP, has a circuit leak (e.g., face mask or bronchopleural fistulae) or is too weak to turn off the inspiratory flow. In these settings spontaneously breathing patients may be more comfortable with the fixed inspiratory time provided by assist-control PCV. The actual inspiratory time needs to be titrated to the needs of the patient (usually between 0.6 and 1.2 seconds). Assist-control PCV may similarly be very useful in non-invasive positive pressure ventilation, especially in those patients with weak inspiratory efforts [33].

PCV in Severe Airway Obstruction

One of the major problems in the ventilation of the patient with severe airway obstruction is the potentially high pressures generated when volume control modes are used. Traditionally two main approaches have been used:
1) high flows to limit inspiratory time, accepting very high airway pressures; and
2) lower flows to limit inspiratory pressure, accepting longer inspiratory time.

Much of the high airway pressure generated during inspiration is assumed to be dissipated in the circuit, endotracheal tube and proximal airways, but the actual pressure seen by the patient's airways has not been examined in detail. Those lung units with a short time constant may well be exposed to pressures considered excessive. At least in theory, in situations with lung units of varying resistances, a more uniform distribution of ventilation occurs with PCV [34].

The use of PCV in asthma allows the upper limit for imposed airway pressure to be set at a level considered acceptable, and relies on the ventilator to optimize the flow pattern. An initially high flow will rapidly increase the circuit pressure to the desired level, then the flow tends to decrease to a constant (very slowly decelerating) profile. The ventilator is therefore able to determine the maximum flow that can be

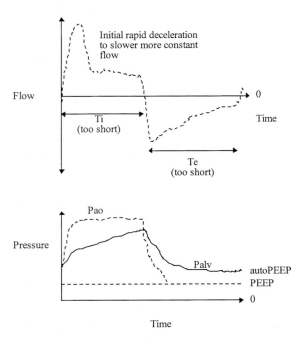

Fig. 1. Schematic representation of pressure and flow versus time graphs in a patient with severe airflow obstruction being ventilated with pressure controlled ventilation. The rapid initial inspiratory flow quickly pressurizes the circuit, and the inspiratory flow falls to an almost constant rate. The pressure at airway opening (P_{ao}) rapidly reaches its pre-set value. In this case there is insufficient inspiratory time (Ti) for the flow to reach zero, resulting in the alveolar pressure (P_{alv}) not reaching the pre-set pressure. During exhalation there is insufficient expiratory time (Te) for the expiratory flow to reach zero. This results in gas trapping and autoPEEP. The presence of autoPEEP also limits the incremental pressure seen by the lung (to a maximum of pre-set pressure – autoPEEP)

provided without increasing the airway pressure above the preset threshold. The resultant tidal volume will be directly proportional to the time allowed for inspiration. Short inspiratory times are not appropriate for this method of ventilation, and the longer inspiratory times need a slow respiratory rate to ensure enough time in expiration to minimize gas trapping (Fig. 1). Even in a patient with no spontaneous efforts, the delivered tidal volumes will increase as the patient improves, as a result of less autoPEEP as the expiratory flow improves (decreasing the ventilator pressure wasted to overcome the autoPEEP), and a greater flow delivered as the inspiratory resistance decreases. In this way, the severity of airways obstruction can be indirectly monitored by the resultant tidal volume.

Spontaneously breathing patients with severe airway obstruction have similar problems in PCV as in more conventional ventilatory approaches. Gas trapping resulting in autoPEEP will make triggering the ventilator difficult. This can be partially overcome by optimizing the trigger sensitivity of the system, and by careful titration of extrinsic PEEP. The use of high levels of PEEP (e.g., <15 cmH$_2$O) to decrease inspiratory work in the ventilated patient with severe airway obstruction and very high levels of autoPEEP has not been evaluated in detail. The use of PCV in the presence of inspiratory resistance is also, of course, consistent with its use in neonates (with small endotracheal tubes), and its reported use for ventilation after cricothyrotomy with a 4 mm tube [35].

Titration of Pressure Control Ventilation

Optimal use of PCV requires a good understanding of the principles of the mode, as well as a familiarity with the appearance and use of pressure and flow waveforms [22]. The way in which the individual parameters are titrated is different depending on whether the patient is breathing spontaneously or not (controlled ventilation).

Controlled Ventilation

Maximizing Volume for a Given Pressure: The tidal volume delivered during PCV depends on two factors: (1) the proportion of the pre-set pressure that is seen by the lung; and (2) the compliance of the respiratory system. On the surface this seems obvious, and the conversion of VCV to PCV is based on this principle [2]. Either insufficient inspiratory time or insufficient expiratory time will result in less than 100% of the pre-set pressure being seen by the lung, and a lower delivered tidal volume. An optimum tidal volume will be achieved by ensuring that enough time is allowed for end-inspiratory and end-expiratory flow to reach zero (Fig. 1). An increase in tidal volume will be seen if the patient's spontaneous efforts increase the transpulmonary pressure. Factors influencing tidal volume in PCV are listed in Table 2.

Inspiratory Time (Zero-Flow): Alveolar pressure can be assumed to be equal to the delivered ventilator pressure if inspiratory flow has declined to zero. The maximum tidal volume for a given pre-set inspiratory pressure will be achieved by increasing the inspiratory time until end-inspiratory flow is zero. If inspiratory time is in-

Table 2. Determinants of tidal volume in pressure-controlled ventilation

Factors determining tidal volume	Factors decreasing tidal volume (i.e., how to decrease tidal volume)	Factors increasing tidal volume (i.e., how to increase tidal volume)

1. Incremental pressure seen by lung	Decreased incremental pressure
	– decrease in pre-set pressure
	– decreased patient's contribution to inspiration
	  – sedation, paralysis, fatigue, dys-synchrony
	– insufficient time for expiration (more autoPEEP)
	  – decrease in expiratory time
	    – increase in respiratory rate
	    – increase in I:E ratio
	– insufficient time for inspiration
	  – decrease in inspiratory time
	    – decrease in set time
	    – decrease in I:E ratio
	    – premature cycling (e.g. high pressure)
	– increase in inspiratory resistance
		Increased incremental pressure
		– increase in pre-set pressure
		– increased patient's contribution to inspiration
		  – increased respiratory drive, arousal
		– sufficient time for expiration (less autoPEEP)
		  – increase in expiratory time
		    – decrease in respiratory rate
		    – decrease in I:E ratio
		– sufficient time for inspiration
		  – increase in inspiratory time
		    – increase in set time
		    – increase in I:E ratio
		    – avoid premature cycling
		– decrease in inspiratory resistance

2. Compliance of lung	Decreased lung compliance	Increased lung compliance

creased beyond this, no further increment in tidal volume will be achieved. Prolonged inspiratory times, resulting in inverse I:E ratio ventilation, have not been consistently associated with any benefits other than increasing mean airway pressure (Fig. 1).

Expiratory Time (Zero Flow): If insufficient time is available in expiration for the lung to empty to its resting volume, and expiratory flow is still occurring at the start of inspiration, then gas trapping is present. The pressure generated within the respiratory system by this trapped gas is known as autoPEEP (or intrinsic PEEP). During inspiration, to inflate the lungs, the ventilator must first overcome any autoPEEP. Increasing the expiratory time to allow the end-expiratory flow to reach zero ensures that no autoPEEP is present, and that the lungs potentially see all of the pre-set pressure (Fig. 1).

Maximizing Minute Ventilation: Once the inspiratory time has been set (easier using a fixed inspiratory time mode), the respiratory rate can be adjusted until the expiratory time is just long enough to avoid autoPEEP. Using a fixed I:E ratio means that changes in respiratory rate result in changes in both inspiratory and expiratory time.

Extrinsic PEEP versus autoPEEP: Increases in respiratory rate or prolongation of the inspiratory time (eg. including inverting the I:E ratio) may lead to insufficient time in exhalation to avoid gas trapping and autoPEEP. The amount of autoPEEP present can be approximated by an end-expiratory hold maneuvre of sufficient duration (e.g., 2 seconds), but this is an average pressure. In the laboratory, simulating lung units with different time constants, the heterogenous distribution of actual end-expiratory pressures with autoPEEP has been confirmed [36]. The amount of auto-PEEP can also change quite dramatically if there are changes in expiratory time, tidal volume, expiratory resistance or expiratory effort. AutoPEEP has all the physiologic effects of extrinsic PEEP on hemodynamics and respiratory mechanics, but requires extra work of breathing to initiate a spontaneous breath (as the alveolar pressure must decrease to below any extrinsically applied PEEP before inspiratory flow can occur).

Unless essential, it seems preferable to use extrinsic PEEP to provide whatever end-expiratory pressure is considered desirable [36], and keep autoPEEP to a minimum (ideally zero).

Spontaneous Ventilation

Inspiratory Time: The inspiratory time needs to be titrated to the patient's needs. Too short an inspiratory time may result in flow starvation or double inspiratory efforts [25, 26], while too long an inspiratory time may result in active exhalation and increased expiratory work [25]. Finding the optimal inspiratory time requires observation of the patient and pressure and flow waveforms for signs of dys-synchrony. Once an inspiratory time has been set (usually between 0.6 and 1.2 seconds) regular review will ensure that the requirements have not changed.

Inspiratory Pressure: Titration of the inspiratory pressure in PCV is similar to that with PSV. The initial setting can be based on the compliance of the respiratory system and the desired tidal volume. A reasonable starting point could be a set-pressure to provide the equivalent of the plateau pressure required in VCV for an acceptable tidal volume. PCV allows setting of the maximal pressure generated within the circuit by the ventilator, and this can be set to ensure that the "safe" levels of pressure are not exceeded. It is essential to know whether the pre-set pressure on the ventilator is in addition to PEEP or includes PEEP.

Pressures within the circuit and the patient can exceed the pre-set pressure if the patient actively exhales. As the patient improves, the level of pre-set pressure can be decreased slowly, as would be done with PSV [26]. Titration of the pressure level should take into account clinical parameters (including tachycardia, diaphoresis, use of accessory muscles) as well as respiratory rate (ideally 30 or less) and possibly other indices of respiratory drive (e.g., P 0.1). The response of tidal volume to changes in PCV is very helpful. Similar to titration of PSV, a decrease in the pre-set pressure without a resultant decrease in tidal volume implies that the patient is doing more inspiratory work.

Limitations of Pressure Control Ventilation

Uncontrolled Initial Flow Rates Causing Damage

The flow rates delivered by the ventilator in PCV are at least theoretically also delivered to the patient's lungs. It has been suggested that this may cause damage to the airways, but this has not been addressed in humans.

The actual peak flow rates delivered by the ventilator are only so high as to enable initial pressurizing of the ventilator circuitry, and then rapidly decline (Fig. 1). Observation of flow waveforms on the Puritan Bennett 7200ae shows that very high initial flows are not seen in PCV (even in extreme conditions), and under many conditions are lower than those that could be set in volume cycled ventilation.

No High Tidal Volume Alarm

The alarms traditionally available on mechanical ventilators are more attuned to the adequacy of delivery of a volume cycled breath. Appropriately set low pressure alarms detect disconnection or decreased respiratory impedance; high pressure alarms detect increased respiratory impedance but result in premature cycling off of the ventilator during the inspiratory phase; and low minute ventilation and tidal volume alarms detect disconnection or decreased patient contribution.

Alarms allowing assessment of changes in tidal volume in PCV are as useful to indicate changes as are pressure alarms in VCV. High tidal volume alarms are not available on the vast majority of currently available mechanical ventilators. Increases in tidal volume during PCV may indicate an improvement in respiratory system impedance, a decrease in autoPEEP, or increased spontaneous effort. The patient's spontaneous efforts augment the ventilator's pre-set pressure and the resultant transalveolar pressure may be much higher than anticipated. The resultant tidal volume may well exceed levels currently considered to be appropriate [15], despite an apparently appropriate externally delivered pressure. There is some concern that this may be harmful [1], and this was addressed by the use of sedation in Amato's clinical protocol [10]. If attempts are made to decrease the pre-set pressure to deal with this problem, the end result will be a decrease in the patient's tidal volume, but at the expense of increased patient work of breathing.

Whether the delivery of high tidal volumes because of spontaneous efforts while on PCV (or of course PSV) is actually a significant clinical problem, with potential harm done to the lung is still not clear. The potential additional negative pressure added to the set pressure in PCV could be estimated from a measurement of esophageal pressure or potentially even central venous pressure.

Patient's Spontaneous Efforts May be Crucial

In traditional VCV, the efforts made by the patient to contribute to assisted breaths result in a similar delivered tidal volume, but at a decreased airway pressure. In this scenario the patient effectively does some of the work of the ventilator, which may be viewed as excessive, necessitating some form of intervention (e.g., increasing flows to improve synchrony, decreasing triggering work, or even sedation and/or muscle relaxation). In contrast, during PCV, spontaneous efforts (especially if associated with large swings in intra-thoracic pressure) tend to augment the delivered tidal volume in the assisted breaths, which increases minute volume above and beyond any increase due to respiratory rate. The resultant higher tidal volumes for the set pressure in PCV overestimate the actual lung compliance. In this situation sedation (and/or muscle relaxation) will still decrease work of breathing, but may also result in a profound (or worsened) respiratory acidosis and worsening oxygenation. The impact on ventilation and its clinical significance should be predictable based on a knowledge of the magnitude of the contribution of the patient's efforts to each breath [e.g., airway pressure fluctuations, or respiratory swings in intra-thoracic pressure measurements (including central venous pressure)].

Variable Tidal Volume

When delivered pressure is pre-set, tidal volume becomes a dependent variable. This variability in tidal volume provides useful information about the patient-ventilator interaction, may be indicative of improvement of respiratory mechanics, and unless volumes increase above levels considered unsafe, is unlikely to be harmful. Observation of tidal volume is as essential in PCV as observation of pressure is in VCV.

"Non-Linear Relationship Between Frequency and Minute Ventilation" [3]

Increases in respiratory rate when using VCV result in a linear increase in minute ventilation (though not necessarily alveolar ventilation), but at the expense of higher airway pressures. Increasing the respiratory rate in PCV with a fixed inspiratory time results in a decrease in expiratory time, and eventually gas trapping with the development of autoPEEP. The presence of autoPEEP decreases the actual driving pressure that can be seen by the lung (pre-set pressure – autoPEEP), and the tidal volume decreases. Minute ventilation reaches a plateau at modest respiratory rates [1]. Just as with VCV, but even more so with PCV, titration of respiratory rate should be performed by assessing response to changes.

The Future of Pressure Controlled Ventilation

The use of PCV in the next decade will increase as practitioners gain a greater understanding of what the mode can provide, and develop their expertise in titrating it. Ventilator manufacturers will need to realize the need for more complex monitoring (including waveforms, and high tidal volume alarms). Modifications of pressure limited breath strategies have been developed including modification of the pressure rise time, provision of a volume guarantee, and airway pressure release ventilation [26, 37]. Clinical studies are needed to confirm which, if any, of these strategies offer clinically significant advantages.

Conclusion

PCV is a mode of ventilation which offers itself as the answer to many of the complex ventilatory problems encountered in intensive care. Proper use of PCV requires an understanding of its principles, an appreciation of its limitations, an understanding of pressure and flow waveforms, and careful titration at the bedside. PCV is an easy way to facilitate the delivery of lung protective strategies (keeping the lung-open, while avoiding high inflation pressures) [10, 12], and may well be the optimal method to encourage spontaneous breathing while avoiding fatigue [28]. In the hands of an experienced practitioner, PCV comes close to being the ideal mode of mechanical ventilation.

References

1. Marini JJ (1994) Pressure-controlled ventilation. In: Tobin MJ (ed) Principles and practice of mechanical ventilation. McGraw-Hill, New York, pp 305–318
2. McKibben AW, Ravenscraft SA (1996) Pressure-controlled and volume-cycled ventilation. Clin Chest Med 17:395–410
3. Davis K Jr, Branson RD, Campbell RS, Porembka DT (1996) Comparison of volume control and pressure control ventilation: is flow waveform the difference? J Trauma 41:808–814
4. Mang H, Kacmarek RM, Ritz R, Wilson RS, Kimball WP (1995) Cardiorespiratory effects of volume- and pressure-controlled ventilation at various I/E ratios in an acute lung injury model. Am J Respir Crit Care Med 151:731–736
5. MacIntyre NR (1995) Breathing comfort during weaning with two ventilatory modes. Am J Respir Crit Care Med 151:254–258
6. Marini JJ (1996) Tidal volume, PEEP, and barotrauma. An open and shut case? Chest 109:302–304
7. Webb HH, Tierney DF (1974) Experimental pulmonary edema due to intermittent positive pressure ventilation with high inflation pressures. Protection by positive end-expiratory pressure. Am Rev Respir Dis 110:556–565
8. Muscedere JG, Mullen JB, Gan K, Slutsky AS (1994) Tidal ventilation at low airway pressures can augment lung injury. Am J Respir Crit Care Med 149:1327–1334
9. Tremblay L, Valenza F, Ribeiro SP, Li J, Slutsky AS (1997) Injurious ventilatory strategies increase cytokines and c-fos m-RNA expression in an isolated rat lung model. J Clin Invest 99:944–952
10. Amato MBP, Barbas CSV, Medeiros DM, et al (1995) Beneficial effects of the "open lung approach" with low distending pressures in acute respiratory distress syndrome. Am J Respir Crit Care Med 152:1835–1846
11. Cereda M, Foti G, Musch G, Sparacino ME, Pesenti A (1996) Positive end-expiratory pressure prevents the loss of respiratory compliance during low tidal volume ventilation in acute lung injury patients. Chest 109:480–485
12. Amato MBP, Barbas CSV, Medeiros DM, et al (1996) Improved survival in ARDS: Beneficial effects of a lung protective strategy. Am J Respir Crit Care Med 153:A531 (Abst)
13. Mergoni M, Volpi A, Rossi A (1997) Inflection point and alveolar recruitment in ARDS. In: Vincent J-L (ed) Yearbook of intensive care and emergency medicine. Springer-Verlag, Berlin, Heidelberg, New York, pp 556–567
14. Morris AH, Wallace CJ, Menlove RL, et al (1994) Randomized clinical trial of pressure-controlled inverse ratio ventilation and extracorporeal CO_2 removal for adult respiratory distress syndrome. Am J Respir Crit Care Med 149:295–305
15. Slutsky AS (1993) Mechanical Ventilation (ACCP consensus conference). Chest 104:1833–1859
16. Marini JJ (1994) Ventilation of the acute respiratory distress syndrome. Looking for Mr. Goodmode. Anesthesiology 80:972–975
17. Papadakos PJ, Apostolakos MJ (1996) High-inflation pressure and positive end-expiratory pressure. Injurious to the lung? Yes. Crit Care Clin 12:627–634

18. Nelson LD (1996) High-inflation pressure and positive end-expiratory pressure. Injurious to the lung? No. Crit Care Clin 12:603–625
19. Brower R, Shanholtz C, Shade D, et al (1997) Randomized controlled trial of small volume ventilation (STV) in ARDS. Am J Resp Crit Care Med 155:A93 (Abst)
20. Brochard L, Roudot-Thoraval F (1997) Tidal volume (Vt) reduction in acute respiratory distress syndrome (ARDS): A multicenter randomized study. Am J Resp Crit Care Med 155:A505 (Abst)
21. Stewart E, Meade MO, Granton J, et al (1997) Pressure and volume limited ventilation strategy (PLVS) in patients at high risk for ARDS – results of a multicenter trial. Am J Resp Crit Care Med 155:A505 (Abst)
22. Nahum A (1995) Use of pressure and flow waveforms to monitor mechanically ventilated patients. In: Vincent J-L (ed) Yearbook of intensive care and emergency medicine. Springer-Verlag, Berlin, Heidelberg, New York, pp 89–114
23. Bolton CF (1996) Neuromuscular conditions in the intensive care unit. Intensive Care Med 22:841–843
24. Morley P (1994) Work of breathing. Intensive Care World 11:117–121
25. Dick CR, Sassoon CSH (1996) Patient-ventilator interactions. Clin Chest Med 17:423–438
26. MacIntyre NR (1996) New modes of mechanical ventilation. Clin Chest Med 17:411–421
27. Branson RD, Campbell RS, Davis K Jr, Johnson DJ (1994) Comparison of pressure and flow triggering systems during continuous positive airway pressure. Chest 106:540–544
28. Giuliani R, Mascia L, Recchia F, Caracciolo A, Fiore T, Ranieri VM (1995) Patient-ventilator interaction during synchronized intermittent mandatory ventilation. Effects of flow triggering. Am J Respir Crit Care Med 151:1–9
29. Esteban A, Frutos F, Tobin MJ, et al (1995) A comparison of four methods of weaning patients from mechanical ventilation. N Engl J Med 332:345–350
30. Brochard L, Rauss A, Benito S, et al (1994) Comparison of three methods of gradual withdrawal from ventilatory suport during weaning from mechanical ventilation. Am J Respir Crit Care Med 150:896-903
31. Fabry B, Guttmann J, Eberhard L, Bauer T, Haberthur C, Wolff G (1995) An analysis of desynchronization between the spontaneously breathing patient and ventilator during inspiratory pressure support. Chest 107:1387–1394
32. MacIntyre NR, Cheng KC, McConnell R (1997) Applied PEEP during pressure support reduces the inspiratory threshold load of intrinsic PEEP. Chest 111:188–193
33. Meduri GU (1996) Noninvasive positive-pressure ventilation in patients with acute respiratory failure. Clin Chest Med 17:513–553
34. Chatburn RL, El Khatib MF, Smith PG (1994) Respiratory system behavior during mechanical inflation with constant inspiratory pressure and flow. Respir Care 39:979–988
35. Gregoretti C, Foti G, Beltrame F, et al (1995) Pressure control ventilation and minitracheotomy in treating severe flail chest trauma. Intensive Care Med 21:1054–1056
36. Kacmarek RM, Kirmse M, Nishimura M, Mang H, Kimball WR (1995) The effects of applied vs auto-PEEP on local lung unit pressure and volume in a four-unit lung model. Chest 108:1073–1079
37. Brochard L (1996) Pressure-support ventilation: still a simple mode? Intensive Care Med 22:1137–1138

The Open Lung Concept

S. H. Böhm, G. F. Vazquez de Anda, and B. Lachmann

Introduction

The imperative: "Open up the lung and keep the lung open" from Lachmann's editorial [1] has been quoted many times. The implied rationale, however, has been a matter of debate: Why should we open the lung? What is an open lung? In addition, questions concerning the methodology were asked: How can we open the lung without risking barotrauma? How should we keep the lung open with the least possible side effects? Today, exactly 20 years after the first description of the open lung concept by Lachmann and colleagues [2, 3], this article will address the physiologic and clinical rationale of the opening procedure, and will explain the steps necessary to open the lung.

What is an Open Lung?

The open lung is characterized by an optimal gas exchange [1]. The intrapulmonary shunt is ideally less than 10%, which corresponds to a PaO_2 of more than 450 mmHg on pure oxygen [4–6]. At the same time, airway pressures are at the minimum to ensure the required gas exchange. Hemodynamic side effects are thus minimized [1, 7].

Why Should We Open the Lung?

The classical paper on the acute respiratory distress syndrome (ARDS) by Ashbaugh and colleagues [8] describes the consequences of closed lung units: Hypoxemia; intrapulmonary shunt and atelectasis with high risk of infection; multi organ dysfunction and finally death [8, 9]. Ashbaugh [8] encouraged clinicians to re-expand collapsed lung units by high tidal volumes and high levels of positive end-expiratory pressure (PEEP). However, it has been known for many years that mechanical ventilation itself can also damage the lung [10–12]. The application of high inspiratory pressures and volumes with overdistension of open alveoli for a long time is associated with an increased risk of barotrauma [9, 13–16]. On the other hand, low levels of PEEP may contribute to ventilation-induced lung injury by allowing alveoli to collapse and re-open during each respiratory cycle [9, 10, 12–19]. Shear forces are the result [20–23] and may be responsible for a massive mediator release into the alveoli and into the pulmonary circulation [24, 25]. If these findings are true, what then is a safe strategy to open atelectatic lungs?

Physiologic Background

The relation between airway pressures and lung volumes has been the focus of basic lung physiology since the mid-180s (for a review see [11]). This relation is determined by the interaction of approximately 300 million individual alveoli and to understand the behavior of the entire lung it is, therefore, helpful to look first at a single alveolus.

The membrane of each alveolus is composed of different layers, starting with the capillary endothelium, the basement membranes, the connective tissue, the epithelial layer and finally the intraalveolar surfactant film. The tissue contains elastic and non-elastic fibers that limit the expansion of an alveolus beyond its elastic properties. The surface tension at the air-liquid interface (see later) adds to the elastance of the alveolar wall. Thus, the surface and the tissue elements containing this surface may be thought of as acting in series [11, 20].

Figure 1 demonstrates a simplified model of alveolar expansion. During the inflation of a collapsed elastic balloon its volume and pressure are measured (A). No external restriction to its expansion is present. Initially, increases in pressure lead to little gain in volume. Once a critical opening pressure is reached, the balloon increases its volume rapidly while the pressure inside it drops. If, however, the same procedure takes place in a closed bottle (B), its expansion is limited. Beyond the opening pressure the increase in volume leads to a parallel increase in pressure. Looking at a model of four balloons with different compliance (C), the composite curve shows the opening characteristics of each individual balloon. To simulate the behavior of the entire lung more appropriately, a mathematical model was used (D). One thousand "alveoli" with opening characteristics similar to those of the balloons described above were used. Each individual unit had an opening pressure that was normally distributed around a mean value. The resulting graphs closely resemble standard pressure-volume curves of healthy and sick lungs. The behavior of true alveoli, however, is more complex than simply inflating elastic balloons.

In 1929, Von Neergard [26] first called attention to the contribution of alveolar surface tension to the retractive forces of the lungs. He considered the formation of a bubble on the end of a capillary tube as an analog for the surface geometry of an alveolus [11]. For this model the law of LaPlace [27] provides a mathematical explanation:

$$P = 2\gamma/r, \tag{1}$$

where P is the pressure inside the bubble, γ the surface tension of the liquid and r the radius of the bubble. Before any pressure is applied, the fluid covers the orifice of the capillary tube as a flat perpendicular film. Increasing the pressure in the capillary will start the formation of a small bubble. The pressure within the system rises until the bubble's shape approaches that of a hemisphere. The bubble now has the same radius as the capillary. Once the pressure within the bubble exceeds a critical pres-

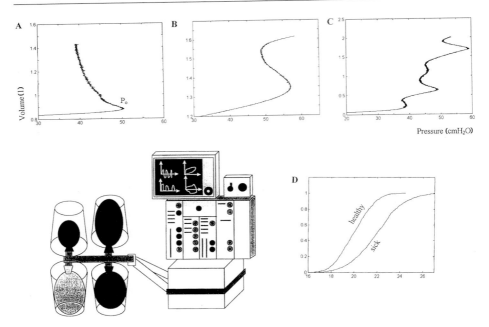

Fig. 1. Experimental set-up for the simulation of alveolar recruitment using a Siemens Servo 300 ventilator and four rubber balloons in glass bottles. With the increase in pressure during inspiration the corresponding volume is calculated by integrating the flow signal. Pressure-volume curves are shown. **A** A single balloon is inflated. At P_O the critical opening pressure is reached. The balloon is "recruited". Despite a reduction in pressure the increase in volume is immediate. **B** The same balloon as in A is placed in a glass bottle. Now, volume expansion is restricted, pressure increase in parallel with the gain in volume. **C** Same measurement as in B but using 4 individual balloons with different compliance. Note the four distinct points at which the balloons open. **D** Mathematical model of a pressure-volume curve. A step function was used to simulate alveolar opening. Opening pressures of 1000 "alveoli" were distributed normally around an assumed mean opening pressure of 20 cmH$_2$O in the healthy and 22 cmH$_2$O in the sick lung. (Provided by courtesy of Per-Göran Eriksson, Irene Lasson and Johanna Larsson at Siemens Elema, Sweden.)

sure, the bubble overcomes the hemispheric state; it opens. Now the bubble can be kept open with a much lower pressure than the critical opening pressure. In an open bubble the pressure changes required to induce certain changes in volume are now significantly lower compared to the closed state [11].

Applying these concepts to the inflation of a surfactant-deficient collapsed alveolus, it becomes apparent that surface forces, as stated in the law of LaPlace [27], act predominantly at a low alveolar radius; they hinder alveolar opening. Once, the alveolus is opened, however, and while maintaining identical opening pressures the volume increases rapidly to about two thirds of the maximal volume up to the point where the tissue forces begin to oppose further expansion. The pressure within this newly expanded alveolus can now be decreased until the bubble reaches its unstable state, and collapses [11, 27]. In a healthy alveolus with a normal surfactant system this collapse pressure is reduced to 3–5 cmH$_2$O. In other words, due to the fact that at end-expiration surface tension decreases almost to zero, the required pressure to stabilize healthy alveoli is only 3–5 cmH$_2$O which is equal to the existing transpulmonary pressure. This, in general, prevents a healthy lung from collapse. However, should the alveolus collapse, active re-expansion, as stated above, is required to open it [1–3]. Thereafter, the pressures are reduced and kept at a value slightly above the previously determined collapsing pressure. This pressure level depends mainly on the function of the surfactant system [7, 23, 28].

In summary, the behavior of alveoli is quantal; they are either open or closed [29]. No stable state in between these endpoints exists. This quantal alveolar physiology was demonstrated by Mead and Staub [11, 30] and was recently confirmed in computer tomography studies by Wegenius et al. [31, 32].

The Need to Open the Lung

The three following statements by Lachmann and colleagues describe the treatment concept in words and in Fig. 2 [7].
1) One must overcome a critical opening pressure during inspiration
2) This opening pressure must be maintained for a sufficiently long period of time
3) During expiration, no critical time that would allow closure of lung units should pass.

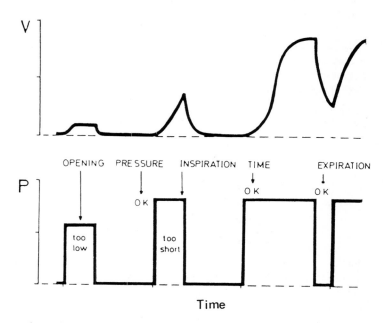

Fig. 2. Schematic diagram showing the improvement of tidal volume (V) during pressure-controlled ventilation of surfactant-deficient lungs, in relation to variations in inflation pressure (P), and inspiratory time.
Note: Choosing an expiratory time which is too short to empty the lung prevents expiratory collapse and results in autoPEEP. (Modified from [7] with permission)

Years later, a consensus document on mechanical ventilation indirectly confirmed these ideas by claiming that the prevention or reversal of atelectasis is one of the clinical treatment objectives of mechanical ventilation [33, 34]. From this statement it is concluded that, it is obligatory to "open up the lung and keep the lung open" [1]. The open lung concept defines the conceptual goals of this treatment strategy which is accomplished by a predetermined sequence of therapeutic phases, each with its specific treatment objective [1–3, 7]. Fig. 3 depicts these different phases schematically. As shown in Fig. 3, the goal of the initial increase in inspiratory pressure is to recruit collapsed alveoli and to determine the critical lung opening pressure. Then, the minimum pressures that prevent the lung from collapse are determined. Finally, after an active re-opening maneuver, sufficient pressure is implemented to keep the lung open.

Procedure to Open the Lung

In the following paragraphs instructions for the clinical application of the method are provided. For details see Figs. 4–6. All interventions discussed below are safe only when used with a pressure-control mode of ventilation; their application with a volume-control mode may even be considered a professional error [1, 29].

Before opening the lungs, the end-expiratory alveolar pressure is set between 15 and 25 cmH$_2$O either as static or as auto PEEP, or as a combination of both. This level will be sufficient to keep those alveoli, which are to be recruited by the peak inspiratory pressures, open [35, 36].

At an I/E ratio which guarantees an end-expiratory flow of zero, peak pressures are successively incremented in steps of 3 to 5 cmH$_2$O until a peak airway pressure between 45 and 60 cmH$_2$O is reached. During the process of opening the lungs the PaO$_2$ helps to guide this effort, because it is the only parameter that reliably correlates with the amount of lung tissue that participates in gas exchange [1–3, 6, 36, 37]. In severe lung disease, frequent measurements of arterial blood gases are required

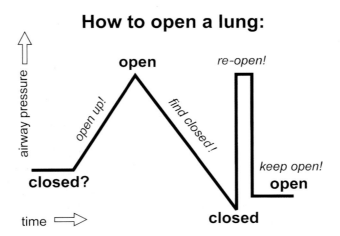

How to open a lung:

airway pressure

open up! — open — find closed! — re-open! — keep open! — open

closed? — closed

time

Fig. 3. Schematic representation of the opening procedure for collapsed lungs. The imperatives (!) mark the treatment goal of each specific intervention. The **bold** words mark the achieved state of the lung. At the beginning the precise amount of collapsed lung tissue is not known

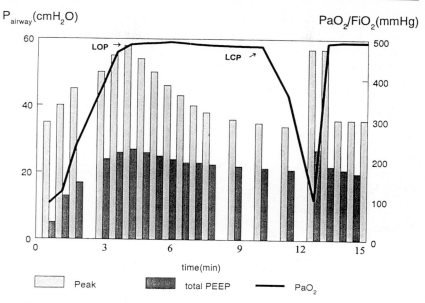

Fig. 4. Schematic representation of the opening procedure for atelectatic lungs. PaO_2/FiO_2, peak inspiratory pressure (PIP) and total PEEP as a result of the I/E ratio and the respiratory rate are displayed over time on the abscissa. PaO_2/FiO_2 increases in parallel with increases in airway pressure. At a certain airway pressure, referred to as lung opening pressure (LOP) the lung is opened fully, indicated by a PaO_2/FiO_2 of almost 500 mmHg. PaO_2/FiO_2 stays high despite a reduction of PIP and total PEEP until pressures reach a critical value where lung areas collapse, referred to as lung closing pressure (LCP). PaO_2/FiO_2 falls immediately. Full recruitment is achieved, again, by setting the airway pressures to the opening values determined before. Airway pressures are then reduced to and maintained at values above the previously determined closing pressures. PaO_2/FiO_2 remains high because the lung is open

during this titration process. A more than proportional increase in the size of the tidal volume following the increase in airway pressure or sometimes in inspiratory time also indicates successful alveolar recruitment (Fig. 2) [38–40].

If the lung disease is inhomogeneous, which is almost always the case [41], there may be a large difference in the pressures needed to open collapsed alveoli; some have always been open while others need further increments in pressure to overcome their closed state [35, 36, 42, 43]. This may result in a transient hemodynamic compromise since open lung units expand further and compress the adjacent capillary bed [7, 29]. Therefore, it is important during the opening procedure to maintain a sufficient intravascular volume. That is why it may even be necessary to administer fluids or to give inotropic support to the right heart before one can finalize the opening procedure. This type of hemodynamic support will be superfluous at lower airway pressures.

If a further increase in airway pressure does not result in a parallel increase in PaO_2, peak inspiratory pressures can carefully be reduced. During this phase the PaO_2 should, however, remain high despite the reduction in airway pressure, until the critical level of pressure is reached at which the least compliant parts of the lung

Oxygenation and Alveolar Collapse

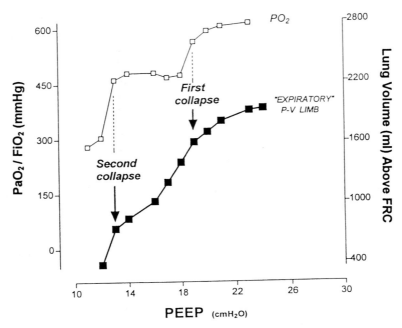

Fig. 5. The deflation limb of a pressure-volume curve (*open squares*) together with on-line arterial oxygen tensions (*solid squares*) from a ventilated patient are displayed as a function of PEEP. The drop in PaO$_2$ corresponds with the drop in lung volumes measured by inductive plethysmography. The pronounced steps in the PaO$_2$ are due to the sudden alveolar de-recruitment (*arrows*). (Figure provided by courtesy of Dr M. Amato, São Paulo, Brazil)

start to collapse [1, 7, 44–48]. Should this occur, the inspiratory pressure is immediately set back to the previously determined opening pressure and is kept there for a short period of 10 to 30 seconds [7, 48]. The lung tissue is yet again fully recruited, and the peak inspiratory pressures should then be reduced to a level which is safely, usually 2 cmH$_2$O, above the closing pressure. If, however, no collapse occurs, the reduction of peak inspiratory pressure continues until alveolar ventilation becomes too low to remove carbon dioxide effectively. PaCO$_2$ increases beyond normal limits. At this point PEEP is reduced too.

As stated before, at the beginning of the opening procedure, PEEP was set to a relatively high value of 15–25 cmH$_2$O to prevent collapse of recruited alveoli. It is, however, not known if this PEEP is really necessary. Therefore, the same procedure as described above for the peak inspiratory pressure, is now performed to find the lowest level of PEEP. After having opened the lungs again, the inspiratory and expiratory pressures are set to levels above the closing pressures and are kept there until the lung condition changes. In the further course of the disease the ventilator can be adjusted carefully to any changes in the patient's respiratory condition. A reduction of the total level of support is generally possible after a successful alveolar recruitment

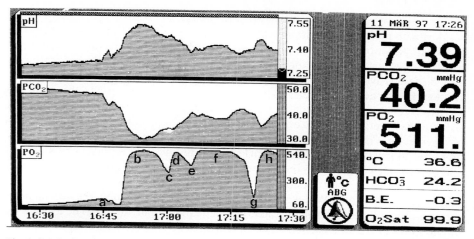

Fig. 6. Original registration of on-line blood gases (Paratrend 7, Diametrix, UK) of an experimental animal model of acute respiratory failure. The lungs of a pig were lavaged and ventilated with settings resulting in a low PaO_2 ($FiO_2 = 1.0$). During the first 15 minutes the animal was ventilated in a volume controlled mode with PEEP of 8 cmH_2O (to maintain a PaO_2 between 60 and 80 mmHg), tidal volume of 7 ml/kg BW and a respiratory rate of 30/bpm (a). $PaCO_2$ rose. Thereafter, the lung was opened by a peak airway pressure of 60 cmH_2O which resulted in a PaO_2 above 500 mmHg (b). The gradual decrease of peak airway pressure from 55 to 28 cmH_2O at a PEEP of 12 cmH_2O led to a decrease in PaO_2 as a sign of alveolar instability (c). The collapsed units were reopened and the peak pressure was set to 30 cmH_2O (d). The increase in peak airway pressure was not enough to keep the entire lung open (e), also the PEEP was increased to 16 cmH_2O (f). Finally, the animal was disconnected from the ventilator and the PaO_2 fell immediately (g). An active opening of the lung leads to full lung function, again, indicated by a final PaO_2 of 511 mmHg and a $PaCO_2$ of 40.2 mmHg (h)

[29]. It is important to realize that the lung has to be kept open at all times [1, 45–47]. Should a renewed collapse of alveoli occur, often caused by intrapulmonary suction or disconnection, a fall in PaO_2 indicates that a recruitment maneuver has to be performed in the same way as previously described. Also, later in the weaning phase, one has to guarantee a sufficient level of PEEP to keep the entire lung open. This can be combined either with pressure or volume support to ensure adequate CO_2 removal. Both levels of support should be reduced according to the improvement of the patient's condition.

After opening the lung and finding the lowest pressures to keep it open, the resulting pressure amplitude is minimized and at the same time pulmonary gas exchange is maximized. The therapeutic steps of the open lung concept help define a ventilatory condition which saves the lung from further damage, allows a reduction of FiO_2, promotes the resorption of interstitial and intrapulmonary edema, and also leads to a reduction of pulmonary artery pressures by overcoming hypoxic pulmonary vasoconstriction.

Alveolar recruitment should almost always be possible during the first 48 hours on mechanical ventilation. Even if not all of the lung tissue may be fully recruited for gas exchange, as in consolidating pneumonia, this ventilatory strategy will prevent further damage to the re-aerated part of the lung [9, 17, 23, 49, 50].

Not every patient with respiratory failure requires an invasive form of respiratory support with prolonged inspiratory times, high levels of PEEP and peak airway pressures. For patients with milder, or even no form of respiratory dysfunction, it is imperative to adjust the ventilator such that further progression or the generation of lung disease is avoided. For this purpose the lung has to be opened. The ventilatory strategy has to achieve normal patient activity; they take deep breaths, sigh and stretch to re-aerate non-ventilated parts of the lung. All considerations for the very sick lung as mentioned above are, without exception, also valid for the milder forms of disease; only the level of support is lower in the latter cases. Increasing airway pressures to levels of around 40 cmH_2O for 2–3 minutes will recruit normal alveoli that become atelectatic when the patient is lying in the supine position, undergoing anesthesia and surgery (unpublished observations), or is disconnected from the ventilator [3, 38–40, 42]. When all lung units have been re-opened, the airway pressures can be reduced to levels that assure an adequate tidal volume. The PEEP level should never be below 5 cmH_2O since all recruited alveoli have to be kept open during expiration.

Conclusion

The basic treatment principles are:
1. Open up the lung with high inspiratory pressures
2. Keep the lung open with PEEP levels above the closing pressures
3. Maintain optimal gas exchange at the smallest possible pressure amplitude to optimize CO_2 removal

With the strict application of these principles, prophylactic treatment is at hand aimed at preventing ventilator-induced lung injury and pulmonary complications. Ongoing and future clinical trials will have to provide further evidence for this treatment concept.

References

1. Lachmann B (1992) Open up the lung and keep the lung open. Intensive Care Med 118:319–321
2. Lachmann B, Bergmann KC, Enders K, et al (1977) Können pathologische Veränderungen im Surfactant-System der Lunge zu einer akuten respiratorischen Insuffizienz beim Erwachsenen führen? In: Danzmann E (ed) Anaesthesia 77, Proceedings of the 6th Congress of the Society of Anaesthesiology and Resuscitation of the GDR Vol. 1 Soc Anesthesiol and Resuscitation of the GDR, Berlin, pp 337–353
3. Haendly B, Lachmann B, Schulz H, Jonson B (1978) Der Einfluß verschiedener Beatmungsmuster auf Lungenmechanik und Gasaustausch bei Patienten während Respiratorbehandlung. Kongreßbericht Anaesthesie 1:665–678
4. Lichtwarck-Aschoff M, Nielsen JB, Sjöstrand UH, Edgren E (1992) An experimental randomized study of five different ventilatory modes in a piglet model of severe respiratory distress. Intensive Care Med 18:339–347
5. Sjöstrand UH, Lichtwarck-Aschoff M, Nielsen JB, et al (1995) Different ventilatory approaches to keep the lung open. Intensive Care Med 21:310–318
6. Kesecioglu J, Tibboel D, Lachmann B (1994) Advantages and rationale for pressure control ventilation. In: Vincent JL (ed) Yearbook of intensive care and emergency medicine. Springer-Verlag, Berlin, Heidelberg, New York, pp 524–533

7. Lachmann B, Danzmann E, Haendly B, Jonson B (1982) Ventilator settings and gas exchange in respiratory distress syndrome. In: Prakash O (ed) Applied physiology in clinical respiratory care. Nijhoff, The Hague, pp 141–176

8. Ashbaugh DG, Bingelow DB, Petty TL, Levine BE (1967) Acute respiratory distress in adults. Lancet 2:319–323

9. Ashbaugh DG, Petty TL, Bigelow DB, et al (1969) Continuous positive pressure breathing (CPPB) in the adult respiratory distress syndrome. J Thorac Cardiovasc Surg 57:31–41

10. Tremblay NL, Slutsky AS (1996) The role of pressure and volume in ventilation induced lung injury. Appl Cardiopulm Pathophysiol 6:179–190

11. Mead J (1961) Mechanical properties of lungs. Physiol Rev 41:281–330

12. Dreyfuss D, Soler P, Basset G, Saumon G (1988) High inflation pressure pulmonary edema. Am Rev Respir Dis 137:1159–1164

13. Dreyfuss D, Basset G, Soler P, Saumon G (1985) Intermittent positive pressure hyperventilation with high inflation pressures produces pulmonary microvascular injury in rats. Am Rev Respir Dis 132:880–884

14. Dreyfuss D, Soler P, Basset G, Saumon G (1988) High inflation pressure pulmonary edema: respective effects of high airway pressure, high tidal volume, and positive end-expiratory pressure. Am Rev Respir Dis 137:1159–1164

15. Dreyfuss D, Saumon G (1993) Role of tidal volume, FRC, and end-inspiratory volume in the development of pulmonary edema following mechanical ventilation. Am Rev Respir Dis 148:1194–1203

16. Webb HH, Tierney DF (1974) Experimental pulmonary edema due to intermittent positive pressure ventilation with high inflation pressures: protection by positive end-expiratory pressure. Am Rev Respir Dis 110:556–565

17. Muscedere JG, Mullen JB, Gan K, Slutzky AS (1994) Tidal ventilation at low airway pressures can augment lung injury. Am J Respir Crit Care Med 149:1327–1334

18. Amato MBP, Barbas CSV, Pastore L, et al (1996) Minimizing barotrauma in ARDS: Protective effects of PEEP and the hazards of driving and plateau pressures. Am J Respir Crit Care Med 153:375A (abst)

19. Froese AB, McCulloch PR, Sugiura M, et al (1993) Optimizing alveolar expansion prolongs the effectiveness of exogenous surfactant therapy in the adult rabbit. Am Rev Respir Dis 148:569–577

20. Mead J, Takishima T, Leith D (1970) Stress distribution in lungs: a model of pulmonary elasticity. J Appl Physiol 28:596–608

21. Schwieler G, Robertson B (1976) Liquid ventilation in immature newborn rabbits. Biol Neonate 29:343–353

22. Bond D, Froese B (1993) Volume recruitment maneuvers are less deleterious than persistent low lung volumes in the atelectasis prone rabbit lung during high-frequency oscillation. Crit Care Med 21:402–412

23. Taskar V, John J, Evander E, et al (1997) Surfactant dysfunction makes the lungs vulnerable to repetitive collapse and reexpansion. Am J Physiol 155:313–320

24. Tremblay L, Valenza F, Ribeiro S, Jingfang L, Slutsky A (1997) Injurious ventilatory strategies increase cytokines and c-fos m-RNA expression in an isolated rat lung model. J Clin Invest 99:944–952

25. Bethmann von A, Brasch F, Müller K, Wndel A, Uhlig S (1996) Prolonged hyperventilation is required for release of tumor necrosis factor-α but not IL-6. Appl Cardiopulm Pathophysiol 6:179–190

26. Von Neergaard K (1929) Neue Auffassungen über einen Grundbegriff der Atemmechanik; Die Retraktionskraft der Lunge, abhängig von der Oberflächenspannung in den Alveolen. Z Ges Exp Med 66:373–394

27. LaPlace PS (1798–1827) Traite de Mecanique Celeste. Crapelet, Courcier, Paris

28. McIntyre R, Laws A, Ramachandran P (1969) Positive expiratory pressure plateau: improved gas exchange during mechanical ventilation. Can Anaes Soc J 16:477–487

29. Böhm S, Lachmann B (1996) Pressure-control ventilation. Putting a mode into perspective. Int J Intensive Care 3:12–27

30. Staub N, Nagano H, Pearce, Spring ML (1967) Pulmonary edema in dogs, especially the sequence of fluid accumulation in lungs. J Appl Physiol 22:227–240

31. Wegenius G (1991) Model simulations of pulmonary edema. Phantom studies with computer tomography. Invest Radiol 26:149–156

32. Wegenius G, Wickerts CJ, Hedenstierna G (1994) Radiological assessment of pulmonary edema. A new principle. Eur J Radiol 4:146–154

33. Slutsky A (1994) Consensus conference on mechanical ventilation January 28–30, 1993 at Northbrook, Illinois, USA. Part 1. Intensive Care Med 20:64–79

34. Slutsky A (1994) Consensus conference on mechanical ventilation January 28–30, 1993 at Northbrook, Illinois, USA. Part 2. Intensive Care Med 20:150–162

35. Gattinoni L, Pelosi P, Crotti S, Valenza F (1995) Effects of positive end-expiratory pressure on regional distribution of tidal volume and recruitment in adult respiratory distress syndrome. Am J Respir Crit Care Med 151:1807–1814

36. Amato MBP, Barbas CSV, Medeiros DM, et al (1995) Beneficial effects of the "Open Lung Approach" with low distending pressures in acute respiratory distress syndrome. Am J Respir Crit Care Med 152:1835–1846

37. Hedenstierna G, Tokics L, Strandberg A, Lundquist H, Brismar B (1986) Correlation of gas exchange impairment to development of atelectasis during anaesthesia and muscle paralysis. Acta Anaesthesiol Scand 30:183–191

38. Rothen HU, Sporre B, Engberg G, Wegenius G, Hedenstierna G (1993) Reexpansion of atelectasis during general anaesthesia: a computed tomography study. Br J Anaesth 71:788–795

39. Hedenstierna G, Lundquist H, Lundh B, et al (1989) Pulmonary densities during anaesthesia. An experimental study on lung morphology and gas exchange. Eur Respir J 2:528–535

40. Hedenstierna G, Tokics L, Strandeberg A, Lundquist H, Brismar B (1986) Correlation of gas exchange impairment to development of atelectasis during anaesthesia and muscle paralysis. Acta Anaesthesiol Scand 30:183–191

41. Gattinoni L, Pesenti A, Avalli L, Rossi F, Bombino M, (1987) Pressure-volume curve of total respiratory system in acute respiratory failure. A computed tomographic scan study. Am Rev Respir Dis 136:730–736

42. Bendixen H, Hedley Whyte J, Chir B, Laver M (1963) Impaired oxygenation in surgical patients during general anesthesia with controlled ventilation. A concept of atelectasis. N Engl J Med 269:991–996

43. Housley E, Louyada N, Becklake M (1970) To sigh or not to sigh. Am Rev Respir Dis 101:611–614

44. Lachmann B, Jonson B, Lindroth M, Robertson B (1982) Modes of artificial ventilation in severe respiratory distress syndrome. Lung function and morphology in rabbits after washout of alveolar surfactant. Crit Care Med 10:724–732

45. Dreyfuss D, Saumon G (1994) Should the lung be rested or recruited? The Charybdis and Scylla of ventilator management. Am Rev Respir Crit Care Med 149:1066–1068

46. McCulloch P, Forkert G, Froese A (1988) Lung volume maintenance prevents lung injury during high frequency oscillatory ventilation in surfactant-deficient rabbits. Am Rev Respir Dis 137:1185–1192

47. Froese A (1997) High-frequency oscillatory ventilation for adult respiratory distress syndrome: let's get it right this time. Crit Care Med 25:906–908

48. Froese A, Bryan Ch (1987) High frequency ventilation. Am Rev Respir Dis 135:1363–1374

49. Amato MBP, Barbas CSV, Medeiros, et al (1996) Improved survival in ARDS: beneficial effects of a lung protective strategy. Am J Respir Crit Care Med 153:A531 (Abst)

50. Snyder JV, Froese A (1987) The open lung approach: Concept and application. In: Snyder JV, Pinsky MR (eds) Oxygen transport in the critically ill. Year Book medical publishers Inc., Chicago, pp 374–395

Lung Stretching and Barotrauma

Inflammatory Consequences of High Stretch Lung Injury

J.-D. Chiche

Introduction

After 30 years of extensive research, the acute respiratory distress syndrome (ARDS) remains a therapeutic challenge for critical care physicians [1]. Clinical management of patients with ARDS involves primarily supportive measures aimed at maintaining cellular and physiologic functions of the lung while the acute injury resolves. Among these measures, mechanical ventilation plays a pivotal role and has been the focus of thorough investigation. It has become increasingly evident that mechanical ventilation *per se* can create lung injury [2, 3]. Ventilatory strategies are now directed toward achievement of acceptable gas exchange as well as the prevention of ventilator-induced lung injury [4].

Despite an overall improvement in the quality of supportive care, mortality from ARDS remains high, although recent data indicate that mortality rates may have slightly fallen over the past 20 years [5]. Concurrently, causes of mortality have gradually shifted. Refractory hypoxemia is no longer the primary cause of mortality, and only a small percentage of patients with ARDS eventually die of respiratory failure [1, 5]. Instead, most non-survivors develop a progressive systemic inflammatory response that results in multiple organ failure (MOF) [6]. One possible explanation for this observation could be that mechanical ventilation, invariably used in acute hypoxemic respiratory failure, triggers and/or amplifies a local inflammatory response in the lung that propagates to the systemic circulation resulting in MOF and death. Supporting this hypothesis are recently reported experimental studies which suggest that injurious ventilatory strategies can increase pulmonary neutrophil infiltration and adhesion, as well as stimulate the production of inflammatory cytokines [7–9]. The goal of this chapter is to review the evidence that led to the recognition of this novel mechanism of injury. Specifically, we propose to:
1) Briefly review the rationale for the current approach to mechanical ventilation in ARDS
2) Present the observations supporting the existence of a ventilator-induced inflammatory response
3) Discuss the pathophysiological mechanisms potentially involved in the inflammatory response to injurious ventilatory strategies

Ventilator-Induced Lung Injury and Lung-Protective Ventilatory Strategies

Over the last decade, intensivists have developed growing scientific and clinical interest in newer approaches to mechanical ventilation of patients with ARDS. These changes have been driven by an evolving knowledge of lung pathoanatomy and respiratory mechanics in ARDS, as well as the recognition of ventilator-induced lung injury. Experimental studies extensively reviewed elsewhere [2] provided unequivocal evidence that mechanical ventilation *per se* can induce or exacerbate a high-permeability type of pulmonary edema. Consequently, research has been mainly directed at understanding the respective roles of large inflation volumes and pressures in the pathogenesis of the functional and anatomic lung alterations associated with mechanical ventilation [3]. It has repeatedly been demonstrated that ventilator-induced lung injury is due to large tidal volumes (V_T) rather than high airway pressures (P_{aw}) [2, 3]. In a series of important studies, Dreyfuss and Saumon [10–13] assessed the respective effects of high P_{aw}, high V_T and positive end-expiratory pressure (PEEP) on edema formation. They convincingly demonstrated that the end-inspiratory volume is a key determinant of what should be named "volutrauma" rather than "barotrauma". On the other hand, many investigators reported that ventilation with low end-expiratory lung volume was also associated with worsening lung injury [11, 14]. The use of PEEP to keep end-expiratory lung volume above the lower inflexion point of the static pressure-volume (P-V) curve (Fig. 1) seems to exert a protective effect [14]. This protective effect may result from the reduction of cyclic lung stretch associated with repetitive opening/collapse of alveoli, and from minimized hemodynamic alterations [2, 4, 14]. Finally, previously injured lungs are more susceptible to ventilator-induced lung injury [10].

In light of the points raised above, ventilatory objectives in ARDS have been redefined. Mechanical ventilation has evolved from a high-V_T, normoxic and normocapnic strategy to a pressure-targeted, lung protective approach aimed at ensuring adequate gas exchange while minimizing transalveolar cycling pressures and volumes [4]. Recent guidelines recommend to target an acceptable SaO_2 ($\geq 90\%$), and to keep the plateau pressure (P_{plat}) below 35 cmH_2O [15]. Finally, several investigators pointed out that strict observance of these guidelines does not decrease the risk

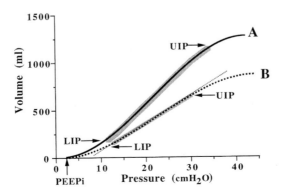

Fig. 1. Static Pressure-Volume (P-V) curves in ARDS. The static P-V curve has a sigmoid shape with a lower inflexion point (LIP) indicating a sudden improvement in compliance, and an upper inflexion point (UIP) above which the P-V curve diverges from a straight line. Tidal ventilation should cycle between LIP and UIP to limit the risk of volotrauma. In patient B, limitation of tidal volume is mandatory to reach this goal (PEEPi = intrinsic PEEP). (From [9] with permission)

of ventilator-induced lung injury in all patients [16, 17]. A significant number of patients are still ventilated with end-inspiratory volumes above the upper inflection point when V_T is titrated on the basis of P_{plat} (Fig. 1) [16]. Reduction of the risk of volotrauma mandates a deliberate reduction of V_T which unavoidably leads to hypercapnia in these patients. Whereas consensus supports the use of physiologically targeted, patient-specific goals to guide ventilator settings, it has become increasingly evident that these goals should also be defined on the basis of lung mechanics [4, 17].

Despite compelling experimental evidence supporting the use of lung protective oxygenation strategies, the benefit of altering traditional approaches to mechanical ventilation has not been clearly demonstrated in the clinical setting. As reported by Milberg and Hudson [5], the overall mortality of ARDS has slowly but steadily decreased over the past 20 years. Since no specific treatment accounts for this improvement in survival [1], it is likely that numerous changes in supportive therapy have had small, but additive effects, resulting finally in a measurable difference in mortality. Among these therapies, implementation of well-reasoned ventilatory strategies has probably contributed significantly to improved outcome. Indeed, Amato and coworkers [18] recently reported the beneficial effects of a ventilatory approach designed to minimize cyclic parenchymal stretch. Using a strategy based on the use of pressure-limited ventilation, low V_T (<6 ml/kg) and permissive hypercapnia with PEEP set according to the P-V curve, these investigators convincingly demonstrated that this rational ventilation approach can markedly improve lung function [18]. In a preliminary report concerning a larger group of patients, this strategy led to a statistically significant reduction in mortality [19].

This work, as other outcome studies designed to evaluate ventilatory modalities in ARDS, should be interpreted with the following points in mind. On one hand, the impact of novel ventilatory strategies on mortality may be obscured by a high incidence of MOF. Since MOF is the leading cause of death in ARDS [1, 6], lung protective strategies are likely to decrease mortality only if such strategies can limit the inflammatory response and prevent the development of MOF. On the other hand, the absence of improvement in mortality rates may imply that suboptimal patterns of mechanical ventilation serve to initiate and exacerbate a ventilator-induced inflammatory response.

Evidence in Support of a Ventilator-Induced Inflammatory Response

Several lines of evidence support the hypothesis that mechanical ventilation *per se* can significantly influence the production of inflammatory mediators. Both clinical [20, 21] and experimental studies have established a link between the development of respiratory physiologic abnormalities and lung inflammatory mediators [7, 22–24]. More than 10 years ago, Hamilton et al. [22] using a surfactant-deficient model of ARDS reported that different ventilatory strategies significantly affected the degree of lung injury. In this study, high-frequency oscillatory (HFO) ventilation maintained excellent gas exchange and avoided hyaline membrane formation. In contrast, rabbits ventilated with conventional mechanical ventilation (CMV) had poor gas exchange, a large number of granulocytes and extensive hyaline membrane formation in their damaged lungs. Subsequently, Kawano and coworkers [23] developed this work and found that these structural changes, initially attributed to barotrauma, were actually mediated by activated leukocytes; granulocyte-depleted animals had good gas exchange, minimal protein leak and no hyaline membranes, and repletion of granulocytes from donor rabbits induced a significant deterioration of lung structure and function.

Concurrently, several studies demonstrated that mechanotransduction plays a pivotal role in determining the structure and function of the lung [25–28]. Pulmonary cells are exposed to an array of physical forces including those generated by tidal ventilation, pulsatile pulmonary blood flow or cell interactions with extracellular matrices. These physical forces can be converted to biochemical signals capable of altering cell phenotype and metabolism [29]. Accordingly, mechanical stretch has been found to induce physiologically relevant molecular alterations which modulate lung growth and development [26, 27, 30, 31], endothelial permeability [32] and surfactant production [33]. The signaling mechanisms through which physical stimuli are transduced may include the release of paracrine or autocrine factors, the modulation of stretch-sensitive ion channels, and direct conformational changes in membrane-bound molecules leading to activation of downstream messengers [29, 34, 35]. Taken together, these data support the hypothesis that mechanical ventilation *per se* can significantly influence the production of inflammatory mediators.

Mechanisms Involved in the Ventilator-Induced Inflammatory Response

Early studies suggested that the presence of neutrophils and their infiltration into the lungs plays a pivotal role in the alteration of lung cellular functions that occur in response to injurious ventilatory strategies. The following sections summarize the role of the different mechanisms that may actually contribute to the inflammatory aspects of ventilator-induced lung damage.

Role of Cellular Factors

Although the pathogenesis of ARDS remains the subject of active debate, an impressive body of evidence has established the critical role of cellular factors in the pathophysiology of ARDS [36]. After a primary insult, the local activation of cells which normally serve a crucial function in host defense, results in a local tissue reponse and in the systemic release of inflammatory cell activators. Neutrophils, macrophages, endothelial cells and platelets all contribute to the release of toxic compounds which mediate lung injury, including pro-inflammatory cytokines, reactive oxygen species, lipid mediators and proteolytic enzymes [36].

A growing body of evidence suggests that injurious ventilatory strategies influence infiltration and activation of neutrophils [7, 8, 23, 24, 37] as well as macrophages [38]. Recent *in vitro* studies demonstrated that mechanical stress affects structure and function of polymorphonuclear neutrophils (PMN), macrophages and endothelial cells [28, 32, 39, 40]. For example, Kitagawa and colleagues [39] recently reported that leukocytes can be activated by mechanical deformation imposed by geometric constraints of the capillaries when they emigrate from the vascular space into the interstitial tissues. Since the conventional approach to mechanical ventilation commonly results in large swings in transpulmonary pressures, physical forces applied on alveolar and intravascular cells during the ventilatory cycle are likely to have a direct effect on their ability to release inflammatory mediators.

To test this hypothesis, Tremblay et al. [9] examined the effect of ventilatory pattern on the production of lung cytokines in an *ex vivo* non-perfused rat lung model. Lungs from normal or lipopolysaccharide (LPS)-challenged rats were excised and randomly allocated to a (a) non-injurious (Ctl), (b) moderate volume, high PEEP (MVHP), (c) moderate volume, zero PEEP (MVZP), or (d) high volume, zero PEEP (HVZP) ventilatory strategy. After 2 hours, levels of pro-inflammatory [tumor necrosis factor (TNF-α), interleukin-1β (IL-1β), IL-6, macrophage inflammatory protein (MIP-2), and interferon-γ (IFN-γ)] and anti-inflammatory (IL-10) cytokines were measured in the bronchoalveolar lavage (BAL) by enzyme-linked immunosorbent assay (ELISA). In saline-treated animals, increasingly injurious ventilatory strategies resulted in a parallel increase in the levels of all cytokines measured, with lowest levels in the Ctl group and highest in the HVZP group (see Fig. 4 in following chapter "Mechanical and Ventilation-Induced Injury"). Interestingly, the authors observed a synergistic effect of large V_T and zero PEEP ventilation (HVZP, 56-fold increase in TNF-α above control values) as compared to strategies with similar end-inspiratory lung volumes (MVHP, 3-fold increase) or with a lesser degree of stretch in the absence of PEEP (MVZP, 6-fold increase). LPS caused a significant increase in the baseline levels of TNF-α and MIP-2. After a LPS challenge, the effect of ventilatory strategy on cytokine levels was similar to that observed in healthy lungs (Ctl < MVHP < MVZP < HVZP) except for MIP-2, whose level was attenuated in the MVHP group as compared to Ctl. Finally, the effect of these ventilatory settings on the activation of pulmonary cells at the transcriptional level was determined for TNF-α and c-*fos*, an immediate-early response gene with a stretch responsive promoter [41]. Northern blot analysis revealed that injurious ventilatory strategies significantly induce both TNF-α and c-*fos* messenger ribonucleic acids (mRNAs) [9].

This model however, which was designed to provide mechanistic information regarding the cytokine response to physical forces applied to the lungs, has several limitations. First, the effect of ventilatory strategies on inflammatory mediators was assessed independently of changes in cardiac output, which regularly occur with different ventilatory settings and can influence both the degree and the pattern of mechanical stretch. Also, intravascular cells and cytokines released in the systemic circulation certainly play a role in the modulation of injury and of the inflammatory response. Finally, a concurrent priming effect of ischemia on lung expression of inflammatory mediators cannot be ruled out. Therefore, changes in the cytokine profile described with this model may differ significantly from those seen *in vivo*.

To better understand the inflammatory aspects of ventilator-induced lung injury *in vivo*, Takata et al. [8] evaluated the effects of CMV and HFO on intraalveolar expression of the TNF-α gene in surfactant-depleted rabbits. Lung lavage was performed in previously saline-lavaged mechanically ventilated rabbits, in order to extract RNA from the lavage cells and quantitate mRNA for TNF-α by reverse-transcription polymerase chain reaction using glyceraldehyde-3-phosphate dehydrogenase (GAPDH) mRNA as an internal standard. After 1 h of ventilation with either

CMV or HFO [inspired fraction of oxygen (FiO$_2$) = 1.0, mean Paw = 13 cmH$_2$O], few physiologic abnormalities were detectable; PaO$_2$ was slightly lower with CMV than HFO, while BAL cell counts and cytology were similar between the two groups. However, the ratio of TNF-α mRNA to GAPDH mRNA increased significantly with CMV but not with HFO (Fig. 2). In a separate series of experiments, the duration of mechanical ventilation was increased to 4 h to evaluate whether clinically relevant physiologic or morphologic changes would take place either with CMV or HFO. As previously described [22, 23], CMV resulted in progressive hypoxemia, decreased lung compliance, increased number of neutrophils in BAL fluid, and in substantial morphologic changes including hyaline membrane formation and neutrophil accumulation (Fig. 3). Minimal changes in such physiologic and morphologic abnormalities were observed in rabbits ventilated with HFO [8]. Taken together, these results indicate that activation of alveolar macrophages and production of pro-inflammatory cytokines may play a central role in the early stage of ventilator-induced lung injury, and that ventilatory settings substantially modulate macrophage activation and hence the degree of lung injury.

Besides cytokines, several potent mediators are involved in the initiation and the propagation of the pulmonary injury [36]. Imai and colleagues [7] assessed the effect of CMV and HFO on the production of platelet activating factor (PAF), thromboxane B$_2$ (TXB$_2$) and 6-ketoprostaglandin F$_{2\alpha}$ (PGF$_{2\alpha}$) in surfactant-depleted rabbit lungs. After 4 h of ventilation, the numbers of PMN and the levels of PAF and TXB$_2$ in lung lavage fluid were significantly greater during CMV than during HFO, even when FiO$_2$ was adjusted to maintain the same PaO$_2$ with both modes. Using a different experimental approach, others found that the concentration of 15-hydroxyeicosatetraenoic acid (15-HETE), a metabolite of the lipoxygenase pathway, was reduced by more than 50% during HFO as compared to suboptimal CMV [42].

It is worth noting that CMV was not optimized in these studies suggesting that HFO could result in a lower incidence of chemically mediated lung injury as compared to CMV [7, 8, 22, 23, 42]. The use of low PEEP levels presumably contributed to initiate the inflammatory events consistently reported in these studies. The respective contribution of high inflation pressures and volumes to the intraalveolar production of inflammatory mediators remains unclear however. The degree and the pattern of mechanical stretch induced by these variables may differ significantly and

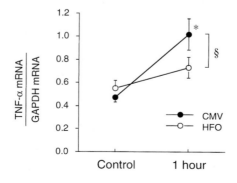

Fig. 2. Changes in intraalveolar expression of TNF-α gene. Changes in the relative amount of TNF-α gene transcripts were expressed by the mRNA ratio of TNF-α to GAPDH. Values are means ± SEM. * P < 0.01 (paired t-tests); § P < 0.05 (2-way ANOVA). (From [8] with permission)

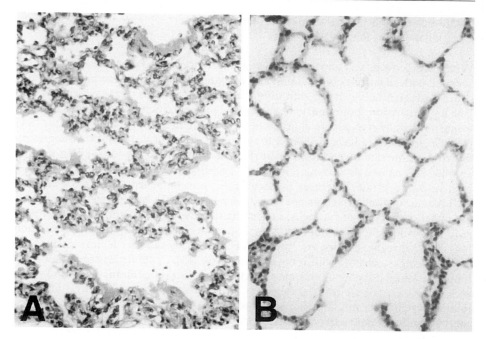

Fig. 3. Pathological changes induced by 4 h of CMV or HFO. Ventilation of surfactant-depleted rabbits with CMV (**A**) induces substantial morphological changes including hyaline membrane formation and neutrophil accumulation as compared to HFO (**B**). (From [8] with permission)

may therefore influence cellular responses [26, 27, 29]. Accordingly, preliminary data from von Bethmann et al. [43] indicate that a high P_{aw} may have a more significant effect on the intraalveolar production of inflammatory mediators than a high V_T. Using an isolated-perfused and ventilated mouse lung preparation, they reported that barotrauma stimulated the production of TNF-α, IL-6 and PGI_2 to a greater extent than volutrauma [43].

Taken together, the data presented in this section suggest that mechanical strain directly induces the production of cytokines and eicosanoids by intraalveolar cells. Yet, the mechanisms involved in the transduction of mechanical load into intracellular signals regulating gene expression are poorly understood. In cardiomyocytes, cell stretch rapidly activates a plethora of second messenger pathways including tyrosine kinases, $p21^{ras}$, mitogen-activated protein (MAP) kinases, S6 kinases, protein kinase C, phospholipase C, phospholipase D, and probably the phospholipase A_2 pathways [25, 41]. Signals generated by these second messengers seems to activate the p67SRF-p62TCF complex via the serum response element, causing induction of c-*fos* [41]. Whether the same pathways are activated in response to lung stretch is unknown. Mechanotransduction in the lung may also involve stretch-sensitive ion channels, G protein-dependent reactions, the action of autocrine or paracrine signals, or a combination of these factors [27, 34].

Inactivation of Surfactant Functions Contributes
to the Inflammatory Response

Ventilation settings that allow tidal closing and re-opening of unstable alveoli are associated with repetitive compression and re-expansion of the surfactant film resulting in both qualitative and quantitative alterations of the surfactant system [44, 45]. During ventilation, pulmonary surfactant is converted within the alveolar space from the surface active large aggregates (LA) to the inactive small aggregates (SA) [46]. Several studies have evaluated the effect of different ventilatory strategies on the conversion rate of endogenous surfactant from LA to SA [45–48]. In normal animals [46] as well as in injured lungs [47], ventilation with high V_T but not with a high respiratory rate, increases the aggregate conversion from LA to SA and the SA/LA ratio of the surfactant phospholipid pool [46, 47]. Interestingly, PEEP does not affect conversion of LA to SA, suggesting that the dynamic amplitude of changes in lung volume is more important for aggregate conversion than static distension [47]. The aggregate conversion rate is also affected by indirect factors such as increased protease activity within the alveolar space [45]. Capillary leakage induced by injurious ventilatory strategies may inactivate surfactant proteins SP-A and SP-B, which both contribute to LA integrity during surface-area cycling by stabilizing tubular myelin and multilamellar structures [45, 46]. Finally, the ventilatory pattern can markedly influence the aggregate conversion of exogenous surfactant preparations, and may consequently compromise the efficacy of such therapies [49]. Together, these data indicate that suboptimal ventilation of normal or injured lungs can alter the structure and function of pulmonary surfactant.

The reduction in functional surfactant probably contributes to the inflammatory response triggered by injurious ventilatory strategies. Specific components of surfactant (proteins and phospholipids) interact with many alveolar cells involved in pulmonary host defense systems [50, 51]. For example, surfactant proteins SP-A and SP-D play a major role in the phagocytosis of various microorganisms. Binding of these molecules to alveolar macrophages via high-affinity specific surface receptors effects the release of reactive oxygen species from resident alveolar macrophages, as well as the chemotaxis of alveolar macrophages [50]. Furthermore, SP-A up-regulates macrophage production of nitric oxide, a highly reactive molecule that plays a role in host defense against pathogens and attenuates reperfusion injury, in a concentration- and time-dependent manner [52]. Hence, inactivation of these components by intralveolar edema may affect the host defense capacities of pulmonary surfactant, and therefore contribute to the increased expression of immunoregulatory cytokines and other pro-inflammatory mediators in the lungs. For instance, Geertsma and coworkers [51] demonstrated that pulmonary surfactant inhibits the production of TNF-α and IL-1β induced by IFN-γ, one of the primary cytokines involved in the activation of phagocytes. The suppressive effects of surfactant on the production of inflammatory cytokines may involve transcriptional regulation through inhibition of nuclear factor-kappa B (NF-κB) activation [53]. In addition, human surfactant significantly attenuates the production of hydrogen peroxide (H_2O_2) by IFN-γ-activated monocytes [51]. Thus, it is reasonable to postulate that high-stretch ventilatory strategies alter not only surfactant's ability to reduce surface tension at the alveolar air-liquid interface, but also its ability to down-regulate the production of inflammatory mediators and to protect the alveolar epithelium against injury caused by reactive oxygen species and pro-inflammatory cytokines.

Role of Structural Injury

Ventilator-induced lung injury has been associated with histologic findings ranging from mild airspace enlargement and alveolar distension, to a complete rupture of the blood-gas barrier [2]. Using transmission and scanning electron microscopy, Fu et al. [54] demonstrated the presence of ultrastructural breaks in endothelial and epithelial cells when either capillary transmural pressure or transpulmonary pressure were increased above 40 mmHg. These breaks are the morphological correlates of the increased microvascular permeability associated with high stretch mechanical ventilation. Recent evidence suggests that the structural injury induced by shear forces also participates in the inflammatory response [55]. Disruption of the blood-gas interface may allow bacterial translocation from the alveoli into the blood stream and thereby propagates lung injury. As demonstrated by Nahum et al. [55] using a dog model of *E. coli* pneumonia, ventilatory strategies allowing atelectasis without tidal recruitment or assuring full recruitment with PEEP prevent bacterial translocation. Conversely, ventilation with low PEEP and large V_T increases the incidence of bacteremia. Besides the propagation of an intrapulmonary infection, high stretch lung injury may also account for the systemic dissemination of a local inflammatory process. Several studies suggest that the lungs may release cytokines into the systemic circulation during pulmonary Gram-negative infection [56–58], but the contribution of ventilator-induced lung injury to the progression of the systemic inflammatory reaction has been overlooked. Tutor and colleagues [57] recently used an isolated-perfused rat lung model to assess whether compartmentalization of alveolar TNF-α is preserved during lung injury. Whereas endogenous or exogenous pulmonary TNF-α remains predominantly compartmentalized in control animals, alveolar-capillary injury results in loss of compartmentalization of alveolar TNF-α [57]. These observations suggest that the injured lung may contribute to a systemic inflammatory response and subsequent MOF. Likewise, high stretch mechanical ventilation is likely to induce the evolution of a primary pulmonary inflammatory process to a generalized inflammatory reaction.

From the Mechanical Insult to the Inflammatory Response: A Vicious Cycle

Injurious ventilatory strategies initiate cellular and molecular biological changes from the very early stages of ventilator-induced lung damage [8, 9]. The mechanical insult is likely to be the triggering signal of a multifactorial process in which all the mechanisms discussed above interact *in vivo* to create and amplify the inflammatory response. The cycle of pathologic events which perpetuate the ventilator-induced inflammatory response is probably more complex than it appears in Fig. 4. Initially, cell stretch resulting from suboptimal ventilatory settings is associated with recruitment and activation of neutrophils, release of inflammatory cytokines and eicosanoids as well as surfactant inactivation. Pulmonary surfactant can in turn modulate

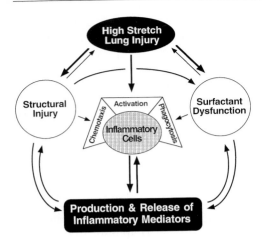

Fig. 4. Inflammatory consequences of high-stretch lung injury: A mechanistic over-view.
See text for further explanation

the secretion of cytokines and the activity of inflammatory cells recruited in response to increased BAL levels of chemokines such as MIP-2 [51, 53]. On the other hand, inflammatory mediators have been shown to inhibit surfactant synthesis and adsorption [59, 60]. Furthermore, structural injury promotes extravasation of intravascular cells and edema fluid, which further inactivates pulmonary surfactant and increases shear forces. Altogether, quantitative and qualitative alterations of the surfactant system compromise the pulmonary host defense system, alter the production of reactive oxygen species and contribute to increase both the production and release of cytokines via direct and indirect mechanisms [50, 51, 53]. In addition, surfactant dysfunction makes lungs more vulnerable to repetitive collapse and reexpansion [44], and may thus play a pivotal role in sustaining the vicious cycle of inflammation initiated by high stretch mechanical ventilation. Finally, the underlying lung disease that sensitizes the lung to ventilator-induced injury may differentially affect the components of this cycle.

Future Directions

Taken together, these experimental studies provide important insights into the processes underlying the inflammatory response to high stretch lung injury. However, several important questions remain unanswered. Do injurious ventilatory strategies effect the inflammatory reaction to the same extent when they are applied in the early or late phases of ARDS? Is the ventilator-induced inflammatory response dependent upon the etiology of ARDS (pulmonary vs extrapulmonary)? Also, further studies are needed to characterize the temporal pattern of the cytokine release, identify the cells involved in mediator production, and clarify the role of specific respiratory parameters (i.e., inflation pressures and volumes) in the modulation of the inflammatory response. Moreover, injurious ventilatory strategies may also impact many other cellular mechanisms which regulate the interplay between inflammatory and anti-inflammatory mediators, including the coagulation and complement systems, neutrophil-endothelial cell interactions or the balance between oxidants and antioxidants. The influence of damaging ventilatory patterns on these systems deserves to be further investigated. Likewise, the effects of injurious ventilatory strategies on the molecular processes involved in lung repair (e.g., apoptosis, extracellular matrix production and destruction, ...) should be the focus of future investigations. Finally, although the actions and interactions of mediator systems in the pathogenesis of ARDS and MOF have been extensively investigated, very few studies have considered the possible contribution of ventilator-induced lung injury to the local and systemic inflammatory reactions. Ventilatory management should be strictly defined and controlled in future studies aimed at defining cellular and molecular changes in ARDS.

Conclusion

A growing body of evidence indicates that the mechanical strain applied to lung structures modulates gene expression and pulmonary cell production of inflammatory mediators. Both mechanical and inflammatory processes play a role in the initiation and the exacerbation of ventilator-induced lung injury, which may in turn result in a systemic inflammatory response that culminates in MOF. Although further studies are needed to better define the inflammatory consequences of injurious ventilatory strategies, the observation that mechanical ventilation *per se* can initiate or amplify the inflammatory response in the lung provides further rationale for the use of patient-specific, physiologically-targeted lung protective strategies. In addition, recognition of this novel mechanism of injury may prompt clinicians to use pharmacologic or immunologic therapies to modulate the inflammatory components of ventilator-induced lung injury. Among these therapies, adjuvants to mechanical ventilation such as nitric oxide, exogenous surfactants or partial liquid ventilation combine appealing anti-inflammatory properties with selective and efficient drug delivery to the primary target organ. These agents may prove useful to support gas exchange, attenuate the inflammatory consequences of ventilation, and improve outcome for patients with acute respiratory failure.

Acknowledgements: The author thanks K. D. Bloch, M. D., R. M. Kacmarek, Ph. D. and M. Takata, M. D., Ph. D. for critical reviews of this manuscript.

References

1. Kollef MH, Schuster DP (1995) The acute respiratory distress syndrome. N Engl J Med 332: 27–37
2. Dreyfuss D, Saumon G (1994) Ventilator-induced lung injury. In: Tobin MJ (ed) Principles and practice of mechanical ventilation. Mc Graw Hill, New York, pp 793–811
3. Parker JC, Hernandez LA, Peevy KJ (1993) Mechanisms of ventilator-induced lung injury. Crit Care Med 21:131–143
4. Marini JJ (1996) Evolving concepts in the ventilatory management of acute respiratory distress syndrome. Clin Chest Med 17:555–575
5. Milberg JA, Davis DR, Steinberg KP, Hudson LD (1995) Improved survival of patients with acute respiratory distress syndrome (ARDS): 1983–1993. JAMA 273:306–309

6. Montgomery AB, Stager MA, Carrico CJ, Hudson LD (1985) Causes of mortality in patients with the adult respiratory distress syndrome. Am Rev Respir Dis 132:485–489
7. Imai Y, Kawano T, Miyasaka K, Takata M, Imai T, Okuyama K (1994) Inflammatory chemical mediators during conventional ventilation and during high frequency oscillatory ventilation. Am J Respir Crit Care Med 150:1550–1554
8. Takata M, Abe J, Tanaka H, et al (1997) Intraalveolar expression of tumor necrosis factor alpha gene during conventional and high-frequency ventilation. Am J Respir Crit Care Med 156:272–279
9. Tremblay L, Valenza F, Ribeiro SP, Li J, Slutsky AS (1997) Injurious ventilatory strategies increase cytokines and c-fos m-RNA expression in an isolated rat lung model. J Clin Invest 99:944–952
10. Dreyfuss D, Soler P, Saumon G (1995) Mechanical ventilation-induced pulmonary edema. Interaction with previous lung alterations. Am J Respir Crit Care Med 151:1568–1575
11. Dreyfuss D, Saumon G (1993) Role of tidal volume, FRC, and end-inspiratory volume in the development of pulmonary edema following mechanical ventilation. Am Rev Respir Dis 148:1194–1203
12. Dreyfuss D, Soler P, Basset G, Saumon G (1988) High inflation pressure pulmonary edema. Respective effects of high airway pressure, high tidal volume, and positive end-expiratory pressure. Am Rev Respir Dis 137:1159–1164
13. Dreyfuss D, Basset G, Soler P, Saumon G (1985) Intermittent positive-pressure hyperventilation with high inflation pressures produces pulmonary microvascular injury in rats. Am Rev Respir Dis 132:880–884
14. Muscedere JG, Mullen JB, Gan K, Slutsky AS (1994) Tidal ventilation at low airway pressures can augment lung injury. Am J Respir Crit Care Med 149:1327–1334
15. Slutsky AS (1994) Consensus conference on mechanical ventilation – Part I. Intensive Care Med 20:64–79
16. Roupie E, Dambrosio M, Servillo G, et al (1995) Titration of tidal volume and induced hypercapnia in acute respiratory distress syndrome. Am J Respir Crit Care Med 152:121–128
17. Brunet F, Jeanbourquin D, Monchi M, et al (1995) Should mechanical ventilation be optimized to blood gases, lung mechanics, or thoracic CT scan? Am J Respir Crit Care Med 152:524–530
18. Amato MB, Barbas CS, Medeiros DM, et al (1995) Beneficial effects of the "open lung approach" with low distending pressures in acute respiratory distress syndrome. A prospective randomized study on mechanical ventilation. Am J Respir Crit Care Med 152:1835–1846
19. Amato MBP, Barbas CSV, Medeiros D, et al (1996) Improved survival in ARDS: beneficial effects of a lung protective strategy. Am J Respir Crit Care Med 153:A531 (Abst)
20. Donnelly TJ, Meade P, Jagels M, et al (1994) Cytokine, complement, and endotoxin profiles associated with the development of the adult respiratory distress syndrome after severe injury. Crit Care Med 22:768–776
21. Meduri GU, Kohler G, Headley S, Tolley E, Stentz F, Postlethwaite A (1995) Inflammatory cytokines in the BAL of patients with ARDS. Persistent elevation over time predicts poor outcome. Chest 108:1303–1314
22. Hamilton PP, Onayemi A, Smyth JA, et al (1983) Comparison of conventional and high-frequency ventilation: oxygenation and lung pathology. J Appl Physiol 55:131–138
23. Kawano T, Mori S, Cybulsky M, et al (1987) Effect of granulocyte depletion in a ventilated surfactant-depleted lung. J Appl Physiol 62:27–33
24. Sugiura M, McCulloch PR, Wren S, Dawson RH, Froese AB (1994) Ventilator pattern influences neutrophil influx and activation in atelectasis-prone rabbit lung. J Appl Physiol 77:1355–1365
25. Sadoshima J, Izumo S (1997) The cellular and molecular response of cardiac myocytes to mechanical stress. Annu Rev Physiol 59:551–571
26. Vandenburgh HH (1992) Mechanical forces and their second messengers in stimulating cell growth in vitro. Am J Physiol 262:R350–R355
27. Rannels DE (1989) Role of physical forces in compensatory growth of the lung. Am J Physiol 257:L179–L189
28. Mattana J, Sankaran RT, Singhal PC (1995) Repetitive mechanical strain suppresses macrophage uptake of immunoglobulin G complexes and enhances cyclic adenosine monophosphate synthesis. Am J Pathol 147:529–540
29. Watson PA (1991) Function follows form: generation of intracellular signals by cell deformation. FASEB J 5:2013–2019

30. Liu M, Xu J, Liu J, Kraw ME, Tanswell AK, Post M (1995) Mechanical strain-enhanced fetal lung cell proliferation is mediated by phospholipase C and D and protein kinase C. Am J Physiol 268:L729–L738

31. Rannels DE, Rannels SR (1989) Influence of the extracellular matrix on type 2 cell differentiation. Chest 96:165–173

32. Waters CM (1996) Flow-induced modulation of the permeability of endothelial cells cultured on microcarrier beads. J Cell Physiol 168:403–411

33. Wirtz HR, Dobbs LG (1990) Calcium mobilization and exocytosis after one mechanical stretch of lung epithelial cells. Science 250:1266–1269

34. Martin DK, Bootcov MR, Campbell TJ, French PW, Breit SN (1995) Human macrophages contain a stretch-sensitive potassium channel that is activated by adherence and cytokines. J Membr Biol 147:305–315

35. Sachs F (1991) Mechanical transduction by membrane ion channels: a mini review. Mol Cell Biochem 104:57–60

36. Demling RH (1993) Adult respiratory distress syndrome: current concepts. New Horizons 1:388–401

37. Matsuoka T, Kawano T, Miyasaka K (1994) Role of high-frequency ventilation in surfactant-depleted lung injury as measured by granulocytes. J Appl Physiol 76:539–544

38. Woo SW, Hedley-Whyte J (1972) Macrophage accumulation and pulmonary edema due to thoracotomy and lung over inflation. J Appl Physiol 33:14–21

39. Kitagawa Y, Van Eeden SF, Redenbach DM, et al (1997) Effect of mechanical deformation on structure and function of polymorphonuclear leukocytes. J Appl Physiol 82:1397–1405

40. Downey GP (1997) Effect of mechanical deformation on structure and function of polymorphonuclear leukocytes. J Appl Physiol 82:1395–1396

41. Sadoshima J, Izumo S (1993) Mechanical stretch rapidly activates multiple signal transduction pathways in cardiac myocytes: potential involvement of an autocrine/paracrine mechanism. Embo J 12:1681–1692

42. Nagase T, Fukuchi Y, Shimizu T, Matsuse T, Orimo H (1990) Reduction of 15-hydroxy-eicosatetraenoic acid (15-HETE) in tracheal fluid by high frequency oscillatory ventilation. Prostaglandins Leukot Essent Fatty Acids 40:177–180

43. von Bethmann AV, Brasch F, Muller KM, Uhlig S (1996) Barotrauma induced cytokin- and eicosanoid-release from the isolated perfused and ventilated mouse lung. Am J Respir Crit Care Med 153:A530 (Abst)

44. Taskar V, John J, Evander E, Robertson B, Jonson B (1997) Surfactant dysfunction makes lungs vulnerable to repetitive collapse and reexpansion. Am J Respir Crit Care Med 155:313–320

45. Veldhuizen RA, Ito Y, Marcou J, Yao LJ, McCaig L, Lewis JF (1997) Effects of lung injury on pulmonary surfactant aggregate conversion in vivo and in vitro. Am J Physiol 272:L872–L878

46. Veldhuizen RA, Marcou J, Yao LJ, McCaig L, Ito Y, Lewis JF (1996) Alveolar surfactant aggregate conversion in ventilated normal and injured rabbits. Am J Physiol 270:L152–L158

47. Ito Y, Veldhuizen RA, Yao LJ, McCaig LA, Bartlett AJ, Lewis JF (1997) Ventilation strategies affect surfactant aggregate conversion in acute lung injury. Am J Respir Crit Care Med 155:493–499

48. Veldhuizen RA, McCaig LA, Akino T, Lewis JF (1995) Pulmonary surfactant subfractions in patients with the acute respiratory distress syndrome. Am J Respir Crit Care Med 152:1867–1871

49. Froese AB, McCulloch PR, Sugiura M, Vaclavik S, Possmayer F, Moller F (1993) Optimizing alveolar expansion prolongs the effectiveness of exogenous surfactant therapy in the adult rabbit. Am Rev Respir Dis 148:569–577

50. Pison U, Max M, Neuendank A, Weissbach S, Pietschmann S (1994) Host defence capacities of pulmonary surfactant: evidence for 'non-surfactant' functions of the surfactant system. Eur J Clin Invest 24:586–599

51. Geertsma MF, Teeuw WL, Nibbering PH, Van Furth R (1994) Pulmonary surfactant inhibits activation of human monocytes by recombinant interferon-gamma. Immunology 82:450–456

52. Blau H, Riklis S, Van Iwaarden JF, McCormack FX, Kalina M (1997) Nitric oxide production by rat alveolar macrophages can be modulated in vitro by surfactant protein A. Am J Physiol 272:L1198–L1204

53. Antal JM, Divis LT, Erzurum SC, Wiedemann HP, Thomassen MJ (1996) Surfactant suppresses NF-kappa B activation in human monocytic cells. Am J Respir Cell Mol Biol 14:374–379

54. Fu Z, Costello ML, Tsukimoto K, et al (1992) High lung volume increases stress failure in pulmonary capillaries. J Appl Physiol 73: 123–133
55. Nahum A, Hoyt J, McKibben A, et al (1996) Effect of mechanical ventilation strategy on E. Coli pneumonia in dogs. Am J Respir Crit Care Med 153: A530 (Abst)
56. Fukushima R, Alexander JW, Gianotti L, Ogle CK (1994) Isolated pulmonary infection acts as a source of systemic tumor necrosis factor. Crit Care Med 22: 114–120
57. Tutor JD, Mason CM, Dobard E, Beckerman RC, Summer WR, Nelson S (1994) Loss of compartmentalization of alveolar tumor necrosis factor after lung injury. Am J Respir Crit Care Med 149: 1107–1111
58. Debs RJ, Fuchs HJ, Philip R, et al (1988) Lung-specific delivery of cytokines induces sustained pulmonary and systemic immunomodulation in rats. J Immunol 140: 3482–3488
59. Vara E, Arias-Diaz J, Garcia C, Hernandez J, Balibrea JL (1996) TNF-alpha-induced inhibition of PC synthesis by human type II pneumocytes is sequentially mediated by PGE2 and NO. Am J Physiol 271: L359–L365
60. Bachurski CJ, Pryhuber GS, Glasser SW, Kelly SE, Whitsett JA (1995) Tumor necrosis factor-alpha inhibits surfactant protein C gene transcription. J Biol Chem 270: 19402–19407

Mechanical Ventilation-Induced Injury

L. N. Tremblay and A. S. Slutsky

Introduction

Mechanical ventilation is an indispensable supportive intervention in intensive care medicine. However, ventilatory support can have a number of adverse sequelae directly on the lung, and indirectly on distal organs. In this review, we examine the manifestations and proposed pathophysiology of ventilator-induced injury, as well as the rationale behind several ventilatory strategies that have been suggested to minimize or prevent ventilator associated morbidity and mortality.

Ventilator-Induced Lung Injury

Classic Barotrauma – Airleaks

Gross barotrauma manifesting as airleaks was one of the earliest recognized complications of ventilatory support. Macklin et al. [1] demonstrated that disruption of the respiratory epithelium at the juncture of the alveolar base and the bronchovascular sheath could occur with high airway pressures, allowing air to escape into the pulmonary interstitium and track along the bronchovesicular sheaths leading to pneumomediastinum, pneumopericardium, pneumoretroperitoneum, subcutaneous emphysema, pneumothorax, and/or pneumoperitoneum.

Although airway pressures are often monitored in clinical practice, and although high airway pressures are thought to be the critical factor leading to gross barotrauma, as Macklin realized, it is the gradient between alveolar pressure and the bronchovesicular pressure which is the likely causative factor. After all, trumpet players can tolerate airway pressures in excess of 150 cmH$_2$O without developing airleaks [2]. Factors that lead to alveolar overdistension [high end inspiratory lung volumes, auto-positive end-expiratory pressure (PEEP)], as well as factors that affect underlying tissue resilience (e.g., lung disease, malnutrition, age) predispose patients to barotrauma [3, 4]. Of note, due to the heterogeneous distribution of lung injury, consolidation and/or pulmonary edema in critically ill patients, it is possible for barotrauma to occur secondary to regional overdistension of alveoli even in the absence of overall lung overdistension. In a recent multivariate analysis of patients requiring ventilation for greater than 24 hours, only the presence of acute respiratory distress syndrome (ARDS), independently correlated with the risk of developing pneumothorax [3]. Thus, the association of airleaks with high ventilatory pressures noted in early studies may have been more a reflection of the severity of the patient's under-lying lung injury necessitating ventilation with high airway pressures, rather than the airway pressures *per se* causing the injury [5l.

Diffuse Lung Injury

In addition to airleaks, mechanical ventilation has been shown to cause diffuse lung injury. Lung injury very similar to that seen in ARDS has been produced by high pressure/high volume ventilation in animals (Fig. 1). In this study, young pigs venti-lated for 22 hours with high peak inspiratory pressures [PIP 40 cmH$_2$O, PEEP 3–5 cmH$_2$O, respiratory rate 20 bpm, inspired oxygen fraction (FiO$_2$) 0.4] developed alveolar hemorrhage, alveolar neutrophil infiltration, alveolar macrophage and type II pneumocyte proliferation, interstitial congestion and thickening, interstitial lym-phocyte infiltration, emphysematous changes, and hyaline membrane formation; histologic findings similar to those of early ARDS. More prolonged ventilation (3–6 days) led to organized alveolar exudate, similar to that found in the later stages of ARDS. However, animals ventilated with lower PIP (18 cmH$_2$O) developed no signif-icant changes in either lung function or histology. In a number of other studies, using a variety of animal species, mechanical ventilation has also been found to pro-duce alterations in alveolar capillary permeability, pulmonary edema, surfactant in-activation, hyaline membrane formation, leukocyte infiltration, and impaired gas exchange [6–11].

Clinically, it is difficult to distinguish ventilator induced injury from injury secon-dary to the underlying disease process or combinations of these factors. Certainly, findings such as hyaline membranes were infrequently seen prior to the introduc-tion of mechanical ventilation into clinical practice [12, 13]. A recent post-mortem examination of the lungs of critically ill ventilated patients found evidence of air-space enlargement (alveolar overdistension in aerated lung areas or intraparenchy-mal pseudocysts in non-aerated lung areas) in 26/30 patients [4]. Severe airspace enlargement, associated with a greater incidence of pneumothorax, correlated with exposure to higher PIP, larger tidal volumes, more prolonged use of high FiO$_2$, and a greater decrease in body weight over the intensive care unit (ICU) stay. Other features of barotrauma were also found, including pleural cysts, bronchiolar dila-tion, alveolar overdistension and intraparenchymal pseudocysts. Using serial high resolution computer tomography, investigators have noted persistent abnormalities of lung structure principally in the anterior lung regions of ARDS survivors who re-quired prolonged ventilation (86 to 97 days) [14], or emphysema-like lesions and cysts predominantly in dependent lung zones, with an apparent relationship between the number and spatial distribution of the lesions, and the duration of ARDS [15].

Pathogenesis of Ventilator-Induced Lung Injury

Structural Disruption

The spectrum of ventilator-induced lung injury extends from subtle ultrastructural breaks, to gross lung disruption. There are a number of mechanisms whereby me-

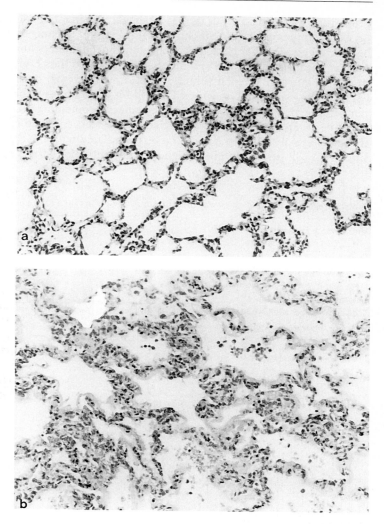

Fig. 1. a) Lung from non-ventilated pig. No histologic abnormalities aside from slight pulmonary congestion and thickening of alveolar septa. **b)** Lung from a pig ventilated with PIP of 40 cmH$_2$O, FiO$_2$ of 0.4 for 42 h. Severe lesions consisting of disruption of epithelial lining, hyaline membrane formation, alveolar hemorrhage, alveolar neutrophil infiltration, alveolar macrophage and type II pneumocyte proliferation, interstitial thickening and fibrosis, and endothelial swelling. (From [8] with permission)

chanical ventilation may generate sufficient stress on the lung to produce structural injury.

Direct force: Mechanical ventilation can exert excessive force directly on the lung tissue. In recent years, the term volutrauma (injury as a result of lung overdistension) has often been substituted for the term barotrauma (injury as a result of excessive pressure). The reason for this is, that although pressure and volume are dependent (as can be appreciated from pressure-volume loops of the lung), airway pressure can be affected by a number of factors completely independent of lung volume (Table 1). And, as has been illustrated by a number of studies, unless high airway pressure is translated into high alveolar volume, significant lung injury does not ensue [16–19]. For example, when rabbits encased in plaster casts to limit chest expansion were ventilated with PIP of 45 cmH$_2$O, neither macroscopic lung injury nor changes in pulmonary capillary filtration coefficients were seen. In sharp contrast, significant changes were observed in normal rabbits ventilated with the same pressures [17]. Similarly, as illustrated in Fig. 2, high volume ventilation of rats (using either posi-

Table 1. Examples where high airway pressures may not reflect high lung volumes

High airway resistance
   e.g., secretions, bronchospasm
Increased endotracheal tube resistance
   e.g., small diameter tube, kinking or partial obstruction
High inspiratory gas flow rates
Increased pleural pressure
   e.g., stiff chest wall, splinting, obesity, pregnancy, ascites, pleural effusions, pneumothorax
Decreased chest wall compliance

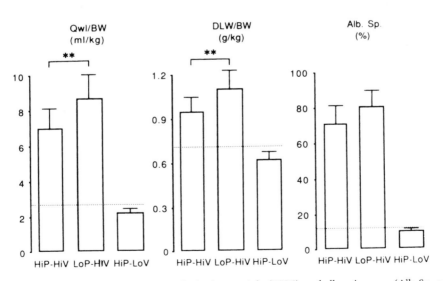

Fig. 2. Extravascular lung water (Qwl), dry lung weight (DLW), and albumin space (Alb. Sp., a reflection of ^{125}I-labeled albumin leakage from the pulmonary vessels) in rats ventilated with high airway pressure and high tidal volume (HiP-HiV), low pressure and high volume (LoP-HiV), and high pressure and low volume (HiP-LoV). Horizontal dotted lines represent the 95% confidence limit for control values. HiP-HiV and LoP-HiV were always different from controls (p<0.001). Differences between groups: ** indicates p<0.01. (From [19] with permission)

tive or negative pressure ventilation) was found to cause significant increases in extravascular lung water, while low volume-high pressure ventilation of rats (chest excursions restricted by thoracoabdominal straps) was comparable to controls [19].

At the ultrastructural level, disruption of alveolar epithelium, capillary endothelium, or sometimes all layers of the alveolar-capillary membrane (associated with increases in physiologic parameters of lung permeability) have been found to occur after brief periods (i.e., 5–10 min) of over-distension with high pressure (45 cmH$_2$O PIP) ventilation in rats [20, 21]. If the ventilatory strategy causing over-distension was continued for more prolonged periods, severe lung injury ensued (e.g., hyaline membranes, profound changes in epithelial integrity). However, the injury was reversible and lung function reverted to normal if the over-distension was discontinued sufficiently early [22].

Fu et al. [23] found that both the transcapillary pressure gradient, as well as lung volume are important in the pathogenesis of these breaks in the alveolar-capillary membrane (Fig. 3). Increased numbers of breaks were seen at higher lung volumes despite similar transcapillary wall pressures. These lesions are thought to be responsible, in part, for the increase in alveolar epithelial permeability and pulmonary edema found during mechanical ventilation at high lung volumes [24–26].

In a series of studies in rats, Dreyfuss and colleagues [16] demonstrated that end-inspiratory lung volume, rather than the tidal volume or functional residual capacity (FRC) appeared to be the major determinant of ventilation-induced edema. In these studies, doubling the tidal volume did not lead to pulmonary edema unless PEEP was added to increase end-inspiratory lung volumes [16], while even small tidal volume ventilation lead to pulmonary edema if combined with sufficiently high PEEP.

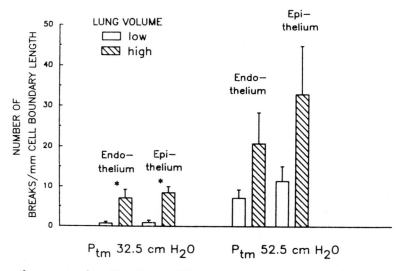

Fig. 3. Histogram of average number of breaks per millimeter boundary length of endothelium and epithelium at 20 (high lung volume) and 5 cmH$_2$O transpulmonary pressure (low lung volume). * Significantly greater (p < 0.05) at high compared to low lung volume at the same capillary Ptm. (From [23] with permission)

Heterogeneity and Interdependence: Regional disparities in ventilation (e.g., secondary to atelectasis) can significantly magnify the forces on adjacent alveoli as a result of the interdependence of alveolar units. Restated, the alveolar walls of the lung form "honeycomb" structures. When uniformly inflated, the force exerted on each alveolar wall by the neighboring alveolar wall can be simplified as a function of the transpulmonary pressure (i.e., P_{alv}-P_{pl}). In the presence of atelectasis, however, the "pull" of surrounding expanded alveoli on the collapsed alveoli increases significantly. Mead et al. [27] postulated that at a transpulmonary pressure of 30 cmH$_2$O, "the pressure tending to expand an atelectatic region surrounded by a fully expanded lung would be approximately 140 cmH$_2$O".

Shear: In an injured lung, there is an increased tendency for alveoli and distal airways to collapse secondary to impaired surfactant function, and the weight of overlying edematous or inflamed lung. At low lung volumes, this tendency to collapse is further increased due to reduced parenchymal tethering forces. As illustrated by computer tomography of patients with early ARDS, the pressure required to re-open the alveoli and distal airways will vary, depending on the position within the lung [28]. The result is that during ventilation, in addition to alveolar regions that are completely open during the ventilatory cycle, or that are completely closed, there are alveoli that repetitively open and collapse with each breath.

The shear forces generated during this repetitive "ripping open" of closed airways and alveoli has been postulated to play a role in the lung injury observed (i.e., hyaline membranes and distal airway epithelial injury) with ventilation strategies using low or no PEEP [29, 30]. For example, in a surfactant deficient *ex vivo* lung model, ventilation with either no PEEP or PEEP less than the lower inflection point (i.e., point 1 in Fig. 5) produced significantly more injury (epithelial necrosis, sloughing, and development of hyaline membranes) than that seen in lungs ventilated with PEEP greater than the inflection point [31]. The distribution of the lesions was dependent upon the level of PEEP used; in the zero PEEP group the injury was more proximal (i.e., respiratory and membranous bronchioli), and in the low PEEP group it was more distal (alveolar ducts). Other studies have shown that lung injury can be reduced if ventilation is carried out using sufficient (but not excessive) end-expiratory volumes [6, 31–33]. Of note, aside from preventing alveolar collapse and allowing more uniform distribution of ventilation, ventilation strategies that maintain FRC (e.g., high PEEP, HFV, lung rest) may also prevent lung injury through hemodynamic effects [16], as well as effects on surfactant function.

Surfactant Dysfunction

Another mechanism by which mechanical ventilation is thought to cause lung injury, is via impairment of normal surfactant function. Aside from maintaining low surface tension in the alveoli and distal airways, surfactant has a number of other important functions including immunomodulatory effects [34].

Studies have shown that mechanical ventilation strategy can have significant effects on both endogenous as well as exogenous surfactant [11, 35–38] For example, mechanical ventilation of healthy dogs with peak inflation pressures of 26–32 cmH$_2$O leads to diffuse atelectasis within 24 hours, accompanied by an increase in the minimum surface tension of lung lavage fluid [10]. The increase in surface tension was found to be directly related to tidal volume and duration of ventilation, and inversely related to end-expiratory lung volume [11].

In vitro, Brown et al. [39] noted that although surfactant films could be reversibly compressed up to 50% of the initial surface area, further compression resulted in rupture on re-expansion. As well, repetitive alveolar collapse has been suggested to result in "pumping" of surfactant out of the alveoli [40]. Thus, the protective effects of ventilatory strategies that maintain FRC, may be due in part to prevention of these two phenomena [11, 40, 41].

Surfactant dysfunction is also known to further increase the susceptibility of the lung to injury by mechanical ventilation [42–44]. Even very mild alterations in surfactant, such as those produced by prolonged anesthesia in rats, have been found to synergistically augment the deleterious effects of high volume ventilation. For example, although only mild injury was found in lungs subjected to either ventilation or surfactant inactivation (with dioctyl succinate), extensive lung injury was found when both insults were combined [42].

"Biotrauma" – Inflammatory Cell and Mediator Induced Injury

More recently, attention has turned to the possible role of inflammatory cells and mediators in the pathogenesis of ventilation induced lung injury. In a surfactant depleted rabbit model, significant lung injury (consisting of poor gas exchange, increased pulmonary permeability and edema, neutrophil infiltration, and hyaline membrane formation), originally attributed to barotrauma, was found to be almost completely abrogated in granulocyte depleted rabbits [33]. Mechanical ventilation strategy was also shown to have significant effects on both neutrophil influx and activation [45, 46]. The effects of ventilation on granulocytes extended beyond the lung, as changes in circulating neutrophil chemotaxis were also found (although no changes in activation as assessed by chemiluminescence were found).

In the same surfactant depleted model, more severe lung injury and higher concentrations of the mediators platelet-activating factor (PAF) and thromboxane-B_2 were found in the lung lavage fluid of rabbits subjected to pressure control ventilation (mean airway pressure of 15 cmH$_2$O, PIP $= 25$ cmH$_2$O, PEEP $= 5$ cmH$_2$O) as compared to high frequency oscillatory ventilation [47]. In normal rat lungs, ventilation strategy was shown to have a significant effect on lavage concentrations of a number of inflammatory mediators (Fig. 4) [48]. In this study, mechanical ventilation with high end-inspiratory pressure/high PEEP (V_T 15 ml/kg, PEEP 10 cmH$_2$O) increased the lung lavage concentration of tumor necrosis factor-α (TNF-α) twofold as compared to control ventilation. Ventilation using the same tidal volume (15 ml/kg) but no PEEP increased lung lavage concentrations of TNF-α three-fold as compared to control ventilation. However, high end-inspiratory lung volume ventilation in combination with zero PEEP (V_T 40 ml/kg) had a synergistic effect, resulting in a 56 fold increase in lavage TNF-α relative to the control ventilation strategy. Narimanbekov et al. [49] demonstrated both reduced lung lavage concentrations of a number of markers of lung injury (i.e., albumin, elastase, neutrophils), as well as reduced structural injury, if an interleukin (IL)-1 receptor antagonist was administered prior to ventilation in a hyperoxia-surfactant deficient rabbit injury model. Of note, no improvement was observed in either lung compliance or oxygenation, suggesting that other mediators (e.g., cytokines, arachidonic acid derivatives, comple-

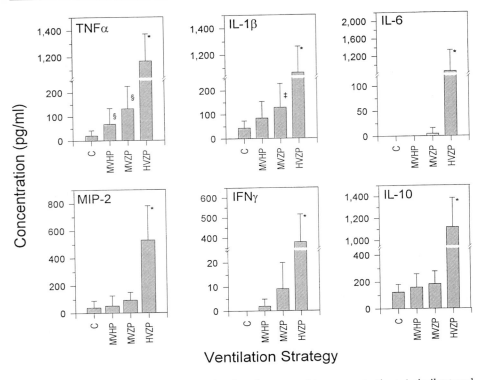

Fig. 4. Effect of ventilation strategy on absolute lung lavage cytokine concentrations. A similar trend was seen for all cytokines, with lowest levels in the control group (C: $V_T = 7$ ml/kg; PEEP = 3 cmH$_2$O) and highest in the high volume-zero PEEP group (HVZP: $V_T = 40$ ml/kg). Second highest levels were seen with moderate volume-zero PEEP ventilation (MVZP: $V_T = 15$ ml/kg). Despite similar end-inspiratory distention, moderate volume-high PEEP ventilation (MVHP: $V_T = 15$ ml/kg; PEEP = 10 cmH$_2$O) had significantly lower lung lavage cytokine concentrations than HVZP ventilation. * $p < 0.05$ vs. Control, MVHP, MVZP; ‡ $p < 0.05$ vs. Control, MVHP; § $p < 0.05$ vs. Control. (From [48] with permission)

ment, reactive oxygen species, cationic proteins, and proteolytic enzymes [50, 51]) as well as physical forces are involved in this lung injury model.

Effect of Underlying Lung Injury

Not unexpectedly, the presence of underlying lung injury significantly increases the risk of ventilator-induced lung injury. Intuitively, it is appreciated that factors that either weaken the lung or increase stress on the lung should lead to greater lung injury. Thus, it is not surprising that in patients with gastric acid aspiration and histologic evidence of tissue necrosis, the incidence of airleaks was significantly higher (50%) than in a patients with normal lungs (4%) [52]; or that a higher incidence of pneumothoraces correlated with pathologic findings of increased numbers of bullae, intraparenchymal pseudocysts, pleural cysts, bronchiolar and alveolar overdistension [4].

Experimentally, lung injury has been found to have a synergistic effect with mechanical ventilation in worsening injury in a variety of animal models. For example, Hernandez et al. [53] demonstrated that low doses of oleic acid or mechanical ventilation alone did not increase capillary filtration coefficients; however, the combination of oleic acid and mechanical ventilation lead to significant lung injury. Other factors that have been found to predispose to barotrauma include underlying lung disease, malnutrition, oxygen toxicity, infection, and age [1, 3, 4].

Another consideration is the heterogeneous distribution of ventilation that may occur in the presence of underlying lung injury. For example, patients with ARDS can have significant collapse of dependent lung regions resulting in a smaller volume of aerated lung which can be as low as 20% of the volume of a normal lung [54]. Thus, delivery of even modest tidal volumes (such as 10 ml/kg), may result in overdistension of the aerated lung units equivalent to what would be observed if healthy lungs were ventilated with tidal volumes of 50 ml/kg.

Role of Mechanical Ventilation in Systemic Morbidity and Mortality

Aside from direct effects on the lung, mechanical ventilation may also have systemic sequelae. First, ventilation strategy is known to have significant effects on cardiac output, as well as to affect both oxygenation and the distribution of blood flow to various organs (e.g., mesenteric, renal and hepatic perfusion) [55–57]. Second, as discussed, mechanical ventilation has been found to have effects on both inflammatory cells and inflammatory mediators. Although in normal lungs such inflammatory mediators would remain largely compartmentalized within the alveolar space [58], in the presence of increased alveolar capillary permeability (as may occur with either ventilator-induced lung injury or ARDS), such compartmentalization may be lost. Utilizing an isolated perfused lung model, Uhlig et al. [59] have demonstrated a significant increase in TNF-α and IL-6 levels in the perfusate of lungs ventilated with transpulmonary pressures of 25 cmH$_2$O versus 10 cmH$_2$O. The presence of inflammatory mediators in the circulation has been shown to be involved in the pathophysiology of multiple organ dysfunction and failure [60, 61]. Third, in dogs which had E. coli instilled into their lungs, mechanical ventilation with higher transpulmonary pressures (35 cmH$_2$O, 3 cmH$_2$O PEEP) had a higher incidence of bacteremia versus those ventilated with either similar transpulmonary pressures with 10 cmH$_2$O of PEEP, or lower transpulmonary pressures (15 cmH$_2$O) [62]. High versus lower tidal volume ventilation (20 ml/kg vs. 10 ml/kg) has also been found to increase distal ileal permeability in rats [63]. Thus, mechanical ventilation may play a role in bacterial translocation into the circulation.

A number of animal studies have also shown that ventilation strategy could have a significant effect on mortality [6, 33, 45–47]. Since many of these studies were designed to look only at the early effects of ventilation (i.e., within a few hours), most deaths were attributed to a progressive deterioration in gas exchange and hypoxia. However, in one study examining mild and severe ventilator-induced lung injury in normal sheep, mechanical ventilation was continued until either successful weaning or death. The cause of death in the group with severe lung injury (and 8/11 sheep with mild lung injury) was progressive hypotension unresponsive to intravenous fluids, and multi-organ failure, the pathophysiology of which was unclear [64].

Clinically, a number of trials assessing the efficacy of certain ventilatory strategies have used mortality as an endpoint. To date, of the prospective randomized trials looking at mechanical ventilation in adults, a significant reduction in mortality was found in one study which utilized a strategy with high PEEP and low end inspiratory pressures [65]. Further confirmation of this exciting observation is needed, however, in light of the high mortality in the control group, and the relatively small number of patients enrolled in this single center trial.

Prevention of Ventilation-Induced Lung Injury

In theory, the risk of injury secondary to mechanical ventilation would be minimized or eliminated, if a ventilatory strategy was used that uniformly maintained alveolar recruitment (i.e., avoided repetitive distal airway/alveolar opening and collapse) without causing alveolar overdistension or adverse hemodynamic changes due to lung inflation (i.e., ventilation taking place on the mid-portion of the pressure volume loop of the lung as depicted in Fig. 5).

There are, however, many controversial issues on how best to achieve this objective. In certain patients, such as some patients with early ARDS, a lower "inflection" point (P_{inf}) on the ascending limb of the pressure-volume curve can be identified, and is thought to represent the opening pressure at which many collapsed alveolar units are recruited. On the descending limb of the pressure-volume loop, another "inflection" point may be seen, and is thought to represent the critical closing volume or pressure for a number of alveoli. It has been suggested, therefore, that to prevent lung injury from alveolar opening and collapse with each breath, the lung should be recruited and kept open with an end-expiratory pressure greater than these points. But, what of those patients in whom no clear lower inflection points are seen? Also, alveolar recruitment can occur over most of the breadth of the P-V curve. Computer tomography of supine patients with early ARDS found an increase in P_{inf} as one progressed from non-dependent to dependent lung zones [28]. Thus, although a given PEEP may be sufficient to splint open some regions of the lung, other regions may either remain collapsed, be subjected to tidal recruitment, or become overdistended.

In other patients, a clearly identifiable upper inflection point is also seen (Fig. 5) and is thought to represent the pressure beyond which few alveoli are recruited, and those already open, become further distended. Thus, to minimize lung injury secondary to overdistension, the tidal volume superimposed on the end-expiratory lung volume should not lead to ventilation on this upper less compliant portion of the P-V curve. For those patients in whom this point is not identifiable, it has been recommended that plateau pressure be limited to less than 35 cmH$_2$O [66]. However, in certain patients with acute lung injury, in whom chest wall compliance is diminished [67], ventilation at higher pressures would not necessarily translate into the same

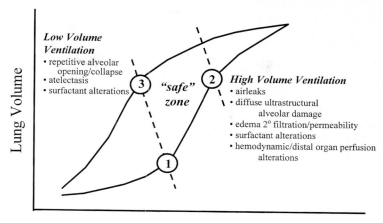

Transpulmonary Pressure (cm H$_2$O)

Fig. 5. Schematic depiction of a static P-V curve of the respiratory system in ARDS. In the early phase of lung injury two "inflection" points (depicted as 1 and 2) are sometimes seen on the inspiratory limb, and one (depicted as 3) on the deflation limb. 1, represents the pressure at which a large number of alveoli open. 2, the point above which a loss of compliance secondary to lung overdistension occurs (i.e. the point at which no further alveoli are recruited, so that those already open must increase in size to accommodate the volume of air). 3, the critical closing pressure of a large number of alveoli. To minimize ventilator induced lung injury, it is suggested that ventilation be carried out on the mid region of the P-V curve

higher, potentially injurious lung volumes as in patients with normal chest wall compliance. In such patients, it may be necessary to measure transpulmonary pressure (P_{alv}-P_{pl}) which is a more appropriate measure of alveolar distention.

Table 2 lists modifications of conventional ventilation strategies, as well as some non-conventional mechanical ventilation strategies, that have been proposed to try and reduce ventilator induced or association morbidity and mortality. To date, no distinct advantage of one technique over another has been identified, although a number of clinical trials are ongoing.

Conclusion

There is no doubt that mechanical ventilation can initiate or exacerbate lung injury. Evidence is also emerging, that how we ventilate the lung may have a number of systemic ramifications and may also have a significant effect on mortality. Experimental studies have shown surfactant dysfunction, changes in inflammatory cells and mediators, as well as structural disruption of the lung at the ultrastructural and macroscopic levels, as a result of mechanical ventilation. These studies have also demonstrated that if extremes of lung volume (overdistension or atelectasis with recurrent opening/collapse) are avoided, lung injury may be abrogated. Practically, in

Table 2. Approaches for limiting ventilator induced lung injury

Avoidance of intubation
- non-invasive positive pressure ventilation
- cuirass negative pressure ventilation

Avoidance of high lung volumes
- pressure and volume limited ventilation
- IVOX, extracorporeal CO_2 removal ($ECCO_2R$) to assist in gas exchange
- Tracheal gas insufflation to minimize tidal volume

Avoidance of low lung volumes (and repetitive opening/collapse)
- sufficient positive end-expiratory pressure (PEEP)
- partial liquid ventilation ("liquid PEEP")
- high frequency ventilation

Improved distribution of ventilation and V/Q matching
- inverse-ratio ventilation
- partial liquid ventilation
- high frequency ventilation
- prone positioning

Adjuvant therapies in combination with mechanical ventilation
- surfactant supplementation
- nitric oxide $\pm$ almitrine

the heterogenously injured lung, applying this objective can be difficult. As such, several novel ventilatory strategies and co-interventions are being explored. However, given the variety of mechanisms thought to be involved in the pathogenesis of ventilator induced lung injury, it is improbable that a single ventilatory strategy will emerge as a panacea for all patients requiring ventilatory assistance.

References

1. Macklin MT, Macklin CC (1944) Malignant interstitial emphysema of the lungs and mediastinum as an important occult complication in many respiratory diseases and other conditions: An interpretation of the clinical literature in the light of laboratory experiment. Medicine 23:281–352
2. Bouhuys A (1969) Physiology and musical instruments. Nature 221:1199–1204
3. Gammon RB, Shin MS, Groves RH, Jr, Hardin MJ, Hsu C, Buchalter SE (1995) Clinical risk factors for pulmonary barotrauma: A multivariate analysis. Am J Respir Crit Care Med 152:1235–1240
4. Rouby JJ, Lherm T, de Lassale EM, et al (1993) Histologic aspects of pulmonary barotrauma in critically ill patients with acute respiratory failure. Intensive Care Med 19:383–389
5. Petersen GW, Baier H (1983) Incidence of pulmonary barotrauma in a medical ICU. Crit Care Med 11:67–69
6. Webb HH, Tierney DF (1974) Experimental pulmonary edema due to intermittent positive pressure ventilation with high inflation pressures. Protection by positive end-expiratory pressure. Am Rev Respir Dis 110:556–565
7. Kolobow T, Moretti MP, Fumagalli R, et al (1987) Severe impairment in lung function induced by high peak airway pressure during mechanical ventilation. Am Rev Respir Dis 135:312–315
8. Tsuno K, Miura K, Takeya M, Kolobow T, Morioka T (1991) Histopathologic pulmonary changes from mechanical ventilation at high peak airway pressures. Am Rev Respir Dis 143:1115–1120
9. Parker JC, Hernandez LA, Longenecker GL, Peevy K, Johnson W (1990) Lung edema caused by high peak inspiratory pressures in dogs. Am Rev Respir Dis 142:321–328

10. Greenfield LJ, Ebert PA, Benson DW (1964) Effect of positive pressure ventilation on surface tension properties of lung extracts. Anesthesiology 25:312–316
11. Faridy EE, Permutt S, Riley RL (1966) Effect of ventilation on surface forces in excised dogs' lungs. J Appl Physiol 21:1453–1462
12. Moon VH (1948) The pathology of secondary shock. Am J Pathol 24:235–273
13. Teplitz C (1976) The core pathobiology and integrated medical science of adult acute respiratory insufficiency. Surg Clin North Am 56:1091–1133
14. Finfer S, Rocker G (1996) Alveolar overdistension is an important mechanism of persistent lung damage following severe protracted ARDS. Anaesth Intensive Care 24:569–573
15. Gattioni L, Bombino M, Pelosi P, et al (1994) Lung structure and function in different stages of severe adult respiratory distress syndrome. JAMA 271:1772–1779
16. Dreyfuss D, Saumon G (1993) Role of tidal volume, FRC, and end-inspiratory volume in the development of pulmonary edema following mechanical ventilation. Am Rev Respir Dis 148:1194–1203
17. Hernandez LA, Peevy KJ, Moise AA, Parker JC (1989) Chest wall restriction limits high airway pressure-induced lung injury in young rabbits. J Appl Physiol 66:2364–2368
18. Carlton DP, Cummings JJ, Scheerer RG, Poulain FR, Bland RD (1990) Lung overexpansion increases pulmonary microvascular protein permeability in young lambs. J Appl Physiol 69:577–583
19. Dreyfuss D, Soler P, Basset G, Saumon G (1988) High inflation pressure pulmonary edema. Respective effects of high airway pressure, high tidal volume, and positive end-expiratory pressure. Am Rev Respir Dis 137:1159–1164
20. West JB, Tsukimoto K, Prediletto R (1991) Stress failure in pulmonary capillaries. J Appl Physiol 70:1731–1742
21. Tsukimoto K, Mathieu-Costello O, Prediletto R, Elliot AR, West JB (1991) Ultrastructural appearances of pulmonary capillaries at high transmural pressures. J Appl Physiol 71:573–582
22. Dreyfuss D, Soler P, Saumon G (1992) Spontaneous resolution of pulmonary edema caused by short periods of cyclic overinflation. J Appl Physiol 72:2081–2089
23. Fu Z, Costello ML, Tsukimoto K, et al (1992) High lung volume increases stress failure in pulmonary capillaries. J Appl Physiol 73:123–133
24. Cooper JA, Van der Zee H, Line BR, Malik AB (1987) Relationship of end-expiratory pressure, lung volume, and ppTc-DTPA clearance. J Appl Physiol 63:1586–1590
25. Marks JD, Luce JM, Lazar NM, Wu JN, Lipavsky A, Murray JF (1985) Effect of increases in lung volume on clearance of aerosolized solute from human lungs. J Appl Physiol 59:1242–1248
26. Nolop KB, Maxwell DL, Royston D, Hughes JMB (1986) Effect of raised thoracic pressure and volume on clearance of aerosolized solute from human lungs. J Appl Physiol 60:1493–1497
27. Mead J, Takishima T, Leith D (1970) Stress distribution in lungs: a model of pulmonary elasticity. J Appl Physiol 28:596–608
28. Gattinoni L, D'Andrea L, Pelosi P, Vitale G, Pesenti A, Fumagalli R (1993) Regional effects and mechanism of positive end-expiratory pressure in early adult respiratory distress syndrome. JAMA 269:2122–2127
29. Gaver DPI, Samsel RW, Solway J (1990) Effects of surface tension and viscosity on airway reopening. J Appl Physiol 69:74–85
30. Robertson B (1984) Lung surfactant. In: Robertson B, Van Golde L, Batenburg J (eds) Pulmonary surfactant. Elsevier, Amsterdam
31. Muscedere JG, Mullen JBM, Gan K, Slutsky AS (1994) Tidal ventilation at low airway pressures can augment lung injury. Am J Respir Crit Care Med 149:1327–1334
32. Argiras EP, Blakely CR, Dunnill MS, Otremski S, Sykes MK (1987) High PEEP decreases hyaline membrane formation in surfactant deficient lungs. Br J Anaesth 59:1278–1285
33. Kawano T, Mori S, Cybulsky M, et al (1987) Effect of granulocyte depletion in a ventilated surfactant-depleted lung. J Appl Physiol 62:27–33
34. Pison U, Max M, Neuendank A, Weibbach S, Pietschmann S (1994) Host defence capacities of pulmonary surfactant: evidence for 'non-surfactant' functions of the surfactant system. Eur J Clin Invest 24:586–599
35. Froese AB, McCulloch PR, Sugiura M, Vaclavik S, Possmayer F, Moller F (1993) Optimizing alveolar expansion prolongs the effectiveness of exogenous surfactant therapy in the adult rabbit. Am Rev Respir Dis 148:569–577

36. Massaro D, Clerch L, Massaro GD (1981) Surfactant aggregation in rat lungs: influence of temperature and ventilation. J Appl Physiol 51:646–653
37. Nicholas TE, Barr HA (1983) The release of surfactant in rat lungs by brief periods of hyperventilation. Respir Physiol 52:69–83
38. Ito Y, Veldhuizen RAW, Yao L, McCaig LA, Bartlett AJ, Lewis JF (1997) Ventilation strategies affect surfactant aggregate conversion in acute lung injury. Am J Respir Crit Care Med 155:493–499
39. Brown ES, Johnson RP, Clements JA (1959) Pulmonary surface tension. J Appl Physiol 14:717–720
40. Faridy EE (1976) Effect of ventilation on movement of surfactant in airways. Respir Physiol 27:323–334
41. Wyszogrodski I, Kyei-Aboagye K, Taeusch W, Avery ME (1975) Surfactant inactivation by hyperventilation: conservation by end-expiratory pressure. J Appl Physiol 38:461–466
42. Coker PJ, Hernandez LA, Peevy KJ, Adkins K, Parker JC (1992) Increased sensitivity to mechanical ventilation after surfactant inactivation in young rabbit lungs. Crit Care Med 20:635–640
43. Bowton DL, Kong DL (1989) High tidal volume ventilation produces increased lung water in oleic acid-injured rabbit lungs. Crit Care Med 17:908–911
44. Bshouty Z, Ali J, Younes M (1988) Effect of tidal volume and PEEP on rate of edema formation in in situ perfused canine lobes. J Appl Physiol 64:1900–1907
45. Sugiura M, McCulloch PR, Wren S, Dawson RH, Froese AB (1994) Ventilator pattern influences neutrophil influx and activation in atelectasis-prone rabbit lung. J Appl Physiol 77:1355–1365
46. Matsuoka T, Kawano T, Miyasaka K (1994) Role of high-frequency ventilation in surfactant-depleted lung injury as measured by granulocytes. J Appl Physiol 76:539–544
47. Imai Y, Kawano T, Miyasaka K, Takata M, Imai T, Okuya K (1994) Inflammatory chemical mediators during conventional ventilation and during high frequency oscillatory ventilation. Crit Care Med 150:1550–1554
48. Tremblay L, Valenza F, Ribeiro SP, Li J, Slutsky AS (1997) Injurious ventilatory strategies increase cytokines and *c-fos* m-RNA expression in an isolated rat lung model. J Clin Invest 99:944–952
49. Narimanbekov IO, Rozycki HJ (1995) Effect of Il-1 blockade on inflammatory manifestations of acute ventilator-induced lung injury in a rabbit model. Exper Lung Research 21:239–254
50. Donnelly SC, Haslett C (1992) Cellular mechanisms of acute lung injury:implications for future treatment of the adult respiratory distress syndrome. Thorax 47:260–263
51. Spragg RG, Smith RM (1992) Biology of acute lung injury. In: Crystal RG, West JB (eds) Lung Injury. Raven Press, New York, pp 243–257
52. de Latorre FJ, Tomasa A, Klamburg J, Leon C, Soler M, Rius J (1977) Incidence of pneumothorax and pneumomediastinum in patients with aspiration pneumonia requiring ventilatory support. Chest 72:141–144
53. Hernandez LA, Coker PJ, May S, Thompson AL, Parker JC (1990) Mechanical ventilation increases microvascular permeability in oleic acid-injured lungs. J Appl Physiol 69:2057–2061
54. Gattinoni L, Pesenti A, Torresin A, et al (1986) Adult respiratory distress syndrome profiles by computed tomography. J Thorac Imag 1:25–30
55. Gammanpila S, Bevan DR, Bhudu R (1977) Effect of positive and negative expiratory pressure on renal function. Br J Anaesth 49:199–204
56. Love R, Choe E, Lippton H, Flint L, Steinberg S (1995) Positive end-expiratory pressure decreases mesenteric blood flow despite normalization of cardiac output. J Trauma Injury Infect Crit Care 39:195–199
57. Bezzant TB, Mortensen JD (1994) Risks and hazards of mechanical ventilation: A collective review of published literature. Disease-a-Month XL:581–640
58. Tutor JD, Mason CM, Dobard E, Beckerman RC, Summer WR, Nelson S (1994) Loss of compartmentalization of alveolar tumor necrosis factor after lung injury. An J Respir Crit Care Med 149:1107–1111
59. Uhlig S, Bethmann AN (1997) Prolonged hyperventilation is required for release of tumor necrosis factor α, but not interleukin-6 from isolated perfused mouse lung. Am J Respir Crit Care Med 155:A320 (Abst)
60. Bone RC (1996) Toward a theory regarding the pathogenesis of the systemic inflammatory response syndrome: What we do and do not know about cytokine regulation. Crit Care Med 24:163–172

61. Roumen RMH, Redl H, Schlag G, et al (1995) Inflammatory mediators in relation to the development of multiple organ failure in patients after severe blunt trauma. Crit Care Med 23:474–480
62. Nahum A, Hoyt J, McKibben A, et al (1996) Effect of mechanical ventilation strategy on E. coli pneumonia in dogs. Am J Respir Crit Care Med 153:A530 (Abst)
63. Guery B, Neviere R, Fialdes P, et al (1997) Mechanical ventilation regimen induces intestinal permeability changes in a rat model. Am J Respir Crit Care Med 155:A505 (Abst)
64. Borelli M, Kolobow T, Spatola R, Prato P, Tsuno K (1988) Severe acute respiratory failure managed with continuous positive airway pressure and partial extracorporeal carbon dioxide removal by an artificial membrane lung. Am Rev Respir Dis 138:1480–1487
65. Amato MB, Barbas CS, Filho GL, et al (1996) Improved survival in ARDS: Beneficial effects of a lung protective strategy. Am J Respir Crit Care Med 153:A531 (Abst)
66. Slutsky AS (1994) Consensus conference on mechanical ventilation. Intensive Care Med 20:64–79
67. Pelosi P, Cereda M, Foti G, Giacomini M, Pesenti A (1995) Alterations of lung and chest wall mechanics in patients with acute lung injury: Effects of positive end-expiratory pressure. Am J Respir Crit Care Med 152:531–537

Barotraumatic Effects of Mechanical Ventilation

L. Puybasset and J.-J. Rouby

Introduction

The crucial and indispensable role of airway maintenance and artificial ventilation in keeping an intensive care patient alive should be appreciated at the outset of this review on barotraumatic effects of artificial ventilation. Though it is extensively used in intensive care patients, the deleterious effects of mechanical ventilation occur only in a minority of patients with severe acute respiratory distress syndrome (ARDS). Mechanical ventilation-induced barotrauma is classically defined as issue of gas outside the alveolar space. Several symptomatic clinical entities familiar to clinicians correspond to this definition: Pneumothorax; pneumomediastinum; pulmonary interstitial emphysema; and subcutaneous emphysema. There is convincing experimental evidence to suggest that there are also other types of mechanical ventilation-induced barotrauma; pulmonary edema caused by "volutrauma" [1, 2] and bronchial lesions caused by "barotrauma" [3]. These lesions, which are easily reproducible in animals, are difficult to observe in humans as they have no histologic specificity. On the contrary, in clinical practice, it is common to find lesions characterized by distension of the pulmonary parenchyma, the origin of which is multifactorial [4]: Mechanical overdistension due to artificial ventilation, emphysema due to malnutrition and/or prolonged hyperoxia; and secondary alveolar destruction due to acute lung injury. The objective of the current review is to focus on these various aspects of barotrauma directly or indirectly related to artificial ventilation.

Pathophysiology

Acute Respiratory Distress Syndrome

In acute lung injury there is a major reduction of lung volume. The loss of volume involves not only the functional residual capacity (FRC) – the ventilated part of the lung – but also the consolidated and atelectatic non-ventilated part of the lung [5–7]. The reduction in lung volume increases progressively along the cephalo-caudal axis of the lung. While the overall volume of the upper lobes is well-preserved, loss of volume predominates in the lower lobes [8]. Such selective loss of volume has a likely explanation based on abnormalities of lung mechanics; supine position, deep sedation and raised intra-abdominal pressure cause a reduction in transpulmonary pressure at the lung base and a collapse of juxta-diaphragmatic pulmonary segments.

Quite often, while the upper lobes remain ventilated, the lower lobes appear non-ventilated and hyperdense on thoracic scan. Ventilated lung zones predominate in the non-dependent part of the lungs. In the supine position, the weight of the over-lying edematous lung "compresses" the lower lung zones and alveolar collapse becomes more and more marked as one moves from sternum to the vertebral plane. This theory was convincingly demonstrated by Pelosi et al. [9]. Thus, the loss of lung volume in ARDS has a dual mechanism: Reduction of ventilated lung volume in dependent zones due to an increase in the anteroposterior pressure gradient; and loss of volume in the lower lobes due to a decrease in the juxta-diaphragmatic transpulmonary pressure gradient.

Alveolar Recruitment Induced by Positive End-Expiratory Pressure (PEEP)

Since mechanical factors contribute to alveolar collapse, it is logical to try to recruit the alveoli by elevating the intrathoracic pressure. In the antero-posterior diameter, PEEP tends to counteract the forces which collapse the lung in the dependent zones; in the cephalo-caudal axis, it tends to re-establish the transpulmonary pressure at the base of the lung, which counteracts the raised intra-abdominal pressure transmitted passively through the diaphragm rendered atonic by muscular paralysis or deep sedation. The administration of PEEP maintains a positive pressure in the thorax at the end of expiration and thereby recruits collapsed alveoli. It has been demonstrated that alveolar recruitment predominates in the non-dependent zones of the lung [10, 11]. It is also to be noted that alveolar recruitment is always associated with a distension of the previously ventilated lung zones (and sometimes overdistension). Under the effects of PEEP, alveolar territories which are already "open" have a volume which correlates directly with the level of PEEP according to the regional static pressure-volume curve while the "recruitable" pulmonary zones open only beyond a certain pressure called the "opening pressure". There are also techniques other than PEEP, which can affect alveolar recruitment: Prolongation of the inspiratory/expiratory (I/E) ratio (inverse I/E ratio ventilation); increasing the mean intrathoracic pressure during high-frequency ventilation; and use of the prone position.

Alterations of Respiratory Mechanics Resulting from the Reduction of Lung Volume

As shown in Fig. 1a the static pressure-volume curve is altered in ARDS. Under physiologic conditions, the pressure-volume relationship is linear in the initial part of the curve with a slope of 100 ml/cmH$_2$O and an upper distending pressure around 35 cmH$_2$O corresponding to a lung volume of 3 litres above the FRC. Three principal abnormalities occur in ARDS [12]. Firstly, there is an inflexion on the initial part of the pressure-volume curve which corresponds to the opening pressure of the collapsed broncho-alveolar territories. This lower inflexion is more a concavity of the initial part of the pressure-volume curve towards the y-axis rather than a definite lower opening pressure. The second abnormality is a decrease in the slope of the initial part of the pressure-volume curve, which is quite often less than 60 ml/cmH$_2$O. Finally, the third abnormality results from the loss of lung volume; the upper dis-

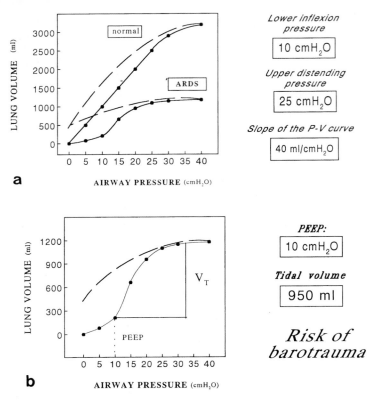

Fig. 1a, b. Pressure-volume curves in a normal subject (Fig. a – *upper curve*) and a patient with acute respiratory distress syndrome (Fig. a – *lower curve*). Pressure-volume curve during inspiration is represented by a continuous line and the pressure volume relation during expiration is represented by a dotted line. In the patient with ARDS, the upper distending pressure is 25 cmH$_2$O, the lower opening pressure 10 cmH$_2$O and the slope of the curve is 40 ml/cmH$_2$O. Figure **b** shows that during each inspiration, the distending pressure is exceeded if a PEEP of 10 cmH$_2$O and a tidal volume of 950 ml are used; two ventilatory settings required to normalize arterial oxygenation and PaCO$_2$ in this particular patient

tending pressure occurs at pressures and volumes which are much lower compared to the normal values. The tidal volumes corresponding to this upper distending pressure vary from one patient to another [13]. As shown in Fig. 2, the upper distending pressure is attained with tidal volumes between 6 and 11 ml/kg and plateau pressures between 18 and 35 cmH$_2$O. There is a risk of barotrauma due to overdistension if this pressure is attained or exceeded during each inspiration (Fig. 2b).

When ventilating patients with severe ARDS, two contradictory requirements need to be taken into account by the clinician: To set a level of PEEP which is above the lower opening pressure to optimize alveolar recruitment; and to avoid end-inspiratory pressures nearing the point of overdistension. In fact, setting a "safe" level of plateau pressure (35 cmH$_2$O as agreed upon in the North American consensus conference in 1993 [14]) appears illusive as the plateau pressure corresponding to

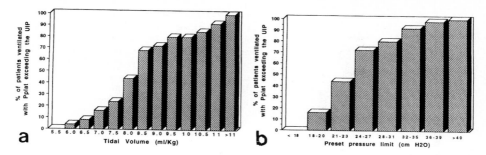

Fig. 2. Figure 2a shows that in more than half of the patients with acute respiratory distress syndrome the upper distending pressure (UIP) is reached or exceeded when tidal volumes equal to or more than 8 ml/kg are used. Figure 2b shows that in 50% of the patients with acute respiratory distress syndrome, the upper distending pressure is reached for a plateau pressure (P_{plat}) above 25 cmH$_2$O. (From [13] with permission)

the upper distending pressure depends on the extent of the pulmonary lesions. To ensure that the plateau pressure has not been exceeded in a given patient, it is necessary to obtain the entire pressure-volume curve to determine:

1) the lower opening pressure which indicates the level of PEEP that allows alveolar recruitment [12].
2) the upper distending pressure which fixes the pressure level not to be exceeded [13].

It is, therefore, highly desirable to have a simple system of determining the pressure-volume curve at the bedside on intensive care ventilators. It is from an analysis of this pressure-volume curve that the clinician should choose the main settings for artificial ventilation: PEEP; plateau pressure; and tidal volume.

The Concept of "Baby Lung"

Schematically, the lungs of a patient with ARDS can be divided into 3 distinct zones: A normally ventilated zone; a zone which is recruitable by PEEP; and a non-recruitable zone, comprising edema or infected alveolar territories [15]. The non-ventilated zones constitute venous admixture (shunt effect). The poorly ventilated zones constitute effective shunt. The zones which are ventilated, but poorly perfused constitute the alveolar dead space. Fig. 3 shows the histogram of the distribution of alveolar dead space in 70 patients with acute respiratory failure. Two-thirds of the patients in this group have an alveolar deadspace above 30%. Because of this increased alveolar deadspace, it is necessary to increase the intrathoracic pressure and the tidal volume to ensure normocapnia. There is a risk of inducing barotrauma if the lung zones accessible to the gas flow from the ventilator represent only 30–40% of the initial lung volume. A tidal volume of 10 ml/kg, apparently "normal" under physiological conditions may represent a tidal volume equivalent to 30 ml/kg if the ventilated lung volume is reduced by two-thirds. A tidal volume of 700 ml, then repre-

Patients (n)

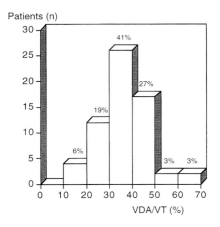

Fig. 3. Distribution of alveolar dead space (V_{DA}/V_T) in 70 patients with acute respiratory failure. The value of V_{DA}/V_T is represented on the x-axis and the number of patients on the y-axis. The numbers above the columns show the percentage of patients within a given range of V_{DA}/V_T. More than two-thirds of the patients with acute respiratory failure have a V_{DA}/V_T above 30%

sents a tidal volume of 2.1 liters in a subject with normal lungs. In other words, with reference to the volume of ventilated lung, an adult patient has a "baby lung" and it can be seen that under these circumstances conventional "adult" ventilation can induce pulmonary barotrauma. "Barotrauma" and "volutrauma" can theoretically interfere one with the other to further deteriorate the lung function in patients with the most severe decrease in lung volume accessible to gas.

Experimental Volutrauma and Barotrauma

Experimental "Volutrauma"

Experimental data over the last 15 years have shown that high tidal volumes with or without elevation of inflation pressures can cause acute pulmonary edema [1, 2, 16–19]. These results have been obtained from both small and large animals (rat, rabbit, pig, dog and sheep). Pulmonary edema was observed twenty minutes after the administration of a tidal volume of 40 ml/kg and an inflation pressure of 40 cmH$_2$O [1]. This pulmonary edema is related to the tidal volume administered and not the inflation pressure used, as similar lung injury also occurred when the animals were placed in an iron-lung which generated the same tidal volume with a negative intrathoracic pressure [16]. This pulmonary edema is due to the so-called "volutrauma".

When experimental acute respiratory failure was produced by injecting α-naphthyl thiourea before hyperventilating the lungs, there was a synergistic and not a simple additive effect between the "toxic" lesions and the lesions produced by mechanical hyperventilation [18, 20, 21]. As shown in Fig. 4, the indices of alveolo-capillary permeability increased in an exponential manner when mechanical hyperventilation was combined with pulmonary lesions induced by α-naphthyl thiourea. If these experimental data are extrapolated to humans, it appears that mechanical hyperventilation is more deleterious when there are pre-existing pulmonary lesions. These data, though not verified in humans, argue in favour of low tidal volumes

Fig. 4. Effect of mechanical hyperventilation on alveolo-capillary permeability in the presence or absence of pre-existing lung injury. Tidal volumes ranging from 25 to 45 ml/kg (HV 25, 33, 45) were administered to two groups of rats: one group without acute respiratory failure (No α-naphthyl thiourea, No ANTU) and another group with acute respiratory failure induced by the administration of α-naphthyl thiourea (ANTU). The index of capillary permeability studied was the diffusion space of labelled albumin (albumin space). When high tidal volumes were combined with toxic pulmonary edema, the diffusion space for labeled albumin increased exponentially. The effects of mechanical hyperventilation and toxic alveolar injury are synergistic and not simply additive. (From [20] with permission)

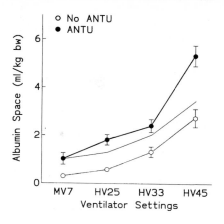

when the indication for artificial ventilation is acute lung injury. They also form the basis of the ventilatory strategy called "permissive hypercapnia" [22].

The mechanisms which initiate this "volutraumatic" lung injury still remain incompletely elucidated. Two explanations have been put forward: Pulmonary edema resulting from the phenomenon of pulmonary-interdependence [23, 24]; and partial inactivation of surfactant resulting in an increase in the alveolar surface tension and pulmonary collapse [25, 26].

Experimental "Bronchotrauma"

Recently, in an alveolar lavage model of acute respiratory failure, it has been demonstrated that conventional mechanical ventilation without alveolar recruitment can cause "barotraumatic" bronchial lesions [3]. In this experimental model of isolated, non-perfused rat lung, different ventilatory strategies were applied after alveolar lavage. One group of lungs were ventilated with a PEEP lower than the lower opening pressure on the pressure-volume curve and a second group with a PEEP higher than the lower opening pressure. As shown in Fig. 5A, when the PEEP applied was higher than the lower opening pressure, there was a normalization of ventilatory mechanics; the pressure-volume curve after the lavage was not different from that of the control lungs. On the contrary, when the applied PEEP was less than the lower opening pressure, there was a progressive deterioration of the pulmonary compliance and histologically, bronchial and bronchiolar lesions characterized by mucosal epithelial necrosis were observed (Fig. 5B). Moreover, in these lungs, pulmonary injury was histologically more severe compared to the lungs ventilated with a higher level of PEEP. These results suggest that the absence of alveolar recruitment could be the cause of "bronchial" barotrauma and aggravation of the lesions induced by the lavage. The most probable pathophysiologic hypothesis is that the opening and closure of the terminal bronchioles with each respiratory cycle causes "bronchotrauma" which manifests itself rapidly as necrosis of the bronchial epithelial lining [3].

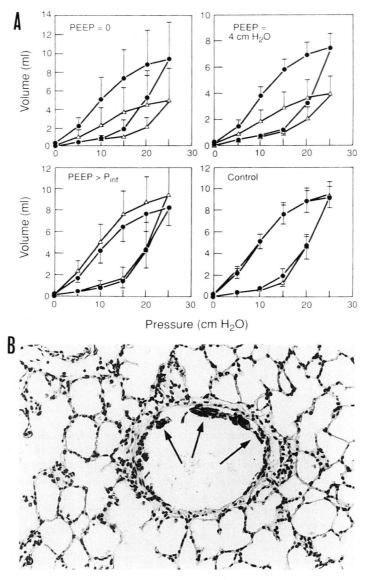

Fig. 5A, B. Barotraumatic effects of artificial ventilation at low pressure in experimental acute respiratory failure. After alveolar lavage, different ventilatory strategies were applied to isolated rat lungs: Conventional ventilation at normal tidal volumes without PEEP (PEEP = 0); conventional ventilation at normal tidal volumes with a PEEP of 4 cmH$_2$O (PEEP value less than the lower opening pressure pressure on the initial part of the pressure-volume curve); conventional ventilation at normal tidal volumes with a PEEP higher than the lower opening pressure (PEEP > P$_{inf}$). The effects of these different ventilatory strategies on pulmonary pressure-volume curves are seen in Fig. 5A – each quadrant shows the P-V curves during inspiration and expiration before and after the alveolar lavage. The right lower quadrant represents a group of control animals. Figure 5B shows a bronchial lesion characterized by epithelial necrosis (*arrows*) in a lung ventilated by a strategy using low PEEP. (From [3] with permission)

Pulmonary Barotrauma in Humans

Accidents of alveolar overdistension due to high intrathoracic pressures have been frequently observed in patients with severe acute respiratory failure on prolonged artificial ventilation [27]. As there is no histologic specificity characterizing the experimental "volutraumatic" pulmonary edema and "barotraumatic" bronchial lesions, it is impossible to know what is the role of artificial ventilation in the observed pulmonary lesions. In fact, alveolar overdistension observed during mechanical ventilation has two distinct clinical patterns: Escape of air outside the alveolar space, exemplified by pneumothorax; and emphysematous or pneumatocele-type lesions which appear on radiologic imaging only when they reach a sufficient size.

Classical Barotraumatic Accidents

The classical barotraumatic accidents occurring in clinical practice, (pneumothorax, interstitial emphysema [28], subcutaneous emphysema, pneumomediastinum [29], rarely pneumoperitonium and exceptionally gaseous emboli [30]) originate from alveolar rupture due to mechanical ventilation. For anatomic reasons, alveolar rupture occurs preferentially around the bronchovascular axis [4]. Alveolar walls fixed to the perivascular sheath at the centre of the secondary pulmonary lobule rupture and release alveolar gas into the peribronchial interstitial tissue (Fig. 6a). The air then follows the bronchovascular axis and may reach the hilum, pleura, extrathoracic subcutaneous space, peritoneum and mediastinum. Pulmonary interstitial emphysema, defined as the presence of air along the bronchovascular axis, is difficult to differentiate from an air bronchogram on a frontal bedside chest x-ray in the adult. Only in children and neonates does it represent an easily identifiable radiologic entity [29].

Pneumothorax is defined as rupture of air into the parietal pleura. Rupture of air into the mediastinal pleura results in pneumomediastinum. Diffusion of air into the subcutaneous planes and the peritoneal cavity causes subcutaneous emphysema and "barotraumatic" pneumoperitoneum. Alveolar ruptures may also occur at the level of septa limiting the secondary pulmonary lobules. Very rarely, air from the alveolar ruptures may gush into the pulmonary veins resulting in air-embolism of the left heart.

Pneumothorax: In the absence of pleural adhesions it is easy to identify a large pneumothorax on a bedside frontal chest radiograph; there is a characteristic line bordering the air. Difficulties in diagnosis arise when the pleura is adherent, which frequently occurs in ARDS. Abnormal hyperluscency on a frontal chest radiograph can also suggest the diagnosis. Only a thoracic scan provides definite evidence of a localized pneumothorax (Fig. 7). Pulmonary echography is also a useful diagnostic tool; absence of pleural sliding is a pathognomonic sign of pneumothorax [31]. Since the communication between the alveolar rupture and the pleural space is most often indirect (Fig. 6b), there is generally no "bubbling" from the thoracic drain. Bronchopleural fistula with continuous "bubbling" of air occurs only when the alveolar rupture is at the periphery and opens directly into the pleural cavity.

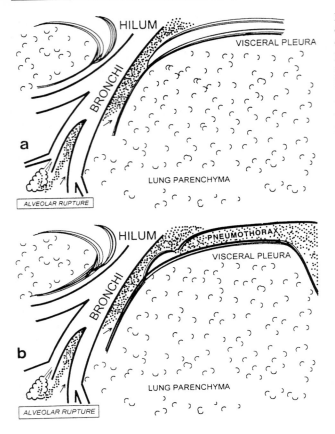

Fig. 6a, b. Rupture of peripheral alveoli causes interstitial emphysema (Fig. 6a) or pneumothorax (Fig. 6b). Alveolar rupture releases air into the perivascular sheath. The air then spreads along the length of the bronchovascular axis producing interstitial emphysema, mediastinal emphysema or pneumothorax

Pneumomediastinum: There is no diagnostic difficulty when the mediastinal separation by air is significant (Fig. 8) and a frontal chest x-ray is suggestive. When the mediastinal separation is minimal, only a thoracic scan will allow a diagnosis with certainty. Very rarely, air may reach the pericardium causing a pneumopericardium.

Subcutaneous emphysema: A frontal chest x-ray is sufficient, in general, to diagnose subcutaneous emphysema, as there is characteristic subcutaneous crepitation which is clinically evident. The subcutaneous emphysema may extend to the distal parts of the lower limbs. One of the classical radiologic signs is the dissection of the muscle fibres of pectoralis major giving an appearance of the spokes of a wheel on a frontal chest radiograph (Figs. 7 and 8).

"Barotraumatic" pneumoperitoneum: The thoracic and abdominal cavities communicate by natural orifices. Occasionally, a pneumoperitoneum can have a barotraumatic origin [27]. If there is no coincidental evidence of barotrauma, the patient may be unnecessarily subjected to a laparotomy. If there is any evidence of associated pneumothorax or pneumoperitonium in a patient ventilated for ARDS, then a diagnosis of barotraumatic pneumoperitonium should be entertained.

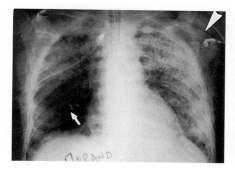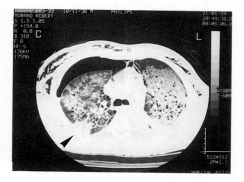

Fig. 7. Right anterior pneumothorax with subcutaneous emphysema in a patient with acute respiratory distress syndrome. On the left, a chest x-ray clearly shows subcutaneous emphysema dissecting the muscle fibres of pectoralis major (*white arrowhead*). There is a hyperluscency of the lung fields on the right (*white arrow*) giving an impression that the right lung is less affected than the left lung. In fact, a thoracic scan (right side of the figure) shows that this appearance is the result of an anterior pneumothorax. It can be noted that the pulmonary parenchyma is subjected to barotrauma and there are a number of pseudocysts (see text) on both sides. The thoracic drain seen on the x-ray is located posteriorly on the scan (*arrowhead*) and was ineffective in draining the anterior pneumothorax

"Barotraumatic" air embolism: Recently, air embolism through pulmonary veins has been reported in patients ventilated for acute respiratory failure [30, 32–34]. It occurred in adults with ARDS [32–34] or pulmonary contusion, and neonates suffering from hyaline membrane disease [30, 33]. As Fig. 9 shows, gaseous emboli, synchronous with the inspiratory phase of the ventilator, are visualized on transesophageal echocardiography, and the flow of these emboli is proportional to the tidal volume administered. Decreasing the intrathoracic pressures by reducing the tidal volumes during conventional ventilation or instituting high frequency ventilation eliminates the gas emboli or at least, reduces their flow rate. Catastrophic visceral accidents related to such gaseous emboli and resulting in patient death have been reported [33].

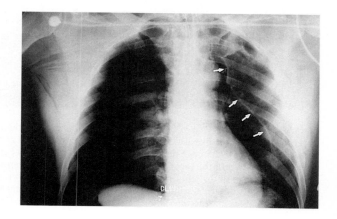

Fig. 8. Mediastinal and subcutaneous emphysema in a patient with bronchopneumonia of the left lower lobe. On the right, muscle fibres of pectoralis major are dissected by air. Separation of the mediastinum from the lung by air can be seen along the left border of the mediastinum which marks the presence of pneumomediastinum (*white arrows*)

Occasionally, gaseous emboli may complicate an extensive subcutaneous emphysema [35].

Histologic Lesions of Distension

Pathophysiology

Barotraumatic lesions of bronchopulmonary distension observed in humans are related to multiple alveolar ruptures occurring at a distance from the bronchovascular axis, and dilatation of terminal bronchioles in consolidated lung zones which are non-recruitable by PEEP. When the confluence of ruptured alveoli occurs in ventilated lung zones, the appearance is one of pulmonary pseudoemphysema [4]. The confluence of ruptured alveoli in a partially ventilated and inflamed lung zone is referred to as a pneumatocele or intraparenchymatous pseudocyst [36]. When the alveolar rupture is associated with extensive fibrosis, it is called bronchodysplasia [37]. In consolidated non-recruitable lung territories, elevated intrathoracic pressures are transmitted totally to the bronchial tree which results in distal bronchial distension with the formation of cystic dilatation of the bronchi or bronchiectasis. These distensive lesions may attain enormous size leading to a destruction of the pulmonary parenchyma.

The size of these lesions depends not only on the ventilatory parameters such as tidal volume, peak inspiratory pressure and the duration of hyperoxic ventilation but also on more general parameters like malnutrition (Fig. 10). These data obtained from humans resemble those from the experimental models of pulmonary emphysema caused by exposure to oxygen [38] and restricted calory intake leading to malnutrition [39, 40]. At present, the most probable hypothesis is that the destructive pulmonary parenchymal lesions caused by toxic processes, inflammation and infec-

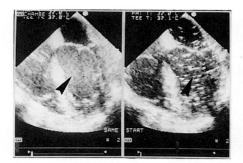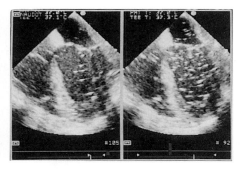

Fig. 9. Gaseous emboli seen in the left atrium of a 27 year old patient admitted to the intensive care unit following a motorbike accident. Each quadrant represents a 4 cavity section on transesophageal echocardiography. The image on the extreme left was obtained when the patient was disconnected from the ventilator. In the second section from the left, gaseous emboli synchronous with inspiration could be seen in the left atrium and left ventricle (*black arrows*). The two right sections show gaseous emboli at two tidal volumes – 350 ml on the left section and 650 ml on the right section. The flow of the bubbles increased with the tidal volume administered. (From [34] with permission)

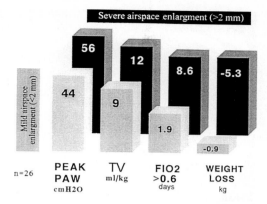

Fig. 10. Effects of mechanical ventilation and malnutrition on the size of barotraumatic lesions. In this human study on 26 young subjects, without any history or antecedent of respiratory illness, who died in the intensive care unit after a long duration of mechanical ventilation for acute respiratory distress syndrome, diameters of the barotraumatic lesions were measured by pulmonary morphometry. The lesions were divided into 2 groups: Those with a mean diameter less than 2 mm and the larger ones with a mean diameter more than 2 mm. The size of the lesions increased with the peak airway pressure (Peak P_{AW}), tidal volume (TV), duration of hyperoxia and loss of weight. (From [4] with permission)

tion are potentiated by mechanical ventilation, hyperoxia and malnutrition. The degree of pulmonary parenchymal overdistension depends directly on the degree of increase in tidal volumes and inspiratory pressures, and the length of exposure to hyperoxia [4].

"Barotraumatic" Pseudoemphysema

In young patients with no past history of respiratory illness, confluence of ruptured alveoli in the ventilated lung produces the appearance of pseudoemphysema [4]. Pulmonary architecture is conserved even though the interalveolar septa are thickened and infiltrated by inflammatory cells. There are also some true emphysematous bullae resulting from the confluence of a number of ruptured alveoli. In the initial stages, it is difficult to diagnose this pulmonary pseudoemphysema either on a chest radiograph or on a thoracic computed tomography (CT) Scan. It is only when they attain a significant size in the inflamed zones of the lung that the "bullae" appear on CT sections (Fig. 11).

Pneumatoceles and Bronchodysplasia

True cystic cavities or pneumatoceles are seen only in the consolidated parts of the lung. Histopathologic examination frequently shows residual bronchial epithelium in the "wall" of the cyst indicating that the bullae might have resulted from disten-

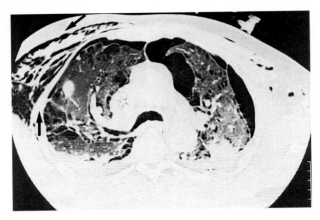

Fig. 11. Extensive pulmonary barotraumatic lesions seen on a computerized tomographic scan in a patient with acute respiratory distress syndrome. Note bilateral subcutaneous emphysema dissecting the muscle fibres of the right pectoralis major (*black arrows*), bilateral anterior pneumothoraces, emphysematous bullae in both right and left upper lobes and intraparenchymal pseudocysts on both the sides. These spectacular barotraumatic lesions were observed after 3 weeks of artificial ventilation delivering tidal volumes resulting in peak airway pressures greater than 45 cmH$_2$O

sion of the distal bronchioles [4]. When intense fibrosis is associated with these pseudocysts, it is referred to as bronchodysplasia of the adult [37] by analogy with what is observed in neonates with hyaline membrane disease [41]. The lesions can attain enormous sizes leading to mutilation of the pulmonary parenchyma and at that stage, it is easy to diagnose them on a thoracic scan. These lesions are normally beyond therapy, and most often result in the death of the patient.

Conclusion

Experimental and clinical data together indicate that artificial ventilation is likely responsible for barotraumatic pulmonary lesions. Such barotraumatic lesions result in a considerable reduction of the residual pulmonary parenchymal volume available for the gas coming from the ventilator, in a situation of already extensive acute lung injury. In this situation, it is critical to reduce tidal volumes to prevent overdistension of the ventilated pulmonary parenchyma and to arrest the formation of "barotraumatic bullae". If the experimental data related to pulmonary edema induced by mechanical hyperventilation apply to humans, artificial ventilation at high tidal volumes could aggravate acute lung injury and precipitate death. This justifies a reduction in tidal volume which culminates in permissive hypercapnia during conventional mechanical ventilation. A ventilatory mode such as high frequency ventilation based on the reduction of tidal volume can also be employed to decrease the risk of barotrauma. Finally, the objective of mechanical ventilation should be to ensure sufficient alveolar recruitment without attaining the plateau pressures causing overdistension of the pulmonary parenchyma. At the bedside, it is essential to measure the pulmonary pressure-volume curve for optimal choice of the ventilator settings in order to minimize the risk of mechanical ventilation-induced barotrauma.

References

1. Dreyfuss D, Basset G, Soler P, Saumon G (1985) Intermittent positive-pressure hyperventilation with high inflation pressures produces pulmonary microvascular injury in rats. Am Rev Resp Dis 132:880–884
2. Kolobow T, Moretti MP, Fumagalli R, et al (1987) Severe impairment in lung function induced by high peak airway pressure during mechanical ventilation. An experimental study. Am Rev Resp Dis 135:312–315
3. Muscedere JG, Mullen JBM, Gan K, Slutsky AS (1994) Tidal ventilation at low airway pressure can augment lung injury. Am J Resp Crit Care Med 149:1327–1334
4. Rouby JJ, Lherm T, Martin de Lassale E, et al (1993) Histologic aspects of pulmonary barotrauma in critically ill patients with acute respiratory failure. Intensive Care Med 20:187–192
5. Falke KJ, Pontoppidan H, Kumar A, Leith DE, Geffin B, Laver MB (1972) Ventilation with end-expiratory pressure in acute lung disease. J Clin Invest 51:2315–2323
6. Petty TL, Silvers GW, Paul GWP, Stanford RES (1979) Abnormalities in lung elastic properties and surfactant function in adult respiratory distress syndrome. Chest 75:571–574
7. Suter PM, Fairley BF, Isenberg MD (1975) Optimum end-expiratory airway pressure in patients with acute pulmonary failure. N Engl J Med 292:284–289
8. Puybasset L, Cluzel P, Chaw N, et al (1997) Distribution of volume reduction in post operative acute lung injury-factors influencing peep-induced alveolar recruitment. Br J Anaesth 78 (suppl 1):A380 (Abst)
9. Pelosi P, D'Andrea L, Pesenti A, Gattinoni L (1994) Vertical gradient of regional lung inflation in adult respiratory distress syndrome. Am J Resp Crit Care Med 149:8–13
10. Gattinoni L, D'Andrea L, Pelosi P, Vitale G, Pesenti A, Fumagalli R (1993) Regional effects and mechanism of positive end-expiratory pressure in early adult respiratory distress syndrome. JAMA 269:2122–2127
11. Gattinoni L, Pelosi P, Crotti S, Valenza F (1995) Effects of positive end-expiratory pressure on regional distribution of tidal volume and recruitment in adult respiratory distress syndrome. Am J Respir Crit Care Med 151:1807–1814
12. Matamis D, Lemaire F, Harf A, Brun-Buisson C, Ansquer JC, Atlan G (1984) Total respiratory pressure-volume curves in the adult respiratory distress syndrome. Chest 86:58–66
13. Roupie E, Dambrosio M, Servillo G, et al (1995) Titration of tidal volume and incuded hypercapnia in acute respiratory distress syndrome. Am J Respir Crit Care Med 152:121–128
14. Slutsky AS (1993) Report of a consensus conference on mechanical ventilation. Chest 104:1833–1859
15. Gattinoni L, Pesenti A, Bombino M, et al (1988) Relationships between lung computer tomographic density, gas exchange, and PEEP in acute respiratory failure. Anesthesiology 69:824–832
16. Dreyfuss D, Soler P, Basset G, Saumon G (1988) High inflation pressure pulmonary edema. Respective effects of high airway pressure, high tidal volume, and positive end-expiratory pressure. Am Rev Respir Dis 137:1159–1164
17. Hernandez LA, Peevy KJ, Moise AA, Parker JC (1990) Chest wall restriction limits high airway pressure-induced injury in young rabbit. J Appl Physiol 66:2364–2368
18. Hernandez LA, Coker PJ, May S, Thompson AL, Parker JC (1990) Mechanical ventilation increases microvascular permeability in oleic-acid injured lung. J Appl Physiol 69:2057–2061
19. Tsuno K, Miura K, Takeya M, Kolobow T, Morioka T (1991) Histopathologic pulmonary changes from mechanical ventilation at high peak airway pressures. Am Rev Respir Dis 143:1115–1120
20. Dreyfuss D, Soler P, Saumon G (1995) Mechanical ventilation-induced pulmonary edema. Interaction with previous lung alterations. Am J Respir Crit Care Med 151:1568–1575
21. Bowton DL, Kuong KL (1989) High-tidal volume ventilation produces increased lung water in oleic acid-injured rabbit lung. Crit Care Med 17:908–911

22. Hickling KG, Henderson SJ, Jackson R (1990) Low mortality associated with low volume pressure limited ventilation with permissive hypercapnia in severe adult respiratory distress syndrome. Intensive Care Med 16:372–377
23. Albert RX, Lakshimarayan KW, Butler J (1980) Lung inflation can cause pulmonary edema in zone I of in situ dog lungs. J Appl Physiol 49:815–819
24. Parker JC, Townsley MI, Rippe B, Taylor AE, Thigpen J (1984) Increased microvascular permeability in dog lung due to high peak airway pressures. J Appl Physiol 57:1809–1816
25. Bredenberg CE, Nieman GF, Paskanik AM, Hart AKE (1986) Microvascular membrane permeability in high surface tension pulmonary edema. J Appl Physiol 60:253–259
26. Parker JC, Hernandez LA, Longenecker GL, Peevy K, Johnson W (1990) Lung edema caused by high peak inspiratory pressures in dogs. Am Rev Respir Dis 142:321–328
27. Haake R, Schlichtig R, Ulstad DR, Henschen RR (1987) Barotrauma. Pathophysiology, risk factors and prevention. Chest 91:608–613
28. Caldwell EJ, Powell RD, Mullooly JP (1970) Interstitial emphysema: a study of physiologic factors involved in experimental induction of the lesion. Am Rev Respir Dis 102:516–525
29. Maunder R, Pierson D, Hudson L (1984) Subcutaneous and mediastinal emphysema: pathophysiology, diagnosis and management. Arch Intern Med 144:1447–1453
30. Blanco CE, Rietveld LA, Ruys JH (1979) Systemic air embolism: a possible complication of artificial ventilation. Acta Paediatr Scand 68:925–927
31. Lichenstein D, Menu Y (1995) A bedside ultrasound sign ruling out pneumothorax in the critically ill: lung sliding. Chest 108:1345–1348
32. Marini JJ, Culver BH (1989) Systemic gas embolism complicating mechanical ventilation in the adult respiratory distress syndrome. Ann Intern Med 110:699–703
33. Bowen FW, Chandra R, Avery GB (1973) Pulmonary interstitial emphysema with gas embolism in hyaline membrane disease. Am J Dis Child 126:117–118
34. Saada M, Goarin JP, Riou B, et al (1995) Systemic gas embolism complicating pulmonary contusion. Diagnosis and management using transesophageal echocardiography. Am J Respir Crit Care Med 152:812–815
35. Morris WP, Buther BD, Tonnesen AS, Allen SJ (1993) Continuous venous air embolism in patients receiving positive end-expiratory pressure. Am Rev Respir Dis 147:1034–1037
36. Lemaire F, Cerrina J, Lange F, Harf A, Carlet J, Bignon J (1982) PEEP-induced airspace overdistension complicating paraquat lung. Chest 81:654–657
37. Churg A, Golden J, Fligiel S, Hogg JC (1983) Bronchopulmonary dysplasia in the adult. Am Rev Respir Dis 127:117–120
38. Riley DJ, Kramer MJ, Kerr JS, Chae CU, Yu SY, Berg RA (1987) Damage and repair of lung connective tissue in rats exposed to toxic levels of oxygen. Am Rev Respir Dis 135:441–447
39. Kerr JS, Riley DJ, Lanza-Jacoby S, et al (1985) Nutritional emphysema in the rat. Influence of protein depletion and impaired lung growth. Am Rev Respir Dis 131:644–650
40. Sahebjami H, Wirman JA (1981) Emphysema-like changes in the lungs of starved rats. Am Rev Respir Dis 124:619–624
41. Taghizadeh A, Reynolds EOR (1976) Pathogenesis of bronchopulmonary dysplasia following hyaline membrane disease. Am J Pathol 82:241–264

Weaning from
Mechanical Ventilation

The Pathophysiology of Weaning Failure

T. Vassilakopoulos, S. Zakynthinos, and C. Roussos

Introduction

Patients who fail to wean pose a great challenge for physicians, since the underlying pathophysiology of weaning failure remains, to a large extent, in the realm of speculation. Clinicians and scientists refer to weaning as an art and/or science. In this review we attempt to discuss, from a scientific standpoint, the pathophysiologic mechanisms of weaning failure, with the belief that their detailed knowledge serves the art of weaning.

Failure to wean has been attributed either to an imbalance between the load faced by the respiratory muscles and their neuromuscular competence, or to an energy supply that is inadequate to meet the muscles' energy demand. Although at first glance these factors seem not to be directly related, we will try to unravel their actual intimate relationship by proposing a "mechanical model" that incorporates the various determinants of energy supply, energy demand and neuromuscular competence that, by fine interplay, create an inappropriate relationship between the ventilatory needs and the neurorespiratory capacity which can lead to the inability to sustain spontaneous breathing, and thus, to weaning failure. Failure to wean can sometimes be attributed to cardiovascular dysfunction that develops on transition from mechanical ventilation to spontaneous breathing. We will explore its pathophysiology and show how this cardiovascular dysfunction is dependent upon the action of the respiratory muscles. We will finally show that the respiratory muscles may potentially "steal" oxygen and blood from other tissues, and that this "stealing effect" occasionally leads to weaning failure through the development of organ dysfuction.

Inappropriate Relation of Ventilatory Needs and Neurorespiratory Capacity

For man to take a spontaneous breath, the inspiratory muscles must generate sufficient force to overcome the elastance of the lungs and chest wall (lung and chest wall elastic loads) as well as the airway and tissue resistance (resistive load). This requires an adequate output from the centers controlling the muscles, anatomic and functional nerve integrity, unimpaired neuromuscular transmission, an intact chest wall and adequate muscle strength. This can be schematically represented by considering the ability to take a breath as a balance between inspiratory load and neuromuscular competence (Fig. 1). Under normal conditions this system is polarized in favour of neuromuscular competence, i.e., there are reserves that permit consider-

Pi / Pimax

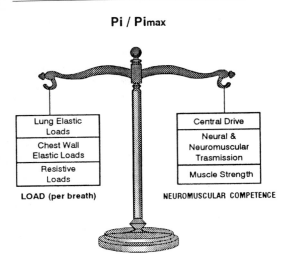

Fig. 1. The ability to take a spontaneous breath is determined by the balance between the load imposed upon the respiratory system (P_i) and the neuromuscular competence of the ventilatory pump (P_{imax}). Normally this balance weighs in favor of competence permitting significant increases in load. However, if the competence is, for whatever reason, reduced below a critical point (e.g., drug overdose, myasthenia gravis, etc.), the balance may then weigh in favor of load, rendering the ventilatory pump insufficient to inflate the lungs and chest wall

able increases in load. However, for a man to breathe spontaneously the inspiratory muscles should be able to sustain the above mentioned load over time and also adjust the minute ventilation in such a way that there is adequate gas exchange. The ability of the respiratory muscles to sustain this load without the appearance of fatigue is called endurance and is determined by the balance between energy supplies (Us) and energy demands (Ud) (Fig. 2).

Energy supplies depend on the inspiratory muscle blood flow, the blood substrate (fuel) concentration and arterial oxygen content, the muscle's ability to extract and utilize energy sources and the muscle's energy stores [1, 2]. Under normal circum-

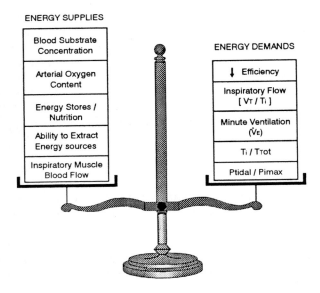

Fig. 2. Respiratory muscle endurance is determined by the balance between energy supplies and demands. Normally, the supplies meet the demands and a large reserve exists. Whenever this balance weighs in favor of demand, the respiratory muscles ultimately become fatigued, leading to inability to sustain spontaneous breathing

stances energy supplies are adequate to meet the demands and a large recruitable reserve exists (Fig. 2). Energy demands increase proportionally with the mean tidal pressure developed by the inspiratory muscles (P_i) expressed as a fraction of maximum ($P_i/P_{i\,max}$), the minute ventilation (V_E), the inspiratory duty cycle (T_i/T_{TOT}) and the mean inspiratory flow rate (V_T/T_i) and are inversely related to the efficiency of the muscles [1, 2]. Fatigue develops when the mean rate of Ud exceeds the mean rate of Us [3] (i.e., when the balance is polarized in favor of demand) [1]

$$Ud > Us \Rightarrow W/E > Us \tag{1}$$

where W is the mean muscle power and E is efficiency.

Bellemare and Grassino [4] have suggested that the product of T_i/T_{TOT} and the mean transdiaphragmatic pressure expressed as a fraction of maximal ($P_{di}/P_{di\,max}$) defines a useful "tension-time index" (TTI_{di}) that is related to the endurance time (i.e., the time that the diaphragm can sustain the load imposed on it). Whenever TTI_{di} is smaller than the critical value of 0.15 the load can be sustained indefinitely; but when TTI_{di} exceeds the critical zone of 0.15-0.18, the load can be sustained only for a limited time period, in other words, the endurance time. This was found to be inversely related to TTI_{di}. The TTI concept is assumed to be applicable not only to the diaphragm, but to the respiratory muscles as a whole [5]:

$$TTI = \frac{P_i}{P_{i\,max}} \cdot \frac{T_i}{T_{TOT}} \tag{2}$$

where P_i is the mean inspiratory pressure per breath, and $P_{i\,max}$ is the maximal inspiratory pressure. Since we have stated that endurance is determined by the balance between energy supply and demand, TTI of the inspiratory muscles has to be in accordance with the energy balance view. In fact as Fig. 3 demonstrates, $P_i/P_{i\,max}$ and T_i/T_{TOT}, which constitute the TTI, are among the determinants of energy demands; an increase in either that will increase the TTI value will also increase the demands. The energy balance may then weigh in favor of demands leading to fatigue. Furthermore, Roussos et al. [6] have directly related $P_i/P_{i\,max}$ with the endurance time. The critical value of $P_i/P_{i\,max}$ that could be generated indefinitely at the functional residual capacity (FRC) was around 0.60. Greater values of the $P_i/P_{i\,max}$ ratio were inversely related to the endurance time in a curvilinear fashion. When lung volume was increased from FRC to FRC + $^1/_2$ inspiratory capacity, the critical value of $P_i/P_{i\,max}$ and the endurance time were diminished to very low values (20–25% of $P_{i\,max}$).

But what determines the ratio $P_i/P_{i\,max}$? The nominator, the mean inspiratory pressure, is determined by the elastic and resistive loads imposed on the inspiratory muscles. The denominator, the maximum inspiratory pressure, is determined by the neuromuscular competence, i.e., the maximum inspiratory muscle activation that can be achieved. It follows, then, that the value of $P_i/P_{i\,max}$ is determined by the balance between load and competence (Fig. 1). But $P_i/P_{i\,max}$ is also one of the determinants of energy demand (Fig. 2); therefore the two balances, i.e., between load and competence and energy supply and demand, are in essence linked, creating a system. Schematically, when the central hinge of the system moves upwards, or is at least at the horizontal level, an appropriate relationship between ventilatory needs and

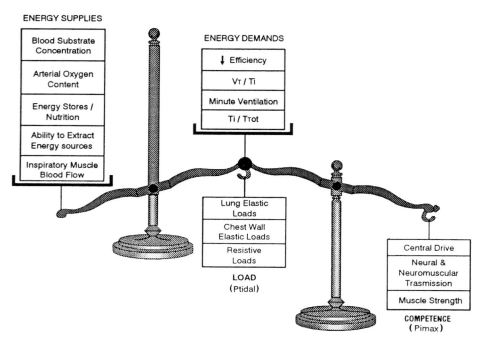

ENERGY SUPPLIES

Fig. 3. The system of two balances, incorporating the various determinants of load, competence, energy supplies and demands is represented schematically. The $P_i/P_{i\,max}$ that was one of the determinants of energy demand (see Fig. 2) is replaced by its equivalent; the balance between load and neuromuscular competence (see Fig. 1). In fact, this is the reason why the two balances are linked. When the central hinge of the system moves upwards or is at least at the horizontal level, an appropriate relationship between ventilatory needs and neuro-respiratory capacity exists and spontaneous ventilation can be sustained. In healthy persons the hinge moves far upwards creating a large reserve

neuro-respiratory capacity exists and spontaneous ventilation can be sustained indefinitely (Fig. 3). One can easily see that the ability of a subject to breathe spontaneously depends on the fine interplay of many different factors. Normally this interplay moves the central hinge far upwards and creates a great ventilatory reserve for the healthy individual. When the central hinge of the system, for whatever reason, moves downward, an inappropriate relation of ventilatory needs to neuro-respiratory capacity develops and spontaneous ventilation cannot be sustained. Consequently, weaning a patient from the ventilator will be successful whenever an appropriate relationship between ventilatory needs and neuro-respiratory capacity exists and will ultimately fail should this relation become inappropriate. Fig. 4 summarizes all possible factors that, by their fine interplay, can lead to this inappropriate balance and then to weaning failure. Evidently, failure to wean is usually multifactorial, with each factor contributing its own percentage. Detailed analysis of each factor is beyond the scope of this paper, and the interested reader should consult our recent review [7].

To validate this theory, we have recently prospectively studied patients who had initially failed to wean from mechanical ventilation (F) but were successfully weaned

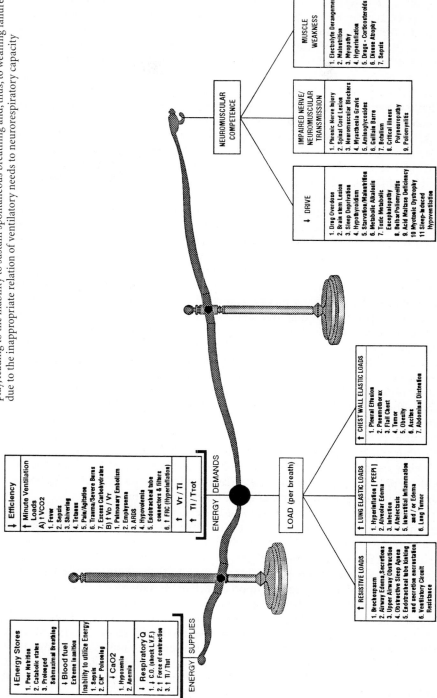

Fig. 4. The various factors that can move the central hinge downwards by their fine inter-play, leading to the inability to sustain spontaneous breathing and, thus, to weaning failure due to the inappropriate relation of ventilatory needs to neurorespiratory capacity

(S) on a later occasion (unpublished data). Compared to S, during F patients had greater intrinsic PEEP (6.10 ± 2.45 vs 3.83 ± 2.69 cmH$_2$O), dynamic hyperinflation (327 ± 180 vs 213 ± 175 ml), total resistance (R$_{max}$, 14.14 ± 4.95 vs 11.19 ± 4.01 cmH$_2$O/l/s), ratio of mean to maximum inspiratory pressure (0.46 ± 0.1 vs 0.31 ± 0.08), tension time index (TTI, 0.162 ± 0.032 vs 0.102 ± 0.023) and power (315 ± 153 vs 215 ± 75 cmH$_2$O/l/min), less maximum inspiratory pressure (42.3 ± 12.7 vs 53.8 ± 15.1 cmH$_2$O) and a breathing pattern that was more rapid and shallow (ratio of frequency to tidal volume, f/V$_T$ 98 ± 38 vs 62 ± 21 b/min/l). Given the obvious multifactorial nature of weaning failure, we performed multiple logistic regression analysis with the weaning outcome as the dependent variable, in order to clarify on pathophysiologic grounds which factors are the major determinants of the inability to wean from mechanical ventilation. The TTI and the f/V$_T$ ratio were the only significant variables in the model. We concluded therefore that the TTI and the f/V$_T$ are the main determinants of the weaning outcome.

The theoretical consideration of the imbalance between energy supply and demand of the respiratory muscles, as well as the finding that TTI is a major determinant of the weaning outcome suggest that inspiratory muscle fatigue is frequently a final common pathway leading to inability to sustain spontaneous breathing and thus to weaning failure. Few data exist in this area. In an important study Cohen et al. [8] studied 12 patients with various disorders leading to hypercapnic respiratory failure after discontinuing mechanical ventilation. To detect diaphragmatic fatigue the power spectrum of diaphragmatic surface electromyographic activity was analyzed. A sustained reduction of the H/L ratio below 80% of the initial value was taken as indicative that diaphragmatic fatigue would ensue. Seven patients showed electromyographic evidence of inspiratory muscle fatigue. Electrical fatigue was followed by respiratory alternans and/or paradoxical inward movement of the abdominal wall during inspiration (abdominal paradox). However, it is possible that these changes may not reflect inspiratory muscle fatigue *per se* but instead, alternations in central drive due to excessive loading response [9]. Nevertheless such high inspiratory loads observed during weaning failure will eventually lead the ventilatory pump to exhaustion and overt fatigue which is, undoubtedly, a terminal event. During weaning trials in clinical practice mechanical ventilation is invariably resumed prior to inspiratory muscle exhaustion in patients failing to wean since many symptoms and clinical signs signal the forthcoming failure.

Some of the controversy regarding the exact role of inspiratory muscle fatigue during weaning failure stems from the fact that fatigue has been defined in dichotomous terms (present or absent) but the impairment in contractility is more likely to exist in the form of a continuum [10]. Furthermore, the bedside clinical diagnosis of fatigue is hampered by the inability to measure the baseline before fatigue and by the lack of a universally agreed upon objective physiologic or clinical test (or set of tests) that is a unique indicator of fatigue [11]. However, recent data offer significant support in favor of fatigue. Respiratory muscle maximum relaxation rate (MRR) has been measured during the weaning process and has been demonstrated to slow in those patients failing to wean; it has also been shown to remain unchanged in those weaning successfully [12]. This suggests that during weaning failure trials a fatigue process is initiated peripherally into the respiratory muscles; associated with the slowing of MRR, it is likely that the central drive is modulated [13].

Furthermore, using similar electrical criteria to Cohen et al. [8] to predict diaphragmatic fatigue, Brochard and co-workers [14] found that seven out of eight patients who met the usual criteria for weaning but who failed to wean, exhibited electromyographic signs of fatigue during spontaneous breathing, followed by a decreased V_T, an increased respiratory rate and the development of hypercapnia. Interestingly all these patients had increased energy demands as evidenced by the VO_2 of the respiratory muscles and the work of breathing per unit of time, WOB, that was always above 8 to 10 l/min. When pressure support was applied, thus reducing the work performed by the muscles, diaphragmatic fatigue was prevented. Impaired diaphragmatic function during weaning was also implicated by Pourriat and co-workers [15] who studied diaphragmatic function and the pattern of breathing in patients with chronic obstructive pulmonary disease (COPD) being weaned from mechanical ventilation after acute respiratory failure. They noted that when P_{di} was expressed as a fraction of the maximal P_{di} ($P_{di\,max}$) this value reached a mean of 46% in the group failing to wean. According to Roussos and Macklem [16] a $P_{di}/P_{di\,max}$ ratio greater than 40% cannot be tolerated for long periods without fatigue of the diaphragm. Appendini and co-workers [17] also studied COPD patients who failed to wean and found that they had a $P_{di}/P_{di\,max}$ ratio of 0.47 and a diaphragmatic TTI averaging 0.17, both greater than the critical fatiguing threshold values. On the contrary, Jubran and Tobin [18] recently reported that only 5 out of their 17 COPD patients who failed to wean had a TTI greater than 0.15. However, the way they calculated TTI (by measuring $P_{i\,max}$ at the beginning of the weaning trial and P_i at the end) might have created an underestimation of the TTI values since $P_{i\,max}$ would have probably decreased at the end of the trial. It was also possible in these patients to measure the load imposed on the respiratory muscles and their capacity. In fact, $P_i/P_{i\,max}$ had an excessively high mean value amounting to 0.42 ± 0.11 in patients failing on discontinuation from mechanical ventilation [19]. Additionally, dynamic hyperinflation amounting to 0.25 ± 0.19 l was present in almost all patients. When the ratio $P_i/P_{i\,max}$ was plotted against the dynamic increase in FRC to account for the effect of hyperinflation, 13 out of 31 patients (42%) were placed above a hypothetical critical line representing the critical inspiratory pressure above which fatigue may occur. In addition, all patients were gathered around the critical line [9] (Fig. 5). Furthermore, the combination of a decrease in inspiratory load and an increase in neuromuscular competence, that resulted in a decrease in the energy demands and a more efficient breathing pattern was adequate to make weaning successful in patients previously unable to wean (unpublished observations). In conclusion, fatigue of the inspiratory muscles frequently seems to be a final common pathway, leading to the inability to sustain spontaneous ventilation and, thus, to weaning failure.

The f/V_T ratio, a measure of rapid shallow breathing introduced by Yang and Tobin [20], has been used as an index for predicting the weaning outcome [21, 22]. Interestingly in our study, the f/V_T ratio measured at the end of the T-piece trial, was one of the two explanatory variables that accounted for the weaning outcome. The adoption of such rapid and shallow breathing may represent the response of the central respiratory control to loaded breathing [23]. Accordingly, Yang and Tobin [20] have reported that patients who fail to wean exhibit rapid shallow breathing on discontinuation of mechanical ventilation. This might also represent the response to inspiratory muscle fatigue [24], as was likely to occur in our patients during weaning

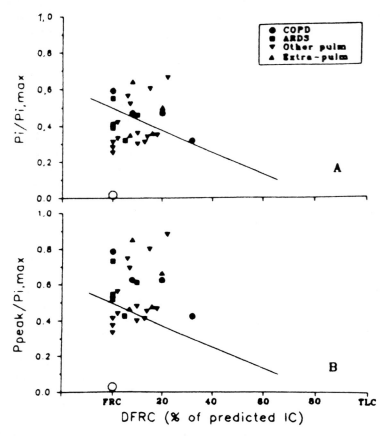

Fig. 5. Pressure-volume diagram similar to that of Roussos and colleagues [6] plotting the ratio $P_i/P_{i\,max}$ (A) and $P_{peak}/P_{i\,max}$ (B) against DFRC expressed as percentage of predicted inspiratory capacity (IC). The ratios $P_i/P_{i\,max}$ and $P_{peak}/P_{i\,max}$ are mean and peak inspiratory pressure per breath, respectively, expressed as a fraction of maximum in 10 normal subjects. The solid line was constructed from data in normal subjects and represents the critical inspiratory pressures above which fatigue may occur. At normal FRC, the critical inspiratory pressure per breath above which fatigue may occur in normal subjects is about 50% of maximum inspiratory pressure, whereas at FRC + $^1/_2$ IC this critical pressure is 25 to 35% of the maximum. All patients had excessively high values of both ratios, clustering around the critical line, rather than remaining away from it, as happens in normal subjects. (From [19] with permission)

failure, or a strategy adopted by the central respiratory control to prevent and/or avoid task failure in the presence of fatiguing loads.

Another possibility is that the rapid, shallow breathing pattern is partly a response of the respiratory center to the dyspnea and anxiety generated during the weaning trial. In fact during weaning trials patients experience substantial degrees of dyspnea [25–27], which is frequently underestimated by their physicians [26]. Accordingly Knebel et al. [26] found substantial degrees of dyspnea in the 21 patients they studied, both before weaning and during weaning trials using partial ventilator support, either in the form of synchronized intermittent mandatory ventilation (SIMV) or in the form of pressure support ventilation (PSV). Interestingly dyspnea levels during the SIMV weaning trials predicted the ability to wean. Convincing data for the role of dyspnea in weaning failure are also provided in a recent study by Stroetz and Hubmayr [27], where seven of the fourteen patients that failed to wean did so because of intense dyspnea. The question now arises: How could dyspnea, a purely sensory modality, contribute to weaning failure? Although no definite answer can be given, some speculations find scientific support. Most patients with chronic pulmonary disease have eliminated from their daily routine strenuous activities and behaviors that are associated with increased shortness of breath, even before they need mechanical ventilation. These patients typically develop a systematic decrease in tolerance to dyspnea and they often exhibit anxiety and avoidance in anticipation of any physical exertion. When starting trials of weaning from mechanical ventilation, many patients display fear and apprehension related to the anticipation of dyspnea rather than the stress of the activity *per se*; a response analogous to the one observed when these "dyspnea intolerant" patients initiate an exercise program [28]. One could speculate that dyspnea may be the limiting factor during weaning trials as is quite often the case during exercise testing. Furthermore, dyspnea seems closely associated with anxiety [29] and this is supported by the results of Knebel et al. [26] where both dyspnea and anxiety were measured using a visual analog scale and were found to be highly correlated [26]. In fact, it seems that in addition to motor output, sensory feedback from peripheral respiratory mechanorecptors contributes importantly to respiratory sensation. When the relationship between effort (motor output) and the anticipated ventilatory consequence (instantaneous change in respired volume) is seriously disturbed neuro-ventilatory dissociation (NVD) ensues, implying awareness of disproportionate or unsatisfied inspiratory effort. The psychophysical basis of NVD probably resides in the complex central processing of integrated sensory information. At a cognitive level NVD may be recognized as a disparity between expectations (whether genetically programmed or learned) and current perceptions of the internal environment. This disparity may elicit patterned psychologic and neurohumoral responses among which anxiety is almost invariably present [30]. Anxiety potentially has important physiologic consequences:

1) Muscle tone is increased and this elevates the chest wall elastic load through its effect on the intercostals [31]. Increased tension in the internal intercostal muscles makes inspiration more difficult since they are expiratory muscles. On the other hand, increased tension in the external intercostals that are inspiratory muscles, opposes expiration. Either effect renders the respiratory muscles less efficient.

2) Anxiety causes muscle deconditioning and this leads to discordinate breathing, again increasing the load. Indirect proof for the above mentioned effects comes from the study of Holiday and Hyers [31] where relaxation biofeedback decreased intercostal muscle tension and improved breathing patterns that became more coordinated. The respiratory muscle efficiency was increased and the weaning time was reduced.

3) Breathing frequency may increase, leading to a rapid, shallow and inefficient breathing pattern. This is indirectly evidenced by various reports [32–34] where biofeedback and/or hypnosis were used to successfully wean patients who had

previously failed at weaning. The beneficial effect of either intervention was mainly attributed to the achieved reduction in the anxiety experienced by the patients during the weaning trials, that resulted in a more efficient pattern of breathing.

Cardiovascular Dysfunction

Patients with underlying ventricular dysfunction may develop increases in pulmonary capillary wedge pressure and sometimes ultimately decreases in cardiac output upon removal from positive-pressure mechanical ventilation [35]. Several factors may be responsible [36, 37] (Table 1). The mechanism leading to weaning failure in these patients might be considered as follows: During spontaneous or diminished support ventilation the increase in respiratory muscle work load as well as anxiety and sympathetic discharge result in an abrupt increase in oxygen and cardiac de-

Table 1. Factors increasing PCWP during unsuccessful weaning from mechanical ventilation. (Modified from [36] with permission)

Increased preload
1) Increased venous return
   - Decreased pleural pressure
   - Sympathetic discharge (stress, hypercapnia)
   - Increased abdominal pressure
2) Reduced LV Compliance (diastolic stiffness)
   - Myocardial ischemia
     - ↓ O_2 supply
       - ↓ PaO_2
       - ↑ LVEDP and ↑ HR, reducing coronary blood flow
       - ↓ Mean arterial pressure
     - ↑ O_2 demands
       - ↑ Catecholamines
       - ↑ HR
       - ↑ Systolic blood pressure
   - LV enlargement
   - RV enlargement (Ventricular interdependence)
     - ↑ Venous return
     - ↑ Pulmonary artery pressure (acute)
     - RV ischemia leading to reduced RV contractility
   - Compression of heart chambers by regionally hyperinflated lung

Reduced contractility
   - Myocardial ischemia
   - Myocardial hypoxia
   - Myocardial acidosis, especially due to hypercapnia
   - Ionized hypocalcemia
   - Drugs

Increased afterload
   - ↑ Systolic blood pressure (hypercapnia, catecholamine discharge)
   - ↓ Pleural pressure

PCWP = Pulmonary capillary wedge pressure; LV = Left ventricle; RV = Right ventricle; LVEDP = Left ventricular end-diastolic pressure

mands. The failing left ventricle then is unable to respond normally and left ventricular end-diastolic pressure (LVEDP) rises causing interstitial, peribronchiolar and alveolar edema. This reduces lung compliance, increases airway resistance and worsens ventilation-perfusion mismatching leading to hypoxemia. Respiratory muscle energy demands are increased while energy supplies are either diminished or not sufficiently increased (inadequate cardiac output, hypoxemia). This eventually leads to an inability to sustain spontaneous ventilation at a level adequate to achieve normocapnia and PCO_2 rises. The abnormal blood gases depress cardiac contractility and, at the same time, respiratory muscle function. This further worsens blood gases and creates a vicious circle that may culminate in failure to wean.

The pivotal role played by the respiratory muscles in the development of left ventricular dysfunction is mediated through the effects of muscle activation on pleural and abdominal pressures. Normally spontaneous inspiration increases abdominal pressure at the same time it decreases pleural pressure due to diaphragmatic contraction and descent. The importance of the decreased pleural pressure for venous return augmentation is easily understood. Furthermore, the negative intrathoracic pressure increases the afterload of both ventricles and this, combined with the increased venous return, may lead to right ventricular distension. Because the two ventricles are constrained by a common pericardial sac and share the interventricular septum, changes in the volume of one ventricle may affect the function of the other; thus, right ventricular distension impedes the filling of the left ventricle [38]. This occurs both through a generalized increase in pericardial pressure and also because of a shift of the interventricular septum toward the left. Left ventricular filling impediment increases its diastolic stiffness at the same time that its afterload is elevated due to the decreased pleural pressure. This combined effect leads to the elevation of LVEDP with the above mentioned sequence of events culminating in weaning failure.

On the contrary, the role of abdominal pressure is not usually considered significant, yet abdominal pressure surrounds the abdominal venous system through which two thirds of the venous return passes [39]. Therefore, an increase in abdominal pressure could theoretically compress the abdominal veins and increase the amount of blood returning to the heart [40]. In order to explain the contradictory results in the literature regarding the effects of diaphragmatic descent on venous return Takata et al. [41, 42] recently expanded the concept of zones of the lung to the abdominal vasculature. According to their model, an increase in abdominal pressure would increase inferior vena cava (IVC) venous return when the transmural IVC pressure at the thoracic inlet (P_{IVC}-P_{ab}) significantly exceeds the critical closing transmural pressure (P_c) i.e.:

$$P_{IVC}\text{-}P_{ab} \geq P_c \text{ (ZONE III condition)}$$

where P_{IVC} is the IVC pressure at the the level of the diaphragm, P_{ab} is the abdominal pressure, and P_c is the critical closing transmural pressure. On the contrary, an increase in abdominal pressure would reduce IVC venous return when the transmural IVC pressure at the thoracic inlet is below the critical closing transmural pressure

$$P_{IVC}\text{-}P_{ab} \leq P_c \text{ (ZONE II condition)}$$

because of the development of vascular waterfall. This concept was successfully tested in animal models [41, 42] and can adequately explain the results of Lemaire and co-workers [35]. In this study, the hemodynamic effects of changing from positive pressure to spontaneous ventilation in 15 patients with combined COPD and coronary artery disease were measured. Spontaneous breathing increased cardiac output and right and left ventricular filling pressures rapidly leading to respiratory failure, while weaning indices had predicted a successful weaning. The increase in venous return and cardiac output was an expected finding since the decrease in pleural pressure associated with spontaneous breathing would increase venous return by lowering right atrial pressure (the downstream pressure for venous return). However, in these patients the right atrial pressure actually rose relative to atmospheric pressure despite the lower pressure surrounding the heart. The increase in venous return could have been due only to either a greater increase in the upstream pressure (P_{ab}) or a reduction in the resistance to venous return. Only the first probability, however, was applicable under those circumstances. Although no patient had clinical evidence of volume overload, all were subsequently forced into diuresis for one week, losing an average of 5 kg. After that, 8 of the 15 patients were successfully weaned. These patients now had cardiac output and filling pressures during spontaneous breathing essentially unaltered from their values during mechanical ventilation. An interesting explanation for these findings is offered by the above mentioned model [43]. Prior to diuresis these patients' abdomens were in ZONE III condition. When they began spontaneous breathing their mean abdominal pressure rose and led to increased venous return; this sudden increase in venous return coupled with elevation of the left ventricular afterload caused by the lowered pleural pressure precipitated heart failure and, in turn, respiratory failure. Afler diuresis the abdomens of many patients were in ZONE II; increased abdominal pressure now did not increase venous return as much, due to the development of vascular waterfall. Although respiratory work and left ventricular afterload initially increased as much as they had the prior week, deterioration of heart function was prevented and these patients were successfully weaned.

The increased left ventricular preload and afterload resulting from the activation of the respiratory muscles upon resumption of spontaneous breathing, may also lead to altered myocardial perfusion and ischemia [44, 45] and thus to the inability to wean successfully. Accordingly, Rasanen et al. [44] found electrocardiographic (EKG) evidence of myocardial ischemia in 6 of their 12 patients with myocardial infarction complicated by respiratory failure on withdrawal of ventilator support. Furthermore, Hurford and co-workers [45] observed new regions of decreased myocardial thallium 201 ([201]TI) uptake and transient left ventricular dilation in 7 of their 15 patients assessed by [201]TI myocardial scintigraphy during discontinuation of mechanical ventilation. Their results suggest that the hemodynamic and ventilatory changes associated with resumption of spontaneous breathing were sufficient to increase myocardial oxygen demands (evidenced by the increased heart rate, arterial blood pressure and left ventricle cavity size during spontaneous ventilation) to such an extent that the available coronary oxygen supply could not meet the demand probably due to coronary atherosclerosis or spasm, thus leading to ischemia. Interestingly, the authors were unable to detect any EKG changes diagnostic of myocardial ischemia, implying that EKG criteria are relatively insensitive and that myocardial ischemia should be suspected in the patient who fails to wean even in the absence of EKG changes.

Recent work [27, 46] lends further credit to the role of cardiac dysfunction in weaning failure. As many as one third of failures in the study of Epstein [46] resulted solely or in part from congestive heart failure whereas 21% of the patients of Stroetz and Hubmayr [27] failed due to the development of cardiovascular dysfunction (7% developed ventricular ectopy and 14% blood pressure changes).

Stealing Effect

In normal subjects who are breathing quietly, the oxygen cost of breathing (VO_{2resp}) is a small proportion of the total oxygen requirement (VO_{2tot}). However, this may not be the case for the patient who fails to wean, whose VO_{2resp} may be significantly elevated at the same time that the available energy may be decreased. In an elegant theoretical analysis, Riley [47] has suggested that patients like these (i.e., who have inappropriate relation of ventilatory needs and neuro-cardiorespiratory capacity) may be severely limited in the extent to which their ventilation may be increased. As ventilation increases, an ever greater proportion of the additional oxygen taken up will have to be diverted to the respiratory muscles at the expense of the oxygen available for non-respiratory work. A point will then be reached beyond which the increase in VO_{2resp} becomes greater than the increase in VO_{2tot} so that oxygen available for non-respiratory work begins to decease and further increases in ventilation are detrimental. This theoretical analysis may be applicable to some patients who fail to wean and in whom VO_{2resp} may increase to such an extent that the working respiratory muscles may steal oxygen and blood from other tissues. Animal studies provide strong support in favor of this "stealing effect". When dogs with cardiogenic or septic shock [48–52] were mechanically ventilated, only 3% of their cardiac output was directed to their respiratory muscles. On the contrary, when these dogs were allowed to breathe spontaneously their respiratory muscles received up to 20% of the cardiac output, stealing blood from other organs such as the brain, liver or other muscles. It has also been shown in animal models that activation of small afferent neural fibers from intensely working respiratory muscles results in active vasoconstriction of vessels supplying other organs [53], further diminishing their nutrient flow which is probably "stolen" in favor of the respiratory muscles. This decrease in the blood flow supplying other organs could theoretically predispose them to dysfunction. Furthermore, at least for the brain, this could also have an impact on the function of the respiratory muscles *per se* by affecting the output of the respiratory center. In fact, in an elegant animal model Nava and Bellemare [54] have shown that when dogs were subjected to shock, thus reducing their carotid blood flow, they gradually developed (after an initial increase) a decline in both P_{di} and the electrical activity of the diaphragm (E_{di}) followed by development of respiratory arrest (apnea). Interestingly, the values of P_{di} measured in response to phrenic nerve stimulation before shock and soon after apnea were not different, suggesting that respiratory failure and apnea resulted from a decrease in central neural output to the respiratory muscles (central fatigue) and not from peripheral contractile failure.

Various studies have tried to address the issue of VO_{2resp} in patients during weaning [14, 55–57]. Their results do not seem at a first glance to provide strong evidence that the respiratory muscles were creating a stealing effect despite the relatively high VO_{2resp} values obtained. However, this holds true as far as the mean values of VO_{2resp} are considered, in the patients studied. When the results are analyzed on a patient by patient basis, the conclusions drawn can be quite different. Accordingly, Field et al. [55] measured the VO_{2resp} in 13 patients with cardiopulmonary disease being weaned from artificial ventilation and found it to be on the average 75 ml O_2/min, representing 24% of VO_{2tot}. However, there were two patients in whom the VO_{2resp} amounted to 286 and 157 ml O_2/min, representing 55% and 44% of VO_{2tot}, respectively. It can be speculated that in these two patients at least, the respiratory muscles were stealing energy from other tissues. Furthermore, Brochard et al. [14] measured the VO_{2resp} in 6 patients during weaning and found similar values: Mean VO_{2resp} was 78 ml O_2/min, representing 27% of the VO_{2tot}; but again, there was a patient whose VO_{2resp} was 59% of his VO_{2tot}. Similarly, Oh and co-workers [56] and Shikora et al. [57] have studied occasional patients with VO_{2resp} amounting to over 40% of their VO_{2tot}. Consequently, it can be assumed that there are patients whose respiratory muscles create a stealing effect during weaning, depriving other organs from oxygen and blood, thus leading to weaning failure.

Interestingly, weaning has been occasionally reported to fail due to the development of organ dysfunction. In the work of Epstein [44], development of encephalopathy was recognized as the etiologic factor and altered mental status appears to be a common cause for delayed weaning from mechanical ventilation [58]. Based on animal models [54] and theoretical considerations, one could speculate that the respiratory muscles were "stealing" blood and oxygen from the brain and that this was the reason for altered mental function.

Conclusion

The etiology of weaning failure is usually multifactorial with each factor contributing its own percentage of the total process. An increase in the TTI and/or the I/V_T ratio, represents the common pathophysiologic pathway culminating in weaning failure.

References

1. Roussos Ch, Macklem PT (1982) The respiratory muscles. N Engl J Med 307:786–797
2. Macklem PT (1986) Respiratory muscle dysfunction. Hosp Prac 21:83–90
3. Monod H, Scherrer J (1965) The work capacity of a synergistic muscular group. Ergonomics 8:329–337
4. Bellemare F, Grassino A (1982) Effect of pressure and timing of contraction on human diaphragm fatigue. J Appl Physiol 53:1190–1195
5. Millic-Emili J (1986) Is weaning an art or a science? Am Rev Respir Dis 134:1107–1108
6. Roussos Ch, Fixley D, Gross D, Macklem PT (1979) Fatigue of inspiratory muscles and their synergic behavior. J Appl Phys 46:897–904
7. Vassilakopoulos T, Zakynthinos S, Roussos C (1996) Respiratory muscles and weaning failure. Eur Respir J 9:2383–2400

8. Cohen CA, Zagelbaum G, Gross D, Roussos Ch, Macklem DT (1982) Clinical manifestations of inspiratory muscle fatigue. Am J Med 73:308–316

9. Tobin M, Perez W, Guenther SM, Lodato RF, Dantzker DR (1987) Does ribcage-abdominal paradox signify respiratory muscle fatigue? J Appl Physiol 63:851–860

10. Slutsky AS (1994) Consensus conference on mechanical ventilation (Part 2). Intensive Care Med 20:150–162

11. NHLBI Workshop (1990) Respiratory muscle fatigue: report of the respiratory muscle fatigue workshop group. Am Rev Respir Dis 142:474–480

12. Goldstone JC, Green M, Moxham J (1994) Maximum relaxation rate of the diaphragm during weaning from mechanical ventilation. Thorax 49:54–60

13. Bigland-Ritchie B, Donovan EF, Roussos CH (1981) Conductions velocity and EMG power spectrum changes in fatigue of sustained maximal efforts. J Appl Physiol 51:1300–1305

14. Brochard L, Hart A, Lorino H, Lemaire F (1989) Inspiratory pressure support prevents diaphragmatic fatigue during weaning from mechanical ventilation. Am Rev Respir Dis 139:513–521

15. Pourriat JL, Lamberto Ch, Hoang Ph, Fournier JL, Vasseur B (1986) Diaphragmatic fatigue and breathing pattern during weaning from mechanical ventilation in COPD patients. Chest 90:703–707

16. Roussos Ch, Macklem PT (1977) Diaphragmatic fatigue in man. J Appl Physiol 43:189–197

17. Appendini L, Purro A, Patessio A, Zanaboni S, Carone M, Spada E, Donner CF, Rossi A (1996) Partitioning of inspiratory muscle workload and pressure assistance in ventilator-dependent COPD patients. Am J Respir Crit Care Med 154:1301–1309

18. Jubran A, Tobin M (1997) Pathophysiological basis of acute respiratory distress in patients who fail a trial of weaning from mechanical ventilation. Am J Respir Crit Care Med 155:906–915

19. Zakynthinos S, Vassilakopoulos T, Roussos C (1995) The load of inspiratory muscles in patients needing mechanical ventilation. Am J Respir Crit Care Med 152:1248–1255

20. Yang KL, Tobin MJ (1991) A prospective study of indexes predicting the outcome of trials of weaning from mechanical ventilation. N Engl J Med 324:1445–1450

21. Epstein SK. Evaluation of the rapid shallow breathing index (RVR) in the clinical setting. Am J Respir Crit Care Med 152:545–549

22. Chatila W, Jacob B, Guaglionone D, Manthous CA (1996) The unassisted respiratory rate-tidal volume ratio accurately predicts weaning outcome. Am J Med 101:61–67

23. Tobin MJ, Perez W, Guenther SM, Semmes BJ, Mador MJ, Allen SJ, Lodato RF, Dantzker DR (1986) The pattern of breathing during successful and unsuccessful trials of weaning from mechanical ventilation. Am Rev Respir Dis 134:1111–1118

24. Yan S, Sliwinski P, Gauthier AP, Lichros I, Zakynthinos S, Macklem PT (1993) Effect of global inspiratory muscle fatigue on ventilatory and respiratory muscle responses to CO_2. J Appl Physiol 75:1371–1377

25. Petrof BJ, Legare M, Goldberg P, Milic-Emili J, Gottfried SB (1990) Continuous positive airway pressure reduces work of breathing and dyspnea during weaning from mechanical ventilation in severe chronic obstructive pulmonary disease. Am Rev Respir Dis 141:281–289

26. Knebel AR, Janson-Bjerklie SL, Malley JD, Wilson AG, Marini JJ (1994) Comparison of breathing comfort during weaning with two ventilatory modes. Am J Respir Crit Care Med 149:14–18

27. Stroetz RW, Hubmayr RD (1995) Tidal volume maintenance during weaning with pressure support. Am J Respir Crit Care Med 152:1034–1040

28. Criner GJ, Isaac L (1994) Psychological problems in the ventilator dependent patient. In: Tobin MJ (ed) Principles and Practice of Mechanical Ventilation. McGraw Hill, New York, pp 1163–1175

29. LaFond L, Horner J (1988) Psychological issues related to long-term ventilatory support. Prob Respir Care 1:241–256

30. O'Donnell DE (1994) Breathlessness in patients with airflow limitation. Mechanisms and management. Chest 106:904–912

31. Holliday JE, Hyers TM (1990) The reduction of weaning time from mechanical ventilation using tidal volume and relaxation biofeedback. Am Rev Respir Dis 141:1214–1220

32. La Riccia PJ, Katz RH, Peters JW, Atkinson GW, Weiss T (1985) Biofeedback and hypnosis in weaning from mechanical ventilators. Chest 87:267–269

33. Gorson JA, Grant JL, Moulton DP, Green RL, Dunkel PT (1979) Use of biofeedback in weaning paralyzed patients from respirators. Chest 76:543–545

34. Yarnal JR, Herrell DW, Sivak ED (1981) Routine use of biofeedback in weaning patients from mechanical ventilation. Chest 79:127
35. Lemaire F, Teboul JL, Cinotti L, Giotto G, Abrouk F, Steg G, Macquin-Mavier I, Zapol WM (1988) Acute left ventricular dysfunction during unsuccessful weaning from mechanical ventilation. Anesthesiology 69:171–179
36. Lemaire F (1993) Difficult weaning. Intensive Care Med 19:69–73
37. Richard Ch, Teboul J-L, Archanbaud F, Herbert J-L, Michaut P, Auzepy P (1994) Left ventricular function during weaning of patients with chronic obstructive pulmonary disease. Intensive Care Med 20:181–186
38. Biondi JW, Schulman DS, Matthay RA (1988) Effects of mechanical ventilation on right and left ventricular function. Clin Chest Med 9:55–74
39. Robotham JL, Becker LC (1994) The cardiovascular effects of weaning: Stratifying patient populations. Intensive Care Med 20:171–172
40. Permutt S (1988) Circulatory effects of weaning from mechanical ventilation: The importance of transdiaphragmatic pressure. Anesthesiology 69:157–160
41. Takata M, Robotham JL (1992) Effects of inspiratory diaphragmatic descent on inferior vena caval venous return. J Appl Physiol 72:597–607
42. Takata M, Wise RA, Robotham JL (1990) Effects of abdominal pressure on venous return. J Appl Physiol 69:1961–1972
43. Fessler HE, Permutt S (1995) Interaction between the circulatory and ventilatory pumps. In: Roussos Ch (ed) The Thorax, 2nd ed. Marcel Dekker, New York, pp 1621–1640
44. Räsänen J, Nikki P, Heikkila J (1984) Acute myocardial infarction complicated by respiratory failure. The effects of mechanical ventilation. Chest 85:21–28
45. Hurford WE, Lynch KE, Strauss WH, Lowenstein E, Zapol WM (1991) Myocardial perfusion as assessed by thallium 201 scintigraphy during the discontinuation of mechanical ventilation in ventilator dependent patients. Anesthesiology 74:1007–1016
46. Epstein SK (1995) Etiology of extubation failure and the predictive value of the rapid shallow breathing index. Am J Respir Crit Care Med 152:545–549
47. Riley RL (1954) The work of breathing and its relation to respiratory acidosis. Ann Intern Med 41:172–176
48. Hussain SNA, Graham R, Rutledge F, Roussos Ch (1986) Respiratory muscle energetics during endotoxic shock in dogs. J Appl Physiol 60:486–493
49. Hussain SNA, Roussos Ch (1985) Distribution of respiratory muscle and organ blood flow during endotoxic shock in dogs. J Appl Physiol 59:1802–1808
50. Hussain SNA, Simcus G, Roussos Ch (1985) Respiratory muscle fatigue: a cause of ventilatory failure in septic shock. J Appl Physiol 58:2033–2040
51. Aubier M, Trippenbach T, Roussos Ch (1981) Respiratory muscle fatigue during cardiogenic shock. J Appl Physiol 51:499–508
52. Viires N, Sillye G, Aubier M, Rassidakis A, Roussos Ch (1983) Regional blood flow distribution in dogs during induced hypotension and low cardiac output. Spontaneous breathing versus artificial ventilation. J Clin Invest 72:935–947
53. Hussain SNA, Chatillon A, Comptois A, Roussos Ch, Magder S (1991) Chemical activation of thin-fiber phrenic afferents: 2 cardiovascular responses. J Appl Physiol 70:77–86
54. Nava S, Bellemare F (1989) Cardiovascular failure and apnea in shock. J Appl Physiol 66:184–189
55. Field S, Kelly SM, Macklem PT (1982) The oxygen cost of breathing in patient with cardiorespiratory disease. Am Rev Respir Dis 126:9–13
56. Oh TE, Bhatt S, Lin ES, Hutchinson RC, Low MJ (1991) Plasma catecholamines and oxygen consumption during weaning from mechanical ventilation. Intensive Care Med 17:199–203
57. Shikora SA, Benotti PN, Johannigman JA (1994) The oxygen cost of breathing may predict weaning from mechanical ventilation better than the respiratory rate to tidal volume ratio. Arch Surg 129:269–274
58. Kelly BJ, Matthay MA (1993) Prevalence and severity of neurologic dysfunction in critically ill patients. Chest 104:1818–1924

What Have We Learned About Weaning Over the Last Five Years?

I. Alia, A. Esteban, and F. Gordo

Introduction

Mechanical ventilation is a lifesaving vital support technique which is not exempt from complications [1]. Some of the risks associated with mechanical ventilation, such as nosocomial pneumonia increase with the duration of ventilatory support. For example, Ruiz-Santana et al. [2] reported, in a prospective study of pneumonias in critically ill patients, a cumulative incidence of pneumonia of 8.5% in the first three days after intubation, 21.1% for day seven, 32.4% for day fourteen and 45.6% for longer than fourteen days.

The best way to prevent the complications associated with mechanical ventilation is reduce ventilatory support duration and extubate patients as quickly as possible. More than 40 percent of the time that a patient receives mechanical ventilation is spent trying to wean the patient from the ventilator [3]. Therefore, measures to reduce weaning duration will decrease total ventilatory time. Over the last five years, several randomized and controlled trials [4–7] have shown that the duration of mechanical ventilation and weaning can be reduced by the implementation of specific strategies including:

1) Identifying, as soon as possible, which patients are capable of breathing spontaneously by means of daily screening of the respiratory function followed by trials of spontaneous breathing
2) Avoiding the use of methods of weaning which may prolong, in difficult to wean patients, the time until extubation
3) Using protocols to wean patients from mechanical ventilation instead of the traditional practice based on personal physician preferences

In this chapter, we would like to provide evidence that the duration of mechanical ventilation can be reduced by standardization of the weaning process. Finally, each of our positions about the weaning process, will be summarized into an algorithm in which the recomendations based on the evidence will be graded according to a published system [8] (Table 1).

How to Assess if Patients are Able to Sustain Spontaneous Breathing

Discontinuation of ventilatory support should be considered when patients have recovered from the cause of their respiratory failure. Numerous indexes indicating the

Table 1. Method of grading levels of evidence and recommendations. (From [8] with permission)

Levels of evidence	
Level I studies	Randomized trials with low false-positive and low false-negative errors
Level II studies	Randomized trials with high false-positive and or high false-negative errors
Level III studies	Non-randomized, concurrent cohort comparisons
Level IV studies	Non-randomized historical cohort comparisons
Level V studies	Case series without controls
Recommendations	
Grade A	Supported by ≥ 1 level I studies or by a meta-analysis in which the lower limit of the confidence interval for the effect of treatment exceeds the minimally clinically significant benefit
Grade B	Supported by either ≥ 1 level II studies or by a meta-analysis in which the estimate of treatment effect exceeds the minimal clinically significant benefit but the lower limit of the confidence interval does not
Grade C	Supported by data other than prospective controlled trials, including secondary analyses of level I or II studies

adequacy of pulmonary gas exchange or the mechanical function of the ventilatory pump, have been evaluated to assess their usefulness in identifying patients who are able to resume and sustain spontaneous breathing and patients who are likely to fail a weaning trial [9–12]. Unfortunately, it is not yet established how these indexes should be used in clinical practice. Should weaning be ruled out in patients with true improvement of respiratory failure but who do not meet weaning criteria? Can those patients who meet the weaning criteria be safely extubated, without a trial of spontaneous breathing? These are unanswered questions despite the extensive research on weaning indexes in the last decade.

The rapid shallow breathing index or ratio of respiratory frequency to tidal volume (f/V_T) was reported by Yang and Tobin [9] as the most accurate predictor of weaning failure. In their study, 95% of patients with a f/V_T ratio higher than 105 failed the trial of weaning. However, recently a lower predictive accuracy for the f/V_T ratio has been reported. Epstein et al. [13, 14] found extubation failure rates ranging from 27 to 40% in patients with f/V_T ratios higher than 100. The studies performed by the Spanish lung collaborative group concerning trials of spontaneous breathing before extubation in mechanically ventilated patients [5, 15, 16] also support the finding that patients with f/V_T ratios higher than 100 have weaning failure rates ranging from 44 to 54% (unpublished data).

In the light of the above results, it seems that an elevated f/V_T ratio does not constitute an indication for delaying trials of weaning and it is possible that patients are ventilated for unnecessarily prolonged periods if the decision to start weaning is based on normal values of the f/V_T ratio. This drawback would be applicable also to other weaning indexes. On the other hand, the general rule is that ventilated patients are not extubated without an attempt at spontaneous breathing even if they have favorable weaning indexes.

Trials of spontaneous breathing are usually performed before extubation, with the aim of adequately evaluating the capacity of patients to sustain their ventilatory demands. Approximately 20% of patients who meet the critera to start weaning show signs of intolerance during the trial of spontaneous breathing [4, 5, 15, 16]. It is possible that patients in whom a trial of spontaneous breathing is considered to have failed might have been successfully weaned if they had been immediately extubated after checking they met favorable weaning indexes, but it seems more likely that some of them would have required re-intubation in the case of performing extubation without a previous spontaneous breathing trial. The general belief is that ventilated patients considered ready to be weaned should undergo a trial of spontaneous breathing before extubation.

The fact that as many as half the patients who have unintentional removal of the endotracheal tube do not require re-intubation [17–19] means that there are some patients able to breathe spontaneously who continue to receive ventilatory support. This undesirable condition could be avoided if physicians made a daily assessment of each ventilated patient with the aim of identifying those capable of breathing spontaneously.

Ely et al. [6] have reported recently that daily screening of the respiratory function of patients receiving mechanical ventilation followed by trials of spontaneous breathing before extubation, can reduce the duration of mechanical ventilation and the cost of intensive care. They conducted a randomized, controlled trial in 300 adult patients receiving mechanical ventilation in medical and coronary ICUs. All the patients underwent daily screening of their respiratory function to determine whether they could breathe without assistance. Five simple weaning criteria were screened: A ratio of the partial pressure of arterial oxygen (PaO_2) to the fraction of inspired oxygen (FiO_2) greater than 200; positive end-expiratory pressure (PEEP) less than 5 cmH_2O; adequate airway reflexes; a ratio of respiratory frequency to tidal volume less than 105 bpm/l; and no infusion of vasopressor agents or sedative drugs. In the patients of the intervention group who met the above criteria, a two-hour trial of spontaneous breathing was performed and physicians were notified when their patients successfully completed such a trial. Patients in the control group were also screened daily, but they did not undergo trials of spontaneous breathing. In both groups, the decision to discontinue mechanical ventilation was made by the attending physician. The percentage of patients who had successful screening tests was not different among groups (76 percent in the intervention group and 68 percent in the control group, $p = 0.14$). The time which elapsed from the initiation of mechanical ventilation until successful screening tests was 3 days (median) in the intervention group and 2 days (median) in the control group ($p = 0.4$). Forty-eight hours after patients had successful screening tests, 57 percent of patients in the intervention group (65 out of 113) had been successfully removed from mechanical ventilation, as compared with 23 percent (24 out of 103 patients) in the control group. The median duration of mechanical ventilation was 4.5 days (25th and 75th centiles, 2–9 days) in the intervention group and 6 days (25th and 75th centiles, 3–11 days) in the control group ($p = 0.003$). The results found by Ely et al. [6] mean that, among ventilated patients who meet criteria for weaning, three patients (95 percent confidence interval, 2–5) need to be treated with the weaning approach used in the interventional group, to successfully extubate one more patient than with a weaning practice based on the physician's judgement.

The report by Ely et al. [6] supports previous studies demonstrating that mechanical ventilation can be safely discontinued in patients who meet weaning criteria and tolerate trials of unassisted breathing. Benito et al. [20] reported a 60% rate of successful discontinuation of mechanical ventilation in 169 patients who met standard weaning indexes and underwent a two hour trial of spontaneous breathing with T-tube. The percentage of patients successfully weaned after a two hour trial of spontaneous breathing with T-tube was 62% in a study performed by Esteban et al. [5] in a population of 546 patients ventilated for a mean time of 7.5 ± 6.1 days, who met standard weaning criteria.

The best technique for performing spontaneous breathing trials before extubation has not been well evaluated. The increase in the work of breathing (WOB) caused by the presence of an endotracheal tube may be an excessive load for some patients breathing through the T-tube circuit, and poor tolerance of the trial can result from this. However, it has been recently demonstrated that the WOB during trials of spontaneous breathing through an endotracheal tube is similar to that after extubation [21, 22]. Pressure support ventilation (PSV) is useful to counteract the extra work imposed by breathing through an endotracheal tube. This task can be accomplished with a level of pressure support of 7 cmH_2O, although the compensatory level ranges from 3 to 15 cmH_2O [23–26]. Sometimes, low levels of pressure support underestimate the work of breathing performed by patients after extubation [22, 26]. Another important feature of PSV is that it improves the efficacy of spontaneous breathing and reduces respiratory work and oxygen consumption by the respiratory muscles during weaning [27, 28].

Esteban et al. [15] have recently reported the results of a randomized study comparing trials of spontaneous breathing performed with either T-tube or pressure support. A population of 484 patients who had received mechanical ventilation for more than 48 hours and who were considered, by their physicians, to be ready for weaning according to clinical criteria and standard weaning parameters, were randomly assigned to undergo a two-hour trial of spontaneous breathing in one of two ways; with a T-tube system or with PSV of 7 cmH_2O. Patients without signs of poor tolerance during the trial of spontaneous breathing were immediately extubated at the end of the two hour period. Of the 246 patients assigned to the T-tube group, 192 successfully completed the trial and were extubated, but 36 of them required re-intubation within 48 hours. Of the 238 patients in the group receiving PSV, 205 were extubated and 38 of them required re-intubation within 48 hours. The results of this study confirm the previously reported finding that ventilator support can be successfully discontinued in two thirds of ventilated patients after a two-hour trial of spontaneous breathing, since the percentage of patients who remained extubated after 48 hours was 63% in the T-tube group and 70% in the PSV group (p = 0.14). The above difference was not statistically significant but it could be considered by some clinicians as clinically relevant, because these results mean an absolute benefit increase of 7% (95 percent confidence interval, −2 to 15) in the percentage of successfully extubated patients and a relative benefit increase of 11% (95 percent confidence interval, −2 to 26), when spontaneous breathing trials were performed with pressure support. In other words, the number of patients who would need to be treated with PSV to successfully extubate one more patient than with a T-tube, is 14.

The percentage of patients failing the trial was significantly higher when the T-tube was used: 22% versus 14% (p = 0.03). This finding suggest that some patients fail spontaneous breathing trials with the T-tube because of the respiratory load imposed by the T-tube circuit, but they can be successfully extubated when this overload is eliminated by the pressure support. Further studies with a higher sample size are needed to confirm that the marginal effect of pressure support on the trial-success rate found by Esteban et al. [15] becomes apparent on the percentage of patients successfully extubated. Meanwhile, the only evidence is that both T-tube and PSV of 7 cmH$_2$O, are suitable methods to perform spontaneous breathing trials before extubation in mechanically ventilated patients.

The duration of spontaneous breathing trials in several studies has been set at two hours, but patients who fail a trial show signs of intolerance at a much earlier time [4, 5, 15, 29, 30]. The optimal duration of such trials is unknown and it is possible that it can be reduced without a higher risk for re-intubation. The Spanish lung failure collaborative group has recently reported that a 30 minute trial of spontaneous breathing is as effective as a 120 minute trial in weaning patients from mechanical ventilation [16]. A total of 526 patients ready to be weaned were randomly assigned to undergo a trial of spontaneous breathing lasting up to 30 minutes (n = 270) or up to two hours (n = 256). The rate of successful weaning was similar for the 30 minute and two-hour groups (75.9% versus 73.0%, p = 0.45). The percentage of patients needing re-intubation within 48 hours after passing the trial of spontaneous breathing was also similar: 13.5% in the 30 minute group and 13.4% in the two hours group (p = 0.26).

In summary, weaning is expedited and the duration of mechanical ventilation is reduced, when a daily screening of ventilated patients is performed with the aim to identify those patients capable of breathing spontaneously. Such a screening should be followed, in appropriate patients, by a trial of spontaneous breathing, and extubation must be immediately performed after a successful trial. Trials of spontaneous breathing are equally efficacious when they are performed with either a T-tube or pressure support of 7 cmH$_2$O. A duration of thirty minutes is enough to evaluate whether patients are able to be extubated.

How to Reduce the Duration of Weaning in Difficult to Wean Patients

While the majority of patients can be easily weaned from mechanical ventilation, a substantial minority pose considerable difficulty. Weaning attempts that are unsuccessful usually indicate incomplete resolution of the illness that precipitated the need for mechanical ventilation or the development of new problems. Every attempt should be made to identify the specific cause of ventilator dependency, and all correctable factors should be corrected. Meanwhile, a gradual withdrawal from mechanical ventilation could be attempted.

In the last few years, two well-designed studies comparing methods of gradual withdrawal of mechanical ventilation have been published [4, 5]. Both of them have shown that strategies of weaning influence the duration of mechanical ventilation and that intermittent mandatory ventilation is the most ineffective method among those studied. However, some conflicting results in these studies have failed to convince the clinicians that one method of weaning is superior to another.

Brochard et al. [4] prospectively evaluated 109 mechanically ventilated patients meeting standard weaning criteria who could not sustain two hours of spontaneous breathing. They were randomly assigned to be weaned with T-piece trials (n = 35), synchronized intermittent mandatory ventilation (SIMV, n = 43) or PSV (n = 31). No statistical difference existed between the groups regarding their characteristics on admission to the intensive care unit, the duration of mechanical ventilation before weaning, the duration of the initial T-piece tolerance test, and the results of pulmonary function tests performed at the onset of the weaning. The main finding reported by the authors was that the probability of remaining on mechanical ventilation over time was significantly lower with PSV than with the two other modalities (cumulative probability for 21 days, p < 0.003 with the log-rank test) (Fig. 1).

Brochard et al. [4] conducted a randomized trial to compare three methods of gradual withdrawal from ventilatory support but, in their paper, they only showed the results of the comparison of two groups of patients; those in the PSV group and those in the T-tube group pooled together with patients in the SIMV group. This suggests that no difference existed when the PSV and T-tube groups were compared. A multivariate analysis was performed to search for factors explaining weaning duration and the Cox proportional-hazards model showed that the length of weaning was first explained by the etiology of the disease (p = 0.01), with patients with chron-

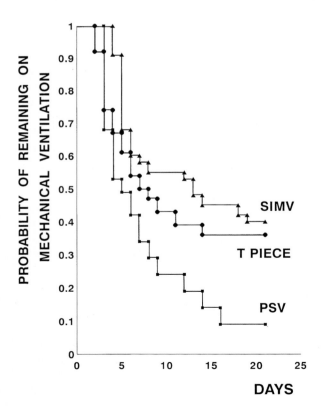

Fig. 1. Probability of remaining on mechanical ventilation in patients with prolonged difficulties in tolerating spontaneous breathing. SIMV: synchronized intermittent mandatory ventilation; PSV: pressure support ventilation. (From [4] with permission)

ic obstructive pulmonary disease (COPD) being the most difficult to separate from the ventilator, and then the mode of weaning (p = 0.03), with PSV allowing the shorter duration. Unfortunately, the authors did not show the adjusted rates of successful weaning with each method and their 95 percent confidence intervals, so it is not possible to know if they compared PSV versus T-tube and SIMV pooled together or separately, nor to estimate the effect of each method on the weaning duration.

Esteban et al. [5] also studied a population of mechanically ventilated patients considered ready for weaning according to standard weaning criteria but who failed a two-hour trial of spontaneous breathing. These patients were randomly assigned to undergo one of four weaning techniques: SIMV (n = 29); PSV (n = 37); intermittent trials of spontaneous breathing with T-tube (n = 33); and a once-daily trial of spontaneous breathing with T-tube (n = 31). The groups were similar with respect to the patients' characteristics, the indication for mechanical ventilation and respiratory function. The only significant difference was in the duration of ventilatory support before weaning was begun, which was shorter in the patients who received SIMV than in the other groups. The relative probablity of weaning success over time was examined by a Cox proportional hazards model. This analysis revealed four factors that predicted the time required for successful weaning, one of them being the weaning technique. The adjusted rate of successful weaning was higher with a once-daily trial of spontaneous breathing than with SIMV (rate ratio, 2.83; 95 percent confidence interval, 1.36 to 5.89, p < 0.006) or PSV (rate ratio, 2.05; 95 percent confidence interval, 1.04 to 4.04, p < 0.04).

There are two main outcomes of interest in studies comparing methods of weaning: The percentage of patients who are successfully weaned with each method; and the duration of the weaning period with each method. Information about these outcomes can be obtained from the Kaplan-Meier curve of the probability of successful weaning in the study by Esteban et al. [5] (Fig. 2) and the Kaplan-Meier curve of the probability of remaining on mechanical ventilation in the study by Brochard et al. [4] (Fig. 1). A common finding in both studies is that discontinuation of mechanical ventilation can be achieved in a short period of time ranging from one to three days in 25% of difficult-to-wean patients. After a few days, the curves for each method separate and the probability of weaning success or the probability of remaining on mechanical ventilation over time are quite different from one method of weaning to another. In patients with difficulties in tolerating spontaneous breathing, the duration of weaning increases two-fold if specific methods of weaning are used. In the study by Esteban et al. [5], 75% of patients were successfully weaned after six days if weaning was performed with either a once-daily trial of spontaneous breathing with T-tube or intermittent trials of spontaneous breathing with T-tube, whereas it took eleven or twelve days to successfully wean 75% of patients in the groups of SIMV or PSV respectively. In the study by Brochard et al. [4], 75% of patients were removed from the ventilator after nine days if PSV was used whereas more than three weeks elapsed until 75% of patients were weaned in either the T-tube group or the SIMV group.

Both studies draw a common conclusion: The use of SIMV as a method of weaning is today clearly unwarranted. With regard to the other methods, the T-tube used in intermittent trials of spontaneous breathing was not superior to PSV in the study by Esteban et al. [5] (adjusted rate of successful weaning 1.66; 95 percent confidence

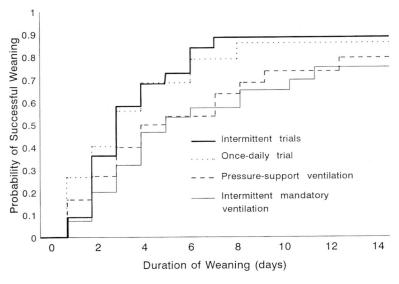

Fig. 2. Kaplan-Meier Curves of the probability of successful weaning with intermittent mandatory ventilation, pressure-support ventilation, intermittent trials of spontaneous breathing, and a once-daily trial of spontaneous breathing. (From [5] with permission)

interval, 0.87 to 3.16; p = 0.13), and it is not clear whether PSV was or was not superior to the T-tube in the study by Brochard et al. [4]. Nevertheless, a trend toward a higher probability of successful weaning with a T-tube was observed in the first study, and a trend toward lower probability of remaining on mechanical ventilation with PSV was observed in the second one. These conflicting results may be explained, at least in part, by the different criteria used to progress in the process of weaning with each of the two aforementioned methods and the criteria used to decide on extubation. On the other hand, it should be borne in mind that physicians taking decisions concerning the progress of weaning were not blinded to the randomization process, so it is also possible that bias existed in favor of the physicians preferred method of weaning in both studies.

In conclusion, it seems that the way in which the weaning strategy is implemented may be as important as the specific method of weaning selected for clinical use. Therefore, it is our contention that until there is sufficient evidence that PSV is truly superior to the intermittent trials of spontaneous breathing with T-tube or *vice versa*, clinicians should use the method they feel most comfortable with and individualize the strategy to the patient's needs. If the T-tube is the chosen method for weaning, we recommend a once-daily trial of spontaneous breathing instead of intermittent trials because both are equally efficacious with respect to speed weaning [5], but the first one simplifies management, since a patient's ability to breathe spontaneously needs to be assessed only once a day.

Reducing Weaning Duration by the Implementation of a Weaning Protocol

Physicians in the ICU have largely practiced weaning as they wished and based the decision to discontinue mechanical ventilation on "judgment and experience". Three recent studies have shown that the implementation of a weaning protocol decreases the duration of mechanical ventilation [6, 7, 31].

Saura et al. [31] compared a group of 51 patients ventilated for more than 48 hours and weaned according to the weaning protocol of the Spanish Society of Intensive Care Medicine, with an historical control group composed of 50 patients weaned in the same ICU in the 13-month period before the implementation of the weaning protocol. Both groups were comparable concerning age, APACHE II score and mortality probability models (MPM) on admission to the ICU, diagnosis and number of days on mechanical ventilation before weaning was started (8.4 ± 7.7 days in the protocol group versus 7.5 ± 5.5 days in the control group). In the protocol group, 41 (80%) patients were extubated after a trial of spontaneous breathing and only 5 (10%) patients were extubated with a weaning technique. In the control group, 5 (10%) patients had direct extubation and 41 (82%) patients were extubated with a weaning technique. The duration of weaning in patients in whom a weaning technique was used was similar in both groups (3.5 ± 3.9 days in the protocol group and 3.6 ± 2.2 days in the control group). There were no significant differences in the reintubation rate (17% in the protocol group versus 14% in the control group). The total duration of mechanical ventilation was shorter in the protocol group (10.4 ± 11.6 days versus 14.4 ± 10.3 days, $p < 0.05$). The authors considered that the major reason for the reduction in mechanical ventilation time was the greater number of patients extubated without any weaning technique in the protocol group. It is likely that, when a weaning protocol does not exist, physicians adopt a conservative weaning approach by gradually reducing ventilatory support. The process of a gradual decrease in ventilatory support could prolong the duration of mechanical ventilation because the physicians may not immediately recognize that the patient is able to breathe spontaneously.

Extubation of the ventilated patient as soon as their recovery and ability to spontaneously breathe are objetively documented should be encouraged, since there is sufficient evidence that 60 to 70% of ventilated patients can be successfully extubated after passing a trial of spontaneous breathing [4–6, 15, 16].

Kollef et al. [7] performed a randomized controlled trial to assess the efficacy and efficiency of using protocols to wean patients from mechanical ventilation compared with a traditional practice of physician-directed weaning. A total of 357 patients were randomly assigned, at the time of ICU admission, to receive protocol-directed weaning implemented by nurses and respiratory therapists (n = 179) or physician-directed weaning (n = 178). Twenty-two (12.3%) patients in the protocol-directed weaning group and 24 (13.5%) patients in the physician-directed weaning group did not undergo any active weaning attempts due to their medical condition, all of them died while receiving mechanical ventilation. The median duration of mechanical ventilation was 35 hours for patients receiving protocol-directed weaning (first quartile, 15 hours; third quartile, 114 hours) compared with 44 hours for patients receiving physician-directed weaning (first quartile, 21 hours; third quartile, 209 hours). The probability of successful weaning over time was significantly higher for the protocol-directed patients. Cox proportional-hazards regression analysis identified five factors that independently predicted the duration of mechanical ventilation before successful weaning, and one of them was the use of a weaning protocol. The adjusted rate of successful weaning was statistically higher with protocol-directed weaning than with physician-directed weaning (risk ratio 1.31; 95 percent confidence interval, 1.15 to 1.50; p = 0.04). The reduction in the duration of mechanical ventilation, for patients in the protocol-directed group, was due both to initiating the weaning process earlier and shortening its duration.

Unlike Saura et al. [31], Kollef et al. [7] employed a randomized controlled design to examine the effect of weaning protocols on the duration of mechanical ventilation. Unfortunately, respiratory therapists and nurses administering patient care could not be blinded to the randomization process, and it is a source of bias because they would want to make the protocol-directed patients wean faster than the physician-directed patients. If the results of the study were explained by this bias, it would indicate that the weaning duration can be safely reduced if people caring for ventilated patients focus their attention on that task.

The effect of weaning protocols on the reduction of the time on mechanical ventilation was also demonstrated in the study by Ely et al. [6], and in this case the aforementioned potential bias did not influence the results because this is the only study about weaning protocols in which all decisions about approaches of weaning, discontinuation of mechanical ventilation and extubation were made by physicians differents from those who enrolled, randomized and screened patients.

In summary, the implementation of a weaning protocol results in an earlier discontinuation of mechanical ventilation and, thus, the duration of ventilatory support shortens.

Conclusion

Ventilatory support can be discontinued without any special weaning technique in three fourths of patients receiving mechanical ventilation. These are patients capable of breathing spontaneously without assistance in which the duration of mechanical ventilation can be reduced if trials of spontaneous breathing are performed as soon as the respiratory failure has resolved. Daily screening of respiratory function is needed to recognize the reversal of respiratory failure, and extubation immediately after successful trials should be encouraged.

Spontaneous breathing trials are safely performed with either T-tube or pressure support of 7 cmH$_2$O. A trial duration of two hours has been extensively evaluated but trials can be reduced to thirty minutes without a higher re-intubation rate.

Patients who fail spontaneous breathing trials need a gradual withdrawal of ventilatory support. The strategy of weaning influences the duration of mechanical ventilation and SIMV is the most ineffective method to successfully wean those patients.

Based on the results of the randomized and prospective trials discussed in this chapter, we recommend the algorithm shown in Fig. 3 as a guideline to discontinuing mechanical ventilation.

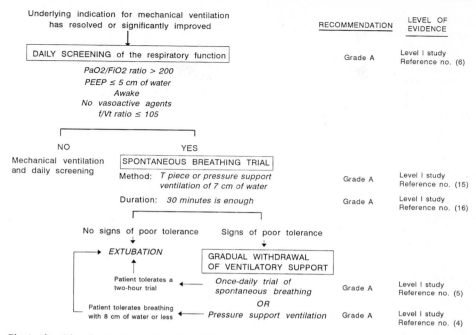

Fig. 3. Algorithm for the discontinuation of mechanical ventilation. The method of grading levels of evidence and recommendations is shown in Table 1

References

1. Pingleton SK (1994) Complications associated with mechanical ventilation. In: Tobin MJ (ed) Principles and practice of mechanical ventilation. McGraw-Hill Inc, New York, pp 775–792
2. Ruiz-Santana S, García A, Esteban A, et al (1987) ICU pneumonias: a multiinstitutional study. Crit Care Med 15:930–932
3. Esteban A, Alía I, Ibañez J, et al (1994) Modes of mechanical ventilation and weaning: a national survey of Spanish hospitals. Chest 106:1188–1193
4. Brochard L, Rauss A, Benito S, et al (1994) Comparison of three methods of gradual withdrawal from ventilatory support during weaning from mechanical ventilation. Am J Respir Crit Care Med 150:896–903
5. Esteban A, Frutos F, Tobin MJ, et al (1995) A comparison of four methods of weaning patients from mechanical ventilation. N Engl J Med 332:345–350
6. Ely EW, Baker AM, Dunagan DP, et al (1996) Effect on the duration of mechanical ventilation of identifying patients capable of breathing spontaneously. N Engl J Med 335:1864–1869
7. Kollef MH, Shapiro SD, Silver P, et al (1997) A randomized, controlled trial of protocol-directed versus physician-directed weaning from mechanical ventilation. Crit Care Med 25:567–574
8. Cook DJ, Guyatt GH, Laupacis A, Sackett DL (1992) Rules of evidence and clinical recommendations on the use of antithrombotic agents. Chest 102:305S–311S
9. Yang KL, Tobin MJ (1991) A prospective study of indexes predicting the outcome of trials of weaning from mechanical ventilation. N Engl J Med 324:1445–1450
10. Sassoon CSH, Mahutte CK (1993) Airway occlusion pressure and breathing pattern as predictors of weaning outcome. Am Rev Respir Dis 148:860–866
11. Mohsenifar Z, Hay A, Hay J, Lewis MI, Koerner SK (1993) Gastric intramural pH as predictor of success or failure in weaning patients from mechanical ventilation. Ann Intern Med 119:794–798

12. Jabour ER, Rabil DM, Truwit JD, Rochester DF (1991) Evaluation of a new weaning index based on ventilatory endurance and the efficiency of gas exchange. Am Rev Respir Dis 144:531–537
13. Epstein SK (1995) Etiology of extubation failure and the predictive value of the rapid shallow breathing index. Am J Respir Crit Care Med 152:545–549
14. Epstein SK, Ciubotaru RL (1996) Influence of gender and endotracheal tube size on preextubation breathing pattern. Am J Respir Crit Care Med 154:459–465
15. Esteban A, Alía I, Gordo F, et al (1997) Extubation outcome after spontaneous breathing trials with T-tube or pressure support ventilation. Am J Respir Crit Care Med 156:459–465
16. The Spanish Lung Failure Collaborative Group (1997) Multicenter, prospective comparison of 30 and 120 minute trials of weaning from mechanical ventilation. Am J Respir Crit Care Med 155:A20 (Abst)
17. Listello D, Sessler CN (1994) Unplanned extubation: clinical predictors for reintubation. Chest 105:1496–1503
18. Tindol GA, DiBenedetto RJ, Kosciuk Y (1994) Unplanned extubations. Chest 105:1804–1807
19. Coppolo DP, May JJ (1990) Self-extubations. A 12-month experience. Chest 98:165–169
20. Benito S, Vallverdú I, Mancebo J (1991) Which patients need a weaning technique? In: Marini JJ, Roussos C (eds) Ventilatory failure. Update in intensive care and emergency medicine. Springer-Verlag, Berlin, Heidelberg, New York, pp 419–429
21. Straus C, Louis B, Isabey D, Lemaire F, Harf A, Brochard L (1997) Work of breathing during T-piece and after extubation: role of the endotracheal tube. Am J Respir Crit Care Med 155:A21 (Abst)
22. Mehta S, Nelson D, Klinger JR, Hill NS, Buczko G, Levy MM (1997) Prediction of post-extubation work of breathing. Am J Respir Crit Care Med 155:A21 (Abst)
23. Fiastro JF, Habib MP, Quan SF (1988) Pressure support compensation for inspiratory work due to endotracheal tubes and demand continuous positive airway pressure. Chest 93:499–505
24. Brochard L, Rua F, Lorino H, Lemaire F, Harf A (1991) Inspiratory pressure support compensates for the additional work of breathing caused by the endotracheal tube. Anesthesiology 75:739–745
25. Nathan SD, Ishaaya AM, Koerner SK, Belman MJ (1993) Prediction of minimal pressure support during weaning from mechanical ventilation. Chest 103:1215–1219
26. Ishaaya AM, Nathan SD, Bulman MJ (1995) Work of breathing after extubation. Chest 107:204–209
27. MacIntyre NR (1986) Respiratory function during pressure support ventilation. Chest 89:677–683
28. Brochard L, Harf A, Lorino H, Lemaire F (1989) Inspiratory pressure support prevents diaphragmatic fatigue during weaning from mechanical ventilation. Am Rev Respir Dis 139:513–521
29. Tobin MJ, Perez W, Guenther SM, et al (1986) The pattern of breathing during successful and unsuccessful trials of weaning from mechanical ventilation. Am Rev Respir Dis 134:1111–1118
30. Jubran A, Tobin MJ (1997) Pathophysiological basis of acute respiratory distress in patients who fail a trial of weaning from mechanical ventilation. Am J Respir Crit Care Med 155:906–915
31. Saura P, Blanch L, Mestre J, Vallés J, Artigas A, Fernández R (1996) Clinical consequences of the implementation of a weaning protocol. Intensive Care Med 22:1052–1056

Non-Invasive
Mechanical Ventilation

Non-Invasive Ventilation in Acute Respiratory Failure: Technological Issues

M. Wysocki

Introduction

Non-invasive mechanical ventilation (NIV) for the treatment of patients suffering from acute respiratory failure and requiring ventilatory support has been investigated extensively during the past decade [1, 2]. Three prospective randomized studies on patients with acute exacerbation of chronic obstructive pulmonary disease (COPD) [3–5] demonstrated that those treated with NIV had less need for endotracheal intubation [4, 5], stayed a shorter time in the intensive care units (ICU) [4] and had a lower in-hospital mortality rate than patients treated conventionally [4]. A recent study [6] in patients with acute respiratory failure without prior chronic pulmonary disease demonstrated that the incidence of pneumonia and the length of ICU stay was reduced by NIV, and we have reported [7] that the need for endotracheal intubation, the time in the ICU and the mortality rate are all reduced when hypercapnic patients are treated in this way. However, several editorials [8] have indicated that further studies are required to better define those patients for whom NIV is of greatest benefit and to determine the most appropriate interface and ventilatory modalities. This report examines the types of ventilation, the ventilators, the exhalation devices, and the interfaces used in NIV.

The Ventilatory Modality

Several ways of generating negative pleural pressures have been tested in patients with acute respiratory failure [9]. While these systems can improve gas exchange [10], the lack of any comparative studies and the size and expense of tank ventilators (the most effective devices) make them suitable only for specialized units. The systems most frequently used for NIV in patients with acute respiratory failure are those generating positive airway pressures by delivering a volume (volume-cycled), or by delivering a pressure (pressure-cycled).

Volume-cycled systems were used first because they were on ventilators for chronically home-ventilated patients [11, 12]. The physiologic effects of volume-cycled non-invasive systems have only recently been thoroughly investigated. Elliot et al. [13] evaluated the effects of NIV using a purpose-built volume-cycled ventilator in five COPD patients. They found an 80% decrease in inspiratory muscle effort (measured by the esophageal pressure-time integral) in four patients and a 50% decrease in one patient. Breath-by-breath analysis of the changes in global inspiratory muscle effort over a period of 60 minutes demonstrated that inspiratory effort was reduced for 95% of the breaths recorded in three patients and for less than 60% in the other two.

By contrast, the physiologic effects of pressure-cycled non-invasive systems, especially pressure-support ventilation (PSV), have been extensively investigated by measuring the electromyograph (EMG) activity of the diaphragm [14, 15] and/or the transdiaphragmatic pressure [16, 17]. Brochard et al. [17] found a 43% reduction in EMG activity of the diaphragm and 50% reductions in the transdiaphragmatic pressure have been reported by others [16–18]. A recent prospective study by Girault et al. [19] compared assist-controlled ventilation (ACV) and PSV in 15 patients with acute hypercapnic respiratory failure. They demonstrated that the inspiratory work of breathing (WOB) was significantly reduced with both modalities but the reduction was greater with ACV (-69%) than with PSV (-55%, $p < 0.05$). Other indexes such as the esophageal pressure-time product (PTP) were also significantly reduced more by ACV than by PSV (Fig. 1). Both methods similarly improved gas exchange but the respiratory comfort, assessed by a visual analog scale, was better in PSV (81 ± 25 mm) than in ACV (57 ± 30 mm, $p < 0.01$). Similar results were suggested by a previous study [20] in which 29 patients suffering from acute exacerbation of COPD and non-invasively ventilated were randomly assigned to ACV ($n = 16$) or PSV ($n = 13$). Both gave the same rate of success, but PSV was better tolerated with fewer side effects. These results [19, 20] suggest that PSV is the first-line system, except in the most severe patients, or in cases of incomplete resolution with PSV. ACV could be tried in this situation before shifting rapidly to PSV to improve tolerance and avoid complications.

Older and newer pressure-cycle systems have also been tested in non-invasively ventilated subjects. Mancebo et al. [21] used three devices delivering assisted NIV with different working mechanisms to compare PSV and intermittent positive pressure breathing (IPPB), while breathing room air or in carbon dioxide (CO_2)-induced

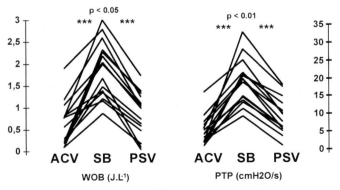

Fig. 1. Values for inspiratory work of breathing (WOB) and the pressure-time product (PTP) during NIV. The decreases in WOB and PTP from spontaneous breathing (SB) to assist-control ventilation (ACV), and pressure support ventilation (PSV) were significant and were significantly greater with ACV ($p < 0.05$). *** p values ACV versus PSV. (From [19] with permission)

hyperventilation. The 7 healthy volunteers were tested with a fixed inspiratory pressure of 10 cmH$_2$O. The WOB was significantly greater with the two IPPB devices (IPPB1: 7.3 ± 5.2 and IPPB2: 7.2 ± 6.2 J·min^{-1}) than with PSV (2.3 ± 3.3 J·min^{-1}) while breathing room air. The IPPB systems were also more uncomfortable. The WOB and PTP were much greater with the two IPPB devices during CO$_2$-induced hyperventilation and the IPPB systems were the most uncomfortable. Thus PSV and IPPB had very different effects on respiratory muscle activity in healthy non-intubated subjects despite their similar operating principles. IPPB machines not only failed to reduce patient effort but they caused significant levels of extra work, demonstrating that one pressure-cycled mode (such as PSV) cannot be replaced by another (such as IPPB).

A new mode of ventilation, proportional assist ventilation (PAV), has been recently investigated in patients on NIV [22]. In PAV the pressure generated by the ventilator is continuously, and breath-by-breath, in proportion with the patient's respiratory effort [23, 24]. Ward et al. [22] tested non-invasive PAV in 11 patients with acute respiratory failure without prior chronic respiratory failure and demonstrated that the respiratory rate and the dyspnea score were significantly reduced after one hour of NIV. We [25] have also compared PSV and PAV generated by a prototype (Respironics, Murrysville, USA) in 7 volunteers at rest and during work (90 watts on a cycle ergometer for 20 minutes). The pressure generated by the ventilator during work was doubled in PAV, while it was unchanged in PSV. The WOB done by the volunteers in PAV was 50% of that in PSV (Fig. 2), suggesting that PAV reduces the patient's WOB during increases in respiratory effort.

Two recent papers [26, 27] have also examined the effects of NIV in volume-cycled mode on the glottis (continuously monitored using a fiber-optic bronchoscope) in a group of 7 volunteers. An increase in delivered minute ventilation (by increasing the delivered tidal volume to 1200 ml and then the respiratory frequency) resulted in a progressive narrowing of the vocal cords, with an increase in inspiratory resistance and a reduction in the percentage of the delivered tidal volume reaching the lungs. This occurred in conscious volunteers [26] and was amplified in sleeping volunteers [27]. The same group did a comparable study using a pressure-cycled system and 6 volunteers [28]. Although the systems were not compared the vocal cords tended to

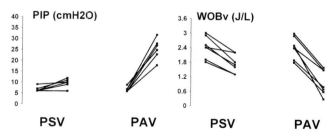

Fig. 2. Changes in the peak inspiratory pressure (PIP) and in work of breathing (WOBv) in pressure support ventilation (PSV) and proportional assit ventilation (PAV) in 7 volunteers non-invasively ventilated while working (cycle ergometer, 90 watts, 20 minutes). PIP increased significantly during effort with PAV but not with PSV. The reduction in WOBv was significantly more in PAV. (From [25] with permission)

narrow less at a given minute ventilation in the pressure-cycled mode than in the volume-cycled mode. The vocal cords of only one of the 6 volunteers narrowed in the pressure-cycled system with an inspiratory pressure of 15 cmH$_2$O [28].

Lastly, only one of the three randomized studies that have compared NIV and conventional ventilation in patients with acute exacerbation of COPD [3-5] used a volume-cycled mode [3] the other two used a pressure-cycled mode [4, 5]. Only these two studies reported a significant reduction in the need for endotracheal intubation. Brochard et al. [4] also reported a significant reduction in the in-hospital mortality.

These studies indicate that the type of ventilation used in NIV should be carefully selected because of the great differences in their physiologic effects. Further studies should be designed to better define the most suitable type of ventilation in specific patients.

The Exhalation Device

This important technological issue has been discussed recently [29–31]. Some ventilators designed for home NIV, use a single inspiration-expiration circuit with a connector between the mask and the circuit which permits venting of expiratory gas to the atmosphere. However, using such a system in an artificial lung [32], in endotracheally intubated patients [32] or those on NIV [29], results in significant re-

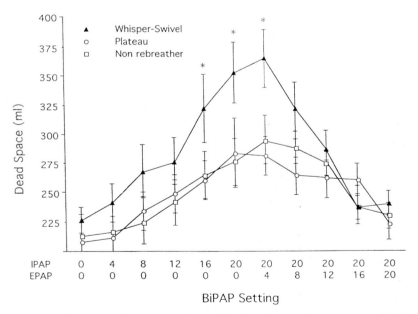

Fig. 3. Dead space ventilation at various positive inspiratory airway pressure (IPAP) and positive expiratory airway pressure (EPAP) during NIV using a BiPAP system (Respironics, Murrysville, PA) and different exhalation devices: Closed triangles, the Whispel-Swivel standard exhalation device; open circle, the non-rebreather plateau valve; open square, the Sanders NRV-2 non-rebreather valve. * indicates p < 0.05 compared with other devices at similar settings. (From [29] with permission)

breathing and an insufficient reduction in $PaCO_2$ [29]. A high (10–12 cmH_2O) positive end-expiratory pressure (PEEP) was required to reduce significantly the amount of exhaled tidal volume that was re-inhaled (Fig. 3). Therefore, patients having acute respiratory failure should use a system with a non-rebreathing valve and a separate circuit for expiration. The exhalation device must also have a low resistance so as not to induce a significant expiratory effort, as occurs with some home-ventilators [32]. Lofaso et al. [32] found that the work imposed by the circuit during exhalation varied up to four-fold across the 6 devices tested from 0.05 ± 0.00 to 0.21 ± 0.00 J/L ($p < 0.05$).

The Ventilator

A frequent question is whether "conventional" ventilators (those used in ICUs for endotracheally intubated patients) or specifically designed ventilators for NIV should be used. The ventilators used by Meduri et al. [33, 34] and by our group [7, 35] were conventional, while those used by Pennock et al. [36, 37] or by Brochard et al. [4, 17] were specifically designed. Both have advantages and limitations (Table 1), while the more recent ventilators have tried to overcome these limitations. Conventional ventilators have been modified by inserting a non-invasive mode in their operating software so that NIV is easily performed while specific ventilators have become more complex.

Studies comparing the efficiency and safety of conventional and specific ventilators have yet to be conducted, while local and financial considerations should be

Table 1. Advantages and limitations of "conventional" and "specific" ventilators designed for NIV

	Advantages	Limitations
Conventional	• Several modes of ventilation available (CPAP, PSV, ACV, PCV, etc. …). • High quality ventilation (sensitive triggering system, high inspiratory flow, fast pressurization, sensitive inspiratory-expiratory cycling, etc) • Precise adjustment of the ventilation (flow, Ti/T_{TOT}, trigger, etc). • Sensitive alarms • Ready to use if the patient needs to be intubated • No acquisition cost if available in the unit	• Too complex for most cases. • Too many alarms or alarms cannot be switched of when there are leaks • Costly • Cannot be used in intermediate care unit or in emergency room.
Specific	• Easy to use • Compact and small • Cheap • Usable in intermediate care units or in emergency room.	• Acquisition cost • Moderate quality ventilation • Not usable if the patient needs to be intubated.

Abbreviations: NIV: non-invasive mechanical ventilation; CPAP: continuous positive airway pressure; PSV: pressure support ventilation; ACV: assist-controlled ventilation; PCV: pressure-controlled ventilation

taken into account when choosing the ventilator used for NIV. A group of six specific pressure-cycled ventilators were recently evaluated using an artificial lung [32]. Of these ventilators, five had been developed for home NIV and one specifically for NIV in patients with acute respiratory failure [4, 17]. There were major differences between the ventilators, such as the minimal PEEP imposed by the ventilator (which was 2–4 fold higher in some home ventilators), but also in the flow acceleration generated (2–4 fold lower in some home-ventilators), and the expiratory work imposed on the lung (2–4 fold higher in some home-ventilators). The authors suggest that ventilators designed for NIV in patients having acute respiratory failure should have a minimal time to generate pressure support and a minimal expiratory resistance as these differences may have a clinical impact [32]. The same group [38] also demonstrated that most continuous positive airway pressure (CPAP) ventilators were unable to maintain the correct pressure when there was a leak in the circuit (Fig. 4). Leaks of varying severity (0.5, 1.0, 1.5 L/s) caused a significant drop in the pressure generated by the ventilators which could be over 50% of the assigned pressure, even in ventilators using leak compensatory systems. Moreover, for the latter ventilators, the time that these ventilators required to compensate for the leaks and to regain the assigned pressure was sometimes very long. This experiment was not

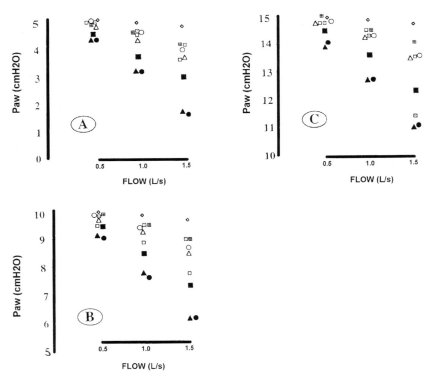

Fig. 4. Airway pressures (P_{aw}) obtained in a steady state after making a leak of 0.5, 1.0 and 1.5 l/s for 5 (A), 10 (B) and 15 cmH$_2$O (C) of pressure assigned. Open symbols indicate ventilators with leak compensatory systems. (From [38] with permission)

done with positive inspiratory airway pressure ventilators but because leaks are frequent in NIV, the ability of the ventilators to maintain inspiratory airway pressure when there is a leak is also important. Most conventional ventilators can increase inspiratory flow to maintain the inspiratory airway pressure, but this may not apply to all specific ventilators.

The Mask

The mask is a critical part of NIV that has been neglected for many years and there has still not been any extensive evaluation of its function, despite the fact that it can be a major cause of NIV failure (poor fit, not-tolerated, patients with facial deformities, etc.,). A recent study on 158 patients non-invasively ventilated for hypercapnic and non-hypercapnic respiratory failure found that 52 patients could not be ventilated with NIV. Of these 52 patients, 9 (17%) could not tolerate the mask or the mask did not fit properly. Several types of mask and patient-ventilator interfaces have been designed for NIV [1, 2, 39], but nasal and facial masks are the most frequently used. Carrey et al. [15] examined 9 patients and demonstrated that nasal masks did not reduce diaphragm EMG activity when the patient's mouth was opened, suggesting that a facial mask would be better for patients breathing with their mouth open (as is frequent in acute respiratory failure). Conversely, we find that the nasal mask is better tolerated than the facial mask and we shift from the facial to the nasal mask as soon as possible in agreement with the report of Putensen et al. [40]. A full face mask was compared recently to a nasal and a naso-buccal mask in a group of 9 patients receiving NIV [41]. Leaks, discomfort and dyspnea were significantly lower using this mask, and gas exchange was improved (as well as with other masks) despite a high internal volume (1500 mL), by maintaining a PEEP level of 5 cmH_2O) and by making two holes in the upper part of the mask. However, to our knowledge, this mask has not yet been investigated further and is not widely available. Clearly, various types of available mask need to be compared for their efficacy, safety and tolerance and at the present a conservative approach is to maintain a wide choice of masks, to look for the mask that is best tolerated and to change it as frequently as possible to avoid discomfort.

Conclusions

Successful NIV can provide substantial benefits to patients and to the rest of society. Therefore technologic issues that may improve the efficacy and tolerance of NIV are of considerable importance. The specific characteristics of this type of ventilation require that all the components (mask, circuit and ventilators) be specifically designed and extensively investigated in patients requiring ventilatory support for acute respiratory failure. This should improve not only efficacy and tolerance but also the ease with which NIV is used in critically ill patients, thus convincing physicians to use it more extensively.

References

1. Ambrosino N (1996) Noninvasive mechanical ventilation in acute respiratory failure. Eur Respir J 9:795–807
2. Meyer TJ, Hill NS (1994) Noninvasive positive pressure ventilation to treat respiratory failure. Ann Intern Med 120:760–770
3. Bott J, Carroll MP, Conway JH, et al (1993) Randomised controlled trial of nasal ventilation in acute ventilatory failure due to chronic obstructive airways disease. Lancet 341:1555–1557
4. Brochard L, Mancebo J, Wysocki M, et al (1995) Noninvasive ventilation for acute exacerbations of chronic obstructive pulmonary disease. N Engl J Med 333:817–822
5. Kramer N, Meyer TJ, Meharg J, Cece RD, Hill NS (1995) Randomized, prospective trial of non-invasive positive pressure ventilation in acute respiratory failure. Am J Respir Crit Care Med 151:1799–1806
6. Antonelli M, Conti G, Rocco M, et al (1997) Non-invasive pressure support ventilation in patients with acute respiratory failure not related to COPD. Intensive Care Med 23 (suppl 1):S5 (Abst)
7. Wysocki M, Tric L, Wolff MA, Millet H, Herman B (1995) Noninvasive pressure support ventilation in patients with acute respiratory failure. A randomized comparison with conventional therapy. Chest 107:761–768
8. Rosenberg JI, Goldstein RS (1997) Noninvasive positive pressure ventilation. A positive view in need of supportive evidence. Chest 111:1479–1481
9. Corrado A, Messori A, Gorini M (1994) Mechanical ventilation. N Engl J Med 331:549
10. Corrado A, Bruscoli G, Messori A, et al. (1992) Iron lung treatment of subjects with COPD in acute respiratory failure. Evaluation of short- and long-term prognosis. Chest 101:692–696
11. Anon. (1959) Historical background to automatic ventilation. In: Mushin WW, Rendell-Baker L, Thompson PW, Mapleson WW (eds) Automatic ventilation of the lungs. 1969th ed. Blackwell, Oxford, pp 185–213.
12. Elliott MW, Simonds AK, Carroll MP, Wedzicha JA, Branthwaite MA (1992) Domiciliary nocturnal nasal intermittent positive pressure ventilation in hypercapnic respiratory failure due to chronic obstructive lung disease: effects on sleep and quality of life. Thorax 47:342–348
13. Elliott MW, Mulvey DA, Moxham J, Green M, Branthwaite MA (1993) Inspiratory muscle effort during nasal intermittent positive pressure ventilation in patients with chronic obstructive airways disease. Anesthesia 48:8–13
14. Ambrosino N, Nava S, Bertone P, Fracchia C, Rampulla C (1992) Physiologic evaluation of pressure support ventilation by nasal mask in patients with stable COPD. Chest 101:385–391
15. Carrey Z, Gottfried SB, Levy RD (1990) Ventilatory muscle support in respiratory failure with nasal positive pressure ventilation. Chest 97:150–158
16. Appendini L, Patessio A, Zanaboni S, et al (1994) Physiologic effects of positive end-expiratory pressure and mask pressure support during exacerbations of chronic obstructive pulmonary disease. Am J Respir Crit Care Med 149:1069–1076
17. Brochard L, Isabey D, Piquet J, et al (1990) Reversal of acute exacerbations of chronic obstructive lung disease by inspiratory assistance with a face mask. N Engl J Med 323:1523–1530
18. Nava S, Ambrosino N, Rubini F, et al (1993) Effect of nasal pressure support ventilation and external PEEP on diaphragmatic activity in patients with severe stable COPD. Chest 103:143–150
19. Girault C, Richard JC, Chevron V, et al (1997) Comparative physiologic effects of noninvasive assist-control and pressure support ventilation in acute hypercapnic respiratory failure. Chest 111:1639–1648
20. Vitacca M, Rubini F, Foglio K, Scalvini S, Nava S, Ambrosino N (1993) Non-invasive modalities of positive pressure ventilation improve the outcome of acute exacerbations in COPD patients. Intensive Care Med 19:450–455
21. Mancebo J, Isabey D, Lorino H, Lofaso F, Lemaire F, Brochard L (1995) Comparative effects of pressure support ventilation and intermittent positive pressure breathing (IPPB) in non-intubated healthy subjects. Eur Respir J 8:1901–1909
22. Patrick W, Webster K, Ludwig L, Roberts D, Wiebe P, Younes M (1996) Noninvasive positive-pressure ventilation in acute respiratory distress without prior chronic respiratory failure. Am J Respir Crit Care Med 153:1005–1011

23. Younes M, Puddy A, Roberts D, et al (1992) Proportional assist ventilation. Results of an initial clinical trial. Am Rev Respir Dis 145:121–129
24. Younes M (1992) Proportional assist ventilation, a new approach to ventilatory support. Theory. Am Rev Respir Dis 145:114–120
25. Richard JC, Arnulf B, Wolff MA, Herman B, Wysocki M (1997) Proportional assist ventilation (PAV) versus pressure support (PSV) during effort in healthy volunteers. Am J Respir Crit Care Med 155:A84 (Abst)
26. Jouniaux V, Aubert G, Dury M, Delguste P, Rodenstein DO (1997) Effects of nasal positive-pressure hyperventilation on the glottis in normal awake subjects. J Appl Physiol 79:176–185
27. Jouniaux V, Aubert G, Dury M, Delguste P, Rodenstein DO (1995) Effects of nasal positive-pressure hyperventilation on the glottis in normal sleeping subjects. J Appl Physiol 79:186–193
28. Parreira VF, Jouniaux V, Aubert G, Dury M, Delguste P, Rodenstein DO (1996) Nasal two-level positive-pressure ventilation in normal subjects. Am J Respir Crit Care Med 153:1616–1623
29. Ferguson GT, Gilmartin M (1996) CO_2 rebreathing during BiPAP ventilatory assistance. Am J Respir Crit Care Med 151:1126–1135
30. Lofaso F, Lorino AM, Duizabo D, et al (1996) Evaluation of an auto-nCPAP device based on snoring detection. Eur Respir J 9:1795–1800
31. Lofaso F, Brochard L, Touchard D, Hang T, Harf A, Isabey D (1995) Evaluation of carbon dioxide rebreathing during pressure support ventilation with airway management system (BiPAP) devices. Chest 108:772–778
32. Lofaso F, Brochard L, Hang T, Lorino H, Harf A, Isabey D (1996) Home versus intensive care pressure support devices. Experimental and clinical comparison. Am J Respir Crit Care Med 153:1591–1599
33. Meduri GU, Abou-Shala N, Fox RC, Jones CB, Leeper KV, Wunderink RG (1991) Noninvasive face mask mechanical ventilation in patients with acute hypercapnic respiratory failure. Chest 100:445–454
34. Meduri GU, Conoscenti CC, Menashe P, Nair S (1989) Noninvasive face mask ventilation in patients with acute respiratory failure. Chest 95:865–870
35. Wysocki M, Tric L, Wolff MA, Gertner J, Millet H, Herman B (1993) Noninvasive pressure support ventilation in patients with acute respiratory failure. Chest 103:907–913
36. Pennock BE, Crawshaw L, Kaplan PD (1994) Noninvasive nasal mask ventilation for acute respiratory failure. Institution of a new therapeutic technology for routine use. Chest 105:441–444
37. Pennock BE, Kaplan PD, Carlin BW, Sabangan JS, Magovern JA (1991) Pressure support ventilation with a simplified ventilatory support system administered with a nasal mask in patients with respiratory failure. Chest 100:1371–1376
38. Lofaso F (1994) Evaluation des ventilateurs en pression type domicile. In: Beydon L, Brochard L, Harf A, Isabey D, Lemaire F (eds) Conference procceedings of the Actualités en ventilation artificielle. Creteil, pp 60
39. Elliott MW, Moxham J (1994) Noninvasive mechanical ventilation by nasal or facial mask. In: Tobin MJ (ed). Principles and practice of mechanical ventilation. McGraw-Hill, New-York, pp 427–454
40. Putensen C, Hormann C, Baum M, Lingnau W (1993) Comparison of mask and nasal continuous positive airway pressure after extubation and mechanical ventilation. Crit Care Med 21:357–362
41. Criner GJ, Travaline JM, Brennan KJ, Kreimer DT (1994) Efficacy of a new full face mask for non-invasive positive pressure ventilation. Chest 106:1109–1115

Non-Invasive Nocturnal Mechanical Ventilation: Is it Feasible for COPD Patients?

L. Appendini and C. F. Donner

Introduction

Nocturnal intermittent mechanical ventilation, using negative or positive pressure devices, improves arterial blood gas tensions during spontaneous ventilation in patients with respiratory failure caused by chest wall deformities or neuromuscular disease. Similar results have been reported in short-term studies of hospitalized patients with chronic obstructive pulmonary disease (COPD). The improvement in arterial blood gas tensions in COPD has usually been ascribed to improved carbon dioxide (CO_2) sensitivity and/or respiratory muscle strength. Nocturnal intermittent mechanical ventilation has been demonstrated to maintain normocapnia during the night and is thought to relieve chronic fatigue by resting respiratory muscles, allowing them to perform more mechanical work with the same amount of load [1]. However, despite these postulations, chronic fatigue has never actually been demonstrated in stable hypercapnic COPD patients. This chapter will explore: 1) Why non-invasive nocturnal mechanical ventilation should be considered for the treatment of COPD patients with chronic hypercapnia; 2) The mechanisms by which it can be effective in reversing chronic ventilatory failure; and 3) The clinical applications of non-invasive nocturnal mechanical ventilation in COPD patients.

The Rationale for Ventilation During Sleep

Polysomnographic studies have shown that oxygen desaturation often occurs in patients with COPD [2]. It is more evident during rapid eye movement (REM) sleep [3], alveolar hypoventilation being the main mechanism. Central apneas and/or partial or complete upper airway obstruction may produce oxygen desaturation in these patients [4, 5]. In addition, breathing pattern abnormalities and impaired respiratory mechanics contribute to oxygen desaturation. In fact, COPD patients have a high physiologic dead space that increases during REM sleep because of the occurrence of a rapid and shallow breathing pattern. Douglas and Flenley [6] considered this last mechanism powerful enough to explain all the hypoxemia occuring during the night. Moreover, hyperinflated COPD patients use the accessory inspiratory muscles more than normal subjects during tidal breathing as the force generating capacity of the diaphragm is impaired by mechanical and geometrical derangements. During REM sleep the physiologic reduction of accessory inspiratory muscle activity prevents the failing diaphragm from maintaining ventilation. This reduction of accessory inspiratory muscle activity also favors costal indrawing of the lower chest wall which might cause a further reduction in ventilation. Finally, several papers have reported that ventilation/perfusion ($\dot{V}/\dot{Q}$) imbalance can be a major cause of hypoxemia during REM sleep in patients with COPD [3, 7, 8].

A summary of possible determinants of night-time oxygen desaturation in COPD patients is presented in Table 1. Whatever the mechanism, it is now widely accepted that important abnormalities of blood gases due to alveolar hypoventilation occur during sleep in patients with COPD.

The daytime effects of arterial blood gas tension abnormalities observed during sleep in COPD patients are summarized in Table 2. COPD patients often show an abnormal ventilatory control during wakefulness detected by reduced minute ventilation and occlusion pressure in response to hypoxia and hypercapnia. This impairment of ventilatory control has been shown to be correlated with sleep-related oxygen desaturation [5, 9–11]. However, it is not clear if the changes in daytime ventilatory control are the cause or the consequence of the changes at night. In fact, many factors such as renal retention of bicarbonate ions in response to nocturnal hypoventilation and acidosis, and sleep disruption [12] may reduce the daytime ventilatory response to both hypercapnia and hypoxia.

The effects of hypoxemia and hypercapnia during sleep on survival and lifestyle during the day are poorly understood. Daytime pulmonary hypertension has been related to nocturnal hypoxemia [13]. Hypoxemia during REM sleep has been reported to be associated to significant night-time increases in pulmonary artery pressures (>20 mmHg) [14]. Hypoxemia during REM sleep was also found in patients with higher daytime pulmonary artery pressures than in COPD patients without REM desaturations [15]. However, significant differences in daytime oxygen saturations were found between these two groups. Respiratory acidosis could strengthen the pulmonary vessel vasoconstrictor response to hypoxia during the period of alveolar hypoventilation occurring during the night, as acidosis has been reported to be a strong vasoconstrictor.

Table 1. Possible determinants of night-time oxygen desaturation in COPD patients

- Central apnea [4, 5]
- Upper airway obstruction [4, 5]
- High physiologic dead space combined with rapid shallow breathing occurring during REM sleep [6].
- $\dot{V}/\dot{Q}$ imbalance [3, 7, 8]
- Impaired respiratory mechanics [39]

Table 2. Daytime effects of arterial blood gas tension abnormalities observed during sleep in COPD patients

- Abnormal ventilatory control [5, 9–12, 20, 24]
- Pulmonary hypertension [13, 14]
- Impaired neuropsychiatric functioning [52]
- Reduced quality of life [52]

The interplay between blood gas derangements and sleep quality in COPD has been considered in the past. It is well known that COPD patients have impaired sleep quality [4]. There is no agreement about the effects of hypoxemia on sleep quality [16, 17] even if acute hypoxemia has been demonstrated to be unable to cause arousal in humans [18]. By contrast, small increases in arterial CO_2 partial pressure ($PaCO_2$) are known to be a potent arousal stimulus [19]. This finding suggests that nocturnal mechanical ventilation, by reducing $PaCO_2$, may improve sleep quality.

In conclusion, the correction of alveolar hypoventilation during the night by means of mechanical ventilation may have important beneficial effects even in COPD patients with impaired gas exchange during sleep. This conclusion can be reached from the above mentioned factors, and from experience in patients with restrictive chest wall disorders in whom the application of nocturnal mechanical ventilation results in improved daytime function.

Role of Non-Invasive Nocturnal Mechanical Ventilation in the Treatment of Chronic Ventilatory Failure

Chronic ventilatory failure is characterized by hypoventilation and hypercapnia that can worsen during the night (see above). Non-invasive mechanical ventilation can control nocturnal hypoventilation, influencing the mechanisms which lead to, and maintain chronic ventilatory failure. First of all, its action on night-time hypercapnia could restore CO_2 sensitivity and improve blood gases during daytime unsupported spontaneous breathing. Second, the reduction of ventilatory load and the eventual improvement of ventilatory pump efficiency operated by mechanical ventilation could contribute to the reversal of chronic ventilatory failure.

There is evidence in the literature that nocturnal mechanical ventilation can increase the daytime ventilatory CO_2 response by avoiding hypercapnia during the night. Berton-Jones and Sullivan [20] demonstrated that, in patients with severe obstructive sleep apnea and daytime hypercapnia, the application of continuous positive airway pressure (CPAP) during the night progressively increased minute ventilation at any given level of alveolar CO_2. By contrast, the ventilatory response to CO_2 did not change in patients who did not show daytime hypercapnia. These data suggest that daytime ventilatory failure could be reversed by night-time treatment of hypoventilation. Similar results were obtained in COPD patients by Elliott and colleagues [19], who found improved daytime blood gases, an increased central responsiveness to CO_2 and no change in airway obstruction or respiratory muscle strength at the end of a six month period of non-invasive nocturnal mechanical ventilation.

The use of nocturnal mechanical ventilation could improve respiratory mechanics, thus ameliorating the balance between the ventilatory load and the force generating capacity of the inspiratory muscles, and lowering hypercapnia. An increase in vital capacity (VC) was reported after prolonged treatment in patients with restrictive chest wall disease [21–23]. An improvement in pulmonary compliance, secondary to reversal of small airway closure and microatelectasis or to reduced stiffness of the rib cage, was advocated as the mechanism leading to the increase in VC. Similar improvements in ventilatory load were reported in COPD patients [24]. They were interpreted as a possible consequence of a reduction in lung water following the application of nocturnal mechanical ventilation. However, a number of studies failed to demonstrate improvements in ventilatory load following successful non-invasive ventilation both in restrictive disease [25–27] and COPD [28] patients. It may be that any reduction in ventilatory load plays a minor role in the reversal of ventilatory failure.

Recently, chronic respiratory muscle fatigue has been hypothesized to be responsible, at least in part, for the development of chronic ventilatory failure. This hypothesis, even if very exciting, is difficult to test as there is still no objective method to assess "chronic fatigue". In theory, the loss of muscle force generating capacity due to fatigue should be reversed by rest. Indeed, there are some data showing improvement of respiratory muscle strength after application of non-invasive mechanical ventilation [29–32]. By contrast, there are also a substantial number of negative reports in patients in whom chronic ventilatory failure was successfully controlled by non-invasive ventilation [24–26, 28]. Several factors can explain these controversial results. Testing respiratory muscle strength requires maximum voluntary effort by the patients. The learning effect due to repeated maneuvers, or a general improvement in patient condition might interfere with the results. Studies based on non-volitional techniques (electrical or magnetic phrenic stimulation) could better define the role of non-invasive mechanical ventilation in improving the force generating capacity of the inspiratory muscles [33]. Furthermore, although non-invasive mechanical ventilation has been demonstrated to be effective in abolishing respiratory muscle electromyograph (EMG) activity [34, 35], this has seldom been confirmed in clinical studies [36, 37]. In conclusion, the role of respiratory muscle fatigue in chronic ventilatory failure remains uncertain [38].

There is, therefore, increasing evidence that the mechanism by which nocturnal mechanical ventilation acts to reverse chronic ventilatory failure depends on its capacity to control nocturnal hypoventilation. The efficiency of nocturnal mechanical ventilation should thus be evaluated by its ability to prevent night-time hypoxia and hypercapnia and not by its ability to provide full support in terms of minute ventilation or muscle rest [39]. However, as the ability to maintain target ventilation for a given level of $PaCO_2$ depends on the interplay between respiratory workload, respiratory muscle contractility and respiratory center output [40], the previous conclusion should be considered with caution.

Clinical Applications

Negative Pressure Ventilation

Clinical studies of long-term negative pressure ventilation (NPV) in patients with COPD have yielded controversial results. Some uncontrolled trials reported significant improvements in inspiratory muscle strength, blood gases and VC [29, 30, 32], whereas two small controlled trials of NPV in COPD patients showed no benefit at all [41, 42]. In a larger double-blind study, from the workers at McGill University, Montreal 184 patients with severe COPD were randomly allocated to active or sham NPV [36]. The authors found no clinically or statistically significant difference in resting lung function, arterial blood gas tensions, exercise tolerance and endurance, maximum inspiratory (P_{imax}) and expiratory (P_{emax}) pressure between active and sham-treated patients. Neither did they find any evidence of a treatment effect in matched sub-groups of patients with whom inspiratory muscle rest by NPV was higher, or in patients with more severe respiratory insufficiency at trial entry. The conflicting results of this study [36] and of previous uncontrolled studies probably reflect differences in patient selection, duration of treatment and placebo effects. Hypercapnia was an entry requirement for most of the uncontrolled trials, but not for the McGill study [36]. A question worth raising concerns the rationale for ventilating normocapnic patients with preserved ventilatory output despite increased workload and respiratory muscle mechanical impairment. Indeed a recent study [43] showed that the inspiratory muscles of COPD patients were able to adapt to the detrimental effects of chronic hyperinflation, being able to generate more negative pressure at increased lung volumes compared with normal subjects. This evidence suggests that fatigue is not an important factor in such patients. Moreover, the McGill study [36] showed that, if mechanical support in patients with hypercapnia is set with the aim of reducing inspiratory muscle effort and not to improve arterial blood gas tensions, ventilatory pump performance does not improve. Alternatively, if levels of ventilation are chosen so as to lower $PaCO_2$ during respiratory muscle rest (RMR) [29, 30, 32], $PaCO_2$ can be kept within normal limits for several hours after RMR withdrawal. In this case, chemoreceptor sensitivity may be reset leading to a consistent decrease in $PaCO_2$ the cost of increased respiratory muscle activity, exactly the opposite one would obtain with mechanical ventilation (i.e., RMR). These data suggest that in addition to RMR, other factors including changes in respiratory drive (response of respiratory centers to PaO_2 and $PaCO_2$), the load placed upon the respiratory muscles, the ventilation-perfusion ratio and sleep quality may also be important determinants of improved arterial blood gas tensions (see also above).

A placebo effect can lead to misleading results with respect to the effectiveness of RMR. For instance, in the McGill study [36] 16% of patients in the sham group had a decrease in the sensation of dyspnea compared to 17% in the active group, and the sham group as a whole had an increase of 7% in the distance walked in a 6 min-walk test (5% in the active group). Finally, NPV is an uncomfortable intervention and as such is poorly accepted by patients. For instance, Shapiro et al. [36], reported that although they had originally planned for their COPD patients to use NPV at night the majority chose to be ventilated during the day because treatment interfered with sleep quality. Only 29% of patients received the target ventilation (average ventilator use of 5 hours per day). It may be concluded that technologic improvements will have to be made to improve patient acceptance, comfort and sleep quality, and that inspiratory muscle rest imposed by NPV cannot be considered the only determinant of improved arterial blood gas tensions.

Positive Pressure Ventilation

Positive pressure ventilators share more sophisticated technology (trigger sensitivity, assisted/spontaneous ventilatory modalities, monitoring capabilities etc.) that allows better patient-ventilation coupling. These features make intermittent positive pressure ventilation (IPPV) delivered by nasal mask widely regarded as more efficient and flexible than negative pressure techniques, having the additional advantage of helping to better preserve the opening of the upper airways. Daytime arterial blood gas improvement has been reported after domiciliary nocturnal nasal IPPV in hypercapnic COPD patients [24, 44]. Although there was no control group in either study, the duration of treatment in both exceeded six months. Multiple factors appeared to contribute to the improvement in arterial blood gas tensions [24]. Tidal volume and minute ventilation increased in patients in whom daytime $PaCO_2$ decreased after treatment, whereas those in whom it rose showed a decrease in both these variables. There was no relationship between arterial blood gas tension improvement and changes in inspiratory muscle strength. Conversely, ventilatory function tended to improve with nocturnal IPPV, and there was a statistically significant relationship between the change in daytime $PaCO_2$ and the change in the amount of gas trapping. Improvements in ventilatory function and mechanics (suggesting reduced small airway obstruction and slightly improved dynamic compliance) seemed to be a true effect of nocturnal IPPV, since patient stability was confirmed before recruitment. There were no changes in therapy during the study. The authors hypothesized that, since all of their patients had previous or current peripheral edema, the aforementioned improvements may have reflected a reduction in lung water following IPPV. Finally, a significant relationship was found between changes in daytime $PaCO_2$ and the increase in minute ventilation and occlusion pressure (P0.1) and an end-tidal CO_2 of 60 mmHg during CO_2 re-breathing, suggesting an adaptation of central chemoreceptors to the reduction in hypercapnia during the night or changes in the quality of sleep [12].

Notwithstanding these positive reports, it has to be mentioned that IPPV in COPD patients is less well tolerated and less effective than in patients with restrictive chest wall disease [39]. In particular, the number of dropouts because of poor comfort, intolerance of the mask, intercurrent illnesses, etc., is significant [44–47]. Moreover, a randomized crossover study by Strumpf and colleagues [47], comparing conventional treatment to IPPV in severe COPD patients, had negative results in terms of pulmonary function, respiratory muscle strength, gas exchange, exercise endurance, sleep efficiency, quality of oxygenation, and dyspnea rating. However, the patients in this study were those in whom the duration of IPPV was the shortest (3 months) and $PaCO_2$ before nocturnal mechanical ventilation was the lowest (47 ± 3 mmHg) in comparison with other studies which showed beneficial effects of IPPV [26, 44–46]. In addition, the patients in the study of Strumpf and colleagues [47] were introduced as outpatients, whereas all the patients in most of the positive studies started IPPV as inpatients [26, 45, 46]. Finally, the choice of ventilator and of the mode of ventilation is crucial [39]. The mode of mechanical ventilation may not ensure adequate alveolar ventilation during the night because of high impedance to inflation (e.g., most of the available domiciliary ventilators that provide pressure-cycled modes cannot deliver inspiratory pressures greater than 20–25 cmH_2O [48]), whereas volume-cycled ventilators seem more efficient in maintaining an adequate alveolar ventilation in hypercapnic COPD patients during the night [26, 44, 46, 49]. Moreover, asynchrony between the patient and the ventilator may be responsible for marked worsening of blood gases with both NPV [50] and IPPV [51] ventilators.

Taking into account all the above mentioned considerations, it can be concluded that IPPV can be used effectively in carefully selected patients with COPD. Well-motivated hypercapnic patients are most likely to benefit from IPPV, provided that adequate education and acclimatization to the technique are supplied [39]. Finally, the efficacy of IPPV in reversing nocturnal hypoventilation should be documented.

Conclusion

In conclusion, long-term mechanical ventilation seems to have no benefit in normo-capnic COPD patients. Controlled studies should be performed in order to confirm improvements obtained in hypercapnic patients. In this latter subgroup, no single factor seems responsible for daytime improvement of $PaCO_2$ and alveolar ventilation following long-term NPV/IPPV. Moreover, convincing evidence of respiratory muscle strength enhancement secondary to chronic fatigue relief has not been found. Changes in load placed upon respiratory muscles and in central chemorecep-tor responsiveness are likely to be mechanisms through which long-term mechani-cal ventilation provides its beneficial effects, if any. However, since load *per se* can influence the respiratory center output [40], and the interaction of other, as yet not investigated, mechanisms (e.g., changes in the ventilation-perfusion ratio) may im-prove arterial blood gas tensions, there is clearly much work to be done to better define the physiologic effects of long-term mechanical ventilation.

References

1. Roussos C (1985) Function and fatigue of respiratory muscles. Chest 88 (suppl 2):124S–131S
2. Douglas NJ, Calverley PMA, Leggett RJE, Brash HM, Flenley DC, Brezinova V (1979) Transient hypoxaemia during sleep in chronic bronchitis ancl emphysema. Lancet 1:1–4
3. Fletcher EC, Gray BA, Levin DC (1983) Nonapneic mechanisms of arterial oxygen desaturation during rapid-eye-movement sleep. J Appl Physiol 54:632–639
4. Arand DL, McGinty DJ, Littner MR (1981) Respiratory patterns associated with hemoglobin desaturation during sleep in chronic obstructive pulmonary disease. Chest 80:183–190
5. Littner NR, McGinty DJ, Arand DL (1980) Determinants of oxygen desaturation in the course of ventilation during sleep in chronic obstructive pulmonary disease. Am Rev Respir Dis 122:849–857
6. Douglas NJ, Flenley DC (1990) Breathing during sleep in patients with obstructive lung disease. Am Rev Respir Dis 141:1055–1070
7. Koo KW, Sax DS, Snider GL (1975) Arterial blood gas tensions and pH during sleep in chronic obstructive pulmonary disease. Am J Med 58:663–670
8. Leitch AG, Clancy LJ, Leggett RJE, Tweeddale P, Dawson P, Evans JI (1976) Arterial blood gas ten-sions, hydrogen ion and electroencephalogram during sleep in patients with chronic ventilatory failure. Thorax 31:730–735
9. Flenley DC, Millar JS (1970) Ventilatory response to oxygen and carbon dioxide in chronic respiratory failure. Clin Sci 33:319–334
10. Tatsumi K, Kimura H, Kunitomo F, Kuriyama T, Watanabe S, Honda Y (1986) Sleep arterial oxygen desaturation and chemical control of breathing during wakefulness in COPD. Chest 90:68–73
11. Fleetham JA, Mezon B, West P, Bradley CA, Anthonisen NR, Kryger M (1980) Chemical control of ventilation and sleep arterial oxygen desaturation in patients with COPD. Am Rev Respir Dis 122:583–589

12. White DP, Douglas NJ, Pickett CK, Zwillich CW, Weil JV (1983) Sleep deprivation and control of ventilation. Am Rev Respir Dis 128:984–986
13. Boysen PG, Block AJ, Wynne JW, Hunt LA, Flick MR (1979) Nocturnal pulmonary hypertension in patients with chronic obstructive pulmonary disease. Chest 76:536–542
14. Coccagna G, Lugaresi E (1978) Arterial blood gases and pulmonary and systemic arterial pressure during sleep in chronic obstructive pulmonary disease. Sleep 1:117–124
15. Fletcher EC, Luckett RA, Miller T, Costarangos C, Kutka N, Fletcher JG (1989) Pulmonary vascular hemodynamics in chronic lung disease patients with and without oxyhemoglobin desaturation during sleep. Chest 95:757–764
16. Calverley PMA, Brezinova V, Douglas NJ, Catterall JR, Flenley DC (1982) The effect of oxygenation on sleep quality in chronic bronchitis and emphysema. Am Rev Respir Dis 126:206–210
17. Fleetham JA, West P, Mezon B, Conway W, Roth T, Kryger M (1982) Sleep, arousals, and oxygen desaturations in COPD. Am Rev Respir Dis 124:429–433
18. Berthon-Jones M, Sullivan CE (1982) Ventilatory and arousal responses to hypoxia in sleeping humans. Am Rev Respir Dis 125:632–639
19. Hedmark L, Kronenberg R (1981) Ventilatory responses to hypoxia and CO_2 during natural and fluorazepam induced sleep in normal adults. Am Rev Resp Dis 123:190 (Abst)
20. Berton-Jones M, Sullivan CE (1987) Time course of change in ventilatory response to CO_2 with long-term CPAP therapy for obstructive sleep apnea. Am Rev Respir Dis 135:144–147
21. Bergovsky EH (1979) Respiratory failure in disorders of the thoracic cage. Am Rev Respir Dis 119:643–669
22. Hoeppner VH, Cockcroft DW, Dosmann JA, Cotton DJ (1984) Nighttime ventilation improves respiratory failure in secondary kyphoscoliosis. Am Rev Respir Dis 129:240–243
23. Simonds AK, Parker RA, Branthwaite MA (1989) The effect of intermittent positive pressure hyperinflation in restrictive chest wall disease. Respiration 55:136–143
24. Elliott MV, Mulvey DA, Moxham J, Green M, Branthwaite MA (1991) Domiciliary nocturnal nasal intermittent positive pressure ventilation in COPD: mechanisms underlying changes in arterial blood gas tensions. Eur Respir J 4:1044–1052
25. Mohr CH, Hill NS (1990) Long term follow-up of nocturnal ventilatory assistance in patients with respiratory failure due to Duchenne-type muscular dystrophy. Chest 97:91–96
26. Gay PC, Patel AM, Viggiano RW, Hubmayr RD (1991) Nocturnal nasal ventilation for treatment of patients with hypercapnic respiratory failure. Mayo Clin Proc 66:695–703
27. Goldstein RS, Molotiu N, Skrastins R, et al (1987) Reversal of sleep-induced hypoventilation and chronic respiratory failure by nocturnal negative pressure ventilation in patients with restrictive ventilatory impairment. Am Rev Respir Dis 135:1049–1055
28. Patessio A, Appendini L, et al (1996) Long-term nocturnal mechanical ventilation in COPD patients: physiological effects of withdrawal. Eur Respir J 9 (suppl 23):112S (Abst)
29. Gutierrez M, Beroiza T, Contreras G, et al (1988) Weekly cuirass ventilation improves blood gases and inspiratory muscle stregth in patients with chronic airflow limitation and hypercarbia. Am Rev Respir Dis 138:617–623
30. Cropp A, DiMarco AF (1987) Effects of intermittent negative pressure ventilation on respiratory muscle function in patients with severe chronic obstructive pulmonary disease. Am Rev Respir Dis 135:1056–1061
31. Scano G, Gigliotti F, Duranti R, Spinelli A, Gorini M, Schiavina M (1990) Changes in ventilatory muscle function with negative pressure ventilation in COPD. Chest 97:322–327
32. Braun NM, Marino WD (1984) Effect of daily intermittent rest of respiratory muscles in patients with severe chronic airflow limitation (CAL). Chest 85:59S–60S (Abst)
33. Moxham J, Goldstone J (1994) Assessment of respiratory muscle strength in the intensive care unit. Eur Respir J 7:2057–2061
34. Carrey Z, Gottfried SB, Levy RD (1990) Ventilatory muscle support in respiratory failure with nasal positive pressure ventilation. Chest 97:150–158
35. Elliott MW, Mulvey DA, Moxham J, Green M, Branthwaite MA (1993) Inspiratory muscle effort during nasal intermittent positive pressure ventilation in patients with chronic obstructive airways disease. Anaesthesia 48:8–13
36. Shapiro SH, Ernst P, Gray-Donald K, et al (1992) Effect of negative pressure ventilation in severe chronic obstructive pulmonary disease. Lancet 2:1425–1429

37. Ambrosino N, Montagna T, Nava S, et al (1990) Short term effect of intermittent negative pressure ventilation in COPD patients with respiratory failure. Eur Respir J 3:502–508
38. Moxham J (1990) Respiratory muscle fatigue: mechanisms, evaluation and therapy. Br J Anaesth 65:43–53
39. Elliott M, Moxham J (1994) Noninvasive mechanical ventilation by nasal or face mask. In: Tobin MJ (ed) Principles and practice of mechanical ventilation, 1st edn. McGraw-Hill, New York, pp 427–453
40. Jounes M (1990) Load responses, dyspnea, and respiratory failure. Chest 97 (suppl 1):59S–68S
41. Zibrak JD, Hill NS, Federman EC, Kwa SL, O'Donnell C (1988) Evaluation of intermittent long-term negative-pressure ventilation in patients with severe chronic obstructive pulmonary disease. Am Rev Respir Dis 138:1515–1518
42. Celli B, Lee H, Criner G, et al (1989) Controlled trial of external negative pressure ventilation in patients with severe chronic airflow obstruction. Am Rev Respir Dis 140:1251–1256
43. Similowski T, Yan S, Gauthier AP, Macklem PT, Bellemare F (1991) Contractile properties of the human diaphragm during chronic hyperinflation. N Engl J Med 325:917–923
44. Elliott MW, Simonds AK, Carroll MP, Wedzicha JA, Branthwaite MA (1992) Domiciliary nocturnal nasal intermittent positive pressure ventilation in hypercapnic respiratory failure due to chronic obstructive lung disease: effects on sleep and quality of life. Thorax 47:342–348
45. Carroll N, Branthwaite MA (1988) Control of nocturnal hypoventilation by nasal intermittent positive pressure ventilation. Thorax 43:349–353
46. Marino W (1991) Intermittent volume cycled mechanical ventilation via nasal mask in patients with respiratory failure due to COPD. Chest 99:681–684
47. Strumpf DA, Millman RP, Carlisle CC, et al (1991) Nocturnal positive-pressure ventilation via nasal mask in patients with severe chronic obstructive pulmonary disease. Am Rev Respir Dis 144:1234–1239
48. Simonds AK, Elliott MW (1991) Use of BiPAP ventilator for noninvasive ventilation: advantages and limitations. Am Rev Respir Dis 143 (suppl):A585 (Abst)
49. Ellis ER, Grunstein RR, Chan S, Bye PTB, Sullivan CE (1988) Noninvasive ventilatory support during sleep improves respiratory failure in kyphoscoliosis. Chest 94:811–815
50. Simonds AK, Brainthwaite MA (1985) Efficiency of negative pressure ventilatory equipment. Thorax 40:213–218
51. Rodenstein DO, Stanescu DC, Delguste P, Liistro G, Aubert-Tulkens G (1989) Adaptation to intermittent positive pressure ventilation applied through the nose during day and night. Eur Respir J 2:473–478
52. Singh B (1984) Sleep apnea: a psychiatric perspective. In: Saunders NA, Sullivan CE (eds) Sleep and breathing. Marcel Dekker, New York, pp 403–422

Lung Perfusion –
Inhaled Nitric Oxide

Distribution of Pulmonary Perfusion in Healthy and Injured Lungs

M. Kleen, B. Zwissler, and K. Messmer

Introduction

The classical concept for understanding the heterogeneity of regional pulmonary blood flow distribution is West's concept of lung zones; Zones have been defined by the relationship of blood pressure in pulmonary arteries and veins to the pressure of air within the alveolar space [1]. Three such zones have been described: Areas of no flow where alveolar pressure exceeds arterial pressure; areas of 'waterfall' flow where alveolar pressure exceeds venous, but not arterial blood pressure; and a zone of continuous flow through arteries and veins where alveolar pressure is lower than both blood pressures. In this article, current data are reviewed that may challenge this model for the *in-vivo* situation. Since West's classical description, much has been learned about the design principle nature uses to create complex trees such as the pulmonary vasculature and bronchial tree. New imaging techniques provide the clinician with overwhelming amounts of data, and progress in this field will continue to enhance resolution of pulmonary structures. We will outline a new concept of distribution of pulmonary blood flow which at the same time gives due credit to the complex structure of the pulmonary vessel tree and can reduce any amount of data on pulmonary perfusion to a single parameter describing heterogeneity.

Gravitational Gradients

The zonal concept of pulmonary blood flow distribution is built on the indisputable fact that pressure increases downward from the pressure source (the right ventricle in this case) and decreases if one moves the point of measurement upward. If one moves upward far enough, eventually a point will be reached where alveolar pressure will be higher than arterial pressure and blood flow will, therefore, cease. This is the basis of the classical zonal concept for understanding heterogeneity of pulmonary blood flow [1]. Among other findings, abolition of perfusion heterogeneity by micro-gravity has been demonstrated for men [2] which provides strong evidence in favor of the zonal perfusion concept. The zonal concept is therefore obviously one possible description of pulmonary perfusion heterogeneity. Very recently, however, a series of reports appeared questioning the role of gravity in the distribution of lung perfusion.

Melsom and colleagues demonstrated that both gravitational and non-gravitational factors govern distribution of pulmonary perfusion in goats [3] and they subsequently confirmed these results in awake animals [4]. Walther et al. [5] found no significant influence of gravity on the distribution of perfusion in the lungs of awake, prone sheep. Treppo and colleagues [6] showed for the anesthetized dog that in the prone position (physiologic for the dog), gravitational forces are balanced out by dorso-ventral differences in vascular conductivity, whereas in the supine position effects of gravity and vascular structural inhomogeneity become additive and produce significant gravitational blood flow gradients. In order to maximize the expected influence of gravity, Hlastala et al. [7] used awake standing horses with 50 cm of distance between the dorsal and the ventral surfaces of the lung. These authors concluded that there is no consistent vertical gradient of pulmonary blood flow which indicates that pulmonary blood flow distribution is not governed by gravity. In awake dogs, it was demonstrated that the pattern of distribution of lung perfusion is stable over days [8]. The basis for all these findings may be regional anatomic differences, namely differences in vascular hindrance of blood flow. Pulmonary vascular conductances are not uniformly distributed in dogs; rather, vessels that are oriented dorsally (anti-gravitational in dogs) have a higher conductance [9]. The assumption that distribution of pulmonary blood flow is dominated only by gravity therefore probably does not fully describe the complexity of pulmonary perfusion.

The Fractal Concept of Pulmonary Blood Flow Heterogeneity

As discussed above, current data indicate that gravity alone is not sufficient to develop a concept which helps to understand the heterogeneity of regional pulmonary blood flow. The anatomical structure of pulmonary vessels may be useful in this situation. Morphometric studies of the canine [10] and human [11] pulmonary vasculature have revealed that the pulmonary arterial and venous vascular beds can be considered as repetitively, dichotomously branching trees. The validity of this concept is supported by the possibility of accurately simulating pulmonary blood flow heterogeneity with a computer-generated model of such a tree [12]. The distribution of several liters of blood per minute to capillaries around more than a hundred square meters of alveolar surface has been solved by nature with a very complex vascular tree which minimizes work force. This complexity can be reduced to simplicity if one considers the basic structural element of the tree; the vascular tree consists of thousands of dichotomous divisions. One simple rule of division has been implemented repeatedly for each generation of vessels. Apart from size, each bifurcation is similar to the next, independent of the generation it belongs to. Self-similarity has been termed a design principle of nature [13] and is one definition of a fractal object [14]. The term 'fractal' was introduced by Mandelbrot [15] to describe objects with a fractional dimension (e.g., 1.2), unlike the integer dimensions (e.g., 1, 2, or 3) in classical geometry. If an object has a fractal dimension above its integer Euclidean dimension, this indicates that the object's structure strives to go beyond the geometric limits but does not quite reach the next higher dimension. For example, the graphical representation of the pulmonary vessel tree is a system of lines that can be drawn on a sheet of paper (Fig. 1). Lines are, by definition, one-dimensional, Euclidean geometric objects. The sheet of paper on which the tree is

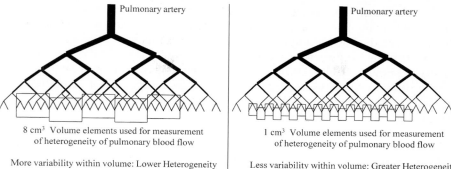

8 cm³ Volume elements used for measurement
of heterogeneity of pulmonary blood flow

1 cm³ Volume elements used for measurement
of heterogeneity of pulmonary blood flow

More variability within volume: Lower Heterogeneity

Less variability within volume: Greater Heterogeneity

Fig. 1. Illustration of the dependence of pulmonary blood flow heterogeneity on resolution of measurement. Left and right panels are schematic drawings of the pulmonary arterial bed. The vascular tree is a fractal, meaning that it is structurally self-similar: The basic structural element, the dichotomous bifurcation, is present many times at different sizes. *Left panel:* Measurement of pulmonary blood flow heterogeneity with low resolution, i.e., large volume elements (symbolized with rectangles). Heterogeneity is low since sources of irregularity, i.e., bifurcations, are hidden within volume elements. *Right panel:* Measurement of pulmonary blood flow heterogeneity with higher resolution, i.e., small volume elements (symbolized with rectangles). Heterogeneity is higher since more arterial bifurcations can be discerned. Therefore, standard heterogeneity data from studies with different resolution of measurement cannot be compared. Fractal dimension relates the increase of heterogeneity to increasing resolution and is therefore a resolution-independent parameter

drawn represents a two-dimensional geometric plane. The drawn vascular tree with all the fine branchings and terminal arterioles will almost, but not completely, fill the two-dimensional plane. In classical geometry, the tree will still be a one-dimensional object, whereas fractal geometry can be used to determine a fractal dimension that will account for the complexity of the tree. The fractal dimension for such a tree will be between 1 (Euclidean dimension of a line) and 2 (Euclidean dimension of the plane).

The fractal 'vascular tree' delivers blood to pulmonary parenchyma. It would be logical to assume that the heterogeneity of regional pulmonary blood flow is governed by the properties of pulmonary vessels. The most striking result of this is the dependence of heterogeneity on resolution. If regional pulmonary blood flow is measured with volume elements of e.g., 8 cm³ (see Fig. 1), a certain heterogeneity (measured with e.g., relative dispersion of perfusion) can be calculated. If such data are then compared to data from studies where perfusion was measured for 1 cm³ volume elements, there may be a huge difference. Heterogeneity of pulmonary perfusion is not a constant phenomenon; it is resolution dependent. This dependence is the consequence of increasing visibility of the complexity of the vascular network by refining the measurement method. For example, an 8 cm³ volume element of pulmonary tissue hides many more generations of vessels and therefore hides more perfusion heterogeneity than a 1 cm³ volume element (Fig. 1). This makes comparison of heterogeneities found in different studies or even in different subjects a difficult task.

Fractal geometry offers a simple solution to this complex situation. By measuring the heterogeneity of pulmonary regional blood flow with a statistical parameter (e.g., coefficient of variation) a one-dimensional 'picture' of perfusion heterogeneity is produced. If blood flow has fractal properties, the fractal dimension of this picture should exceed the Euclidean dimension 1. The determination of the fractal dimension for this case has been shown to be easily feasible [16–18]; the change of heterogeneity of pulmonary blood flow is related to changing resolution through a power law. By fitting a linear regression equation to the logarithms of resolution and heterogeneity data, the fractal dimension of heterogeneity can be derived as 1 minus the slope of the regression line.

An Example of Application of the Fractal Concept to Research in Intensive Care Medicine

After demonstration of the fractal properties of regional pulmonary blood flow in healthy lungs by e.g., Glenny et al. [16] and Walther et al. [5], we first applied fractal geometry to the investigation of experimental lung injury [19]. We hypothesized that the fractal dimension of regional pulmonary perfusion would change in experimental lung injury. Furthermore, we speculated that the beneficial effects of positive end-expiratory pressure (PEEP) therapy would accompany reversal of injury-induced alterations of fractal dimensions.

In eight anesthetized dogs in the left lateral decubitus position, lung injury was produced by combination of oleic acid infusion and glass bead embolization. Regional pulmonary perfusion was assessed quantitatively with radioactive microspheres. The lungs were dried and dissected into 384 ± 77 samples after sacrifice of animals. At baseline, the fractal dimension was 1.25 ± 0.06. In five of eight animals lung injury resulted in a reduction of fractal dimension by 28 to 58% of the total possible range (1.0–1.5). In one animal the fractal dimension remained essentially unchanged and in two animals an increase by 12–14% of the maximal range occurred. Ventilation with increasing PEEP between 10 and 20 cmH_2O produced small changes with no difference between the levels of PEEP. PEEP-induced changes were small but predominantly positive in most animals such that the fractal dimension during PEEP of 20 cmH_2O was greater than at baseline in six of eight animals. However, infusion of 0.2–1.0 µg/kg/min norepinephrine at 20 cmH_2O PEEP reduced fractal dimension by 4 to 38% of the maximal range in six of eight animals. In two animals, 10 and 14% increases of the maximal range were seen. The coefficient of variation as the standard parameter of heterogeneity of pulmonary perfusion was not correlated with the fractal dimension ($r = 0.06$).

It is important to note that at baseline there were anti-gravitational blood flow gradients. Only after induction of severe lung injury, were gradients reversed and displayed the pattern that would be predicted by the zonal concept. PEEP therapy did not completely restore the physiologic pattern of distribution but there was a significant reduction of injury-induced alterations. From these data we conclude that pulmonary blood flow distribution in a model of lung injury is poorly described by the classical zonal concept. Observed gravitational gradients where in contrast to what was predicted by this concept. Only after induction of severe lung pathology, did dependent lung regions received more perfusion than non-dependent parts.

Our study is the first which includes fractal geometric data in a model of lung pathology. The trend towards reduction of fractal dimension (i.e., homogenization) in lung injury is consistent with findings of reduced fractal dimension of myocardial perfusion in shock [20]. A certain degree of disorder in blood flow distribution in the lung is obviously physiologic, whereas lung injury is accompanied by reduction of disorder. PEEP ventilation induced an increase of fractal dimension as our hypothesis predicted. Our data are not sufficient to elucidate the full potential of fractal analysis of pulmonary perfusion in critical care medicine research. However, the usefulness of fractal geometry for assessing blood flow heterogeneity in models of lung injury should be investigated further for several reasons:

1) The parameter fractal dimension is directly related to the anatomical structure of the pulmonary vessel tree and has been extensively validated in the healthy lung
2) We have shown that fractal dimension is sensitive to alterations in pulmonary physiology
3) By using fractal analysis, comparison of heterogeneities from different imaging or measurement methods, different studies, and different individuals is possible since resolution independence is one property of fractal dimension
4) This analysis can reduce any amount of data from high resolution pulmonary diagnostic studies to a single parameter of heterogeneity

Conclusion

In numerous studies, the presence of gravitational gradients of pulmonary perfusion has been demonstrated. The usefulness of this concept for understanding the heterogeneity of pulmonary blood flow has stood the test of time. However, a considerable amount of very recent data indicates that gravitation is less important than generally assumed. Anatomical studies of the pulmonary vasculature show that the lung vessel tree is a self-similar, fractal structure. This makes the concept of analyzing regional pulmonary blood flow with fractal geometry very appealing. Many studies have demonstrated fractal properties of physiologic lung perfusion. We applied fractal methods of analysis to a model of lung injury and found not completely consistent effects in a small group of animals. The new concept of understanding heterogeneity of pulmonary perfusion is undisputed for normal lungs. There is a convincing theoretic basis for this concept and further studies on the usefulness of fractal geometry for investigations in pulmonary pathology are warranted. In the future, incorporation of fractal geometric analysis methods in computer-assisted clinical pulmonary diagnosis may provide more comparability between studies and aid the clinician in interpreting increasing amounts of data.

References

1. Hughes JM, Glazier JB, Maloney JE, West JB (1968) Effect of lung volume on the distribution of pulmonary blood flow in man. Respir Physiol 4:58–72
2. Michels DB, West JB (1978) Distribution of pulmonary ventilation and perfusion during short periods of weightlessness. J Appl Physiol 45:987–998

3. Melsom MN, Flatebo T, Kramer-Johansen J, et al (1995) Both gravity and non-gravity dependent factors determine regional blood flow within the goat lung. Acta Physiol Scand 153:343–353
4. Melsom MN, Kramer-Johansen J, Flatebo T, Muller C, Nicolaysen G (1997) Distribution of pulmonary ventilation and perfusion measured simultaneously in awake goats. Acta Physiol Scand 159:199–208
5. Walther SM, Domino KB, Glenny RW, Polissar NL, Hlastala MP (1997) Pulmonary blood flow distribution has a hilar-to-peripheral gradient in awake, prone sheep. J Appl Physiol 82:678–685
6. Treppo S, Mijailovich SM, Venegas JG (1997) Contributions of pulmonary perfusion and ventilation to heterogeneity in V(A)/Q measured by PET. J Appl Physiol 82:1163–1176
7. Hlastala MP, Bernard SL, Erickson HH, et al (1996) Pulmonary blood flow distribution in standing horses is not dominated by gravity. J Appl Physiol 81:1051–1061
8. Glenny RW, McKinney S, Robertson HT (1997) Spatial pattern of pulmonary blood flow distribution is stable over days. J Appl Physiol 82:902–907
9. Beck KC, Rehder K (1986) Differences in regional vascular conductances in isolated dog lungs. J Appl Physiol 61:530–538
10. Gan RZ, Tian Y, Yen RT, Kassab GS (1993) Morphometry of the dog pulmonary venous tree. J Appl Physiol 75:432–440
11. Huang W, Yen RT, McLaurine M, Bledsoe G (1996) Morphometry of the human pulmonary vasculature. J Appl Physiol 81:2123–2133
12. Glenny RW, Robertson HT (1991) Fractal modeling of pulmonary blood flow heterogeneity. J Appl Physiol 70:1024–1030
13. Weibel ER (1991) Fractal geometry: a design principle for living organisms. Am J Physiol 261:L361–L369
14. Glenny RW, Robertson HT, Yamashiro S, Bassingthwaighte JB (1991) Applications of fractal analysis to physiology. J Appl Physiol 70:2351–2367
15. Mandelbrot BB (1983) The fractal geometry of nature. Freeman, New York
16. Glenny RW, Robertson HT (1990) Fractal properties of pulmonary blood flow: characterization of spatial heterogeneity. J Appl Physiol 69:532–545
17. Bassingthwaighte JB, King RB, Roger SA (1989) Fractal nature of regional myocardial blood flow heterogeneity. Circ Res 65:578–590
18. Kleen M, Habler O, Hutter J, et al (1998) Hemodilution and hyperoxia locally change distribution of regional pulmonary perfusion in dogs. Am J Physiol (in press)
19. Kleen M, Zwissler B, Messmer K (1998) Positive end-expiratory pressure only partly restores disturbed distribution of regional pulmonary blood flow in lung injury. Am J Physiol (in press)
20. Kleen M, Welte M, Lackermeier P, Habler O, Kemming G, Messmer K (1997) Myocardial blood flow heterogeneity in shock and small-volume resuscitation in pigs with coronary stenosis. J Appl Physiol 83:1832–1841

The Administration and Measurement of Nitric Oxide During Mechanical Ventilation

R. M. Kacmarek

Introduction

Although the use of inhaled nitric oxide (NO) is currently still experimental, it is being used increasingly during mechanical ventilation to treat diseases characterized by hypoxemia and pulmonary hypertension [1–10]. Numerous approaches have been designed by researchers to administer NO via the mechanical ventilator [7–36] (Table 1), however few of these experimental approaches are capable of providing accurate, precise and consistent concentrations of inhaled NO without the potential for the formation of nitrogen dioxide (NO_2) at concentrations up to 80 ppm NO and

Table 1. Nitric oxide delivery systems

Type	Description	Examples (Reference numbers)
Internal mixing	Blends NO, O_2 and air to provide the desired [NO] and FiO_2 (e.g., Servo 300)	[7, 8, 9]
Pre-mixing	Mixes a high [NO] with N_2 (or air) proximal to the ventilator and delivers it to the high or low pressure gas inlet of the ventilator	[8, 10–19]
Injection		
Continuous into inspiratory limb	Continuous injection of NO mixture into the inspiratory circuit distal to the ventilator outlet	[17, 20–28]
Continuous into Y-piece	Continuous injection at the Y-piece proximal to the endotracheal tube	[26–28]
Inspiratory phase into inspiratory limb	Inspiratory phase injection into the inspiratory circuit distal to the ventilator outlet	[7, 29–34]
Inspiratory phase into Y-piece	Inspiratory phase injection at the Y-piece proximal to the endotracheal tube	[15, 34]
Servo-controlled to inspiratory flow	Flow measured by pneumotachometer and NO gas mixture servo-controlled to inspiratory flow with a mass flow controller	[35]
Directly into endo-tracheal tube	Flow of NO directly into the endotracheal tube	[36]

NO: nitric oxide; [NO]: NO concentration; FiO_2: inspired oxygen fraction. (From [37] with permission)

during all modes of ventilatory support regardless of their being assist or control [37]. In this chapter, information is presented regarding the technical limitations (precision/bias) and measurement capabilities of current commercially available NO/NO$_2$ analyzers, as well as a detailed analysis of the various NO delivery systems in use, both developed by researchers and commercially available.

Nitric Oxide – The Gas

Concern regarding precise and accurate concentrations of delivered NO during mechanical ventilation should be foremost in the minds of all researchers for not only do high concentrations of NO carry the risk of methemoglobin [16] formation but even more importantly the formation of NO$_2$ [14] and subsequent formation of nitric acid (NHO$_3$) [38].

NO is a highly active molecule that chemically reacts with oxygen to form NO$_2$ which in turn reacts with water to form HNO$_3$:

$$2\,NO + O_2 \rightarrow 2\,NO_2 \tag{1}$$

$$3\,NO_2 + H_2O \rightarrow 2\,HNO_3 + NO \tag{2}$$

The Occupational Safety and Health Administration in the United States has set safety limits for inhaled NO$_2$ at 5 ppm [39] however, airway hyperreactivity [40] and parenchymal lung injury [41] have been reported at levels ≤ 2 ppm. The rate of conversion of NO to NO$_2$ is determined by the concentrations of NO and O$_2$, the time the two gases are in contact, and the temperature of the system [14]. Increases in any of these variables accelerates the conversion of NO to NO$_2$. The kinetics of this reaction have been previously described [42] by the following relationship:

$$-\,d\,[NO]/dt = k \cdot [O_2] \cdot [NO]^2 \tag{3}$$

where [] represents gas concentration and t time. We found k to be 1.46×10^{-9} ppm^{-2} min^{-1} when NO was blended with N$_2$ prior to entry into the Puritan Bennett 7200 ventilator and 1.17×10^{-8} ppm^{-2} min^{-1} when NO was blended with air [14]. The effect of NO and O$_2$ concentrations on the production of 2 ppm NO$_2$ is shown in Fig. 1 [14]. Note that at high concentrations of NO (80 ppm) and high concentrations of O$_2$ (90%) it takes only seconds to generate 2 ppm NO$_2$.

NO$_2$ can be removed from the ventilator circuit by the insertion of a soda lime absorber into the inspiratory limb [43]. However, soda lime does not completely remove NO$_2$, it also removes NO, reducing delivered concentration, and it loses its effectiveness to remove either over time [18]. In addition, soda lime canisters increase system resistance to flow, modify the gas delivery pattern, increase the potential for system leaks and increase the difficulty of patient triggering [44].

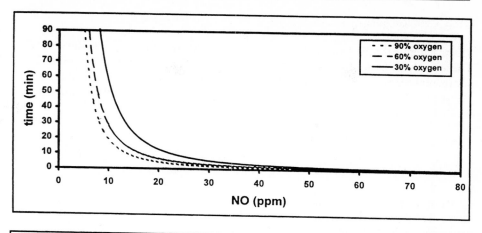

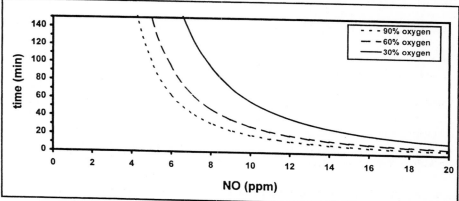

Fig. 1. Time required to generate 2 ppm nitrogen dioxide (NO₂) in systems with varying FiO₂ and NO concentration ([NO]). *Top:* [NO] up to 80 ppm. At 80 ppm and 90% O₂ 2 ppm NO₂ is formed in seconds. *Bottom:* [NO] up to 20 ppm. A relatively long time (20 min) is required to generate 2 ppm NO₂ when [NO] is ≤ 10 ppm. (From [14] with permission)

Nitric Oxide Analyzers

Although there are many methods of analyzing the gases NO and NO_2, the two approaches that are currently used clinically/experimentally are chemiluminescence and electrochemical analysis. Each has distinct advantages and disadvantages for use in clinical settings, with both groups of analyzers capable of accurately monitoring the precision and accuracy of NO/NO_2 delivered during mechanical ventilation [45, 46].

Electrochemical Analyzers

Electrochemical cells have recently become available to measure both NO and NO_2. These analyzers are small, portable, rugged, and less expensive than chemilumines-cence analyzers. The electrochemical cell consists of sensing, counter, and reference electrodes. To detect NO, the following reactions occur at the sensor and counter electrodes, respectively:

$$NO + 2H_2O \rightarrow HNO_3 + 3H^+ + 3e^- \tag{4}$$

$$O_2 + 4H^+ + 4e^- \rightarrow 2H_2O \tag{5}$$

Current is proportional to NO concentration because each NO molecule consumes three electrons at the sensor electrode. Balancing these reactions yields the overall reaction for the NO cell:

$$4NO + 2H_2O + 3O_2 \rightarrow 4HNO_3^- \tag{6}$$

The NO_2 sensing electrode causes reduction of NO_2 to NO, producing a current pro-portional to the concentration of NO_2:

$$NO_2 + 2H^+ + 2e^- \rightarrow NO + H_2O \tag{7}$$

Oxidation of water occurs at the counter electrode:

$$2H_2O \rightarrow 4H^+ + 4e^- + O_2 \tag{8}$$

Balancing the reactions at each electrode yields the overall reaction for the NO_2 cell:

$$2NO_2 \rightarrow 2NO + O_2 \tag{9}$$

For both the NO and NO_2 cells, a reference electrode provides a bias voltage by applying an external potential to keep the sensing electrode at the correct operating voltage.

A number of evaluations have been performed on electrochemical analyzers [45, 47–53] all of which have found these analyzers suitable for clinical use. As indicated in Tables 2 and 3 there are differences in precision and bias for both NO and NO_2 analyzers [45]. NO analyzers are particularly sensitive to the inspired oxygen frac-tion (FiO_2) and system pressure, although the differences do not seem to be clini-cally significant. One of the major limitations of electrochemical analyzers is the fact that they are affected by water vapor in a manner similar to that of oxygen analyzers [49–53]. Continual analysis in the presence of water vapor markedly shortens the life of electrodes and increases the likelihood of inaccurate measurement if water con-denses on the electrode. Problems associated with the effects of humidification can be avoided if analysis is performed proximal to the system humidifier or if analysis is only performed on a periodic basis [45]. In addition, when one considers the accuracy of electrochemical analyzers it becomes obvious that the accuracy of these

Table 2. Bias ± precision (ppm) for agreement of electrochemical analyzers with Eco-Physics chemiluminescence analyzer

Analyzer	Overall	FiO$_2$		NO level (ppm)		Ventilator pressure level		
		<0.50	>0.5	≤20	>20	Low	Moderate	High
Bedfont	−0.8±1.0	−1.0±1.1	−0.5±0.6	−0.3 ±0.5	−1.4 ±1.1	−1.4±1.3	−0.7±0.6	−0.3±0.5
B&W	−0.4±0.6	−0.7±0.6	−0.1±0.4	−0.2 ±0.4	−0.7 ±0.7	−0.5±0.7	−0.5±0.6	−0.3±0.5
Dräger	−1.0±0.7	−1.1±0.6	−0.8±0.7	−0.8 ±0.6	−1.2 ±0.7	−1.2±0.7	−0.9±0.7	−0.9±0.7
EIT	−0.7±1.7	−0.8±1.9	−0.5±1.2	−1.3 ±1.3	−0.02±1.8	−1.1±0.5	−0.5±1.8	−0.5±1.7
Pulmonox	1.8±1.9	2.3±2.2	1.1±0.9	0.9 ±0.7	2.9 ±2.2	1.2±1.3	1.5±1.3	2.8±2.4
Saan	0.1±0.7	0.1±0.7	0.1±0.6	−0.04±0.4	0.3 ±0.9	0.1±0.9	0.1±0.6	0.1±0.4

Bedfont: Bedfont NOxBox, Bedfont Scientific, Kent, England; B+W: B+W Medimax, B+W Technologies, Calgary, Alberta, Canada; Dräger: Dräger Inc. Pittsburgh, PA; EIT: EIT Sensor Stik, Exton, PA; Pulmonox: Pulmonox II, Pulmonox Research and Development, Topfield, Alberta, Canada; Saan: Saan TM-100, Taiyo Sanso, Tokyo, Japan. NO: nitric oxide; FiO$_2$: fraction of inspired oxygen. (From [45] with permission)

Table 3. Bias ± precision for nitrogen dioxide (NO$_2$) between electrochemical analyzers and Eco-Physics chemiluminescence analyzer

Analyzer	Bias ± precision
Bedfont NOxBox	0.01 ± 0.12
Dräger	0.04 ± 0.10
EIT Sensor Stik	0.34 ± 0.22
Pulmonox II	−0.14 ± 0.13
Saan	0.18 ± 0.12

Bedfont NOxBox: Bedfont Scientific, Kent, England; Dräger: Pittsburgh, PA; EIT Sensor Stik: Exton, PA; Pulmonox II: Pulmonox Research and Development, Topfield, Alberta, Canada; Saan: Saan TM-100, Taiyo Sanso, Tokyo, Japan. (From [45] with permission)

analyzers markedly decreases as the NO concentration approaches 1 ppm, making it impossible to measure NO concentrations in the ppb range [45]. A final concern regarding these analyzers is response time. With all of these units response time is greater than 30 seconds, again similar to that observed with oxygen analyzers [47–51]. This, of course makes it impossible to measure the concentration of NO in a system where the NO level changes during a single breath. Specifically, it is impossible to analyze inhaled NO concentrations when NO is injected in an uncontrolled manner into the inspiratory limb (see later sections) or to measure exhaled NO concentration. In spite of these limitations, electrochemical analyzers are very useful and accurate with specific NO delivery systems.

Chemiluminescence

Chemiluminescent analyzers operate by the photochemical detection of electro-magnetically emitted radiation [45]. Specifically the gas to be sampled is drawn into a reaction chamber where it reacts with ozone to produce activated NO that changes its ground state by emitting electromagnetic radiation, which is detected photo-electrically [54].

$$NO + O_3 \rightarrow NO_2^* + O_2 \tag{10}$$

$$NO_2^* \rightarrow NO_2 + hv \tag{11}$$

where O$_3$ is ozone, * indicates a highly excited state and hv is electromagnetic radiation. To measure NO$_2$ the analyzer converts NO$_2$ to NO in a thermal chamber,

$$3\,NO_2 + Mo + 325\,^\circ C \rightarrow 3\,NO + MoO_3 \tag{12}$$

where Mo is molybdenum. The sum of NO and the converted NO$_2$ is referred to as NO$_x$ (NO$_x$ = NO + NO$_2$) [45]. Most analyzers measure NO and NO$_x$ simultaneously and display NO$_x$, NO and NO$_2$. Chemiluminescent analyzers are very accurate and precise but they are large, expensive and cumbersome to use.

Originally, chemiluminescent NO analyzers were developed for the identification of NO as an industrial pollutant [54]. As a result transport delay and response time were not considered important attributes of the function of the analyzer. However, when measurement of exhaled gas is slow or for measurement of NO in systems where concentration changes, both of these characteristics are critical for accurate measurement [46]. Transport delay is the time delay between the initial signal being received by the analyzer and the initial display of NO concentration, whereas response time is normally referred to as the time necessary to identify a specific percent of the maximum signal. That is, the 95% response time is the amount of time from the initial recognition of the signal to a display of 95% of the maximal signal (Fig. 2) [46]. Transport delay of an analyzer is critical in determining the phase delay of NO analysis for comparison with other signals from the ventilating system (e.g., flow, pressure, CO_2). The 95% response time indicates if the system is capable of providing an accurate analysis when NO concentration is changing. For example an analyzer with a 95% response time of longer than the length of the expiratory phase would not provide an accurate measurement of exhaled CO_2. Figure 3 illustrates the NO concentration waveforms from a system where NO concentration varied from 0 to 8 ppm. The Sievers Instruments 270B NOA analyzer (95% response time 0.22±0.04 sec) was the only analyzer to provide an accurate continuous measurement of NO concentration. The Horiba Industries CLA 510S (95% response time 9.74±0.24 sec), the ECO Physics CLD 700 AL (95% response time 3.92±0.63 sec) and the Thermo Environmental Industries Model 42 (95% response time 40.03±0.00 sec) analyzers were all unable to accurately measure the changing NO levels. As noted all tended to underestimate peak, and overestimate minimal, NO concentrations [46]. The long 95% response time on the model 42 resulted in a constant reading of NO concentrations in spite of the concentration changing between 0 and 8 ppm.

Two other factors can affect the accuracy of chemiluminiscence analyzers; "quenching" and the "mass transport effect", although these effects are minimal compared

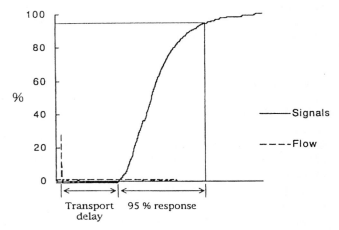

Fig. 2. Illustrations of transport delay and 95% response time. Dashed line indicates generation of flow in measuring system. Solid line indicates signal recognition by analyzer. Horizontal axis is time. (From [46] with permission)

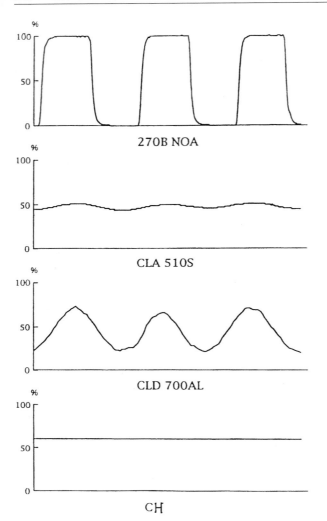

Fig. 3. Representative signal outputs, from various chemiluminescence analyzers during measurement of a NO signal that varied from zero to 8 ppm. 270 B NOA: Sievers Instruments Inc. Boulder, Co; CLA 510S: Noriba, Kyoto, Japan; CLD 700 AL-ECO Physics AG, Postfach, CH; Model 42: Thermo Environmental Instruments Inc., Franklin, MA. (From [46] with permission)

to the response time [54, 55]. Chemiluminescence analyzers measure photoemissions from electronically excited NO molecules produced by the reaction of NO and ozone. The existence of a third molecule in the gas decreases the intensity of the photoemission through collisional energy transfer [55]. This is "quenching" and the presence of O_2, CO_2 and H_2O may influence the measured NO concentration. To minimize quenching the chamber is maintained at a very low pressure through high resistance tubing. However, the use of high resistance tubing can cause a mass transport effect [55]. That is, the concentrations of individual gases may vary across the resistor because of viscosity differences. The use of a molybdenum reaction chamber, drying of gas prior to analysis and the efficient formation of ozone all decrease the quenching effect [54, 55].

NO Delivery Systems

Table 1 lists the various methods currently available for delivering NO via a mechanical ventilator. As you will note the methods employed to date fall into two general categories: Those in which NO is pre-mixed with oxygen and air, with the mixture of these three gases being delivered as the inspired tidal volume; those in which NO is injected into the inspiratory limb of the ventilator/airway circuit mixing with the tidal volume as gas is delivered.

Pre-mixing Systems

Generally two approaches can be used to pre-mix NO with O_2 and air, either prior to entry of gas into the ventilator itself or within the ventilator.

Internal Mixing: To date only one ventilator manufacturer has designed a ventilator with the capability of mixing NO with O_2 and air within the ventilator itself. The Servo 300 ventilator from Seimens has this capability [9, 56, 57]. In an *in vitro* evaluation using a lung model this system was able to deliver accurate and precise concentrations of NO without significant NO_2 production regardless of ventilator settings [56]. When the system was evaluated in an animal model similar results were observed, however concern was raised regarding monitoring of NO levels in the expiratory as opposed to the inspiratory limb of the system [57]. As a result of uptake of NO by the patient, expiratory limb monitoring may result in the delivery of higher than set NO levels.

Pre-mixing: Figure 4 illustrates the method we and others have used to deliver NO via a mechanical ventilator [8–19]. NO is pre-mixed by a standard air/O_2 blender with either N_2 or air and the mixture is delivered to the high pressure (or low pressure) air inlet of the ventilator. The precise concentration of NO delivered to the patient is determined by the actual setting of the blender and the setting of the delivered FiO_2. As shown in Fig. 5, Imanaka et al. [37] have shown that this approach to NO delivery results in a precise and constant concentration of delivered NO regardless of mode, waveform or patient interaction. However, this method of delivery is not without problems. Of major concern is the production of NO_2. As discussed earlier the higher the NO and O_2 concentrations, and the longer the time the gases are in contact, the greater the production of NO_2 [14]. Nishimura et al. [14] using the Puritan Bennett 7200 have shown that <2 ppm NO_2 is formed if N_2 is mixed with NO by the pre-mixing blender or if the NO concentration is <20 ppm when NO is pre-mixed with air. NO_2 formation is a bigger problem with the Servo 900 C during pre-mixing because of the large internal reservoir of the 900 C [14]. Although pre-mixing is possible with any ventilator, ventilators with large internal reservoirs present a marked problem with NO_2 production. In addition, because of the inaccuracies of standard blenders, careful monitoring of delivered NO is required especially at low NO levels where the blender inaccuracies are marked.

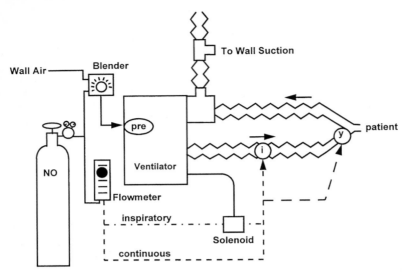

Fig. 4. Illustration of various approaches used to deliver NO during adult mechanical ventilation. Pre: Pre-mixing prior to entering the ventilator; i: injection (continuous or intermittent) into the inspiratory limb of the ventilator circuit; y: injection (continuous or intermittent) at the Y-piece of the ventilator circuit. (From [37] with permission)

Injection Systems

As illustrated in Fig. 4 and Table 2 a number of approaches to injection into the ventilator circuit or airway itself have been described. Essentially these systems inject continuously or intermittently into the inspiratory limb of the circuit or at the circuit Y-piece.

Continuous Injection into the Inspiratory Limb: This approach has been used by numerous groups [17–25]. Since NO is continuously injected, estimation of the mean inspired NO concentration can only be made based on the NO flow and minute ventilation [37].

$$\text{Desired [NO]} = \text{NO flow} \times \text{[NO] source}/\dot{V}_E \qquad (13)$$

However, as illustrated in Fig. 5, the peak NO concentration can markedly exceed the mean estimated level. Unfortunately this data would be unavailable to the researcher if a slow response analyzer were used or if an electrochemical analyzer were used. Only if measurements were made with a fast response chemiluminescence analyzer would the marked differences between estimated and actual delivered NO be obvious. These systems are of particular clinical concern for as shown by Tibballs et al. [17] in patients with a long expiratory time a significant volume of oxygen-lacking gas can accumulate in the inspiratory limb prior to a breath. As with all injection systems, tidal volume (V_T) may be increased and FiO_2 decreased. As a result this delivery method cannot be recommended [17].

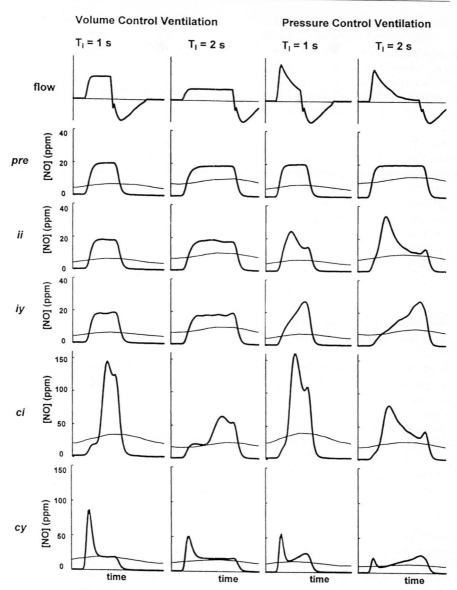

Fig. 5. Nitric oxide levels sampled at simulated mid-trachea in a lung model during volume controlled ventilation (VCV) and pressure controlled ventilation (PCV) with target NO concentration ([NO]) 20 ppm. Thick lines represent [NO] measured using a fast-response analyzer (NOA 280 Sievers Instruments, Boulder Co.) and thin lines represent [NO] measured using a slow-response analyzer (CLD 7000 AL_{MED}, ECO Physics, AG, Switzerland). Pre: pre-mixing of NO; ii: inspiratory injection into the inspiratory limb; iy: inspiratory injection at the circuit y-piece; ci: continuous injection into the inspiratory limb; cy: continuous injection at the circuit y-piece. Since the lung model establishes 100% NO uptake exhaled NO levels are zero. (From [37] with permission)

Continuous Injection at the Y-Piece: If NO is added continuously to the Y-piece of the circuit it does not accumulate during exhalation, but it is impossible to measure inhaled NO because of contamination with exhaled gas. As a result only the mean inhaled NO concentration can be calculated. However, as illustrated in Fig. 5 (with a system demonstrating 100% NO uptake) the actual delivered NO is much higher than calculated. Delivered V_T is normally increased and FiO_2 decreased. As a result this system cannot be recommended [26–28].

Inspiratory Phase Injection – Inspiratory Limb: With this approach NO is injected into the inspiratory limb only during the inspiratory phase. This has most commonly been accomplished with ventilator/nebulizer systems designed to activate only during inspiration. As noted in Fig. 5 during volume ventilation with a square wave flow pattern a constant and precise NO concentration can be delivered with this approach. However, this is not true with flow patterns that are not square (i.e., pressure control or volume control decelerating flow). With these patterns NO concentration increases toward the onset of the inspiratory phase, although the spikes in NO concentration are not as large as with continuous flow NO injection. As with all injection systems tidal volume (V_T) may be increased and FiO_2 decreased. NO_2 formation is not normally a problem with this approach.

Inspiratory Phase Injection – Circuit Y-Piece: Issues with this approach are the same as with injection into the inspiratory limb. A constant NO concentration can be delivered with constant flow ventilation but not during variable flow ventilation (Fig. 5). As discussed earlier, measurement of NO concentration is different because of contamination with exhaled gas. Problems of increased V_T and decreased FiO_2 are also present with this approach.

Tracheal Injection: Injection of NO into the trachea can be accomplished either intermittently or continuously and the problems with these approaches are similar to those with injection at the Y-piece. In addition, accumulation of a large volume of O_2 free gas in the lung can occur during continuous injection with prolonged expiratory phases.

FDA Regulations

In November 1996 the Food and Drug Administration (FDA) proposed that NO administration devices, NO analyzers, and NO_2 analyzers be classified as class II devices for purposes of regulation and identified a number of risks and special controls for NO administration apparatus. The specific risks include loss of NO, incorrect NO concentrations, ventilator malfunction, excessive NO_2 formation and catastrophic release of NO [44]. Table 4 lists the primary special controls required by the FDA.

Table 4. Special FDA controls required on nitric oxide (NO) delivery systems [44]

- NO gas analysis with alarms
- NO_2 gas analysis with alarms
- O_2 gas analysis with alarms
- NO cylinder pressure monitoring
- Reserve NO delivery system
- Battery back-up power
- Specifications and testing for accuracy and stability of NO delivery
- Specifications and testing of [NO] profile within a breath
- Identification of compatible ventilators and other gas delivery systems
- Testing and instruction for flushing NO_2 from the device

NO_2: nitrogen dioxide; [NO]: NO concentration

Commercially Available Systems

In addition to the NO delivery system available with the Servo 300, three other companies worldwide have developed NO delivery systems that may be used with mechanical ventilators: I-NOvent, Ohmeda Madison, WI; NOdomo, Dragerwerk, Germany; Pulmonox, Messer Griesheim, Austria. All three of these units inject NO into the inspiratory limb of the ventilator circuit in proportion to the inspiratory flow. The I-NOvent and the Pulmonox measure the inspiratory flow directly and inject NO in proportion to the measured flow. The NOdomo is designed for use only with Dräger ventilators and proportionally adjusts flow delivery based on data from the ventilator regarding delivered flow. As a result all three of these units should be able to deliver consistent and precise NO concentrations regardless of the gas flow pattern or the mode of ventilation. All three of these devices monitor NO and NO_2 with electrochemical analyzers and are alarmed. The level of NO available with each is primarily dependent on the NO concentration of the cylinder attached to the ventilator. Only the I-NOvent has been systemically evaluated and appears to provide a precise and consistent NO concentration [58].

Conclusion

The three commercially available NO delivery systems discussed above in general fit the description of an ideal NO delivery system. In order to avoid NO_2 formation, NO should be injected into the inspiratory limb of the ventilator circuit but in proportion to delivered flow regardless of waveform or mode and at a sufficient distance from the patient's airway to ensure appropriate gas mixing. Analysis of NO, NO_2 and O_2 with alarms must be available as well as secondary manual delivery systems with NO backup in the case of system failure. The system must limit NO_2 formation and not interfere with the function of the mechanical ventilator.

The knowledge gained over the last 7 years of experimental use of inhaled NO has allowed us now to design and develop systems that provide safe, consistent and accurate delivery of NO regardless of the ventilator or mode of ventilation.

References

1. Manktelow C, Bigatello LM, Hess D, Hurford WE (1997) Physiologic determinate of the response to inhaled nitric oxide in patients with acute respiratory distress syndrome. Anesthesiology 87:297–307
2. Roberts JD Jr, Fineman JR, Morin FC, et al (1997) Inhaled nitric oxide and persistent pulmonary hypertension of the newborn. The inhaled nitric oxide Study Group. N Engl J Med 336:605–610
3. Neonatal Inhaled Nitric Oxide Study Group (1997) Inhaled nitric oxide in full-term and nearly full-term infants with hypoxic respiratory failure. N Engl J Med 336:597–604
4. Chollet-Martin S, Gatecel C, Kermarrec N, Gougerot-Pocidalo MA, Payen DM (1996) Alveolar neutrophil functions and cytokine levels in patients with the adult respiratory distress syndrome during nitric oxide inhalation. Am J Respir Crit Care Med 153:985–990
5. Cheifetz IM, Craig DM, Kern FH, et al (1996) Nitric oxide improves transpulmonary vascular mechanics but does not change intrinsic right ventricular contractility in an acute respiratory distress syndrome model with permissive hypercapnia. Crit Care Med 24:1554–1561
6. Skimming JW, Bender KA, Hutchison AA, Drummond WH (1997) Nitric oxide inhalation in infants with respiratory distress syndrome. J Pediatr 130:225–230
7. Rossaint R, Gerlach H, Schmidt-Ruhnke H, et al (1995) Efficacy of inhaled nitric oxide in patients with severe ARDS. Chest 107:1107–1115
8. Gerlach H, Pappert D, Lewandowski K, Rossaint R, Falke KJ (1993) Long-term inhalation with evaluated low doses of nitric oxide for selective improvement of oxygenation in patients with adult respiratory distress syndrome. Intensive Care Med 19:443–449
9. Gerlach H, Rossaint R, Pappert D, Falke KJ (1993) Time-course and dose-response of nitric oxide inhalation for systemic oxygenation and pulmonary hypertension in patients with adult respiratory distress syndrome. Eur J Clin Invest 23:499–502
10. Channick RN, Newhart JW, Johnson FW, Moser KA (1994) Inhaled nitric oxide reverses hypoxic pulmonary vasoconstriction in dogs. A practical nitric oxide delivery and monitoring system. Chest 105:1842–1847
11. Bigatello LM, Hurford WE, Kacmarek RM, Roberts JD Jr, Zapol WM (1994) Prolonged inhalation of low concentrations of nitric oxide in patients with severe adult respiratory distress syndrome. Effects on pulmonary hemodynamics and oxygenation. Anesthesiology 80:761–770
12. Blomqvist H, Wickerts CJ, Andreen M, Ullberg U, Ortqvist A, Frostell C (1993) Enhanced pneumonia resolution by inhalation of nitric oxide? Acta Anaesthesiol Scand 37:110–114
13. McIntyre RC, Jr., Moore FA, Moore EE, Piedalue F, Haenel JS, Fullerton DA (1995) Inhaled nitric oxide variably improves oxygenation and pulmonary hypertension in patients with acute respiratory distress syndrome. J Trauma 39:418–425
14. Nishimura M, Hess D, Kacmarek RM, Ritz R, Hurford WE (1995) Nitrogen dioxide production during mechanical ventilation with nitric oxide in adults. Effects of ventilator internal volume, air versus nitrogen dilution, minute ventilation, and inspired oxygen fraction. Anesthesiology 82:1246–1254
15. Putensen C, Rasanen J, Thomson MS, Braman RS (1995) Method of delivering constant nitric oxide concentrations during full and partial ventilatory support. J Clin Monit 11:23–31
16. Wessel DL, Adatia I, Thompson JE, Hickey PR (1994) Delivery and monitoring of inhaled nitric oxide in patients with pulmonary hypertension. Crit Care Med 22:930–938
17. Tibballs J, Hochmann M, Carter B, Osborne A (1993) An appraisal of techniques for administration of gaseous nitric oxide. Anaesth Intensive Care 21:844–847
18. Stenqvist O, Kjelltoft B, Lundin S (1993) Evaluation of a new system for ventilatory administration of nitric oxide. Acta Anaesthesiol Scand 37:687–691
19. Lowson SM, Rich GF, McArdle PA, Jaidev J, Morris GN (1996) The response to varying concentrations of inhaled nitric oxide in patients with acute respiratory distress syndrome. Anesth Analg 82:574–581
20. Day RW, Guarin M, Lynch JM, Vernon DD, Dean JM (1996) Inhaled nitric oxide in children with severe lung disease: results of acute and prolonged therapy with two concentrations. Crit Care Med 24:215–221
21. Lu Q, Mourgeon E, Law-Koune JD, et al (1995) Dose-response curves of inhaled nitric oxide with and without intravenous almitrine in nitric oxide-responding patients with acute respiratory distress syndrome. Anesthesiology 83:929–943

22. Watkins DN, Jenkins IR, Rankin JM, Clarke GM (1993) Inhaled nitric oxide in severe acute respiratory failure-its use in intensive care and description of a delivery system. Anaesth Intensive Care 21:861–866
23. Young JD, Brampton WJ, Knighton JD, Finfer SR (1994) Inhaled nitric oxide in acute respiratory failure in adults. Br J Anaesth 73:499–502
24. Krafft P, Fridrich P, Fitzgerald RD, Koc D, Steltzer H (1996) Effectiveness of nitric oxide inhalation in septic ARDS. Chest 109:486–493
25. Samama CM, Diaby M, Fellahi JL, et al (1995) Inhibition of platelet aggregation by inhaled nitric oxide in patients with acute respiratory distress syndrome. Anesthesiology 83:56–65
26. Rich GF, Murphy GD Jr, Roos CM, Johns RA (1995) Inhaled nitric oxide. Selective pulmonary vasodilation in cardiac surgical patients. Anesthesiology 78:1028–1035
27. Levy B, Bollaert PE, Bauer P, Nace L, Audibert G, Larcan A (1995) Therapeutic optimization including inhaled nitric oxide in adult respiratory distress syndrome in a polyvalent intensive care unit. J Trauma 38:370–374
28. Wysocki M, Delclaux C, Roupie E, et al (1994) Additive effect on gas exchange of inhaled nitric oxide and intravenous almitrine bismesylate in the adult respiratory distress syndrome. Intensive Care Med 20:254–259
29. Puybasset L, Stewart T, Rouby JJ, et al (1994) Inhaled nitric oxide reverses the increase in pulmonary vascular resistance induced by permissive hypercapnia in patients with acute respiratory distress syndrome. Anesthesiology 80:1254–1267
30. Puybasset L, Rouby JJ, Mourgeon E, et al (1994) Inhaled nitric oxide in acute respiratory failure: dose response curves. Intensive Care Med 20:319–327
31. Puybasset L, Rouby JJ, Mourgeon E, et al (1995) Factors influencing cardiopulmonary effects of inhaled nitric oxide in acute respiratory failure. Am J Respir Crit Care Med 152:318–328
32. Rossaint R, Falke KJ, Lopez F, Slama K, Pison U, Zapol WM (1993) Inhaled nitric oxide for the adult respiratory distress syndrome. N Engl J Med 328:399–405
33. Abman SH, Griebel JL, Parker DK, Schmidt JM, Swanton D, Kinsella JP (1994) Acute effects of inhaled nitric oxide in children with severe hypoxemic respiratory failure. J Pediatr 124:881–888
34. Benzing A, Geiger K (1994) Inhaled nitric oxide lowers pulmonary capillary pressure and changes longitudinal distribution of pulmonary vascular resistance in patients with acute lung injury. Acta Anaesthesiol Scand 38:640–645
35. Young JD (1994) A universal nitric oxide delivery system. Br J Anaesth 73:700–702
36. Fierobe L, Brunet F, Dhainaut JF, et al (1995) Effect of inhaled nitric oxide on right ventricular function in adult respiratory distress syndrome. Am J Respir Crit Care Med 151:1414–1419
37. Imanaka H, Hess D, Kirmse M, et al (1997) Inaccuracies of nitric oxide delivery systems during adult mechanical ventilation. Anesthesiology 86:676–688
38. Austin AT (1967) The chemistry of the higher oxides of nitrogen as related to the manufacture, storage and administration of nitrous oxide. Br J Anaesth 39:345–350
39. NIOSH recommendations for occupational safety and health standards (1988) MMWR 37 (suppl 7):1–29
40. Bauer MA, Utell MJ, Morrow PE, et al (1986) Inhalation of 0.30 ppm nitrogen dioxide potentiates exercise-induced bronchospasm in asthmatics. Am Rev Respir Dis 134:1203–1205
41. Shiel FO (1967) Morbid anatomical changes in the lungs of dogs after inhalation of higher oxides of nitrogen during anaesthesia. Br J Anaesth 39:413–424
42. Glasson WA, Tuesday CS (1963) The atmospheric thermal oxidation of nitric oxide. J Am Chem Soc 85:2901–2904
43. Aida M, Miyamoto K, Saito S, et al (1995) Effects of temperature and humidity on the stability of nitric oxide, and efficiency of soda lime as a selective absorber of nitrogen dioxide. Nippon Kyobu Shikkan Gakkai Zasshi 33:306–309
44. Hess D, Ritz R, Branson RD (1997) Delivery systems for inhaled nitric oxide. Resp Care Clinics North Am 3:371–410
45. Purtz EP, Hess D, Kacmarek RM (1997) Evaluation of electrochemical nitric oxide and nitrogen dioxide analyzers suitable for use during mechanical ventilation. J Clin Monit 13:25–34
46. Nishimura M, Imanaka H, Uchiyama A, Tashiro C, Hess D, Kacmarek RM (1997) Nitric oxide (NO) measurement accuracy. J Clin Monit 13:241–248
47. Mercier JC, Zupan V, Dehan M, Renaudin MH, Bouchet M, Raveau C (1993) Device to monitor concentration of inhaled nitric oxide. Lancet 342:431–432

48. Petros AJ, Cox PB, Bohn D (1992) Simple method for monitoring concentration of inhaled nitric oxide. Lancet 340:1167
49. Petros AJ, Cox P, Bohn D (1994) A simple method for monitoring the concentration of inhaled nitric oxide. Anaesthesia 49:317–319
50. Etches PC, Harris ML, McKinley R, Finer NN (1995) Clinical monitoring of inhaled nitric oxide: comparison of chemiluminescent and electrochemical sensors. Biomed Instrum Technol 29:134–140
51. Moutalis M, Hatahet Z, Castelalti M, Renaudin M, Monnot A, Fiscider M (1995) Validation of a simple method assessing nitric oxide and nitrogen dioxide concentrations. Intensive Care Med 21:537–541
52. Betit P, Grenier B, Thompson J (1995) Evaluation of four nitric oxide therapy analyzers using known concentratons of nitrogen dioxide. Respir Care 40:1186 (Abst)
53. Betit P, Grenier B, Thompson J, Wessel DL (1996) Evaluation of four analyzers used to monitor inhaled nitric oxide therapy and nitrogen dioxide concentrations during inhaled nitric oxide administration. Resp Care 41:817–825
54. Matthews RD, Sawyer RF, Schefer RW (1977) Interferences in chemiluminescent measurement of NO and NO_2 emissions from combustion systems. Environ Sci Tech 11:1092–1096
55. Zabielski MF, Seery DJ, Dodge LG (1984) Influence of mass transport and quenching on nitric oxide chemiluminescent analysis. Environ Sci Tech 18:88–92
56. Lindberg L, Rydgren G, Larsson A, Olsson SG, Nordstrom L (1997) A delivery system for inhalation of nitric oxide evaluated with chemiluminescence, electrochemical fuel cells, and capnography. Crit Care Med 25:190–196
57. O'Hare B, Betit P, Thompson J (1997) In-vivo evaluation of a composite pediatric nitric oxide delivery monitoring system. Crit Care Med 25 (suppl 1):A54 (Abst)
58. Kirmse M, Hess D, Fujino Y, Kacmarek RM, Hurford WE (1998) Delivery of inhaled nitric oxide using the Ohmeda I-NOvent delivery system. Chest (In press)

Inspiratory NO Concentration Fluctuation During Inhalational NO Administration

M. Sydow, J. Zinserling, and S. J. Allen

Introduction

In the presence of pulmonary hypertension inhalation of nitric oxide (NO) in low concentrations produces selective pulmonary vasodilation without an effect on the systemic vasculature [1]. Inhaled NO is delivered predominantly to well ventilated lung areas. Thus, in lung diseases with severe mismatching of ventilation and perfusion (e.g., acute lung injury) pulmonary vasodilation occurs selectively in ventilated alveoli. This is in contrast to other vasodilators such as intravenous prostacyclin or nitroglycerin. Inhaled NO causes a redistribution of the pulmonary blood flow from non- or poorly ventilated areas to ventilated areas of the lung, and consequently improves oxygenation by a reduction of the intrapulmonary right-to-left shunt [2]. The selectivity of NO's effects are mainly caused by its short action of only a few seconds. NO binds quickly to hemoglobin which is then rapidly converted via nitrosyl Fe(II)-hemoglobin to methemoglobin. Owing to its attractive properties inhalational NO has been proposed as a therapeutic agent in many cardiopulmonary diseases. However, due to its potential chemical reactivity and toxicity the delivery of inhaled NO requires special equipment and techniques.

Impact of Accurate Delivery and Mixing of Inhaled NO

In high concentrations NO can cause methemoglobinemia, pulmonary injury, and death [3, 4, 5]. Therefore, precise control of the inspired NO concentration is essential. The conversion of NO into the toxic compound, nitrogen dioxide (NO_2), by exposure to oxygen is of particular interest during inhalational NO application [6, 7, 8]. As NO_2 production depends on NO and oxygen concentration as well as the duration of NO's exposure to oxygen, contact with oxygen in the ventilatory system must be minimized. Furthermore, NO has to be administered in an exact and constant dose because an inadvertently low dose might result in rebound hypoxemia and pulmonary hypertension [9, 10]. This limited therapeutic range of NO demands continuous and accurate monitoring. Exact analysis of the inspiratory NO concentration is even more important in dose finding studies. At present NO and NO_2 concentrations are usually measured during clinical use either by slow-response chemiluminescence or electrochemical analyzers. These analyzers usually have a response time of about 30–60 secs and display values which are time-weighted averages. Thus, NO concentration fluctuations during an individual breath will be missed with this method. Moreover, inspiratory NO concentration variation by inadequate gas mixing can affect the accuracy of slow response time chemiluminescence analyzers [11, 12, 13] and thus influence accurate monitoring (Table 1 and Fig. 1). As NO is stored and administered in 99.9% nitrogen the simplest solution to analyze

Table 1. Influence of the sampling site and mixing on NO values measured by slow response chemiluminescence. NO concentration values measured by slow response chemiluminescence at different sites of the breathing circuit (see Fig. 1) during NO administration with two different delivery systems (see text for explanations). Note that the measurement is markedly influenced by an overlapping effect of the sampling site with fluctuations of the concentration (i.e. with no added mixing volume). By better mixing of the inspired gas with a mixing chamber in the inspiratory circuit this effect is abolished. (Data adapted in part from [12] with permission)

NO delivery system	Sampling site (see Fig. 1)	Added mixing chamber	Ventilatory mode	
			Constant flow NO [ppm]	Decelerating flow NO [ppm]
Constant NO	1	0	43.5	32.3
flow into the	2	0	31.6	46.2
inspiratory limb	3	0	39.8	39.8
	1	3.2 L	40.8	40.3
	2	3.2 L	40.4	40.3
	3	3.2 L	40.2	40.3
Inspiratory NO	1	0	30.7	94.5
injection via	2	0	39.9	52.8
a medication	3	0	40.2	40.1
nebulizer				
(Servo 900c and	1	3.2 L	39.2	40.1
nebulizer)	2	3.2 L	39.8	39.9
	3	3.2 L	40.0	40.2

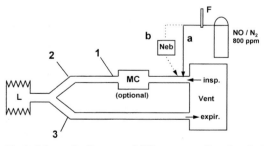

Fig. 1. Schematic diagram of different sampling sites for NO analysis during NO administration with two custom designed delivery systems: (**a**) constant NO flow into the inspiratory limb; (**b**) inspiratory NO injection via a medication nebulizer (neb) [Servo 900c and nebulizer]. The numbers indicate the various capillary positions of the chemiluminescence analyzer. (1) 102 cm after NO gas inlet; (2) 188 cm after NO gas inlet; (3) 22 cm after the Y-piece in the expiratory limb (after gas mixing in the test lung). An optional mixing chamber (MC) was installed directly before (1). L: lung; Vent: ventilator. (Adapted from [12] with permission)

inspiratory NO concentration fluctuation breath by breath is to monitor the carrier gas [13]. This can be performed either with a fast response nitrogen analyzer or a mass spectrometer.

Custom Designed NO Delivery Systems

Several different custom designed systems have been described to administer NO during mechanical ventilation. One of the simplest technical solutions is the addition of a continuous flow of NO into the inspiratory limb of the ventilator circuit [12, 14]. This system is inexpensive, easy to design and is applicable to all types of mechanical ventilator which may explain its widespread use, at least in the United Kingdom [13]. However, continuous NO injection into the inspiratory circuit during phasic flow mechanical ventilation results in considerable fluctuation of inspiratory NO concentration because NO accumulates in the inspiratory circuit during expiration [12] (Fig. 2). This is enhanced by both decelerating flow and increasing minute ventilation (Table 2). Moreover, the marked concentration fluctuation affects the accuracy of slow response NO analyzers (Table 1). The concentration fluctuation can be effectively decreased with the incorporation of progressively larger mixing chambers such that the addition of at least a 21 mixing chamber results in a relatively stable inspiratory NO concentration. However, such a system has several shortcomings. First, the influence of any additional breathing circuit volumes (e.g., mixing chamber) on the system compliance has to be taken into account. Compared to a setting with less volume, any additional circuit volume increases the compressible volume and may decrease lung ventilation. This delivery system provides constant mean NO concentrations for a given NO flow meter rate only if the minute ventilation is kept constant. Any change in minute ventilation requires adjustment of the

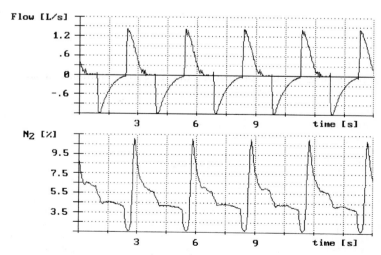

Fig. 2. Inspiratory N_2 concentration and gas flow during decelerating flow ventilation (Evita I (Dräger, Germany); minute ventilation 14 L/min; respiratory rate 20/min; FiO_2 1.0; NO 40 ppm)

Table 2. Fluctuation of inspiratory NOx (NO + NO$_2$) concentration during volume controlled and pressure controlled ventilation

Delivery	$\dot{V}_E$ system [l/min]	Ventilatory mode	Insp. peak flow [l/s]	NOx$_{Cl}$ [ppm]	NOx$_{max}$ [ppm]	NOx$_{min}$ [ppm]	NO$_2$ [ppm]
Continuous	14	VCV	0.71	43.0	97.9	22.2	3.3
NO flow	14	PCV	1.41	44.2	91.2	12.1	3.3
Inspiratory	12	VCV	0.42	29.5	41.9	11.4	5.1
injection via	12	PCV	1.58	30.1	66.2	16.5	5.2
nebulizer							
Servo 300	12	VCV	0.85	28.7	28.5	28.5	1.49
	12	PCV	1.74	28.2	28.0	28.0	1.18
NOdomo	12	VCV	0.62	29.8	31.8	27.8	1.67
	12	PCV	1.42	31.0	37.5	27.4	1.77
Pulmonox	12	VCV	0.61	30.6	31.1	29.2	1.2
mini	12	PCV	1.10	30.1	31.2	28.1	1.1

$\dot{V}_E$, minute ventilation; insp. peak flow, inspiratory peak flow; NOx$_{Cl}$, NOx (i.e., NO + NO$_2$) concentration measured by chemiluminescence in the test lung; NOx$_{max}$, maximal inspiratory NOx concentration calculated from N$_2$ as the carrier gas of NO; NOx$_{min}$, minimal inspiratory NOx concentration calculated from N$_2$; VCV, volume controlled ventilation (constant flow); PCV, pressure controlled ventilation (decelerating flow). Data on the continuous NO flow and the NOdomo system are adapted with permission from [12] and [23]; data on NO injection via medication nebulizer, the Servo 300 and Pulmonox mini system are unpublished data. Delivery systems are described in the text

NO flow into the circuit. Therefore, it can only be used during controlled ventilatory modes with a constant minute ventilation in a patient without spontaneous breathing activity. However, in pediatric ventilators which have a continuous gas flow round the circuit, continuous flow administration of NO into the inspiratory limb can successfully be used. Nevertheless, as the FiO$_2$ of the ventilator does not reflect the true inspiratory oxygen concentration in the circuit the additional installation of an external oxygen monitor is mandatory.

Another technique for phasic-flow ventilators is the injection of NO/N$_2$ into the inspiratory circuit via a medication nebulizer [2, 15]. As the ventilator allows the nebulizer to deliver gas flow only during inspiration, a phasic injection of NO is ensured. Such a system allows NO application close to the Y-piece which should minimize NO$_2$ formation by reduced contact time with O$_2$ in the inspiratory limb. However, this custom designed system has certain drawbacks. As the nebulizer is working with a constant gas flow this method theoretically provides a stable NO dose only in constant flow modes. Thus, during variable flow conditions (pressure controlled or pressure support ventilation) a stable NO dose cannot be provided and NO analysis by slow response chemiluminescence is markedly influenced by the concentration fluctuation (Table 1). However, even during constant flow ventilation a considerable fluctuation of the inspiratory NO concentration occurs (Table 2, unpublished data). If NO is directly administered at the Y-piece during inspiration, the concentration cannot be accurately monitored with slow-response analyzers because the measurements will be influenced by expiratory NO concentrations which are lower than inspiratory concentrations [16, 17]. As the nebulizer provides only one flow level the NO dose has to be readjusted after a change in the respiratory pattern. Thus an additional blender system is required before the nebulizer to adjust the NO source gas concentration. This system works only with a few ventilators that have nebulizers with separate gas delivery systems (e.g., Servo 900C or Bird 8400) and the ability to have them in use permanently during mechanical ventilation.

A custom-designed technique to provide stable NO delivery during various ventilatory modes is to inject NO into the high-pressure gas inlet of the ventilator which is actually reserved for room air [8, 18, 19]. The primary NO/N_2 concentration is first diluted with pure N_2 in a gas blender originally designed for mixing oxygen and air. The final NO concentration in the inspiratory circuit is controlled by the FiO_2 setting of the ventilator as well as by the concentration at the external blender. This system allows NO delivery in any ventilatory mode provided by the ventilator, independent of changes in minute ventilation or flow pattern. In controlled, as well as in spontaneous breathing modes with variable inspiratory flows stable NO concentration administration has been demonstrated by chemiluminescence [8,18]. However, changes in FiO_2 result in changes in the NO concentration [20]. This might be critical particularly in a situation when a sudden increase in the FiO_2 is necessary. Additionally, we recently demonstrated that even with this system NO concentration fluctuation occurs which can influence the accuracy of concentration measurements by slow-response chemiluminescence [12] (Fig. 3). Furthermore, because NO has corrosive properties and could damage some elastomeric ventilator components [21] this delivery technique may not be acceptable for long-term NO application.

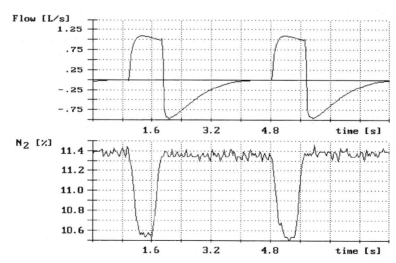

Fig. 3. Nitrogen (N_2) concentration and gas flow during constant flow ventilation (Bennett 7200a, Chula Vista, CA, USA), NO/N_2 inlet at the air high pressure connector as described in [8]. (From [12] with permission)

Commercially Developed Delivery Systems

An optimal NO delivery system should deliver a constant NO concentration during inspiration that is independent of changes in minute ventilation, inspiratory flow rate, and FiO_2. It should be equipped with a monitoring device which allows the setting of upper and lower alarm limits for NO and NO_2. Recently several manufacturers have developed different systems which are either inbuilt in a mechanical ventilator (e.g., Servo 300, Siemens-Elema, Sweden) [22], used as an "add-on" device (e.g., NOdomo, Dräger, Germany) [23] or designed as a "stand-alone" apparatus which can be connected to any mechanical ventilator (e.g., Pulmonox mini, Messer-Griesheim, Austria). Some of these systems are still prototypes and for investigational use only, while others are approved in several countries and are now available on the market.

One device that achieves optimal gas mixing is the Servo 300 system [22] (Table 2, unpublished data), where a third gas inlet enables controlled blending of NO with the basic gas mixture (i.e., air and oxygen). Thus, the chosen NO concentration is automatically adjusted to changes in flow and minute volume. As gas mixing is performed in the ventilator, NO is not just added to the air/oxygen mixture but is an integral part of the selected tidal volume. Furthermore, the O_2 concentration is monitored accurately by the oxygen analyzer of the ventilator. NO and NO_2 is monitored electrochemically in the expiratory limb of the circuit. Although the NO and NO_2 analysis is accurate in a lung model, this might be crucial in patients because NO and NO_2 uptake will result in differences between inspired and expired concentration [24, 25]. However, this delivery system is restricted to this mechanical ventilator.

Flow proportional administration of NO is performed with the Dräger NOdomo [23]. As this system is designed as an optional "add-on" apparatus, it is more flexible than the Servo system. However, this device can exclusively be used with the Evita or Babylog ventilator by the same manufacturer. The NO delivery module is driven by the analog inspiratory flow signal of the ventilator to provide an additional gas flow (i.e., NO/N_2) into the inspiratory limb of the breathing circuit proportional to the actual inspiratory flow. The gas flow of the NOdomo is controlled by a set of valves and orifices arranged in binary steps. Each gas flow level is related to a certain combination of open valves. The valve combinations are calculated from the source gas concentration, the desired NO concentration in the inspiratory gas and the inspiratory flow signal. The administration of NO into the circuit by an external module should result in a delayed delivery. This delay is caused by flow signal processing time and external valve response time. Consequently, the higher the initial inspiratory flow, the higher the resulting inspiratory volume portion without added NO. Moderate inspiratory NO concentration fluctuation can be demonstrated, which increases as inspiratory flow rates increase [23]. However, the mean inspiratory NO concentrations are stable and accurate regardless of the flow level and flow pattern. NO and NO_2 is monitored electrochemically in the inspiratory limb near the Y-piece. The monitoring is accurate during pressure and volume controlled, as well as during pressure support, ventilation. However, it can be slightly affected by the NO concentration fluctuation during an irregular gas flow pattern as occurs during airway pressure release ventilation.

The Pulmonox system uses a mass flow controller to administer NO proportionally to the inspiratory flow. The actual flow is measured independent of the ventilator by a separate pneumotachometer which is an integrated part of the device. Therefore this delivery device can be used with most mechanical ventilators and is more versatile than the others. Owing to the comparable technique, inspiratory NO concentration fluctuation is similar to the NOdomo (Table 2, unpublished data). However, since accurate administration of the chosen NO concentration depends on the precision of the calibration and the flow range of the pneumotachometer, the NO concentration has to be adapted according to the measured inspiratory values. NO and NO_2 are monitored electrochemically in the inspiratory limb with the same accuracy as the NOdomo system. In both systems NO is injected downstream of the oxygen monitoring of the ventilator. The O_2 concentration displayed on the ventilator differs from the final inspired O_2 concentration. Therefore, separate inspiratory O_2 monitoring is mandatory.

Conclusion

Although stable inspiratory NO concentration delivery is recommended [20, 26], it is unknown whether physiologically significant effects occur if the inspiratory NO concentration fluctuates. However, inspiratory NO concentration fluctuations should be avoided for the following reasons. Due to ventilation inequalities inspiratory NO concentration fluctuation might cause different alveolar NO concentrations and possibly result in increased local NO_2 production if the alveolar NO concentration is high. Moreover, it has been demonstrated that NO concentration fluctuation results in differences in the measured NO concentration by slow response time analyzers at various sampling sites in the breathing circuit [11, 12]. This occurred although the mean inspiratory NO concentration calculated by the measured nitrogen concentration was identical to the chemiluminescence values which represent mean concentrations. These concerns support the recommendation for stable inspiratory NO delivery.

References

1. Frostell C, Fratacci MD, Wain JC, Jones R, Zapol WM (1991) Inhaled nitric oxide. A selective pulmonary vasodilator reversing hypoxic pulmonary vasoconstriction. Circulation 83:2038–2047
2. Roissant R, Falke KJ, Lopez F, Slama K, Pison U, Zapol WM (1993) Inhaled nitric oxide for the adult respiratory distress syndrome. N Engl J Med 328:399–405
3. Austin A (1967) The chemistry of higher oxides of nitrogen as related to the manufacture, storage and administration of nitrous oxide. Br J Anaesth 39:345–350
4. Clutton-Brock J (1967) Two cases of poisoning by contamination of nitrous oxide with higher oxides of nitrogen during anaesthesia. Br J Anaesth 39:388–392
5. Stavert DM, Lehnert BE (1990) Nitric oxide and nitrogen dioxide as inducers of acute pulmonary injury when inhaled at relatively high concentrations for brief periods. Inhal Toxicol 2:53–67
6. Meyer M, Piper J (1989) Nitric oxide, a new test gas for study of alveolar-capillary diffusion. Eur Respir J 2:494–496
7. Guidotti TL (1978) The higher oxides of nitrogen. Environ Res 15:443–473

8. Nishimura M, Hess D, Kacmarek RM, Ritz R, Hurford WE (1995) Nitrogen dioxide production during mechanical ventilation with nitric oxide in adults. Anesthesiology 82:1246–1254
9. Petros AJ (1994) Down-regulation of endogenous nitric oxide production after prolonged administration. Lancet 344:191–198
10. Grover R, Murdoch I, Smithies M, Mitchell I, Bihari D (1992) Nitric oxide during hand ventilation in patient with acute respiratory failure. Lancet 340:1038–1039
11. Betit P, Adatia I, Benjamin P, Thompson JE, Wessel DL (1995) Inhaled nitric oxide: Evaluation of a continuous titration delivery technique for infant mechanical and manual ventilation. Resp Care 40:706–715
12. Sydow M, Bristow F, Zinserling J, Allen SJ (1997) Variation of nitric oxide concentration during inspiration. Crit Care Med 25:365–371
13. Young JD, Dyar OJ (1996) Delivery and monitoring of inhaled nitric oxide. Intensive Care Med 22:77–86
14. Watkins DN, Jenkins IR, Rankin JM, Clarke GM (1993) Inhaled niric oxide in severe respiratory failure – its use in intensive care and description of a delivery system. Anaesth Intensive Care 21:861–875
15. Puybasset L, Stewart T, Rouby, et al (1994) Inhaled nitric oxide reverses the increase in pulmonary vascular resistance induced by permissive hypercapnia in patients with adult respiratory distress syndrome. Anesthesiology 80:1254–1267
16. Lu Q, Mourgeon E, Law-Koune JD, et al (1995) Dose-response curves of inhaled nitric oxide with and without intravenous almitrine in nitric oxide-responding patients with acute respiratory distress syndrome. Anesthesiology 83:929–943
17. Stenquist O, Nathorst-Westfelt, Lundin S (1995) Pulmonary uptake of inhaled nitric oxide. Brit J Anaesth 74 (suppl 1):S123 (Abst)
18. Putensen C, Räsänen J, Thomsen MS, Braman RS (1995) Method of delivering constant nitric oxide concentrations during full and partial ventilatory support. J Clin Monit 11:23–31
19. Wessel DL, Adatia J, Thompson JE, Hickey PR (1994) Delivery and monitoring of inhaled nitric oxide in patients with pulmonary hypertension. Crit Care Med 22:930–938
20. Hess D, Kacmarek RM, Ritz R, Bigatello LM, Hurford WE (1995) Inhaled nitric oxide delivery systems: A role for respiratory therapists. Resp Care 40:702–705
21. Kain ML (1967) Higher oxides of nitrogen in anaesthetic circuits. Br J Anaesth 39:382–387
22. Lindberg L, Rydgren G, Larsson A, Olsson SG, Nordstrom L (1997) A delivery system for inhalation of nitric oxide evaluated with chemiluminescence, electrochemical fuel cells, and capnography. Crit Care Med 25:190–196
23. Sydow M, Bristow F, Zinserling J, Allen SJ (1997) Flow proportional administration of nitric oxide with a new delivery system: Inspiratory NO concentration fluctuation during different flow conditions. Chest 112:496-504
24. Borland DC, Higenbottom TW (1989) A simultaneous single breath measurement of pulmonary diffusing capacity with nitric oxide and carbon monoxide. Eur Respir J 2:56–63
25. Overton JH, Miller FJ (1988) Absorption of inhaled reactive gases. In: Gardner DE, Crapo JD, Massaro EJ (eds) Toxicology of the lung. Raven Press, New York, pp 47–507
26. Skimming JW, Cassin S, Blanch PB (1995) Nitric oxide administration using constant-flow ventilation. Chest 108:1065–1072

Effects of Inhaled Nitric Oxide on Circulating Blood Cells

C. Adrie and A. T. Dinh-Xuan

Introduction

Endothelium-derived relaxing factor (EDRF), an endogenous vasodilator released from vascular endothelium, was identified as nitric oxide (NO) in 1987 [1]. Subsequent studies have demonstrated that exogenous nitrosovasodilators such as nitroglycerin or sodium nitroprusside dilate vascular smooth muscle (VSM) through the release of NO (or a closely related substance) which readily crosses the underlying cell membrane. The resulting activation of VSM soluble guanylate cyclase increases intracellular levels of the second messenger guanosine 3',5'-cyclic monophosphate (cGMP). As NO is rapidly bound to, and therefore inactivated by oxyhemoglobin, most of the biological effects of NO occur in the vicinity of its sites of release [2,3]. This explains why inhaled NO causes selective pulmonary vasodilation and hence its therapeutic use in primary pulmonary hypertension and acute respiratory distress syndrome (ARDS) [4–6]. Because inhaled NO preferentially diffuses to well ventilated alveoli, it also improves ventilation-perfusion matching by diverting blood flow from poorly ventilated to well ventilated lung areas contrasting with the deleterious effect of intravenous vasodilators on gas exchange (such as NO donors or prostacyclin) [6].

In vitro studies suggest that the antiplatelet effect of NO is mediated by activation of intraplatelet soluble guanylate cyclase and the resulting increase of platelet cGMP. The latter stimulates cGMP-dependent protein kinase which, through a complex phosphorylation reaction, reduces intracellular calcium-ion concentration. This, in turn, inhibits fibrinogen binding to the glycoprotein IIb/IIIa receptor on the surface of the platelet membrane, which is required for platelet aggregation [7].

Despite the rapid inactivation of inhaled NO by oxyhemoglobin, and a high selectivity for the pulmonary vascular system, recent data suggest that inhaled NO also exerts systemic effects through its action on platelets, red and white blood cells (Table 1).

Inhaled NO and Platelets

A slight prolongation of bleeding time has been observed in rabbits and in normal humans breathing NO, suggesting that inhaled NO can alter platelet transit in the pulmonary circulation [8, 9]. Inhibition of platelet aggregation was also observed during the administration of inhaled NO in patients with ARDS [10]. After random

Table 1. Putative effects of inhaled nitric oxide (NO) on circulating blood cells

	Biological activity	Molecular targets	Authors [ref.]
Red blood cells	NO inactivation by hemoglobin	Heme moiety	Gibson et al. [2]
	Endocrine effect	SH-cysteine β93 of hemoglobin β subunit	Jia et al. [30]
Polymorpho-nuclear cells	Modulator of leukocyte adherence	Soluble guanylate cyclase	Kubes et al. [27]
	Inhibition of oxidative burst		Chollet-Martin et al. [29]
Platelets	Inhibition of platelet adhesion and aggregation	Soluble guanylate cyclase	Radomski et al. [7]
	Disaggregation of aggregated platelets		Samama et al. [10]

administration of inhaled NO (1 to 100 ppm), *ex vivo* platelet aggregation induced by adenosine diphosphate, collagen, and ristocetin was decreased with a maximal effect at 3 ppm. This was, however, not followed by any effect on bleeding time. This inhibitory effect of NO is supported by experimental studies in pigs showing that inhaled NO decreased platelet sequestration in the lungs during extracorporeal circulation [14]. Platelet inhibition induced by inhaled NO may be deleterious due to a higher risk of bleeding. This particularly applies to patients with pre-existing coagulation disorders such as disseminated intravascular coagulation (DIC) or thrombocytopenia. On the other hand, platelet inhibition induced by NO may be beneficial as it might alleviate both the early and late stage pulmonary hypertensive response seen in ARDS [12]. The early vasoconstriction, responsive to vasodilators, has been attributed to platelet and leukocyte aggregation and the subsequent release of vasoconstrictors such as thromboxane A_2, endoperoxides, leukotrienes and vasoactive prostaglandins. The sustained increase in pulmonary vascular resistance during the later stages of ARDS, unresponsive to vasodilators, probably results from mechanical obstruction of pulmonary vessels by thrombi [12]. It can be assumed therefore that inhaled NO, by preventing platelet aggregation and thrombi formation in the pulmonary circulation, may at least in part prevent the pulmonary hypertension during both early and late stages of ARDS.

The effect of inhaled NO in experimental pulmonary embolism has been investigated recently in pigs [13]. Pulmonary embolism was induced by stepwise injection of 300 µm microspheres until mean pulmonary arterial pressure increased to 45 mmHg. In this setting, inhaled NO significantly decreased pulmonary artery pressure and inhibited platelet aggregation. Platelet activation may also play a pivotal role in the pathogenesis of pulmonary hypertension and hypoxemia during acute massive pulmonary embolism. For example, platelet activation may aggravate right ventricular afterload and cardiac ischemia, and eventually contribute to right ventricular failure. Inhaled NO inhibits platelet activation and prevents the subsequent release of vasoactive substances, thus reducing the pulmonary hypertension associated with mechanical obstruction caused by pulmonary emboli.

Platelets contribute to normal hemostasis by adhering to the damaged subendo-thelial surfaces of blood vessels, and amassing additional platelets at the site through platelet interactions. This event can lead to, or enhance, activation of the coagulation cascade, resulting in the deposition of fibrin. In disease, thrombogenic surfaces such as ruptured atherosclerotic plaques act as the initial site of platelet deposition. If the subsequent platelet aggregation is unchecked, larger aggregates can develop, result-ing in distal embolization of platelet-fibrin thrombi and occluding vessels. There-fore the use of antiplatelet agents has become increasingly important in the treat-ment of coronary ischemic disease [15]. The antithrombic effect of inhaled NO has prompted its use as a therapeutic drug in different cardiovascular disorders. Chro-nic inhalation of low concentrations of NO gas has been shown to inhibit neointimal formation after balloon-induced arterial injury in rats [16]. Breathing 80 ppm NO decreased neointimal formation one and two weeks after carotid injury. This effect is thought to be mediated by platelet inhibition. However, there was no prolongation of the tail-transection bleeding time which reflects both platelet and coagulation function. Moreover, inhaled NO at concentrations of 20 and 80 ppm increased coro-nary patency and decreased cyclic flow variation frequency in a canine model of pla-telet-mediated coronary reocclusion observed after thrombosis and thrombolysis [17]. This effect was, not associated with any decrease in systemic blood pressure unlike intravenous NO donors that are known to induce systemic vasodilatation at the doses used to inhibit platelet activation [18–20]. This lack of antithrombotic effect of high dose (200 ppm) inhaled NO may be explained by the formation of peroxynitrite ($ONOO^-$) and the pro-aggregatory effect of the latter on human pla-telets.

This effect may last well beyond the expected half-life of NO in biological fluids [21] since the increase in coronary artery patency was sustained for at least 45 minutes after discontinuation of NO (80 ppm) [17]. Furthermore, the inhibition of platelet aggregation observed *ex vivo* needed at least 20 minute preparation time to obtain the final plasma rich platelet [10, 13].

A modest effect of inhaled NO on bleeding time was observed by some [8, 9] but not all authors [10, 16, 17]. The clinical value of bleeding time is still controversial as this test is neither sensitive nor specific for predicting the risk of bleeding [11].

Inhaled NO and White Blood Cells

Although there is some evidence to suggest that tissue injury can occur even with neutropenia, neutrophils are probably key cells in causing tissue injury and organ dysfunction in systemic inflammatory response syndrome (SIRS), ARDS, and multi-ple organ dysfunction syndrome (MODS). Neutrophils release a wide variety of mediators such as enzymes (protease, elastase, etc.), oxygen metabolites, bioactive lipids, and cytokines that induce lung injury [25, 26]. A few years ago, Kubes et al. [27] showed that endothelium-derived NO is an important endogenous modulator of leukocyte adherence which may be related to its ability to inactivate the super-oxide anion [28].

NO inhalation has been shown to have potential beneficial effects by attenuating the polymorphonuclear neutrophil (PMN) oxidative burst and adhesion as well as cytokine release (IL-6, IL-8) within the alveolar space of the lungs in patients with ARDS [29]. Moreover inhaled NO can alter PMN activation within the pulmonary circulation when administered to neonates and infants with pulmonary hypertension [22]. Neutrophil respiratory burst has been evaluated by assessing superoxide anion production after neutrophil priming with *Escherichia coli* or with N-formyl-methionyl-leucyl-phenylalanine (fMLP). Superoxide anion production was determined by a flow cytometric method using dihydrorhodamine (DHR)-123 as an oxidative probe and results were expressed as mean relative fluorescence intensity (mRFI). Respiratory burst was decreased after more than 24 h of NO inhalation, an effect which lasted up to 96 h after the end of NO inhalation.

Bloomfield et al. [23] studied the effect of the administration of NO gas in a porcine model of ARDS induced by Gram-negative sepsis. Septic animals treated with inhaled NO exhibited no significant increase in bronchoalveolar lavage content and no increase in neutrophil transendothelial migration as compared with untreated septic animals. Furthermore, breathing 20 ppm NO significantly attenuated the increase of CD18 expression observed in septic animals not receiving NO gas. Pretreatment with inhaled NO may therefore attenuate acute lung injury associated with Gram-negative sepsis by disrupting events associated with neutrophil migration and/or neutrophil respiratory burst.

However, the inhibitory effect of inhaled NO on neutrophils is like a two edged sword: On the one hand, impairment of neutrophil function may weaken the host defense mechanism as suspected in other experimental models [24]; however, such impairment is likely to be beneficial in SIRS, ARDS or MODS as these disorders are thought to be adversely affected by leukocyte activation.

Inhaled NO and Red Blood Cells

Until recently, oxyhemoglobin was thought to be only a scavenger of NO explaining the restriction of the effects of inhaled NO to the pulmonary circulation [1–4]. This concept has been questioned by Jia et al. [30] showing that hemoglobin may in some cases carry NO and release it in the peripheral blood stream with a potential role as a blood pressure regulator [31, 32].

Earlier studies done by Stamler's group investigated compounds such as S-nitrosothiols, or RSNOs, as observed with the serum albumin (33). These compounds may act as a reservoir and carrier of NO and may play a role as regulator for the maintenance of vascular tone [33–35]. RSNOs form in the body when oxidized NO reacts with the highly reactive thiol group on the amino acid cysteine. Cysteines are widely distributed on proteins, including serum albumin and hemoglobin which has a pair of cysteinyl residues (Cysβ93).

NO in any form is expected to rapidly react with oxygenated heme groups, which inactivate NO, thus leaving a positive charge on the hemoglobin. However after incubating hemoglobin in a bath of RSNOs, these compounds rapidly react with the hemoglobin's cysteine, forming SNO-hemoglobin [32]. Thus the free RSNOs are able to transfer NO groups to cysteine without reacting with the hemes. Erythrocyte access of RSNOs is thiol group specific; exposure of oxygenated red blood cells to NO produces mainly methemoglobin. Hemoglobin gives up its oxygen and mops up carbon dioxide when, upon reaching oxygen-poor tissues, it undergoes an allosteric change that reduces its affinity for oxygen. The same conformational change of this protein also releases RSNO. The reverse effect takes place in the lungs, enabling hemoglobin to take on RSNO at the same time as it binds oxygen and releases carbon dioxide [31, 32].

It seems reasonable to think that inhaled NO may induce the formation of such compounds as RSNOs which secondarily act with hemoglobin to form SNO-hemoglobin. This hypothesis is strengthened by a recent report showing an increased oxygen affinity of sickle erythrocytes in patients breathing 80 ppm NO without significant methemoglobin production [36]. This supports the hypothesis that NO gas is able to react with the amino-acid cysteine of the hemoglobin S.

Conclusion

The effect of inhaled NO on circulating platelets is well established. Many studies show an inhibition of platelet activity when breathing NO, which could be deleterious in patients with pre-existing coagulation disorders, but could also be beneficial in patients with coronary artery disease. Data on the effects of inhaled NO on red and white blood cells are still sparse. They suggest, however that both cell types may critically affect both the physiology and the pharmacology of inhaled NO. Further studies are certainly needed to investigate these hypotheses.

References

1. Palmer RMJ, Ferige AG, Moncada S (1991) Nitric oxide release accounts for the biological activity of endothelium-derived relaxing factor. Nature 327:524–526
2. Gibson QH, Roughton FJM (1957) The kinetics and equilibria of the reactions of nitric oxide with sheep haemoglobin. J Physiol 136:507–526
3. Rimar S, Gillis N (1993) Selective pulmonary vasodilation by inhaled nitric oxide is due to hemoglobin inactivation. Circulation 88:2884–2887
4. Frostell C, Fratacci M-D, Wain JC, Jones R, Zapol WM (1991) Inhaled nitric oxide: A selective pulmonary vasodilator reversing hypoxic pulmonary vasoconstriction. Circulation 83:2038–2047
5. Pepke-Zaba J, Higenbottam TW, Dinh-Xuan AT, Stone D, Wallwork J (1991) Inhaled nitric oxide as a cause of selective vasodilatation in pulmonary hypertension. Lancet 338:1173–1174
6. Rossaint R, Falke K, Lopez F, Slama K, Pison U, Zapol WM (1993) Inhaled nitric oxide for the adult respiratory distress syndrome. N Engl J Med 328:399–405
7. Radomski MW, Moncada S (1993) Regulation of vascular hemostasis by nitric oxide. Thromb Haemost 70:36–41
8. Högman M, Frostell C, Arnberg H, Sandhagen B, Hedenstierna G (1993) Bleeding time prolongation and nitric oxide inhalation. Lancet 341:1664–1665
9. Högman M, Frostell C, Arnberg H, Sandhagen B, Hedenstierna G (1994) Prolonged bleeding time during nitric oxide inhalation in the rabbit. Acta Physiol Scand 151:125–129
10. Samama CM, Diabi M, Fellahi J-L, et al (1995) Inhibition of platelet aggregation by inhaled nitric oxide in patient with acute respiratory distress syndrome. Anesthesiology 83:56–65
11. Rodgers C, Levin J (1990) A critical reappraisal of the bleeding time. Semin Thromb Hemost 16:1–20
12. Heffner JE, Sahn SA, Repine JE (1987) The role of platelets in the adult respiratory distress syndrome: culprit or bystanders? Am Rev Respir Dis 135:482–492

13. Gries A, Bottiger BW, Dorsam J, et al (1997) Inhaled nitric oxide inhibits platelet aggregation after pulmonary embolism in pigs. Anesthesiology 86:387–393

14. Malmros C, Blomquist S, Dahm P, Martensson L, Thorne J (1996) Nitric oxide inhalation decreases pulmonary platelet and neutrophil sequestration during extracorporeal circulation in the pig. Crit Care Med 24:845–849

15. Stein B, Fuster V, Israel DH, et al (1989) Platelet inhibitor agents in cardiovascular disease: an update. J Am Coll Cardiol 14:813–836

16. Lee JS, Adrie C, Jacob HJ, Roberts JD, Zapol WM, Bloch KD (1996) Chronic inhalation of nitric oxide inhibits neointimal formation after balloon-induced arterial injury. Circ Res 78:337–342

17. Adrie C, Bloch KD, Moreno PR, et al (1996) Inhaled nitric oxide increases coronary artery patency after thrombolysis. Circulation 94:1919–1926

18. Loscalzo J (1992) Antiplatelet and antithrombotic effects of organic nitrates. Am J Cardiol 70:18B–22B

19. Folts JD, Stamler J, Loscalzo J (1991) Intravenous nitroglycerin infusion inhibits cyclic blood flow responses caused by periodic platelet thrombus formation in stenosed canine coronary arteries. Circulation 83:2122–2127

20. Rovin JD, Stamler J, Loscalzo J, Folts JD (1993) Sodium nitroprusside, an endothelium derived relaxing factor congener, increases platelet cyclic GMP levels and inhibits epinephrine-exacerbated in vivo platelet thrombus formation in stenosed canine coronary arteries. J Cardiovasc Pharmacol 22:626–631

21. Ignarro LJ (1989) Biological actions and properties of endothelium-derived nitric oxide formed and released from artery and vein. Circ Res 65:1–21

22. Gessler P, Nebe T, Birle A, Mueller W, Kachel W (1996) A new side effect of inhaled nitric oxide in neonates and infants with pulmonary hypertension: functional impairment of the neutrophil respiratory burst. Intensive Care Med 22:252–258

23. Bloomfield GL, Holloway S, Ridings PC, et al (1997) Pretreatment with inhaled nitric oxide inhibits neutrophil migration and oxidative activity resulting in attenuated sepsis-induced acute lung injury. Crit Care Med 25:584–593

24. Eichacker PQ (1997) Inhaled nitric oxide in adult respiratory distress syndrome: Do we know the risks versus benefits? Crit Care Med 25:563–565

25. Fujishima S, Aikawa N (1995) Neutrophil-mediated tissue injury and its modulation. Intensive Care Med 21:277–285

26. Weiss SJ (1989) Tissue destruction by neutrophils. N Engl J Med 320:365–376

27. Kubes P, Suzuki M, Granger DN (1991) Nitric oxide: An endogenous modulator of leukocyte adhesion. Proc Natl Acad Sci USA 88:4651–4655

28. Gaboury J, Woodman RC, Granger DN, Reinhardt P, Kubes P (1993) Nitric oxide prevents leukocyte adherence: role of superoxide. Am J Physiol 265:H862–H867

29. Chollet-Martin S, Gatecel C, Kermarrec N, Gougerot-Pocidalo MA, Payen DM (1996) Alveolar neutrophil functions and cytokine levels in patients with the adult respiratory distress syndrome during nitric oxide inhalation. Am J Respir Crit Care Med 153:985–990

30. Jia L, Bonaventura C, Bonaventura J, Stamler JS (1996) S-nitrosohaemoglobin: a dynamic activity of blood involved in vascular control. Nature 380:221–226

31. Glanz J (1996) Hemoglobin reveals new role as blood pressure regulator. Science 271:1670–1674

32. Stamler JS, Jia LJ, Eu JP, et al (1997) Blood flow regulation by S-nitrosohemoglobin in the physiological oxygen gradient. Science 276:2034–2037

33. Stamler JS, Jaraki O, Osborne J, et al (1992) Nitric oxide circulates in mammalian plasma primarily as an S-nitroso adduct of serum albumin. Proc Natl Acad Sci USA 89:7674–7677

34. Sharfstein JS, Keaney JF, Slivka A, et al (1994) In vivo transfer of nitric oxide between a plasma protein-bound reservoir and low molecular and low molecular weight thiols. J Clin Invest 94:1432–1439

35. Keaney JF, Simon DI, Stamler JS, et al (1993) NO forms adduct with serum albumin that has endothelium-derived relaxing factor-like properties. J Clin Invest 91:1582–1589

36. Head CA, Brugnara C, Martinez-Ruiz R, et al (1997) Low concentrations of nitric oxide increase oxygen affinity of sickle hemoglobin in vitro and in vivo. J Clin Invest 100:1193–1198

Acid-Base – Lactate Metabolism

Recent Advances in Acid-Base Physiology Applied to Critical Care

J. A. Kellum

Introduction

Unlike most other aspects of critical care medicine, the management of metabolic dysfunction has not seen any major innovations in many years. Although acid-base imbalance is as integral an aspect of sepsis or severe trauma as hemodynamic instability or acute lung injury, the management of acidosis and alkalosis has not evolved as other areas have. There are no analogies in acid-base to norepinephrine and pressure controlled ventilation. However, what is perhaps even more disturbing, and what is, no doubt, behind this stagnation, is that our understanding of the pathophysiology of acid-base disturbances has also failed to keep pace with the advancements in other areas of critical care.

Yet, the field has not been completely barren of new thought. It has, regrettably, been slow to appreciate what few innovations have occurred. Little more than 15 years ago Peter Stewart published his revolutionary physical chemical analysis of acid-base physiology [1, 2]. Although originally praised [3], the revolution it was to have started has been slow in coming. Indeed, there has been relatively little interest in this approach until quite recently [4–12]. It would seem that the disinterest was due mainly to the fact that the approach, while conceptually simple and elegant, is operationally complicated and unwieldy. Most clinicians retreat from the sight of complex polynomial equations and few can be easily convinced that "relearning" acid-base physiology is worth while when the traditional approach works so well.

It is this last issue that deserves closer scrutiny, particularly in the critically ill. For patients in the intensive care unit (ICU), extreme derangements in physiology are common and traditional methods are often inadequate to explain the severe acid-base disorders present in some of these patients. Although there are at least three valid approaches to acid-base physiology (base excess, the "bicarbonate" approach and the Stewart approach), these approaches are vastly different. Indeed, all three have merit and utility. However, both base excess and the bicarbonate approach are essentially phenomenologic, while the Stewart approach is actually mechanistic. Put another way, only the Stewart approach starts with the accepted principles of physical chemistry and then predicts the resulting physiology. The other two methods are simply mathematical manipulations of measured variables. Neither the base excess nor the bicarbonate can tell us how a disturbance came about, only that it exists and to what degree.

Though "newer", the Stewart approach has now been validated in a wide variety of patient types [6, 7, 10, 11] and experimental conditions [5, 12–15]. With the assistance of a personal computer or even a programmable calculator, one can easily discern that the equations are correct and will yield the same results as using base excess or the traditional six equations [9, 15]. So then, if this "new" approach yields the same results as traditional approaches why should it be used? Clearly, base excess is faster and easier [9, 16] and besides "everyone understands it". Of course, these were the same arguments facing Copernicus when he declared that the Earth was not the center of the universe. Prior to this knowledge it was still quite possible to "understand" the universe and it is very unlikely that the life of the average person living in those times was altered in any way by this understanding [17]. The understanding that bicarbonate (HCO_3^-) and hydrogen ions (H^+) are not at the center of the acid-base universe produces as violent a change in our concepts of physiology as did Copernicus change our concepts of astronomy.

In this review, I will explain the fundamental aspects of the Stewart approach, review the implications for clinical medicine, particularly in the ICU, and consider some of the more practical aspects of acid-base management from this perspective. Several more detailed treatments of the Stewart approach are available in the literature [1, 2, 4, 8, 18]; the purpose of this discussion is to provide the reader with a general understanding of the approach and its implications. However, the interested reader is advised to seek out these other sources as well.

Fundamental Principles of Hydrogen Ion Regulation

Large living organisms seek to maintain plasma pH within strict tolerance limits. In fact, H^+ concentration ($[H^+]$) is maintained within the nmol/L range (36–43 nmol/L). By contrast, most other ions are regulated in the mmol/L range. One reason $[H^+]$ is so closely regulated is that these ions have very high charge densities and consequently very large electric fields, and the strength of H^+ bonds (ubiquitous in biologic systems) are very sensitive to local $[H^+]$. Biochemical reactions as well as interactions of hormones and drugs with plasma proteins and cell surface receptors are also influenced by changes in $[H^+]$. In addition, fluctuations in intracellular $[H^+]$ have major effects on cellular performance presumably by altering protein charge, thereby affecting structure and enzymatic function. Obviously then, in order to understand how the body regulates plasma $[H^+]$, we must first understand the physical chemical determinants of $[H^+]$.

Biochemistry of Aqueous Solutions

Virtually all solutions in human biology contain water, and aqueous solutions provide a virtually inexhaustible source of H^+. In these solutions, $[H^+]$ is determined by the dissociation of water into H^+ and OH^- ions. Put another way, changes in $[H^+]$ occur not as a result of how much H^+ is added or removed but as a consequence of water dissociation. What then determines the dissociation of water? Answer: the laws of physical chemistry. Two in particular apply here: Electroneutrality (which dictates that, in aqueous solutions, the sum of all positively charged ions must equal the sum of all negatively charged ions); and conservation of mass (which means that the amount of a substance remains constant unless it is added or generated, or removed or destroyed). In pure water, according to the principle of electroneutrality, the concentration of H^+ must always equal the concentration of OH^-. In more complex solutions, we have to consider other determinants of water dissociation, but still, the source of H^+ remains water. Fortunately, even in a solution as complex as blood plasma, the determinants of $[H^+]$ can be reduced to three. If we know the value of these three determinants, the $[H^+]$ can be predicted under any condition. These three determinants are the strong ion difference (SID), pCO_2, and total weak acid concentration (A_{TOT}).

SID, pCO_2 and A_{TOT}

The SID is the net charge balance of all strong ions present, where a "strong" ion is one that is completely (or near completely) dissociated. For practical purposes this means $(Na^+ + K^+ + Ca^{++} + Mg^{++}) \cdot (Cl^- + lactate)$. This is often referred to as the "apparent" SID (SIDa) with the understanding that some "unmeasured" ions might also be present [5]. In healthy humans, this value is 40–42 mEq/L, though it is often quite different in critically ill patients. Of note, neither H^+ nor HCO_3^- are strong ions. The pCO_2 is an independent variable assuming that there is an open system (i.e., ventilation is present). Finally, the weak acids (A^-) which are mostly proteins and phosphates, contribute the remaining charges to satisfy the principle of electroneutrality (Fig.1). A^- however, is not an independent variable because it changes with alterations in SID and pCO_2. A_{TOT}, $(AH + A^-)$ is the third independent variable because its value is not determined by any other. The essence of the Stewart approach (and indeed what is revolutionary) is the understanding that only these three variables are important. Neither H^+ nor HCO_3^- can change unless one or more of these three variables change. The principle of conservation of mass makes this point more than semantics. Strong ions cannot be created or destroyed to satisfy electroneutrality but H^+s are generated or consumed by changes in water dissociation. Hence, in order to understand how the body regulates pH we need only ask how it regulates these three independent variables (SID, pCO_2 and A_{TOT}).

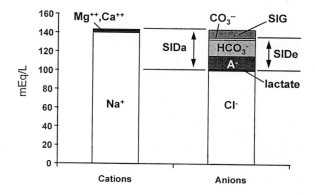

Fig. 1. Total charge balance in blood plasma. The strong ion difference (SID) is always positive (in plasma) and SID-SIDe (effective) must equal zero. Any difference between SID apparent (SIDa) and SIDe is the strong ion gap (SIG) and must represent unmeasured anions

Clinical Implications

Naturally, when one views acid-base balance from this perspective, several aspects of patient management are affected. We will discuss some of the more common examples here, but there are many others which will become obvious as one ponders the various implications of this approach. First, let us consider one of the most common forms of metabolic alkalosis seen in the ICU; loss of gastric secretions. The loss of hydrochloric acid (HCl) from the stomach results in a hypochloremic metabolic alkalosis sometimes severe enough to require therapy. Of course, this is the loss of H^+, isn't it? But, isn't H^+ also lost with every molecule of water removed from the body? Moreover, gastric secretions may reach a pH of 1.0, or a $[H^+]$ of 10^8 nmol/L. If one liter of gastric fluid is lost, this would mean that 10^8 nmols (0.1 moles!) of H^+ would be removed. If one considers that plasma $[H^+]$ is 40 nmol/L (or 4×10^{-8} mol/L), and if the majority of body fluids are at, or near, this concentration, one sees that the amount of total body free H^+ is only about 1.6×10^{-7} moles. If physiology were just simple accounting, a patient with pyloric stenosis would rapidly run out of H^+. Of course the $[H^+]$ decreases by a much smaller amount, but why? The answer is that the plasma SID is increased because Cl^- (a strong anion) is lost without loss of a strong cation. This increased SID forces a decrease in the amount of water dissociation and hence a decrease in the plasma $[H^+]$. When H^+ is "lost" as water (HOH) rather than HCl, there is no change in the SID and hence no change in the plasma $[H^+]$. Next, consider the treatment for a hypochloremic metabolic alkalosis. Aside from preventing further Cl^- loss, the therapy is to give back Cl^-. Saline works in this regard because even though one is giving equal amounts of Na^+ and Cl^-, the plasma $[Cl^-]$ is always much lower than the plasma $[Na^+]$ and thus Cl^- increases more than Na^+ when large amounts of saline are administered. KCl works better for this indication because, with a metabolic alkalosis, much of the K^+ goes intracellular leaving much of the Cl^- in the plasma to decrease the SID. From this vantage point, one sees no need to invoke complex renal tubular or hormonal mechanisms to account for the restoration of normal plasma pH; the principles of physical chemistry are quite sufficient.

"Dilutional" Acidosis

From the example above, one can easily understand not only how administration of 0.9% saline can correct a hypochloremic metabolic alkalosis but also how massive amounts would lead to a decreased plasma SID and thus a hyperchloremic metabolic acidosis. Although dilutional acidosis was first described over 40 years ago [19–20], it has more recently been likened to Lewis Carroll's Cheshire cat in that it is more imaginary than real [21]. In healthy animals, large doses of NaCl have been demonstrated to produce only a minor hyperchloremic acidosis [22]. These studies have been interpreted to show that if dilutional acidosis occurs it is only in the extreme case and even then it is only mild. This line of reasoning cannot be applied to many critically ill patients for two reasons. First, large volume resuscitation is commonly required in patients with sepsis and trauma. These patients may receive crystalloid infusions of 5–10 times their plasma volumes in a single day. The second

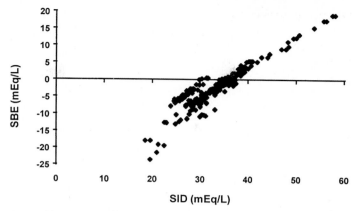

Fig. 2. Scattergram of strong ion difference (SID) versus standard base excess (SBE) for 266 arterial blood samples from patients in the ICU. Note that the intercept for SBE = 0 mEq/L is at a SID of 30–35 mEq/L rather than 40–42 mEq/L as seen in healthy individuals

problem with this line of reasoning is that it fails to consider the fact that critically ill patients are frequently not in normal acid-base balance to begin with. These patients may have lactic acidosis or renal insufficiency. Furthermore, critically ill patients might not be able to compensate normally by increasing ventilation and may have abnormal buffer capacity owing to hypoalbuminemia [23]. In ICU patients [24] as well as in animals with experimental sepsis [25], dilutional acidosis does occur and can produce significant acid-base derangements.

From the preceding discussion, it is obvious how so called "dilutional" acidosis occurs. However, it may be less obvious why critically ill patients are more susceptible. What appears to happen is that many critically ill patients have a significantly lower SID than do healthy individuals even when they have no evidence of a metabolic acid-base derangement [26] (Fig. 2). This is not surprising given that the positive charge of the SID is balanced by the negative charges of A^- and total CO_2 (Fig. 1). Since many critically ill patients are hypoalbuminemic, A^- tends to be reduced. Because the body defends pCO_2 for other reasons, a reduction in A^- leads to a reduction in SID by the body in order to maintain normal pH. Thus a typical ICU patient might have a SID of 30 mEq/L rather than 40–42 mEq/L. If this same patient then developed a metabolic acidosis (e.g., lactate) the SID would decrease further. If we then resuscitated this patient with a large volume of normal saline we would find that it produces a significant metabolic acidosis. These effects are demonstrated by the example in Table 1. Note that as the SID decreases, so does the pH despite the "compensatory" hyperventilation. Also, note that the fall in pH is greater when the SID changes from 20 to 14 mEq/L than when it changes from 30 to 20 mEq/L. This relationship is further illustrated in Fig. 3 and demonstrates that a patient with a lower baseline SID is more susceptible to a subsequent acid load.

The clinical implication for management of patients in the ICU is that when large volumes of fluid are used for resuscitation they should be more physiologic than saline. One alternative is lactated Ringer's solution. This fluid contains a more physiologic difference between Na^+ and Cl^- and thus the SID is closer to normal

Table 1. Effects of lactic acidosis and resuscitation with saline

	SID (mEq/L)	pH	pCO$_2$ (mmHg)	SBE (mEq/L)
Baseline	30	7.40	38	− 2.0
Lactic acidosis	20	7.29	29	−11.4
10 L 0.9% saline	14	7.13	25	−20.1

Results of lactic acidosis (arterial whole blood lactate 10 mmol/L) and subsequent resuscitation with 10 L of 0.9% saline in a 70 kg man with no urine output and before any change in lactate concentration. Baseline [Na$^+$] and [Cl$^-$] are 130 mEq/L and 100 mEq/L respectively. SID = strong ion difference, SBE = standard base excess

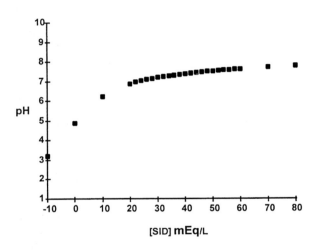

Fig. 3. pH at various concentrations of strong ion difference ([SID]). For these curves, A$_{TOT}$ and pCO$_2$ were held constant at 18 mEq/L and 40 mm-Hg respectively. Assumes a water dissociation constant for blood of 4.4×10^{-14} (Eq/L). Note how steep the pH curve becomes at [SID] < 40 mEq/L

(roughly 28 mEq/L compared to saline which has an SID of 0 mEq/L). Of course this assumes that the lactate in lactated Ringer's is metabolized, which as we will discuss below is almost always the case.

Lactate and Lactic Acidosis

Lactate is a strong ion by virtue of the fact that at pH within the physiologic range, it is almost completely dissociated (i.e., the pK of lactate is 3.9; at a pH of 7.4, 3162 ions are dissociated for every one that is not). Because the body can produce and dispose of lactate rapidly, it functions as one of the most dynamic components of the SID. Lactic acid therefore can produce significant acidemia. However, often critically ill patients have hyperlactatemia that is much greater than the amount of acidosis seen. Physical chemistry also allows us to understand how hyperlactatemia may exist without metabolic acidosis. First, acid is not being "generated" apart from lactate such as through "unreversed ATP hydrolysis" as some have suggested [27]. Phosphate is a weak acid and does not contribute substantially to metabolic acidosis even under extreme circumstances. Furthermore, the [H$^+$] is not determined by how much H^+ is produced or removed from the plasma but rather by changes in one of the three independent variables (SID, pCO_2 or A_{TOT}). Virtually anywhere in the body, the pH is above 6.0 and lactate behaves as a strong ion. Its generation will then decrease the SID and result in increased water dissociation and thus increased $[H^+]$. How then might plasma [lactate] be increased and $[H^+]$ not? There are two possible answers. First, if lactate is added to the plasma, not as lactic acid but rather as the salt of a strong acid (i.e., sodium lactate), there will be little change in the SID. This is because a strong cation (Na^+) is being added along with a strong anion. In fact, as lactate is then removed by metabolism, the remaining Na^+ will increase the SID resulting in metabolic alkalosis. Hence it would be possible to give enough lactate to increase the plasma [lactate] without any change in $[H^+]$. However, the amount of exogenous lactate required would be very large. This is because normal metabolism results in the turnover of approximately 1500–4500 mmol of lactic acid per day. Thus, only very large amounts of lactate infused rapidly will result in appreciable increases in the plasma [lactate]. Levraut et al. [28] infused 1 mmol/kg of lactate over 15 min in 10 patients with acute renal failure on continuous renal replacement therapy. Their mean plasma [lactate] increased from 1.4 to 4.8 mmol/L after the infusion but normalized rapidly. Under such conditions it is possible (if transiently) to produce hyperlactatemia without acidemia. Unfortunately, these authors do not report the acid-base status of their patients. However, in another recent study, Morgera et al. [29] showed that lactate-based hemofiltration resulted in increased plasma $[HCO_3^-]$ and pH as well as hyperlactatemia.

A more important mechanism whereby hyperlactatemia exists without acidemia (or with less acidemia than expected) is where the SID is corrected by the elimination of another strong anion from the plasma. This was demonstrated by Madias et al. [30]. In the setting of sustained lactic acidosis induced by lactic acid infusion, these investigators found that Cl^- moves out of the plasma space to normalize pH. Under these conditions, hyperlactatemia may persist but base excess may be normalized by compensatory mechanisms to restore the SID.

Nonetheless, given that lactate is a strong ion, and that lactic acidosis is a marker for mortality in many forms of critical illness, it is reasonable to search for the anatomic sources and pathophysiologic mechanisms that are responsible for increases in plasma [lactate]. Conventional wisdom suggests that the gut and the muscle are the sources of this increased lactate. However, the results of a recent study suggest that in sepsis, neither the muscle nor the gut release lactate [31]. In fact, studies in animals as well as humans have shown that the lung may be a prominent source of lactate in the setting of acute lung injury [31–33].

While studies such as these do not address the underlying pathophysiologic mechanisms of hyperlactatemia in sepsis, they do suggest that the conventional wisdom regarding lactate as evidence of tissue dysoxia is an oversimplification at best. Indeed, many authors have begun to offer alternative interpretations of hyperlactatemia in this setting [33–36]. First, metabolic dysfunction from mitochondrial to enzymatic derangements can, and do, lead to lactic acidosis. In particular, pyruvate dehydrogenase (PDH), the enzyme responsible for moving pyruvate into the Krebs cycle is inhibited by endotoxin [37]. However, data from recent studies suggest that increased aerobic metabolism may be more important than metabolic defects or anaerobic metabolism. Gore et al. [38] observed increased glucose and pyruvate production and oxidation in patients with sepsis. Furthermore, when PDH was stimulated by dichloroacetate there was a further increase in oxygen consumption but a decrease in glucose and pyruvate production. Their results suggest that hyperlactatemia in sepsis occurs as a result of increased aerobic metabolism rather than tissue hypoxia or PDH inhibition. Day et al. [39] reminds us that catecholamine use, especially epinephrine, also results in lactic acidosis presumably by stimulating cellular metabolism. Whether one of these mechanisms or lung lactate release accounted for the findings of hyperlactatemia in a study of cardiac surgery patients by Raper et al. [40] is unknown. However, these patients had no evidence of inadequate oxygen delivery and mortality was extremely low.

Unexplained Anions

Another important application of the Stewart approach is the investigation of unmeasured anions in the blood of patients with critical illness. As one can see from Fig. 1, the principle of electroneutrality can be used to detect the presence of unmeasured anions in the blood. By definition the SID must be equal and opposite to the negative charges contributed by A^- and total CO_2. This latter value is termed effective SID (SIDe) [5]. Thus, if SIDa > SIDe unmeasured anions must exist and if SIDa < SIDe there must be unmeasured cations present. This difference has been termed the strong ion gap (SIG) to distinguish it from the anion gap (AG) [7]. Unlike the AG, the SIG is normally zero and does not change with changes in pH or [albumin] as does the AG. Thus, the accuracy of the AG is questionable in certain clinical situations [41], particularly in critically ill patients who are frequently hypoalbuminemic and acidotic. This has prompted some authors to adjust the "normal range" for the AG by the patient's albumin [42] or even phosphate [26] concentration. Each g/dl of albumin has a charge of 2.8 mEq/L at pH 7.4 (2.3 mEq/L at 7.0 and 3.0 mEq/L at 7.6) and each mg/dl of phosphate has a charge of 0.59 mEq/L at pH 7.4 (0.55 mEq/L at 7.0 and 0.61 mEq/L at 7.6). Except in cases of abnormal paraproteins, globulin does not contribute to the AG [5]. Thus a convenient way to estimate the "normal" AG for a given patient is by use of the following formula:

$$\text{"normal" AG} = 2\,(\text{albumin g/dl}) + 0.5\,(\text{phosphate mg/dl}) \tag{1}$$

Or for international units:

$$\text{"normal" AG} = 0.2\,(\text{albumin g/L}) + 1.5\,(\text{phosphate mmol/L}) \tag{2}$$

However, Salem and Mujais [41] found routine reliance on the traditional AG to be fraught with numerous other pitfalls in addition to those mentioned above. These problems are largely omitted by the SIG calculation [17] and this is the preferred method for quantifying unexplained anions when precision is required. In recent years, unmeasured anions have been reported in the blood of patients with sepsis [6, 43] and liver disease [7, 44]. These anions may be the source of much of the unexplained acidosis seen in patients with critical illness [45]. The presence of unexplained anions in the blood of patients with sepsis and liver disease was investigated further in an animal model of sepsis using endotoxemia [13]. In this study, it was found that during control conditions, the liver cleared unmeasured anions from the circulation (mean flux -0.34 mEq/min). With early endotoxemia, however, the liver switched to release of anions (0.12 mEq/min, $p < 0.005$). These data suggest that the liver has a role in systemic acid-base balance by way of regulating anion fluxes apart from metabolism of lactate.

Treatment of Metabolic Acid-Base Disorders

This physical chemical approach also provides more logical basis for treatment of metabolic acid-base disorders. In metabolic acidosis the SID is narrowed and there is either an increased strong ion such as lactate, or the normal difference between $[Na^+]$ and $[Cl^-]$ is reduced. The AG is a reasonable screening test to distinguish these, provided that the patient's [albumin] and [phosphate] are near normal or one corrects the AG as described above. The distinction is very important since non-AG metabolic acidoses are the result of the body's inability to maintain the normal $[Na^+]$ and $[Cl^-]$. Treatment, therefore, must include an assessment of the $[Na^+]$ and $[Cl^-]$ and the reasons for their abnormality must be sought. If the disorder is characterized by a decreased (or at least normal) $[Na^+]$, administration of sodium bicarbonate ($NaHCO_3$) can prove effective. From the discussion above, it should be clear that it is the $[Na^+]$ we are trying to influence not the $[HCO_3^-]$. HCO_3^- is not an independent variable. Its concentration is determined by the three independent variables we have discussed. Therefore, only by increasing the $[Na^+]$ relative to the $[Cl^-]$ can $NaHCO_3^-$ repair a metabolic acidosis. When the $[Na^+]$ is already increased, there is no room for $NaHCO_3^-$ therapy. In such a condition it would be necessary to consider other options. These include a greater removal of Cl^- than Na^+ perhaps by use of renal replacement therapy (e.g., hemofiltration) or administration of a weak base such as THAM (trishydoxymethyl-aminomethane). Theoretically, it would also be possible to remove Cl^- from the stomach via a nasogastric tube, but this is rarely done.

When the acidosis is from an anion which can be metabolized (e.g., lactate, ketones) the goal of therapy should be to augment metabolic removal and reduce production. In the case of lactate, hypoperfusion should be reversed when present and other metabolic triggers (e.g., epinephrine) should also be removed. In keto-acidosis, insulin repairs the metabolic defect and results in the metabolism of keto-nes. If therapies are given which increase the SID by increasing $[Na^+]$ or decreasing $[Cl^-]$, the result will be overshoot alkalosis when the causative anion is removed. Rarely, partial treatment is necessary in order to improve metabolic removal of the anions or to stabilize the patient until metabolic removal can occur. Severe acidemia impairs normal hepatic lactate metabolism, for example, [46] and therapy to increase the pH above perhaps 7.20 may be useful in some cases.

We have already examined the treatment of metabolic alkalosis and the principles are the same. The repair of the $[Cl^-]$ can be achieved by NaCl, KCl or HCl. In all cases however, our goal is the same; to increase the $[Cl^-]$ relative to the $[Na^+]$. The $[HCO_3^-]$ will then be returned to the point set by the SID, pCO_2 and A_{TOT}.

Conclusion

The Stewart approach is merely another perspective; a third vantage point from which to view acid-base physiology. From this position, it is possible to understand the causes of, and treatments for, acid-base derangements which are common in the ICU. Metabolic acidemia results from a decrease in the plasma SID usually brought about by the addition of strong anions (lactate, Cl^-, other "unknown" anions). Conversely, metabolic alkalemia occurs when the plasma SID is increased either as a result of the addition of strong cations without strong anions (e.g., $NaHCO_3$) or by the removal of strong anions without strong cations (e.g., gastric suctioning).

Hyperlactatemia may occur with or without acidemia depending on the balance of other ions. In some forms of critical illness, most notably sepsis, hyperlactatemia may not indicate tissue hypoxia but may instead reflect hypermetabolism or PDH inhibition. In acute lung injury, lactate may be released from the lung.

References

1. Stewart PA (1981) How to understand acid-base. In: Stewart PA (ed) A quantitative acid-base primer for biology and medicine. Elsevier, New York, pp 1–286
2. Stewart PA (1983) Modern quantitative acid-base chemistry. Can J Physiol Pharmacol 61: 1444–1461
3. Reeves RB (1983) Commentary on review article by Dr. Peter Stewart. Can J Physiol Pharmacol 61:1442–1443
4. Fencl V, Leith DE (1993) Stewart's quantitative acid base chemistry: Applications in biology and medicine. Resp Physiol 91:1–16
5. Figge J, Mydosh T, Fencl V (1992) Serum proteins and acid base equilibria: a follow-up. J Lab Clin Med 120:713–719
6. Gilfix BM, Bique M, Magder S (1993) A physical chemical approach to the analysis of acid-base balance in the clinical setting. J Crit Care 8:187–197
7. Kellum JA, Kramer DJ, Pinsky MR (1995) Strong ion gap: A methodology for exploring unexplained anions. J Crit Care 10:51–55
8. Jones NL (1990) A quantitative physicochemical approach to acid-base physiology. Clin Biochem 23:189–195
9. Schlichtig R (1996) Base Excess: a powerful clinical tool in the ICU. Critical Care Symposium. Society of Critical Care Medicine 1:1–30
10. Jabor A, Kazda A (1995) Modeling of acid-base equilibria. Acta Anaesth Scand 39 (suppl 107): 119–122
11. Alfaro V, Torras R, Ibanez J, Palacios L (1996) A physical-chemical analysis of the acid-base response to chronic obstructive pulmonary disease. Can J Physiol Pharmacol 74:1229–1235
12. Rozenfeld RA, Dishart MK, Tonnessen TI, Schlichtig R (1996) Methods for detecting local intestinal ischemic anaerobic metabolic acidosis by pCO_2. J Appl Physiol 81:1834–1842
13. Kellum JA, Bellomo R, Kramer DJ, Pinsky MR (1995) Hepatic anion flux during acute endotoxemia. J Appl Physiol 78:2212–2217
14. Lindinger MI, Heigenhauser GJF, McKelvie RS, Jones NL (1992) Blood ion regulation during repeated maximal exercise and recovery in humans. Am J Physiol 262:R126–R136
15. Kellum JA, Bellomo R, Kramer DJ, Pinsky MR (1997) Splanchnic buffering of metabolic acid during early endotoxemia. J Crit Care 12:7–12
16. Severinghaus JW (1993) Siggard Andersen and the "great trans-Atlantic acid-base debate". Scand J Clin Lab Invest 53 (suppl 214):99–104
17. Magder S (1997) Pathophysiology of metabolic acid-base disturbances in patients with critical illness. In: Ronco C, Bellomo R (ed) Critical care nephrology. Kluwer Academic Publishers, Dordrecht, pp 279–296

18. Leblanc M, Kellum JA (1997) Biochemical and biophysical principles of hydrogen ion regulation. In: Ronco C, Bellomo R (eds) Critical care nephrology. Kluwer Academic Publishers, Dordrecht, pp 261–277

19. Cheek DB (1956) Changes in total chloride and acid-base balance in gastroenteritis following treatment with large and small loads of sodium chloride. Pediatrics 17:839–847

20. Shires GT, Tolman J (1948) Dilutional acidosis. Ann Intern Med 28:557–559

21. Garella S, Chang BS, Kahn SI (1975) Dilution acidosis and contraction alkalosis: review of a concept. Kidney Int 8:279–283

22. Garella S, Tzamaloukas AH, Chazan JA (1973) Effect of isotonic volume expansion on extracellular bicarbonate stores in normal dogs. Am J Physiol 225:628–636

23. Kellum JA, Kramer DJ (1997) Water, electrolyte, and acid-base balance in hepatic cirrhosis. In: Park G, Pinsky MR (ed) Critical care management: Case studies – tricks and traps, W. B. Saunders Company Ltd, London, pp 124–128

24. Mathes DD, Morell RC, Rohr MS (1997) Dilutional acidosis: Is it a real clinical entity? Anesthesiology 86:501–503

25. Kellum JA, Bellomo R, Kramer DJ, Pinsky MR (1995) Etiology of metabolic acidosis during saline resuscitation in endotoxemia. Am J Resp Crit Care 151:A318 (Abst)

26. Kellum JA, Kramer DJ, Pinsky MR (1996) Closing the GAP: A simple method of improving the accuracy of the anion gap. Chest 110:18S (Abst)

27. Zilva JF (1978) The origin of acidosis in hyperlactatemia. Ann Clin Biochem 15:40–43

28. Levraut J, Ciebiera JP, Jambou P, Ichai C, Labib Y, Grimaud D (1997) Effect of continuous venovenous hemofiltration with dialysis on lactate clearance in critically ill patients. Crit Care Med 25:58–62

29. Morgera S, Heering P, Szentandrasi T, et al (1997) Comparison of a lactate-versus acetate-based hemofiltration replacement fluid in patients with acute renal failure. Renal Failure 19:155–164

30. Madias NE, Homer SM, Johns CA, Cohen JJ (1984) Hypochloremia as a consequence of anion gap metabolic acidosis. J Lab Clin Med 104:15–23

31. Bellomo R, Kellum JA, Pinsky MR (1996) Visceral lactate fluxes during early endotoxemia in the dog. Chest 110:198–204

32. Brown, S, Gutierrez G, Clark C, Nelson C, Tiu A (1996) The lung as a source of lactate in sepsis and ARDS. J Crit Care 11:2–8

33. Kellum JA, Kramer DJ, Lee KH, Mankad S, Bellomo R, Pinsky MR (1997) Release of lactate by the lung in acute lung injury. Chest 111:1301–1305

34. Stacpoole PW (1997) Lactic acidosis and other mitochondrial disorders. Metabolism 46:306–321

35. Fink MP (1996) Does tissue acidosis in sepsis indicate tissue hypoperfusion? Intensive Care Med 22:1144–1146

36. Gutierrez G, Wolf ME (1996) Lactic acidosis in sepsis: A commentary. Intensive Care Med 22:6–16

37. Kilpatrick-Smith L, Dean J, Erecinska M, Silver IA (1983) Cellular effects of endotoxin in vitro. II Reversibility of endotoxic damage. Circ Shock 11:101–111

38. Gore DC, Jahoor F, Hibbert JM, DeMaria EJ (1996) Lactic acidosis during sepsis is related to increased pyruvate production, not deficits in tissue oxygen availability. Ann Surgery 224:97–102

39. Day NP, Phu NH, Bethell DP, et al (1996) The effects of dopamine and adrenaline infusions on acid-base balance and systemic haemodynamics in severe infection. Lancet 348:219–223

40. Raper RF, Cameron G, Walker D, Bowey CJ (1997) Type B lactic acidosis following cardiopulmonary bypass. Crit Care Med 25:46–51

41. Salem MM, Mujais SK (1992) Gaps in the anion gap. Arch Intern Med 152:1625–1629

42. Gabow PA (1985) Disorders associated with an altered anion gap. Kidney Int 27:472–483

43. Mecher C, Rackow EC, Astiz ME, Weil MH (1991) Unaccounted anion in metabolic acidosis during severe sepsis in humans. Crit Care Med 19:705–711

44. Kirschbaum B (1997) Increased anion gap after liver transplantation. Am J Med Sci 313:107–110

45. Mehta K, Kruse JA, Carlson RW (1986) The relationship between anion gap and elevated lactate. Crit Care Med. 14:405–414

46. Cohen RD (1979) The production and removal of lactate. Lactate in acute conditions. International Symposium. Karger, Basel, pp 10–19

Pivotal Role of Lactate in Aerobic Energy Metabolism

X. M. Leverve, I. Mustafa, and F. Peronnet

Introduction

A defect in the energy status of the cell is believed to play a central role in the pathophysiology of shock and possibly also of other less severe acute disorders. It has been known for a long time that defects in oxidative energy metabolism could be accompanied by increases in blood lactate concentration, and many efforts have been made during the last decades to use blood lactate levels in acutely ill patients to better understand the pathophysiology and the prognosis of the disease as well as the effects of therapeutic approaches [1–9]. However, the metabolic significance of the lactate anion is very broad and an increase in blood lactate concentration cannot be considered only as a marker of a defect in oxidative energy metabolism.

The large number of studies devoted to the pathophysiology of shock or related pathologic states has improved our understanding of the sequence of events [10–14] and has unraveled the major role played by macrophages, endothelial cells and the gut. However, among several questions which remained unanswered, the possible role of energy defects is still a matter of debate [3]. The metabolic response to stress can be described as a shift in priorities in order to better cope with the new threatening situation. This shift may affect various major physiologic parameters (e.g., body-temperature set point, loss of lean body mass, etc.), and organ functions (e.g., decrease of the perfusion and metabolism of the skin, subcutaneous tissue, muscles, kidneys or gut according to the severity of the illness), as well as several biochemical pathways (e.g., increased and decreased protein synthesis in the liver and muscle, respectively, increased liver gluconeogenesis; decreased insulin action because of insulin resistance). As a consequence, changes in some functions or metabolic pathways might be considered not only as deleterious events responsible for increased morbidity, but rather as adaptative changes which re-direct the metabolism towards new priorities and organs (such as the brain, heart or liver) as well as mechanisms which limit or repair damage resulting from the disease. Thus, an impaired energy status of the cell could be either a major deleterious event or an adaptative change, depending on the organ and/or the stage of the disease. In this respect, changes in lactate metabolism, although related to changes in the energy status, do not simply reflect changes in anaerobic energy production associated with impairments in aerobic metabolism. In fact, as shown in the present chapter, lactate could play a central role in aerobic metabolism.

Mechanisms of Defense:
Comparison Between Patient in Shock and Cellular Apoptosis

Interesting similarities exist between the patient in shock and the cell in apoptosis, the programmed pathway of cell suicide [14–18]. On one hand, humans and cells both have in common the ability to repair themselves. Examples of this include the spontaneous healing of wounds or recovery from sepsis in humans, and the deoxyribonucleic acid (DNA) self-repairing system in response to damage from various causes. However, under certain circumstances depending on the duration and/or severity of the disease, the metabolic changes are no longer adaptive (i.e., favoring the self-repair processes), but become deleterious and lead to a state of multiorgan failure (MOF) [19–23]. Similarily, although the cell can tolerate and repair some damage, when this damage is beyond repair a program of self-destruction is triggered which eventually leads to the death of the cell [15, 18, 24, 25]. A better understanding of the mechanism of apoptosis is of major importance since pharmacologic interventions might be beneficial on both sides of the process; activation to prevent abnormal cell selection, or inhibition leading to increased cell survival. Recent findings have shown that mitochondria play a central role in the triggering of apoptosis [26–29] not simply via a decrease in the energy state of the cell. It has been shown, for example, that hypoxia may have some protective effect on apoptosis induction [17, 30–32]. In addition, certain energy consuming processes with lower priorities, could be temporarily turned off, thus allowing the cell to fully use its resources against the threatening situation and to restore its integrity and function [33].

Lactate and Energy: Aerobic or Anaerobic Metabolism?

Classically, the basic statements concerning energy and lactate metabolism can be summarized as follows:
(1) Adenosine triphosphate (ATP) production in the body is mainly sustained from aerobic metabolism with only about 10% of the energy yield provided from anaerobic energy sources.
(2) Anaerobic ATP re-synthesis results in lactate production.
(3) An increase in blood lactate concentration reflects an energy deficit, the level of lactate concentration being proportional to the defect in oxidative metabolism.

Although these statements are roughly true, in clinical practice a more detailed analysis of the significance of blood lactate concentration should be made.

Aerobic or Anaerobic Metabolism: Role of Lactate as a Shuttle of Reducing Equivalents

Under anaerobic conditions ATP is re-synthesized in the absence of oxygen. In humans this is only possible to a significant degree by two pathways: ATP re-synthesis from creatine phosphate via creatine kinase; and the glycolytic pathway. The creatine kinase reaction is of major importance in muscle metabolism. However, this pathway will not be discussed here since the amounts of creatine phosphate stored in the body remain limited. Hence, in the steady state, anaerobic ATP re-synthesis is only possible from the energy released by the glycolytic pathway, in which glucose is utilized and lactate is produced. Actually, net ATP production in the glycolytic pathway occurs at the pyruvate kinase step. However, under anaerobic conditions, pyruvate must be converted into lactate in order to avoid accumulation of reducing equivalents which cannot be oxidized in the mitochondrion matrix (Fig. 1) [34]. Therefore, anaerobic energy metabolism is characterized by: (i) the absence of respiration; (ii) glucose utilization; and (iii) lactate production and release or accumulation. This occurs, for instance, in the erythrocyte where all of these three conditions are met. In contrast, for the whole body, in humans, except in certain situations, such as intense short-duration exercise, lactate excretion is almost negligible and lactate does not accumulate. As a consequence, the energy is entirely derived from aerobic metabolism. Taken as a whole, the organism, is thus 100% aerobic in steady state conditions! When lactate accumulates in the body, e.g., during short duration high intensity exercise, anaerobic metabolism does contribute to the energy yield. However, during the recovery process, lactate is metabolized and disappears from the body. Accordingly, when both the exercise and recovery periods are taken into account, the organism works under complete aerobic conditions. In the same way, erythrocyte energy metabolism is entirely anaerobic but the lactate produced is finally metabolized by the liver in such a way that the erythrocyte/liver system works as a whole in fully aerobic conditions; the liver "respires" for the red blood cells (Fig. 2). This important point has two main consequences: (1) Except when lactate is accumulating or being excreted, energy metabolism is entirely aerobic what-

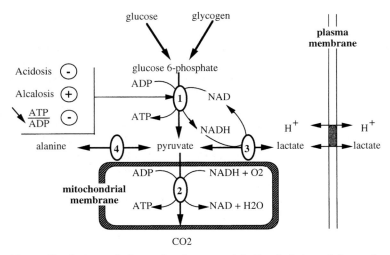

Fig. 1. Glycolysis regulation and redox potential. Glycolysis is mainly regulatated at two steps: phosphofructokinase and pyruvate kinase. Phosphate potential (ATP/ADP.Pi), redox potential (NADH + H$^+$/NAD) and pH play a major role in this regulation (1). When oxidative metabolism is impaired (2), conversion of lactate to pyruvate (3) is the main way to eliminate the excess reducing equivalent. Cytosolic pyruvate concentration is dependent on glycolysis rate, redox potential and alanine metabolism via transamination [4]

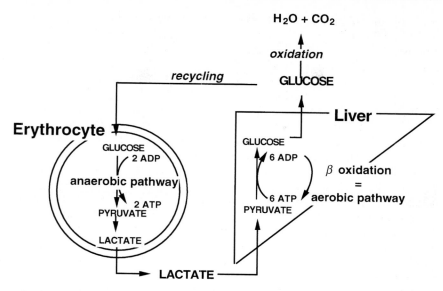

Fig. 2. Glucose lactate cycling: Cori cycle. The glucose re-cycling via lactate creates a futile cycle between 3 and 6 carbon compounds. On one hand it dissipates directly 2/3 of the energy (6 ATP are needed to build one glucose from 2 lactate whereas 2 ATP only are produced when splitting glucose into lactate), but on the other hand, the source of energy in the liver mainly comes from fatty acids. Hence, glucose re-cycling provides "glycolytic ATP" to several peripheral cells (erythrocytes for instance) while this ATP is formed from energy coming actually from lipid store oxidation. In other words, one can say that the "liver respires for anaerobic tissues such as erythrocytes"

ever the lactate concentration; and (2) lactate plays a pivotal role in aerobic metabolism by providing substrates from one organ to another for the respiratory chain (reducing equivalents coming from the conversion of lactate to pyruvate). Lactate-pyruvate serves as a shuttle for transporting reducing equivalents from one organ to another (Fig. 3) [35] as has been described during prolonged submaximal exercise [36]. In fact, any reduced compounds released from the cell, such as 3-hydroxybutyrate, can play the role of a redox shuttle between organs and tissues. Furthermore, this redox shuttle is probably not limited to inter-organ exchange (Fig. 3A) but also to intra-organ metabolism (Fig. 3B). For example, it has been recently reported that a large increase in the interconversion of both lactate-to-pyruvate and pyruvate-to-lactate was present in type II diabetes [37]. Such a phenomenon could explain the regional lactate production or utilization in critically ill patients, in the lung for instance [38].

Mitochondrial Oxidation of Carbohydrate: Glucose or Lactate as Pyruvate Source?

Aerobic carbohydrate oxidation via the Krebs cycle is mainly controlled at pyruvate dehydrogenase, a key enzyme which is tightly regulated by four main cellular metabolic parameters: Phosphate potential (ATP/ADP.Pi); redox potential (NADH/NAD);

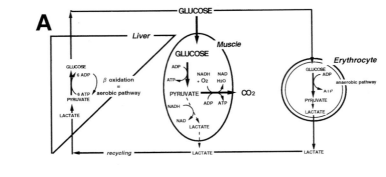

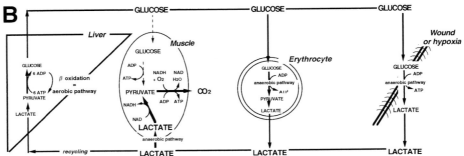

Fig. 3. Competition between glucose and lactate as pyruvate source. **A** In aerobic metabolism, glucose is the main source for pyruvate oxidation. Lactate is mainly metabolized through liver gluconeogenesis. **B** In the case of high plasma lactate concentrations (for instance from injured tissues), there is a competition between lactate and glucose for substrate supply to mitochondrial oxidation. Due to its high plasma concentration, lactate is oxidized preferentially. Hence, the injured tissues "benefit from the 2 glycolysis (non aerobic) ATP" whereas the oxidative tissue only have access to the lower fully oxidative part of the pathway (i.e., from pyruvate to CO_2)

free/esterified CoA ratio; and pH [34, 39]. This enzyme could play a major role in the pathogenesis of metabolic disorders during sepsis and lactic acidosis [3, 4, 40–44] and it is the target in the use of dichloroacetate [4, 45]. In addition to the above mentioned factors regulating the activity of pyruvate dehydrogenase, pyruvate concentration in the mitochondria also controls the oxidation of pyruvate [46]. Since pyruvate can be supplied from many sources including glucose, lactate and alanine, depending on the respective concentrations of these precursors and on the regulation of the glycolytic pathway (Fig. 1), carbohydrates can be oxidized in a tissue either directly from glucose or via lactate or alanine produced from glucose in other organs or tissues (Fig. 4) [35, 47]. In this situation where reducing equivalents are shuttled from one organ to the other, the utilization of lactate instead of glucose as a source of pyruvate increases with blood lactate concentration. In other words, glucose could be oxidized directly in the cell into CO_2, and H_2O. Alternately, glucose could be broken down in one cell to pyruvate and/or lactate according to the redox-state (see above and Fig. 3); lactate and/or pyruvate are then released from the cell and completely oxidized into CO_2 and H_2O in another cell from a different organ or

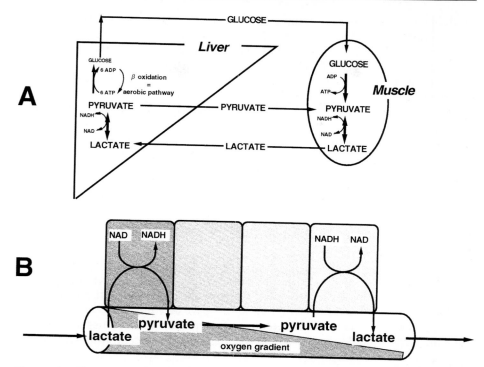

Fig. 4. Role of lactate/pyruvate interconversion as reducing equivalent shuttle. Lactate-to-pyruvate exchange and *vice versa* could be viewed as a reducing equivalent shuttle either from one organ to another (**A**) or within one organ (**B**) depending, for instance, on the oxygen tension in the immediate cell vicinity. NADH can be transported from one cell to another

within the same organ or tissue (Fig. 4). The main difference between these two different pathways for glucose oxidation is that, in the first case, anaerobic ATP (glycolytic or non-aerobic ATP) is provided together with aerobic ATP (mitochondrial ATP) in the same cell, while in the second case different cells gain anaerobic versus aerobic ATP. As discussed above, for the entire organism, energy metabolism is almost always completely aerobic. However, energy metabolism could be anaerobic, entirely or in part, in some cells, organs or tissues, while it could be predominantly (if not entirely) aerobic in other cells, organs or tissues. In this respect, the steady state blood lactate concentration plays a major role in determining the source of carbons for mitochondrial oxidation in the tissues with oxidative metabolism (Fig. 4). For example, we have shown that hypoxia *in vivo* results in an inhibition of the transcription of phosphoenolpyruvate carboxykinase (PEPCK), one of the key enzymes which regulates lactate utilization for gluconeogenesis in the liver [48]. In addition, high lactate concentration could be responsible for a decrease in glucose oxidation through the development of insulin resistance [49, 50]. We therefore propose that the increase in blood lactate concentration observed in shock is actually a key metabolic event which favors lactate rather than glucose oxidation in tissues where oxygen is available, thus preserving blood glucose for non-aerobic ATP re-synthesis through glycolysis in those tissues where oxidative metabolism is limited (Fig. 4) [48]. Recent findings in healthy volunteers at rest (unpublished observations) or during exercise [51], or in patients after cardiac bypass surgery (unpublished data), or in cardiogenic shock (unpublished data) receiving an exogenous lactate load, indeed indicate that this lactate is almost completely oxidized and not converted into glucose.

Interestingly, a compartmentation of glucose/lactate metabolism between different types of cells in the same organ has recently been reported by Magistretti and his group [52–54] in the brain, with lactate being produced from glucose in glial cells before being oxidized in neurones. Taken as a whole, the brain, thus, remains a fully aerobic organ, which utilizes glucose and produces CO_2 and H_2O. However, lactate production and release by the glial cells could be a key factor in the regulation of neurone metabolism [52–54].

Conclusion

It is clear that most of these considerations allow a better understanding of the mechanisms underlying the pathophysiology of shock, rather than direct clinical application. Blood lactate concentration in intensive care practice remains a useful metabolic marker to monitor the evolution of the patient and the effects of therapy. Nevertheless, it should be kept in mind that high lactate concentrations can be due to an increase in lactate production or to a decrease in lactate utilization, or both, and that it is not possible from routine biochemical determination to draw conclusion about these mechanisms. Simultaneous measurement of both lactate and pyruvate provides an estimation of the deficit in oxidative metabolism since the lactate/pyruvate ratio directly reflects the accumulation of reducing equivalents in the cell. Moreover, although this is only a crude estimate, a very high lactate/pyruvate ratio is probably associated with a large interorgan flux of reducing equivalents via the lactate/pyruvate shuttle. However, the respective contributions of liver versus peripheral tissues, and of liver gluconeogenesis versus lactate/pyruvate oxidation, in plasma lactate clearance remain to be clarified. Finally, lactate could also be a metabolic signal between different organs or different cells in a given organ or tissue, as shown in the brain. In this respect, a better understanding of the functional significance, not only of high, but also of modest increases in blood lactate concentration, could help explain the underlying mechanisms which allow a shift in metabolic priorities in acutely ill patients.

References

1. Groeneveld AB, Kester AD, Nauta JJ, Thijs LG (1987) Relation of arterial blood lactate to oxygen delivery and hemodynamic variables in human shock states. Circ Shock 22:35–53
2. van Lambalgen AA, Runge HC, van den Bos GC, Thijs LG (1988) Regional lactate production in early canine endotoxin shock. Am J Physiol 254:E45–E51
3. Hotchkiss RS, Karl IE (1992) Reevaluation of the role of cellular hypoxia and bioenergetic failure in sepsis. JAMA 267:1503–1510

4. Barron JT, Parrillo JE (1995) Production of lactic acid and energy metabolism in vascular smooth muscle: effect of dichloroacetate. Am J Physiol 268:H713–H719
5. Vincent J-L, De Backer D (1995) Oxygen uptake/oxygen supply dependency: fact or fiction? Acta Anaesthesiol Scand Suppl 107:229–237
6. Vincent J-L (1995) Lactate levels in critically ill patients. Acta Anaesthesiol Scand Suppl 107:261–266
7. Marecaux G, Pinsky MR, Dupont E, Kahn RJ, Vincent J-L (1996) Blood lactate levels are better prognostic indicators than TNF and IL-6 levels in patients with septic shock. Intensive Care Med 22:404–408
8. Takala J, Uusaro A, Parviainen I, Ruokonen E (1996) Lactate metabolism and regional lactate exchange after cardiac surgery. New Horizons 4:483–492
9. Vincent J-L (1996) End-points of resuscitation: arterial blood pressure, oxygen delivery, blood lactate, or …? Intensive Care Med 22:3–5
10. Parrillo JE, Parker MM, Natanson C, et al (1990) Septic shock in humans. Advances in the understanding of pathogenesis, cardiovascular dysfunction, and therapy. Ann Intern Med 113:227–242
11. Parrillo JE (1993) Pathogenetic mechanisms of septic shock. N Engl J Med 328:1471–1477
12. Thijs LG (1994) Regional or organ blood flow and oxygen consumption: observations in septic shock. Curr Top Intensive Care 1:101–123
13. Chaudry IH, Zellweger R, Ayala A (1995) The role of bacterial translocation on Kupffer cell immune function following hemorrhage. Prog Clin Biol Res 392:209–218
14. Ayala A, Chaudry IH (1996) Immune dysfunction in murine polymicrobial sepsis: mediators, macrophages, lymphocytes and apoptosis. Shock 6 (suppl 1):S27–S38
15. Hinshaw VS, Olsen CW, Dybdahl-Sissoko N, Evans D (1994) Apoptosis: a mechanism of cell killing by influenza A and B viruses. J Virol 68:3667–3673
16. Richter C, Gogvadze V, Laffranchi R, et al (1995) Oxidants in mitochondria: from physiology to diseases. Biochim Biophys Acta 1271:67–74
17. Beilharz EJ, Williams CE, Dragunow M, Sirimanne ES, Gluckman PD (1995) Mechanisms of delayed cell death following hypoxic-ischemic injury in the immature rat: evidence for apoptosis during selective neuronal loss. Mol Brain Res 29:1–14
18. Krams SM, Egawa H, Quinn MB, et al (1995) Apoptosis as a mechanism of cell death in liver allograft rejection. Transplantation 59:621–625
19. Grootendorst AF (1990) Hemodynamic aspects of multiple organ failure. Intensive Care Med 16 (suppl 2):S165–S167
20. Lekander BJ, Cerra FB (1990) The syndrome of multiple organ failure. Crit Care Nurs Clin North Am 2:331–342
21. Deitch EA (1992) Multiple organ failure. Pathophysiology and potential future therapy. Ann Surg 216:117–134
22. Reilly E, Yucha CB (1994) Multiple organ failure syndrome. Crit Care Nurse 14:25–26, 28–31
23. Baue AE (1996) MOF/MODS, SIRS: an update. Shock 6 (suppl 1):S1–S5
24. Chinnaiyan AM, Dixit VM (1997) Portrait of an executioner: the molecular mechanism of FAS/APO-1-induced apoptosis. Semin Immunol 9:69–76
25. Yuan J (1997) Genetic control of cellular suicide. Reprod Toxicol 11:377–384
26. Kroemer G, Petit P, Zamzami N, Vayssière JL, Mignotte B (1995) The biochemistry of programmed cell death. FASEB J 9:1277–1287
27. Bernardi P (1996) The permeability transition pore. Control points of a cyclosporin A-sensitive mitochondrial channel involved in cell death. Biochim Biophys Acta 1275:5–9
28. Marchetti P, Castedo M, Susin SA, et al (1996) Mitochondrial permeability transition is a central coordinating event of apoptosis. J Exp Med 184:1155–1160
29. Kroemer G, Zamzami N, Susin SA (1997) Mitochondrial control of apoptosis. Immunol Today 18:44–51
30. Graeber TG, Osmanian C, Jacks T, et al (1996) Hypoxia-mediated selection of cells with diminished apoptotic potential in solid tumours. Nature 379:88–91
31. Long X, Boluyt MO, Hipolito ML, et al (1997) p53 and the hypoxia-induced apoptosis of cultured neonatal rat cardiac myocytes. J Clin Invest 99:2635–2643
32. Yun JK, McCormick TS, Judware R, Lapetina EG (1997) Cellular adaptive responses to low oxygen tension: apoptosis and resistance. Neurochem Res 22:517–521

33. Harkness RA (1997) Is post-hypoxic-ischemic cell damage associated with excessive ATP consumption rather than a failure of ATP production? Acta Paediatr 86:1–5
34. Newsholme EA, Leech AR (1990) Control of gluconeogenesis and glycolysis. In: Newsholme EA, Leech AR (eds) Biochemistry for the medical sciences, John Wiley & Sons, Chichester, pp 450–460
35. Leverve X (1995) Amino acid metabolism and gluconeogenesis. In: Cynober L (ed) Amino acid metabolism and therapy in health and nutritional disease. CRC Press, New York, pp 45–56
36. Brooks GA (1986) Lactate production under fully aerobic conditions: the lactate shuttle during rest and exercise. Fed Proc 45:2924–2929
37. Avogaro A, Toffolo G, Miola M, et al (1996) Intracellular lactate- and pyruvate-interconversion rates are increased in muscle tissue of non-insulin-dependent diabetic individuals. J Clin Invest 98:108–115
38. Douzinas EE, Tsidemiadou PD, Pitaridis MT, et al (1997) The regional production of cytokines and lactate in sepsis- related multiple organ failure. Am J Respir Crit Care Med 155:53–59
39. Pilkis SJ (1991) Hepatic gluconeogenesis/glycolysis: regulation and structure/function relationships of substrate cycle enzymes. Annu Rev Nutr 11:465–515
40. Vary TC, Siegel JH, Nakatani T, Sato T, Aoyama H (1986) Effect of sepsis on activity of pyruvate dehydrogenase complex in skeletal muscle and liver. Am J Physiol 250:E634–E640
41. Lewandowski ED, White LT (1995) Pyruvate dehydrogenase influences postischemic heart function. Circulation 91:2071–2079
42. Medina JM, Tabernero A, Tovar JA, Martìn-Barrientos J (1996) Metabolic fuel utilization and pyruvate oxidation during the postnatal period. J Inherit Metab Dis 19:432–442
43. Shangraw RE, Jahoor F, Wolfe RR, Lang CH (1996) Pyruvate dehydrogenase inactivity is not responsible for sepsis-induced insulin resistance. Crit Care Med 24:566–574
44. Gore DC, Jahoor F, Hibbert JM, DeMaria EJ (1996) Lactic acidosis during sepsis is related to increased pyruvate production, not deficits in tissue oxygen availability. Ann Surg 224:97–102
45. Stacpoole PW, Greene YJ (1992) Dichloroacetate. Diabetes Care 15:785–791
46. Carter TC, Coore HG (1995) Effects of pyruvate on pyruvate dehydrogenase kinase of rat heart. Mol Cell Biochem 149:71–75
47. Felig P (1973) The glucose-alanine cycle. Metabolism 22:179–207
48. Pison CM, Chauvin C, Fontaine E, et al (1995) Mechanism of gluconeogenesis inhibition in rat hepatocytes isolated after in vivo hypoxia. Am J Physiol 268:E965–E973
49. Lovejoy J, Newby FD, Gebhart SS, DiGirolamo M (1992) Insulin resistance in obesity is associated with elevated basal lactate levels and diminished lactate appearance following intravenous glucose and insulin. Metabolism 41:22–27
50. Vettor R, Lombardi AM, Fabris R, et al (1997) Lactate infusion in anesthetized rats produces insulin resistance in heart and skeletal muscles. Metabolism 46:684–690
51. Péronnet F, Burelle Y, Massicotte D, Lavoie C, Hillaire-Marcel C (1997) Respective oxidation of 13C-labeled lactate and glucose ingested simultaneously during exercise. J Appl Physiol 82:440–446
52. Tascopoulos M, Magistretti PJ (1996) Metabolic coupling between glia and neurons. J Neurosci 16:877–885
53. Magistretti PJ, Pellerin L (1996) Cellular bases of brain energy metabolism and their relevance to functional brain imaging: evidence for a prominent role of astrocytes. Cereb Cortex 6:50–61
54. Magistretti PJ, Pellerin L (1996) Cellular mechanisms of brain energy metabolism. Relevance to functional brain imaging and to neurodegenerative disorders. Ann NY Acad Sci 777:380–387

Metabolism

Skeletal Muscle In Critical Illness

R. Keays

Introduction

In critical illness profound changes in protein metabolism occur. Skeletal muscle proteins are broken down in order to provide amino acids for alternative protein synthesis, most notably the acute phase proteins which are synthesized by the liver in large quantities. Muscle protein is also an energy reserve and the amino acids made available by proteolysis are used as oxidizable fuels. In whole body terms there is an increase in protein synthesis accompanied by an even greater increase in protein breakdown [1] reflected by a negative nitrogen balance.

The concept of nitrogen balance reflects the dominance of synthesis or degradation but not the underlying metabolic processes. This chapter will explore some of those processes and discuss some more recent perspectives on the problem of skeletal muscle catabolism in the critically ill.

Skeletal Muscle Protein Turnover

Skeletal muscle constitutes 45–60% of the total body protein pool in a healthy male [2] and, as with all proteins, there is constant turnover. This protein turnover is merely the balance between protein synthesis and protein degradation and the precise cellular mechanisms governing these processes in the myocyte are far from clear. It has been estimated that the rate of muscle protein catabolism in healthy individuals is between 1.5–2.2% per day [3] which is matched by a similar level of protein synthesis in the steady state. In situations where insufficient nutrients are supplied, the early adaptive response by skeletal muscle is to release amino acids. This is due to a marked rise in proteolysis accompanied by a fall in protein synthesis. A rise in urinary nitrogen excretion is noted within 24–48 hours. These changes are a response to falling insulin levels in the presence of glucocorticoids.

The problem of skeletal muscle loss and negative nitrogen balance is commonly encountered in intensive care unit (ICU) patients where a variety of promoters of catabolism are held to be responsible [4]. The most consistent finding in a study of muscle biopsies from ICU patients is that intracellular free glutamine and muscle protein concentrations fall [5]. Some studies have characterized different patterns of disruption of muscle protein balance. Trauma, whether surgical or accidental, results in decreased muscle protein synthesis [6], which is reflected in the reduction in polyribosomal content [7], whereas protein degradation is unaffected unless sepsis supervenes [8]. Losses of 4–8 g are common in septic or trauma patients and may even approach up to 20 g of nitrogen per day – which equates to 600 g of lean tissue mass [9]. This reduction in lean tissue mass, when sustained, is associated with diminished immune responsiveness, increased infection rates, delayed tissue healing and, inevitably, reduced skeletal muscle function [10]. Furthermore, in contrast to the fasting state, nutritional support does not lead to a reversal in the catabolic state [11]. Whilst early enteral feeding is undoubtedly beneficial in terms of improving gut blood flow and reducing mucosal permeability [12], and various feed modifications may promote greater immunocompetence [13], little evidence exists for successful prevention of protein catabolism by dietary means in the critically ill.

Functional Role of Muscle Proteolysis

Skeletal muscle protein degradation may have an important physiologic function in the context of critical illness, although this assumption is by no means proven. Amino acids are made available to the liver for hepatic gluconeogenesis or are used as oxidizable substrates themselves. This capacity to provide energy from muscle-derived amino acids may be of crucial importance, particularly to the rapidly dividing cells of the immune system and the gastrointestinal tract. Whether this is an important function is difficult to demonstrate. Intuitively a lack of available energy substrate would seem to be detrimental, however, exogenous provision of the appropriate amino acids does not dramatically improve the outcome in critical illness, as discussed in the previous section.

Amino acids mobilized from muscle are also used in the synthesis of other proteins, particularly the acute phase proteins. However, acute phase proteins contain a high proportion of aromatic amino acids whereas skeletal muscle proteins contain comparatively little. Therefore, in order to provide sufficient substrate for an acute phase response, a disproportionate degree of skeletal muscle protein may be degraded. If this is indeed a physiologically useful response by the body to severe sepsis or inflammation some features of the acute phase response need to be borne in mind.

Firstly, it is a highly preserved response in endothermic animals, albeit phylogenetically more primitive than the evolution of immunoglobulins [14]. This implies that it must confer some survival advantage; no examples of gene deletions for C-reactive protein (CRP) have been discovered. Secondly, CRP binds to phosphocholine-containing molecules, which include lipoproteins, membrane phospholipids and microbial products, and this binding is believed to aid phagocytosis. In addition, complexed CRP effectively activates the classical pathway of the complement cascade as well as modulating the function of phagocytic leukocytes. These properties are demonstrable but no definite *in vivo* function has been attributed to CRP [15], which begs the question as to whether the acute phase response is a help or, in view of the capacity for tissue damage, a hindrance? [14]. Finally, if skeletal muscle breakdown in acute illness does indeed occur, in part to provide substrate for alternative protein synthesis, then how is the effector mechanism activated? This last question requires knowledge of the intracellular mechanisms of protein breakdown.

Protein Degradation

Protein degradation involves lysosomal and non-lysosomal enzyme systems [16] (Fig. 1). Lysosomal enzymes such as the cathepsins are activated by a variety of stimuli. Falling insulin levels result in enhanced activity and cathepsin B and D degrade actin and myosin when stimulated to do so by an acidotic milieu [17]. Calcium activated proteases may also play a part in the proteolysis encountered in the critically ill but increasingly the predominant pathway for protein breakdown is recognized as being the ATP-dependent ubiquitin proteasome pathway [18].

When proteins are destined for degradation they become covalently linked to a small protein co-factor, ubiquitin. The ubiquitin-tagged proteins are then attached to a large tubular protein called the proteasome which contains a proteolytic core. The protein is first unfolded and then fed through the tunnel of the proteasome. The proteolytic core then cleaves the protein into small peptide fragments which are released and rapidly hydrolyzed by cytosolic peptidases. It is of interest that protein ubiquitinization requires energy whereas protease hydrolysis of peptide bonds does not, so the reliance on energy-dependent proteolysis may be a mechanism for controlling the degree of protein degradation.

In animal models of fasting, denervation atrophy or acidosis, blocking lysosomal enzymes or the calcium activated proteases did not prevent proteolysis but inhibitors of adenosine triphosphate (ATP) production did [19]. In fasting states, ubiquitin messenger ribonucleic acid (mRNA) levels rise and this rise is synchronous with the rise in protein breakdown [20]. These observations demonstrate that the energy-dependent ubiquitin proteolytic pathway is the most important mechanism determining muscle protein breakdown under these pathophysiologic conditions. Additionally, proteasome subunit mRNA levels are also increased, as is the level of ubiquitin conjugated intracellular proteins. Ubiquitin is a heat-shock protein and the rise appears independently as other heat-shock proteins are not induced. Up-regulation of the ubiquitin pathway, such as has also been observed in animal models of sepsis and cancer, seems to be a specific, common genetic-programmed response to different causes of muscle atrophy.

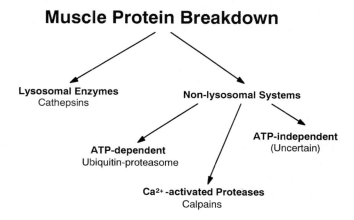

Fig. 1. Pathways of muscle protein breakdown

Hormonal Signals

How this up-regulation of proteolysis is triggered is still unclear, although various hormones and cytokines have been implicated in differing pathologic states. In denervation or disuse atrophy the trigger must either come from within the myocyte or, as is discussed below, the withdrawal of some nerve-derived trophic factor.

The absence of glucocorticoids prevents increased muscle protein breakdown in fasted rats [21]. Therefore, it seems that glucocorticoids display a permissive role in proteolysis and are capable of ubiquitin activation. In addition, they reduce DNA and protein synthesis as well as reducing amino acid uptake by muscle. These catabolic effects are inhibited by the presence of insulin but this inhibition can be overcome if sufficient levels of glucocorticoid are attained. Thyroid hormones also promote proteolysis by maintaining intracellular proteasome and lysosomal enzyme levels. However, thyroid hormones exhibit opposite effects on the body at high or low doses. A minimal level of tri-iodothyronine (T_3) is essential for normal muscle growth but excessive amounts lead to severe muscle wasting.

Cytokine Signals

There is conflicting data on the effects of cytokines on skeletal muscle protein degradation. It has been demonstrated that endotoxin is capable of stimulating proteolysis via the ubiquitin ATP-dependent pathway and this was thought to be as a result of interleukin-1 (IL-1) production. Indeed, some workers have demonstrated that infused IL-1 appears to cause enhanced proteolysis [22] and that tumor necrosis factor (TNF) activates the ubiquitin system [23]. Other work has failed to show increased protein breakdown by IL-1α, IL-1β or TNF, or even combinations of IL-1 and TNF [24, 25].

In spite of this confusion, *in vivo* studies suggest that both IL-1 and TNF infusions can cause protein breakdown in intact animals [26, 27], and can induce increased ubiquitin mRNA levels in much the same way as endotoxin can. The case for cytokine activation of the ubiquitin proteolytic system is therefore good, although other accompaniments of critical illness and sepsis can cause proteolysis independently, such as metabolic acidosis [28] and pyrexia [29].

Whatever the signal pathways may be, cytokines and hormones are not the only factors involved. A recent paper has observed that even in non-septic head injured patients there was an increase in mRNA expression for components of all skeletal muscle proteolytic enzyme systems very soon after the initial injury when catabolic hormone and cytokine production are unlikely to have become significant [30].

Protein Synthesis

The factors responsible for enhanced protein synthesis are discussed below. Obviously the initial requirement for anabolism is the provision of suitable nutrient substrate in sufficient amounts. How the muscle is then able to utilize that substrate is a complex interaction of hormonal factors, muscular activity and nerve-derived trophic factors.

Hormones

Critically ill patients have a higher basal secretion of growth hormone (GH) but re-duced levels of insulin-like growth factor-1 (IGF-1) [31] which implies a relative re-sistance to the effects of growth hormone as IGF-1 is the effector molecule of the GH/IGF-1 axis. IGF acts to stimulate myofibrillar synthesis and inhibit lysosomal enzymes.

Insulin stimulates amino acid transport into muscles and promotes initiation of protein synthesis, predominantly of myofibrillar proteins. In addition insulin in-hibits protein degradation, but only in the presence of the appropriate amino acid substrates [32]. These effects are independent of insulin enhanced glucose uptake [33]. In the critically ill, these anabolic effects are antagonized by the presence of stress induced counter-regulatory hormones, particularly glucocorticoids.

However, in normal physiologic circumstances the most important stimulus to skeletal muscle development is activity [34]. How this is translated into a stimulus for protein synthesis is not known but several investigators have postulated non-cholinergic nerve-derived trophic factors. The background to this hypothesis and the effect of neuromuscular activity on muscle maintenance is discussed below.

Activity-Dependent Phenotypic Expression in Skeletal Muscle

The fact that muscle bulk is dependent on activity has been appreciated for a long time. It is well known that an immobilized limb results in significant muscle wastage in a relatively short period of time [35]. Even in normal individuals, enforced im-mobilization will result in a negative balance for nitrogen, calcium, phosphorus, potassium and sulfur despite adequate nutritional intake [36]. Not only does activ-ity maintain muscle bulk but the activity characteristics of the nerve determine the properties of the target skeletal muscle. Experiments where nerves from slow twitch muscles were made to innervate a fast twitch muscle, resulted in profound changes to the myofilament and other cell structures [37]. Therefore the activity imposed by the motoneurone determines the physiologic and biochemical properties of the muscle [34], and a lack of activity, as in denervation, results in classic changes. It was shown in the early 1970s that maintaining muscular activity by using direct electri-cal stimulation prevented these changes from occurring in denervated muscle [38].

Non-Activity-Dependent Trophic Mechanisms

Nevertheless, in spite of this compelling evidence, it is not solely activity that is re-sponsible for maintaining muscle properties. Other mechanisms of trophic regula-tion exist as is evidenced by the observation that changes to muscle after denerva-tion occur less rapidly the further away from the muscle the nerve is transected. In other words, the longer the transected nerve stump left attached to the muscle, the longer the muscle properties are maintained [39]. Blocking cholinergic transmis-sion by using the action potential blocking tetrodotoxin to ensure complete inactiv-ity leads to much attenuated denervation changes in the muscle which develop more slowly than after surgical nerve transection [40]. Similarly, blocking axonal transport with colchicine results in denervation changes even though neuromuscular transmission is unaffected [41]. This suggests that some nerve-derived, non-cholinergic trophic factor must exist.

What this trophic factor or factors may be is, as yet, unknown although there have been extensive attempts at isolation. Some possible candidates have emerged in recent years; certainly, ciliary neurotrophic factor has been shown to counteract some of the morphologic and functional changes that occur in muscles after denervation [42]. More recently, a family of proteins called the neuregulins, caused by alternative splicing of a single gene transcript, have been demonstrated to have myotrophic properties [43].

Treating the Catabolic State in the Critically Ill

Traditionally, attempts at limiting the catabolic effects of critical illness have involved various feeding regimes to preserve lean muscle mass and other tissues. These attempts have been unsuccessful [11] and the focus of therapeutic efforts has been to manipulate feed constituents to provide supplementation of nutrients more appropriate to the catabolic state encountered in the critically ill.

Before highlighting these newer strategies it is worth noting that hormonal therapy has shown some success in reducing negative nitrogen balance. In spite of the raised levels of GH in the critically ill, it has been observed that GH treatment can attenuate muscle protein breakdown or indeed, under some circumstances, abolish negative nitrogen balance [44]. To date, no evidence of improved skeletal muscle function has yet been revealed and studies are currently being conducted to determine whether improvement can be achieved. Potential disadvantages of GH treatment include hyperglycaemia, insulin resistance, and sodium and water retention. Benign intracranial hypertension was also noted in a group of patients receiving GH to enhance somatic growth [45]. The effect of IGF-1 in critically ill patients has yet to be evaluated.

Insulin is the major anabolic hormone of the body. Reductions in nitrogen losses have been observed in burn and trauma patients treated with insulin [46, 47]. But the risks of hypoglycemia and the unpredictable intracellular shift of certain electrolytes has no doubt made physicians cautious in its use.

Skeletal muscle is the major reservoir of glutamine in the body and this is mobilized during times of physiologic stress, when glutamine becomes a conditionally essential amino acid. It is a necessary component for protein and nucleotide synthesis and acts as a fuel substrate in rapidly dividing cells; one mole of glutamine oxidized generates 30 mmols of ATP as compared with 36 mmols ATP generated by an equimolar amount of glucose. There is conflicting evidence on the nitrogen retaining effects of feeds supplemented with glutamine. In an animal model, glutamine levels correlated positively with muscle protein synthesis and prevented protein breakdown [48]. In the critically ill, supplemental glutamine reverses small bowel atrophy and reduces bacterial translocation but these enteral feeds showed no extra advantage in nitrogen retention over standard enteral feeds [49]. In normals, parenteral glutamine is similarly unable to reduce the normal rate of proteolysis [50].

However, recent work has demonstrated shortened ICU stays and an improvement in long-term survival in critically ill patients who received glutamine supplemented feeds [51].

Branched chain amino acids (BCAA) are degraded in skeletal muscle at a rate greater than that in the liver. The rate of oxidation of these amino acids increases markedly in muscle in catabolic states. These amino acids have been shown to reduce protein breakdown in isolated skeletal muscle [33] and this effect is separate from the glucose sparing effect. Unfortunately, reduced protein breakdown has not been demonstrated in patient trials with BCAA-supplemented feeds and there was no improvement in outcome as a result of such a regime [52].

Arginine has been shown experimentally to enhance protein retention [53] as have medium chain fatty acids [54]. Other supplements, such as omega-3 fatty acids and nucleotides are primarily directed at improving immune function but the former may have some effect on reducing protein breakdown by reducing the levels of catabolic cytokines. A recent trial did not address the problem of protein breakdown but was able to demonstrate some shortening of ICU and hospital stay when using the immunologically designed enteral formula feed [13].

Conclusion

Protein catabolism in the critically ill patient is initiated as a consequence of cytokine and counter-regulatory hormone production, although the effects of muscular disuse and a variety of other factors may also play a part (Fig. 2). In other physiologic and pathologic states characterized by muscle wasting, such as ageing, cancer, human immunodeficiency virus (HIV) disease and steroid therapy, exercise regimes can ameliorate the degree of skeletal muscle loss. Exercise is impractical in the critically ill, but some mechanism of maintaining neuromuscular continuity and activity may be able to reverse the catabolic trend. It has been shown that disuse atrophy can be prevented by electrical Faradic stimulation [35]. Work by a French group [55] has shown that in a population of stable ICU patients, 9 out of 10 of whom were requiring mechanical ventilation, electrical stimulation significantly reduced the magnitude of muscle breakdown and creatinine excretion. This suggests that skeletal muscle loss is partly a result of muscle not being stimulated to retain its protein content.

Another strategy may be to block the ubiquitin system. Recent work suggests tripeptide aldehydes can be used to partially block the ubiquitin proteasome [56, 57]. As a variety of pathologic processes, including sepsis, result in protein breakdown via the ubiquitin-ATP-dependent pathway, blocking the proteasome may prevent this. In the isolated skeletal muscle preparation protein breakdown was prevented with a resultant increase in intracellular ubiquitin-conjugated protein levels. However, although these blocking agents themselves are relatively non-toxic, complete proteasome blocking is undesirable as mitotic cyclins will not be degraded, abnormal proteins may accumulate and class I antigen presentation is inhibited.

The catabolic state has remained resistant to treatment in the critically ill for as long as the problem has been appreciated. Recent developments offer some encouragement that this situation may be about to change. This conclusion has highlighted

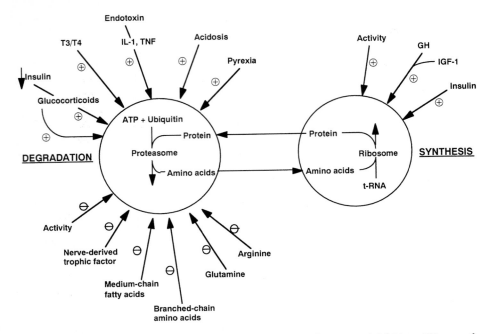

Fig. 2. Factors involved in muscle protein turnover. +: stimulation; −: inhibition; GH: growth hormone; IGF: insulin-like growth factor; IL: interleukin; TNF: tumor necrosis factor; T₄: thyroxine; T₃: tri-iodothyronine

two approaches that have yet to be studied, although greater understanding of the underlying physiology suggests that a multi-therapy approach may offer the best hope.

References

1. Long CL, Jeevandam M, Kim BM, Kinney JM (1977) Whole body protein synthesis and catabolism in septic man. Am J Clin Nutr 30:1340–1344
2. Young VR (1970) The role of skeletal and cardiac muscle in the regulation of protein metabolism. In: Munro H (ed) Mammalian protein metabolism. Academic Press, New York, pp 585–674
3. McKeran RO, Halliday D, Purkiss P (1978) Comparison of human myofibrillar protein catabolic rate derived from 3-methylhistidine excretion with synthetic rate from muscle biopsies during L-[a15N]Lysine infusion. Clin Sci Mol Med 54:471–475
4. Smeets HJ, Kievit J, Harinck HI, Frolich M, Hermans J (1995) Differential effects of counterregulatory stress hormones on serum albumin concentrations and protein catabolism in healthy volunteers. Nutrition 11:423–427
5. Gamrin L, Essen P, Forsberg AM, Hultman E, Wernerman J (1996) A descriptive study of skeletal muscle metabolism in critically ill patients: free amino acids, energy-rich phosphates, protein, nucleic acids, fat, water and electrolytes. Crit Care Med 24:575–583
6. Rennie MJ, Bennegard K, Eden E, Emery PW, Lundholm K (1984) Urinary excretion and efflux from the leg of 3-methylhistidine before and after major surgical operation. Metabolism 33:250–256

7. Vinge O, Edvardsen L, Jensen F, et al (1996) Effect of transcutaneous electrical muscle stimulation on postoperative muscle mass and protein synthesis. Br J Surg 83:360–363

8. Sjolin J, Stjernstrom H, Friman G, Larsson J, Wahren J (1990) Total and net muscle protein breakdown in infection determined by amino-effluxes. Am J Physiol 258:E856–E863

9. Birkhahn RH, Long CL, Fitkin D, Geiger JW, Blakemore WS (1980) Effects of major skeletal trauma on whole body protein turnover in man measured by L-[1,^{14}C]-leucine. Surgery 88:294–300

10. Ziegler TR, Gatzen C, Wilmore DW (1994) Strategies for attenuating protein-catabolic responses in the critically ill. Annu Rev Med 45:459–480

11. Streat SJ, Beddoe AH, Hill GL (1987) Aggressive nutritional support does not prevent protein loss despite fat gain in septic intensive care patients. J Trauma 27:262–266

12. Zaloga GP, Roberts PR (1997) Early enteral feeding improves outcome. In: Vincent JL (ed) Yearbook of intensive care and emergency medicine. Springer-Verlag, Berlin, Heidelberg, New York, pp 701–714

13. Bower RH, Cerra FB, Bershadsky B, et al (1995) Early administration of a formula (Impact) supplemented with arginine, nucleotides and fish oil in intensive care unit patients: Results of a multicenter, prospective, randomized clinical trial. Crit Care Med 23:436–449

14. Ballou SP, Kushner I (1992) C-reactive protein and the acute phase response. Adv Int Med 37:313–336

15. Vigushin DM, Pepys MB, Hawkins PN (1993) Metabolic and scintigraphic studies of radioiodinated human C-reactive protein in health and disease. J Clin Invest 91:1351–1357

16. Hasselgren PO, Fischer JE (1997) The ubiquitin-proteasome pathway: review of a novel intracellular protein breakdown during sepsis and other catabolic conditions. Ann Surg 225:307–316

17. Bird JWC, Schwartz WN, Spanier AM (1977) Degradation of myofibrillar proteins by cathepsins B and D. Acta Biol Med Ger 36:1587–1604

18. Tiao G, Fagan JM, Samuels N, et al (1994) Sepsis stimulates nonlysosomal, energy-dependent proteolysis and increases ubiquitin mRNA levels in rat skeletal muscle. J Clin Invest 94:2255–2264

19. Mitch WE, Goldberg AL (1996) Mechanisms of muscle wasting. N Engl J Med 335:1897–1905

20. Medina R, Wing SS, Haas A, Goldberg AL (1991) Activation of the ubiquitin-ATP-dependent proteolytic system in skeletal muscle during fasting and denervation atrophy. Biomed Biochim Acta 50:347–356

21. Wing SS, Goldberg AL (1993) Glucocorticoids activate the ATP-ubiquitin-dependent proteolytic system in skeletal muscle during fasting. Am J Physiol 264:E668–E676

22. Dinarello CA, Clowes GHA, Gordon AH, Saravis CA, Wolff SM (1984) Cleavage of human interleukin-1: Isolation of a peptide from plasma from febrile humans and activated monocytes. J Immunol 133:1332–1338

23. Garcia-Martinez C, Agell N, Llovera M, Lopez-Soriano FJ, Argiles JM (1993) Tumor necrosis factor-α increases the ubiquitinization of rat skeletal muscle proteins. FEBS Lett 323:211–214

24. Goldberg AL, Kettelhut EC, Furuno K, Fagan JM, Baracos V (1988) Activation of protein breakdown and prostaglandin E2 production in rat skeletal muscle in fever is signaled by a macrophage product distinct from interleukin-1 or other known monokines. J Clin Invest 81:1378–1383

25. Moldawer LL, Svaninger G, Gelin G, Lundholm KG (1987) Interleukin-1 and tumor necrosis factor do not regulate protein balance in skeletal muscle. Am J Physiol 253:C766–C773

26. Zamir O, Hasselgren PO, von Allmen D, Fischer JE (1991) The effect of interleukin-1 alpha and the glucocorticoid receptor blocker RU 38486 on total and myofibrillar protein breakdown in skeletal muscle. J Surg Res 50:579–583

27. Hall-Angeras M, Angeras U, Zamir O, Hasselgren PO, Fischer JE (1990) Interaction between corticosterone and tumor necrosis factor stimulated protein breakdown in rat skeletal muscle, similar to sepsis. Surgery 108:460–466

28. Mitch WE, Medina R, Grieber S, et al (1994) Metabolic acidosis stimulates muscle protein degradation by activating the adenosine triphosphate-dependent pathway involving ubiquitin and proteasomes. J Clin Invest 93:2127–2133

29. Baracos V, Wilson EJ, Goldberg AL (1984) Effects of temperature on protein turnover in isolated rat muscle. Am J Physiol 246:C125–C130

30. Mansoor O, Beaufrere B, Boirie Y, et al (1996) Increased mRNA levels for components of the lysosomal, Ca2+-activated, and ATP-ubiquitin-dependent proteolytic pathways in skeletal muscle from head trauma patients. Proc Natl Acad Sci USA 93:2714–2718

31. Ross RJM, Miell J, Feeman E, et al (1991) Critically ill patients have high basal growth hormone levels with attenuated oscillatory activity associated with low levels of insulin-like growth factor-1. Clin Endocrinol 35:47–54

32. Goodman MN, Gomez MD (1987) Decreased myofibrillar proteolysis after refeeding requires dietary protein or amino acids. Am J Physiol 253:E52–E58

33. Fulks RM, Li JB, Goldberg AL (1975) Effects of insulin, glucose and amino acids on protein turnover in rat diaphragm. J Biol Chem 250:290–298

34. Pette D, Vrbova G (1985) Neural control of phenotypic expression in mammalian muscle fibres. Muscle Nerve 8:676–689

35. Gibson JNA, Smith K, Rennie MJ (1988) Prevention of disuse muscle atrophy by means of electrical stimulation: maintenance of protein synthesis. Lancet 8614:767–770

36. Deitrick JE, Whedon GD, Shorr E (1948) Effects of immobilization upon various metabolic and physiological functions of normal men. Am J Med 4:3–36.

37. Buller AJ, Eccles JC, Eccles RM (1960) Interactions between motoneurones and muscles in respect of the characteristic speeds of their responses. J Physiol 150:417–439

38. Lomo T (1976) The role of activity in the control of membrane and contractile properties of skeletal muscle. In: Thesleff S (ed) Motor innervation of muscle. Academic Press, New York, pp 289–321

39. Davey B, Younkin SG (1978) Effect of nerve stump length on cholinesterase in denervated rat diaphragm. Exp Neurol 59:168–175

40. Pestronk A, Drachman DB, Griffin JW (1976) Effect of muscle disuse on acetylcholine receptors. Nature 260:352–353

41. Tiedt TN, Wisler PL, Younkin SG (1977) Neurotrophic regulation of resting membrane potential and acetylcholine sensitivity in rat extensor digitorum longus muscle. Exp Neurol 57:766–791

42. Helgren ME, Squinto SP, Davis HL, et al (1994) Trophic effects of ciliary neurotrophic factor on denervated skeletal muscle. Cell 76:493–504

43. Florini JR, Samuel DS, Ewton DZ, Kirk C, Sklar RM (1996) Stimulation of myogenic differentiation by neuregulin, glial growth factor 2. J Biol Chem 271:12699–12702

44. Voerman HJ, Strack van Schijndel RJM, Groeneveld ABJ, et al (1992) Effects of recombinant human growth hormone in patients with severe sepsis. Ann Surg 216:648–655

45. Malozowski S, Tanner LA, Wysowski D, Fleming GA (1993) Growth hormone, insulin-like growth factor-1 and benign intracranial hypertension. N Engl J Med 329:665–666

46. Hinton P, Allison SP, Littlejohn S, Lloyd J (1971) Insulin and glucose to reduce catabolic response to injury in burned patients. Lancet 703:767–769

47. Woolfson AMJ, Heatley RV, Allison SP (1979) Insulin to inhibit protein catabolism after injury. N Engl J Med 300:14–17

48. MacLennan PA, Brown RA, Rennie MJ (1987) A positive relationship between protein synthetic rate and intracellular glutamine concentration in perfused rat skeletal muscle. FEBS Lett 215:187–191

49. Long CL, Nelson KM, DiRienzo DB, et al (1995) Glutamine supplementation of enteral nutrition: Impact on whole body protein kinetics and glucose metabolism in critically ill patients. J Parenter Enteral Nutr 19:470–476

50. Hankard RG, Haymond MW, Darmaun D (1996) Effect of glutamine on leucine metabolism in humans. Am J Physiol 271:E748–E754

51. Griffiths RD, Jones C, Palmer TEA (1997) Six-month outcome of critically ill patients given glutamine-supplemented parenteral nutrition. Nutrition 13:295–302

52. Bower RH, Muggia-Sullam M, Vallgren S, et al (1986) Branched chain amino acid-enriched solutions in the septic patient: a randomized prospective trial. Ann Surg 203:13–20

53. Kirk SJ, Barbul A (1990) Role of arginine in trauma, sepsis and immunity. J Parenter Enteral Nutr 14:226S–229S

54. Maiz A, Yamazaki K, Sobrado J, et al (1984) Protein metabolism during total parenteral nutrition in injured rats using medium-chain triglycerides. Metabolism 33:901–909

55. Bouletreau P, Patricot MC, Saudin F, Guiraud M, Mathian B (1987) Effects of intermittent electrical stimulations on muscle catabolism in intensive care patients. J Parenter Enteral Nutr 11:552–555

56. Rock KL, Gramm C, Rothstein L, et al (1994) Inhibitors of the proteasome block the degradation of most cell proteins and the generation of peptides presented on MHC class 1 molecules. Cell 78:761–771

57. Tawa NE, Odessey R, Goldberg AL (1997) Inhibitors of the proteasome reduce the accelerated proteolysis in atrophying rat skeletal muscle. J Clin Invest 100:197–203

Metabolic Requirements of the Neurosurgical Patient

J. Piek and M. Piek

Introduction

Feeding the critically ill neurosurgical patient is a unique challenge in neurosurgical intensive care management. Although it is not an initial priority in the first hours after an acute lesion of the central nervous system (CNS), it becomes more and more important in the later course of the illness. As the clinical course of these patients is difficult to predict, they, as a rule, should not be allowed to remain in unopposed starvation for prolonged periods of time. Early, adequate, and aggressive nutritional support will help to overcome the adverse effects of catabolism, and will improve wound healing and immunological competence, resulting in a better outcome.

Patients with acute CNS lesions have to overcome both central and systemic insults. Adverse metabolic effects of such lesions are mediated both neuronally and chemically. They have been studied extensively during the last 20 years and include increased energy expenditure, increased protein turn-over with increased renal nitrogen loss and negative nitrogen balance, as well as altered glucose metabolism, and increased lipolysis. Nutritional support in this situation must meet the patient's requirements and create a normal 'internal milieu' to minimize secondary brain injury.

Preoperative Nutritional Status

The two variables that determine the rate at which malnutrition will develop are the pre-existing nutritional status and the degree of hypermetabolism. Nutritional assessment is the first step in the treatment of malnutrition, and once the decision to commence nutritional support has been made, an initial patient evaluation should be performed. As no single indicator can characterize the nutritional status of an individual patient, a number of tests have been developed to characterize the nutritional profile of the patient. We performed a battery of tests (Table 1) in 42 patients with brain tumors and found no nutritional risk in these patients (unpublished data).

Energy Expenditure

Hypermetabolism is the uniform response to trauma in general, as well as to acute lesions of the CNS. In patients with midline lesions, hypermetabolism may even con-

Table 1. Pre-operative nutritional status in 42 patients with supratentorial brain tumors.

Parameter	Mean	Median	± Std.
Body Weight (% opt. BW)	84.17	83.61	14.77
Total Plasma Protein (g/l)	71.21	71.50	4.84
Serum Albumin (g/l)	41.47	40.48	4.94
Pre-Albumin (g/l)	0.378	0.4	0.13
Retinol-Binding Protein (g/l)	0.057	0.054	0.018
α1-Globulin (g/l)	3.025	2.970	0.762
α2-Globulin (g/l)	10.22	10.07	3.05
β-Globulin (g/l)	13.01	12.50	2.73
γ-Globulin (g/l)	14.61	14.47	2.95
Renal Nitrogen-loss (g/day)	11.06	9.87	6.56
Total Free Plasma Amino Acids (µmol/l)	3155.50	3183.90	528.08

tinue for years after trauma [1]. During the sixties, energy requirements in patients with multiple trauma (especially with additional head injuries) were frequently overestimated resulting in excessive nutrient administration [2]. Excessive nutritional support, however, may lead to severe disturbances of metabolism with hyperglycemia, hyperosmolarity, fluid and electrolyte imbalance, and increased CO_2 production. Since Wesemann's studies in 1975 [3] it is beyond doubt that "energy requirements of most neurosurgical patients rarely exceed 3000 kcal/day and are comparable to those of other traumatised patients".

Numerous studies have measured resting energy expenditure (REE) in patients with head injuries [1, 3–15]. REE levels of 30–50% above normal have been found in these patients for approximately two weeks post-injury. It has been suggested that sedated patients have the lowest metabolic rates, whereas those with decerebrate activity have the highest ones [7, 8, 10, 12, 13].

The influence of steroid administration on REE has also been studied. Greenblatt et al. [16] suggested that steroid administration in patients with head injuries increases REE, but Robertson et al. [17] could not demonstrate a significant difference.

Our own studies suggest that not only the depth of coma (Fig. 1) but also the underlying disease itself (Fig. 2) significantly influence REE [18, 19]. Patients with head injuries show a higher REE than patients with spontaneous intracranial hemorrhages, whereas REE is lowest after brain tumor surgery. Deeper coma usually results in lower REE values in patients with head injuries.

The cause for REE increase in these patients has not been yet explained. Bucci et al. [20] found a strong correlation between raised intracranial pressure and increased REE. It remains unclear whether this is an indirect or a direct effect as hormonal changes are frequently observed after head injuries [21], and may be caused by direct lesions of the hypothalamus and the pituitary gland itself [22].

All authors who have measured energy expenditure by indirect calorimetry agree that the individual REE of a patient with an acute CNS lesion varies extremely. Standard formulas usually under- or over-estimate energy expenditure in such situations [23]. Currently, this increased metabolic rate is best managed by providing

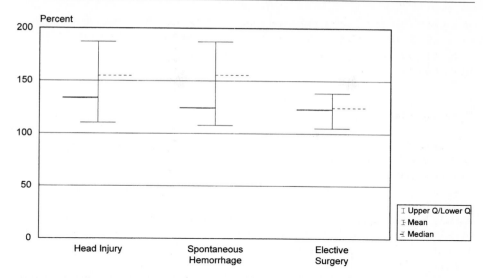

Fig. 1. Resting energy expenditure in various neurosurgical patient groups (values are given in percent of calculated basal metabolic rate): With wide individual variation, comatose patients with head-injuries or spontaneous hemorrhages show comparable REE values, whereas the REE in comatose patients after elective surgery is significantly lower

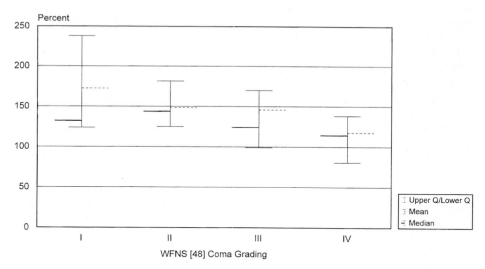

Fig. 2. Resting energy expenditure (REE) in comatose patients (values are given in percent of calculated basal metabolic rate): Patients in deeper coma have lower REE values

nutrition in amounts matched to measured energy expenditure. Clifton et al. [24] developed a nomogram for estimation of energy expenditure in patients with head injuries including the Glasgow Coma Scale score and the number of days since injury as most predictive variables. From our own studies, we conclude that calculating REE from sex, weight, depth of coma, and diagnosis gives adequate results for routine clinical use, with an energy balance ranging from $-2\%-+16\%$ compared to measured REE (unpublished data).

Nitrogen Balance

Among the many metabolic changes seen in the critically ill, the most important are those involving amino acid nitrogen. Protein is mobilized from the skeletal muscle, the gut mucosa, short-lived serum proteins, and the connective tissue into the extracellular amino acid pool. It is then mainly used for the hepatic synthesis of acute-phase proteins (immune regulation, wound healing) and of gluconeogenetic precursors. Efflux of skeletal muscle amino acids may result in muscle weakness with difficulties in weaning and mobilizing a patient. Severe catabolism, characterized by increased protein turnover, depressed levels of short-lived serum proteins, efflux of skeletal amino-acids, increased renal nitrogen loss, and disturbances in free plasma amino-acids is usually also observed after isolated head injuries [4-6, 8, 10, 12, 25-28], spontaneous intracranial hemorrhages [29], and elective intracranial surgery (unpublished data). Daily renal nitrogen loss is highest on days 2-4. Catabolism is also present in patients with spontaneous intracranial hemorrhages and after elective surgery (Fig. 3). A positive nitrogen balance in the acute phase can usually not be attained. The goal of nutritional support in this situation is to minimize negative nitrogen balance in order to maintain organ function and structure. This can be achieved by administration of non-protein together with protein calories. Administration of recombinant growth hormone may improve immunological compe-

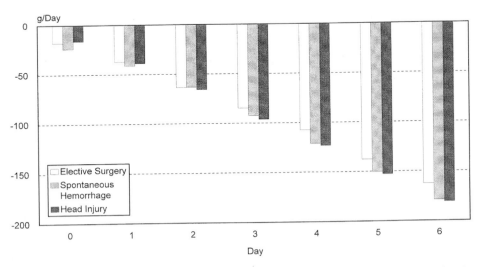

Fig. 3. Cumulative renal nitrogen loss in various neurosurgical patient groups: Renal nitrogen-loss is identical in all groups regardless of the underlying disease

tence both in patients fed parenterally [30] and enterally [31] but may fail to improve negative nitrogen balance [30]. Clifton et al. [24] found that the level of calorie and protein intake influences nitrogen excretion stronger than any other variable. Similar changes for patients with multiple injuries have been found by Behrendt et al. [32]. This study also showed that the level of protein intake had a much higher influence on the cumulative nitrogen balance than the caloric intake. The authors concluded that a daily administration of 0.2 g nitrogen/kg body weight (i.e., 1.25 g amino-acids/kg body weight) is the optimum in this situation. However, administration of amino acids is limited by the renal capacity for nitrogen transport: if daily administration of amino acids exceeds 1.75 mg/kg body weight, serum nitrogen can accumulate. This dose is also safe in most neurosurgical patients (unpublished observations).

Amino Acids

Even preoperatively, patients with brain tumors can show individual disturbances of their free amino acid pattern [33], especially when receiving steroids. In the post-operative/post-traumatic period a variable pattern is found. We measured free plasma amino acids for six days in patients with head injuries, spontaneous hemorrhages, and following elective surgery who received total parenteral nutrition. The changes can be summarized as follows:

Free Amino Acids in Elective Surgery: On day 0 (day of surgery) most plasma amino acids were normal except elevated levels for glutamine (GLU) and phenylalanine (PHE). This was followed by an increase of all amino acids until day 6 [exception: tyrosine (TYR) and histidine (HIS)].

Free Amino Acids in Head Injury: Patients with head injuries also showed significant changes in the pattern of free plasma amino acids. Initially an elevation of leucine (LEU), arginine (ARG), GLU, and PHE was observed followed by an additional increase of threonine (THR) and serine (SER) on day 2 and 4. Gross changes were observed on day 6 with elevated levels of 8 amino acids [lysine (LYS), THR, ARG, TYR, ORN, GLU, PHE, methionine (MET)].

Free Amino Acids in Spontaneous Intracranial Hemorrhage: Patients with spontaneous intracranial hemorrhages had only minor changes in the pattern of free plasma amino acids. On admission only valine (VAL) was depressed and PHE was elevated. On days 2 and 4 elevated levels of PHE and THR were observed. All amino acids showed normal levels on day 6.

Glucose Metabolism

Glucose is an obligate energy source for the brain as well as for red blood cells, and the renal medulla. Under normal conditions, the liver produces glucose either by glycogenolysis or gluconeogenesis from glucose precursors such as lactate, glycerol, and amino acids. Depending on the oxygen tension of the tissue glucose is metabolized either aerobically or anaerobically to produce adenosine triphosphate (ATP).

Hypoxic areas of the brain metabolize glucose by anaerobic pathways resulting in intracellular lactacidosis with secondary insult to the injured areas. Hyperglycemia is a common observation following acute CNS lesions. Although doubted in some studies [34] most clinical and experimental studies have shown that hyperglycemia increases post-traumatic brain edema and worsens outcome. Robertson et al. [35] randomized patients with head-injuries into a saline/amino acid versus a glucose 5%/amino acid group. From their findings (increased brain oxidation of ketone bodies and decreased oxidation of glucose) they concluded that a nutritional regimen with amino acids and saline during the first 5 post-traumatic days should be preferred. In our opinion these preliminary findings need further evaluation by major outcome studies. Our current procedure is to apply an amount of non-protein energy (70% glucose, 30% fat) that matches the patient's energy expenditure. Blood glucose levels should not exceed 200 mg/dl and should be checked every 4 hours.

Fat

Fat is the major energy source during illness and injury. Unlike protein and glucose, fat metabolism has been hardly studied in patients with acute CNS lesions. According to Little and coworkers [36] fat is the predominant source of energy during the first 6 post-traumatic hours in traumatized patients. Our studies were performed during the later course of injury and showed RQ values around 0.8 demonstrating that fat as well as glucose serve as energy sources (unpublished data).

Problems resulting from overfeeding patients with glucose alone have prompted the use of mixed-fuel systems for parenteral nutrition. Emulsions of long-chain, polyunsaturated triglycerides (LCT) were developed in Sweden in the early sixties. Concern over reticulo-endothelial system dysfunction with improper use of these emulsions has led to the development of medium-chain triglyceride (MCT) emulsions which are now widely used in Europe. Our studies showed no side effects in patients with spontaneous intracranial hemorrhages when given as part of a mixed-fuel system in approximately 20–30% of total calories (unpublished data). Calon et al. [37] could even demonstrate some positive effects on short-lived serum protein levels with LCT/MCT mixtures, Adolph et al. [38] demonstrated beneficial effects on the pattern of fatty acids itself.

Parenteral versus Enteral Nutrition

Nutritional support may be administered either enterally, parenterally peripherally, or parenterally via a central line [total parenteral nutrition (TPN)]. Administering nutritional support via a peripheral vein is usually limited by its osmotic tolerance (max. 600–900 mOsm/l). Given this consideration and the high energy requirements of most neurosurgical patients, the alternative TPN versus enteral nutrition remains. There is a long-lasting debate whether TPN or enteral nutrition is preferred for neurosurgical patients in the immediate postoperative/post-traumatic period. Obviously, the enteral route is the more physiologic, is less expensive, and has a lower risk, compared to TPN via a central venous catheter. It may also be associated with an accelerated normalization of nutritional status [39].

While gastrointestinal absorption is usually not altered in neurosurgical patients, gastric emptying is often delayed [40] partly due to prolonged sedation [41]. Gastric feeding is often not well tolerated in this group and it is difficult to apply an amount of nutrition that matches the patient's needs [41–44]. A significant risk of aspiration and pneumonia must also be taken into account [45]. Rapp and co-workers [42] even suggested that TPN may improve outcome in neurosurgical patients. Since the majority of acute patients usually have central venous catheters in place for monitoring purposes, we prefer TPN in the early post-traumatic/postoperative period and start enteral feeding from the 4th post-traumatic day.

Nutritional assessment in the early period is extremely difficult. Adaequate nutritional support is best achieved by measuring energy expenditure (indirect calorimetry) and calculating daily nitrogen balance. If a patient receives artificial nutritional support, close metabolic monitoring is necessary to avoid side-effects such as hyperglycemia and ketoacidosis.

Conclusion

Patients with acute CNS lesions sustain a systemic response to stress which may cause a secondary injury to the already severely traumatized brain. There is good evidence that this systemic response usually lasts longer than that occurring in multiple trauma patients without head injury. In some cases (midline lesions), it may even last for months or years. Nutrient support alone cannot completely counteract this response but, as important supportive therapy, it will help to create a normal 'milieu interne' for CNS regeneration and repair.

Nutritional assessment in the early post-injury period is extremely difficult. Adequate nutritional support is best achieved by measuring energy expenditure (indirect calorimetry) and calculating daily nitrogen balance. If a patient receives artificial nutritional support, close metabolic monitoring is necessary to avoid side effects such as hyperglycemia and ketoacidosis.

Future studies should concentrate on the question of enteral versus parenteral feeding, the role of modulating the hormonal stress response and the metabolism of fat in these patients.

References

1. Frowein RA, Harrer G (1948) Über Grundumsatzsteigerungen und deren Beziehung zur Größe des 3. Ventrikels und zum Commotionssyndrom. Wein Klin Wochenschr 60:79–81
2. Dudrick SJ, Wilmore DW, Vars HM, et al (1968) Long-term total parenteral nutrition with growth, development, and positive nitrogen balance. Surgery 64:134–142
3. Wesemann W (1975) Permanent registration of the energy transformation in patients with skull-brain injuries and brain tumors. Infusionsther Klin Ernähr 2:365–376
4. Clifton GL, Robertson CS, Grossman RG, et al (1984) The metabolic response to severe head injury. J Neurosurg 60:687–696

5. Deutschman CS, Konstantinides FN, Raup S, et al (1986) Physiological and metabolic response to isolated closed-head injury. Part 1: Basal metabolic state: correlations of metabolic and physiological parameters with fasting and stressed controls. J Neurosurg 64:89–98

6. Deutschman CS, Konstantinides FN, Raup S, et al (1987) Physiological and metabolic response to isolated closed-head injury. Part 2: Effects of steroids on metabolism. Potentiation of protein wasting and abnormalities of substrate utilization. J Neurosurg 66:388–395

7. Fruin AH, Taylon C, Pettis MS (1986) Caloric requirements in patients with severe head injuries. Surg Neurol 25:25–28

8. Gadisseux P, Ward JD, Young HF, et al (1984) Nutrition and the neurosurgical patient. J Neurosurg 60:219–232

9. Long CL, Schaffel N, Geiger JW, et al (1979) Metabolic response to injury and illness: estimation of energy and protein needs from indirect calorimetry and nitrogen balance. J Parenter Enteral Nutr 3:452–456

10. Robertson CS, Clifton GL, Grossman RG (1984) Oxygen utilization and cardiovascular function in head-injured patients. Neurosurgery 15:307–314

11. Touho H, Karasawa J, Nakagawara J, et al (1987) Measurement of energy expenditure in the acute stage of head injury. No To Shinkei 39:739–744

12. Young B, Ott L, Norton J, et al (1985) Metabolic and nutritional sequelae in the non-steroid treated head injury patient. Neurosurgery 17:784–791

13. Dempsey DT, Guenter P, Mullen JL, et al (1985) Energy expenditure in acute trauma to the head with and without barbiturate therapy. Surg Gynecol Obstet 160:128–134

14. Moore R, Najarian MP, Konvolinka CW (1989) Measured energy expenditure in severe head trauma. J Trauma 29:1633–1636

15. Borzotta AP, Pennings J, Papasadero B, et al (1994) Enteral versus parenteral nutrition after severe closed head injury. J Trauma 37:459–468

16. Greenblatt SH, Long CL, Blakemore WS, et al (1989) Catabolic effect of dexamethasone in patients with major head injuries. J Parenter Enteral Nutr 13:373–376

17. Robertson CS, Clifton GL, Goodman JC (1985) Steroid administration and nitrogen excretion in the head-injured patient. J Neurosurg 63:714–718

18. Piek J, Brachwitz K, Bock WJ (1988) The energy consumption of patients with craniocerebral trauma and spontaneous intracranial hemorrhage in the early postoperative/post-traumatic phase. Anästh Intensivther Notfallmed 23:325–329

19. Piek J, Zanke T, Sprick C, et al (1989) Resting energy expenditure in patients with isolated head injuries and spontaneous intracranial haemmorrhages. Clin Nutr 8:347–351

20. Bucci MN, Dechert RE, Arnoldi DK, et al (1988) Elevated intracranial pressure associated with hypermetabolism in isolated head trauma. Acta Neurochir Wien 93:133–136

21. Chiolero R, Schutz Y, Lemarchand T, et al (1989) Hormonal and metabolic changes following severe head injury or noncranial injury. J Parenter Enteral Nutr 13:5–12

22. Crompton MR (1971) Hypothalamic lesions following closed head injury. Brain 94:165–172

23. Sunderland PM, Heilbrun MP (1992) Estimating energy expenditure in traumatic brain injury: comparison of indirect calorimetry with predictive formulas. Neurosurgery 31:246–252

24. Clifton GL, Robertson CS, Choi SC (1986) Assessment of nutritional requirements of head-injured patients. J Neurosurg 64:895–901

25. Miller SL (1984) The metabolic response to head injury. S Afr Med J 65:90–91

26. Ott L, Young B, McClain C (1987) The metabolic response to brain injury. J Parenter Enteral Nutr 11:488–493

27. Piek J, Lumenta CB, Bock WJ (1985) Protein and amino acid metabolism after severe cerebral trauma. Intensive Care Med 11:192–198

28. Young B, Ott LG, Beard D, et al (1988) The acute-phase response of the brain-injured patient. J Neurosurg 69:375–380

29. Hersio K, Vapalahti M, Kari A, et al (1990) Impaired utilization of exogenous amino acids after surgery for subarachnoid haemorrhage. Acta Neurochir Wien 106:13–17

30. Kudsk KA, Mowatt Larssen C, Bukar J, et al (1994) Effect of recombinant human insulin-like growth factor I and early total parenteral nutrition on immature depression following severe head injury. Arch Surg 129:66–70

31. Behrman SW, Kudsk KA, Brown RO, et al (1995) The effect of growth hormone on nutritional markers in enterally fed immobilized trauma patients. J Parenter Enteral Nutr 19:41–46

32. Behrendt W, Bogatz V, Giani G (1990) Influence of posttraumatic calorie and nitrogen supply upon the cumulative nitrogen balance. Infusionstherapie 17:32–39
33. Piek J, Mahlke L, Bock WJ (1989) Preoperative nutritional status of neurosurgery patients. Infusionstherapie 16:102–105
34. Shapira Y, Artru AA, Cotev S, et al (1992) Brain edema and neurologic status following head trauma in the rat. No effect from large volumes of isotonic or hypertonic intravenous fluids, with or without glucose. Anesthesiology 77:79–85
35. Robertson CS, Goodman JC, Narayan RK, et al (1991) The effect of glucose administration on carbohydrate metabolism after head injury. J Neurosurg 74:43–50
36. Little RA, Stoner HB, Frayn KN (1981) Substrate oxidation shortly after accidental injury in man. Clin Sci 61:789–791
37. Calon B, Pottecher T, Fray A, et al (1990) Long-chain versus medium and long-chain triglyceride-based fat emulsion in parental nutrition of severe head trauma patients. Infusionstherapie 17:246–248
38. Adolph M, Hailer S, Echart J (1995) Serum phospholipid fatty acids in severely injured patients on total parenteral nutrition with medium chain/long chain triglyceride emulsions. Ann Nutr Metab 39:251–260
39. Suchner U, Senftleben U, Eckart T, et al (1996) Enteral versus parenteral nutrition: effects on gastrointestinal function and metabolism. Nutrition 12:13–22
40. Ott L, Young B, Phillips R, et al (1991) Altered gastric emptying in the head-injured patient: relationship to feeding intolerance. J Neurosurg 74:738–742
41. Zielman S, Grote R (1995) The effects of long-term sedation on intestinal function. Anaesthesist 44 (suppl 3):S549–S558
42. Rapp RP, Young B, Twyman D, et al (1983) The favorable effect of early parenteral feeding on survival in head-injured patients. J Neurosurg 58:906–912
43. Twyman D, Young AB, Ott L, et al (1985) High protein enteral feedings: a means of achieving positive nitrogen balance in head injured patients. J Parenter Enteral Nutr 9:679–684
44. Clifton GL, Robertson CS, Contant CF (1985) Enteral hyperalimentation in head injury. J Neurosurg 62:186–193
45. Young B, Ott L, Twyman D, et al (1987) The effect of nutritional support on outcome from severe head injury. J Neurosurg 67:668–676

Enteral Nutrition in the Critically Ill Patient: A Practical Approach

H. L. Chee and D. Bihari

Introduction

It is now well recognized that there is an association between a poor nutritional status and a poor clinical outcome. So while a healthy individual will succumb only after 60 to 80 days of food deprivation [1], it is obvious that starvation as an additional insult in the setting of an episode of critical illness is not an option. What is less obvious however, is how nutritional support should be best provided in critical care practice.

Why Enteral Nutrition?

The problem is further complicated by a scarcity of evidence that nutritional support improves survival. The Veterans Affairs (VA) perioperative total parenteral nutrition (TPN) study [2] is the largest prospective randomized trial of nutrition support conducted to date. It included 395 malnourished patients and demonstrated that 33 severely malnourished patients (weight loss greater than 10% in the preceding 3 months, albumin less than 28 g/l on admission to hospital) undergoing elective surgical procedures benefited from 10 days of perioperative intravenous nutrition. However, the vast majority of patients (362 patients) were not severely malnourished on entry into the study and overall there was a significant increase in the incidence of infectious complications in patients receiving TPN (14% compared to 6% in the control group; relative risk 2.20, 95% confidence interval 1.19–4.05). It is important to remember that this was a study of perioperative parenteral nutrition and hence, its relevance to intensive care practice is questionable.

In contrast, more data are available comparing parenteral nutrition with enteral nutrition in a specific group of patients requiring intensive care, those suffering an episode of severe trauma [3–5]. These studies have demonstrated better outcomes in those patients who are fed enterally, septic morbidity being significantly less than those who are fed parenterally. Yet this specific diagnostic group are distinguished by their relatively young age (average age less than 40 years) and their good prognosis making it difficult to apply these results more widely to the general intensive care unit (ICU) population.

There are a number of reasons why enteral nutrition may be beneficial in reducing septic complications. Firstly, gut mucosal mass and function is better maintained with enteral nutrition [6]. Gut mucosal atrophy may result in bacterial translocation

[7] although at present there is insufficient evidence for this phenomenon occurring to any great extent in humans. Enteral feeding may also be needed for the gut to secrete immunoglobulin A [8]. Hypermetabolism, secondary to the stress response, seems to be attenuated by early enteral feeding [9]. Finally, gut feeding may simply stimulate peristalsis, maintain gut flora and prevent overgrowth of pathogens [10].

When to Start Enteral Feeding?

Having determined that enteral nutrition is the preferred route of feeding critically ill patients, it appears that one should start early in order to reap the full benefits. Moore et al. [11] demonstrated in a meta-analysis that early enteral nutrition in postoperative patients was associated with fewer complications than early parenteral nutrition. But how early is "early"? Grahm et al. [12] found that starting small bowel feeds within 36 hours of severe head injury reduced the frequency of sepsis, while feeding made no difference if it was commenced 4 to 5 days after injury. It therefore seems that feeding should begin within 48 hours of injury but only after the patient has been fully resuscitated and cardiovascular stability has been achieved [13].

How to Start?

In a survey by Heyland et al. [14], only 74% of patients eligible to receive enteral nutrition in the ICU were started on it. The reasons for this were varied and included: Absence of bowel sounds; high nasogastric aspirates; other supposed contraindications to enteral nutrition; and tolerance of oral nutrition. Lack of any apparent reason accounted for 5% of the cases not started on enteral nutrition. Widespread misconceptions still remain about perceived contraindications to starting feeds. The absence of bowel sounds is commonly interpreted as indicating the presence of an adynamic bowel. Bowel sounds are produced by movement of intraluminal gas and fluid from the stomach into the small bowel during gastric emptying and peristalsis. Patients who are intubated and ventilated, sedated or paralyzed, do not swallow air and therefore may not have bowel sounds in the presence of a functioning gut [15]. Free drainage of the stomach by a nasogastric tube is another factor preventing the movement of gas from the stomach into the small bowel. It has also been thought that early feeding (within 4 hours of return from the operating room) is contraindicated in patients who have undergone bowel surgery even though there is little evidence for this and now several studies suggest the opposite [16, 17]. Acute pancreatitis is also not a contraindication to early enteral nutrition [18], such patients having been fed enterally with less complications than with parenteral nutrition. In fact, absolute contraindications to enteral nutrition are few with gastrointestinal obstruction, high output enterocutaneous fistulae, and unprotected, recent bowel anastomosis being the most commonly encountered cases.

Failure to establish patients on enteral nutrition using the nasogastric route is usually related to gastroparesis, the causes of which include medications (such as opioids), hyperglycemia [19] and brain injury [20]. Prokinetic agents which can be used to overcome gastroparesis include macrolides, for example, erythromycin. This drug has been shown to be very effective in the treatment of diabetic gastroparesis but data on its use in the ICU is scarce. An alternative prokinetic is cisapride, which increases the physiologic release of acetylcholine from postganglionic nerve endings of the myenteric plexus. It should be remembered that there have been reports of torsades de pointes or prolonged QT intervals in patients who were simultaneously taking cisapride and medications of the imidazole class or macrolide antibiotics [21].

ICUs which have an established protocol for enteral feeding are usually much more successful in getting their patients established early on enteral nutrition and achieving the required nutritional goals. In a recent study, Adam and Batson [22] surveyed 5 ICUs and found that the percentage of optimal enteral feed delivered was $78 \pm 31\%$ in ICUs with a feeding protocol compared with $66 \pm 34\%$ in those without. Other reasons preventing delivery of feeds were gut dysfunction and elective stoppage for procedures. It should be emphasized that meeting conventional nutritional goals (for example, achieving a certain energy or protein intake over a 24 hour period) is not the prime aim of "early enteral nutrition" [23]. Rather, it is the provision of specific nutrients within the lumen of the gut early on in critical illness in order to maintain splanchnic blood flow and prevent repeated episodes of ischemia and reperfusion. In terms of specific nutrients having pharmacologic or immunologic effects, then the issue of "dosing" becomes important and it is not unreasonable to assume that unless a critical amount of the compound is absorbed relatively early on in the natural history of the illness, then that compound is unlikely to have any specific effect.

There are many ways to establish the access route. Most patients begin by having a nasogastric tube inserted at the time of admission. Alternative routes for delivery of enteral nutrition are shown in Table 1. As in all things, there are complications associated with these techniques of access (Table 2) but with appropriate care and attention, complication rates can be kept very low. In our experience it is possible to feed the vast majority of patients via the nasogastric route providing care is taken in avoiding over sedation with opiates, and prokinetics are liberally prescribed.

Bolus versus Continuous Feeding

There is no evidence to show which method of enteral feeding is superior. Bolus feeding into the stomach is more physiologic but requires a more time-consuming

Table 1. Routes of access for delivery of enteral nutrition

Route	Methods of Placement
Nasogastric	via nasopharynx
Nasojejunal	endoscopy, image intensification at time of laparotomy
Percutaneous endoscopic gastrostomy/jejunostomy	endoscopic, through anterior abdominal wall
Feeding gastrostomy/jejunostomy	open surgical procedure or via laparoscope

Table 2. Complications of feeding conduits

- inability to pass tube to stomach or duodenum
- perforation of pharynx, oesophagus, trachea, bronchus
- misplacement of tube into trachea, bronchi, pleural space
- erosion of nostril, pharynx, and esophageal, gastric, duodenal mucosa
- migration of tube proximally or distally
- tracheo-esophageal fistula
- knotting and blockage

Gastrostomy/jejunostomy tubes
- dislodgement of tube
- leakage around the tube
- non-healing of fistula tract

feeding schedule. Other problems include greater intolerance in patients with short bowel and malabsorption syndromes and a greater risk of pulmonary aspiration of regurgitated feeds. Patients on jejunostomy feeding are not free of the risk of aspiration [24]. Elevation of the head of the bed can help reduce but not eliminate the risk of aspiration.

Continuous nasogastric feeding is easier to manage and reduces the incidence of abdominal distention, pain and discomfort, and vomiting. There is a danger of bacterial overgrowth of the feed if it is left hanging at room temperature for long periods [25]. It is therefore recommended that feeds be discarded after 12 hours, and that the feeding bags and connection tubing be changed at least once a day.

What to Give?

There are a number of enteral nutrition formulae on the market, each with slightly varying compositions of nutrients, purportedly designed for different nutritional requirements (Table 3).

Special Supplements

In recent years, a number of nutrients have been investigated for their effects on specific metabolic functions. Their effects are still being evaluated in doses that exceed those used in general nutritional support. Opinions differ concerning the quality of the evidence available suggesting that various proprietry feeds unequivocally improve patient outcome in the ICU setting (Table 4). For example, a recent report [26] described a controlled clinical trial of glutamine enriched TPN in critically ill patients. The glutamine treated group had an increased six month survival rate ($p = 0.49$) but the differences described were small and most commentators believe that this requires further confirmation. Immune enhancing enteral feeds (Impact, Novartis Nutrition; Immun Aid, McGraw; Shriner's Modular Tube Feed, Shriner's Burn Institute) have been more extensively studied and a metaanalysis of the various randomized controlled clinical trials has recently been presented [27].

Table 3. Some commonly used enteral nutrition formulae

Formula	Usage	kcals/l	g protein/l	CHO: fat: protein (energy source)
Ensure	general purpose	1060	37	64: 22: 14
Ensure Plus	high calorie when volume limited	1500	55	53: 32: 15
Isocal	general purpose	1100	35	50: 36: 13
Osmolite	general purpose	1060	37	55: 32: 14
Glucerna	low carbohydrate, modified fat, fibre-containing, for better sugar control	1000	42	34: 49: 17
Jevity	high nitrogen, fibre-containing	1060	44	54: 29: 17
Nepro	moderate protein, for patients with renal failure on dialysis	2000	70	43: 43: 14
Osmolite	low osmolality	1060	37	57: 29: 14
Pulmocare	high fat, low carbohydrate, to reduce CO_2 production	1500	63	28: 55: 17
Traumacal	high protein, low carbohydrate, to reduce protein breakdown	1500	82	38: 41: 22
Vivonex	elemental	1000	38	82: 3: 15
Impact	arginine, purine nucleotides and omega$_3$ fatty acids	1000	56	53: 27: 20
ImmunAid	arginine, glutamine, branched chain amino acids, nucleic acids, omega$_3$ fatty acids	1000	80	48: 21: 31
Shriner's Burn Modular Tube Feed	arginine, histidine cysteine, omega$_3$ fatty acids	1016	53.5	66: 13: 21

Table 4. Evidence for nutritional supplements

Nutrient	Study outcomes
Branched-chain amino acids	Intravenous infusion in postoperative and septic patients inhibits the release of endogenous amino acids from muscle, possibly improving nitrogen balance and decreasing muscle protein [36, 37]
Glutamine	Human studies suggest that parenteral administration improves nitrogen balance in patients with sepsis [38], after bone marrow transplant [39], and after surgery [40]
Arginine	Rats fed an arginine-enriched diet survived longer after an intraperitoneal bacterial challenge [41]
Omega-3 fatty acids	Improved survival, reduced infectious complications and reduced immunosuppression secondary to blood transfusion in burns patients [42]
Nucleotides	Nucleotide-enriched diet improved survival of mice with bacterial infections [43]
Growth hormone	Reduced septic complications in burns patients [44]

Polymeric versus Elemental Formulas

Elemental formulas have been recommended in cases of short bowel and malabsorption syndrome. While luminal feeding stimulates mucosal growth of the gastrointestinal tract and therefore prevents translocation of bacteria, animal studies have shown that elemental diets promote bacterial overgrowth and result in greater degrees of translocation [28]. They have not been found to have any advantage over standard polymeric formulas in critically ill patients [29].

CO_2 Retention

In patients with CO_2 retention, who are difficult to wean from mechanical ventilation, Pulmocare (Abbott Laboratories) may be indicated. This is a feed with a high fat:carbohydrate ratio in terms of calorie provision so as to reduce the production of CO_2. Theoretically, such a feed will lead to a reduction in respiratory quotient and thus result in a lower requirement for a given minute ventilation. This effect is both measurable and reproducible and although there is little evidence that it makes a great difference to clinical outcome [30], some would advocate its use in the occasional "difficult" patient.

Immunonutrition

The real interest concerns diets enhanced with nutrients that have been found to boost immune function. Impact (Novartis Nutrition) is an enteral nutrition formula enhanced with omega-3 fatty acids, arginine, and purine nucleotides in the form of ribonucleic acid (RNA). Bower et al. [31] in a multicenter study of 279 evaluable patients (of whom 235 had suffered an episode of trauma) suggested that this formula may have beneficial effects, especially in that group of patients who were septic on study admission. There was a reduction in the length of hospital stay and a significant reduction in the frequency of acquired infections. Atkinson et al. [32] found that this form of immunonutrition did not affect overall mortality in a group of 390 general ICU patients in an intent-to-treat analysis. Nevertheless, in those 50 patients who managed to achieve early enteral nutrition with Impact (the feeding commencing within 48 hours of admission, and successful early enteral nutrition defined *a priori* as the absorption of at least 2.5 L of feed in 72 hours) there was a significant reduction in requirement for mechanical ventilation and an associated reduction in the length of hospital stay compared with 51 patients fed with an isocaloric, isonitrogenous control feed.

Immun Aid (McGaw) is a formula enriched with glutamine, arginine and branch-chain amino acids and as a consequence has a very high nitrogen content. Improved survival has been reported in mice that have been pre-treated with 7 days of Immun Aid after intraperitoneal bacterial challenge [33]. Moore et al. [34] performed a multicenter prospective controlled trial of 114 patients sustaining major torso trauma comparing feeding with Immun Aid versus feeding with Vivonex. Patients receiving the immune enhancing feed had significantly greater increases in their total lymphocyte counts and they developed significantly fewer intrabdominal abscesses and significantly less multiple organ failure. One criticism of this study was the much greater amount of protein administered in the trial feed group which by itself might have accounted for the beneficial effects. A more recent study [35] in 35 trauma patients addressed this issue and confirmed the beneficial effect of Immun Aid (fewer infectious complications, a reduction in the use of antibiotics and a shorter length of stay) as compared with patients fed with a standard isonitrogenous isocaloric control feed and others who were given no feeding at all in the first seven days of their illness.

A meta-analysis of the clinical effects of immunonutrition in intensive care patients was presented at the 1997 European Congress on Intensive Care Medicine in Paris [27]. 13 double blind, prospective, randomized controlled clinical trials were assessed including 705 patients receiving an immune enhancing feed (Impact or Immun Aid) and 688 control patients. Using an intent-to-treat analysis, immunonutrition patients had a significant reduction in ICU infection risk (relative risk 0.8, 95% CI 0.6–1.0) and a shorter ICU (2.3 days 95% CI 0.2–4.5) and hospital (2.6 days 95% 1.2–3.8) length of stay; mortality was unaffected. The strength of this evidence in support of immune enhancing feeds seems impressive compared with the evidence for many other well accepted practices in the ICU (e.g., mechanical ventilation with PEEP) and continued skepticism is difficult to maintain.

Conclusion

While there are still some unanswered questions on how to best provide nutrition to the critically ill patient, a few points have become clear. Enteral nutrition is preferred over parenteral nutrition and should be the route chosen for delivery of nutrition whenever possible. This is because the bulk of the evidence suggests that enteral nutrition is associated with a reduced incidence of septic complications and development of multiorgan failure. Various manipulations of enteral nutritional formulae have been investigated and there is a growing body of evidence that specific combinations of essential nutrients may make a clear difference to the long-term outcome of the critically ill patient. Of course it may be possible to improve the available formulations by the judicious addition of other pharmaconutrients but it seems likely in our opinion that since, after all, "we are what we eat", immunonutrition is here to stay.

References

1. Zimmerman MD, Appadurai K, Scott JG, et al (1997) Survival. Ann Intern Med 127:405–409
2. The Veterans Affairs Total Parenteral Nutrition Cooperative Study Group (1991) Perioperative total parenteral nutrition in surgical patients. N Engl J Med 325:525–532
3. Moore EE, Jones TN (1989) Benefits of immediate jejunostomy feeding after major abdominal trauma – A prospective randomised study. J Trauma 26:874–881
4. Moore FA, Moore EE, Jones TN, et al (1989) TEN versus TPN following major abdominal trauma – Reduced septic morbidity. J Trauma 29:916–923

5. Kudsk KA, Croce MA, Fabian TC, et al (1992) Enteral versus parenteral feeding – effects on septic morbidity after blunt and penetrating abdominal trauma. Ann Surg 215:503–511
6. Lo CW, Walker WA (1989) Changes in the gastrointestinal tract during enteral or parenteral feeding. Nutr Rev 47:193–198
7. Alexander JW (1990) Nutrition and translocation. J Parent Enteral Nutr 14 (suppl 5):170S–174S
8. Alverdy JC, Chi HS, Sheldon GF (1985) The effect of parenteral nutrition on gastrointestinal immunity – The importance of enteral stimulation. Ann Surg 202:681–684
9. Chiarelli A, Enzi G, Casadei A, et al (1990) Very early nutrition supplementation in burned patients. Am J Clin Nutr 51:1035–1039
10. Deitch EA (1988) Does the gut protect or injure patients in the ICU? Perspect Crit Care 1:1–32
11. Moore FA, Feliciano DV, Andrassy RJ, et al (1992) Early enteral feeding, compared with parenteral, reduces postoperative septic complications: The results of a metaanalysis. Ann Surg 216:172–183
12. Grahm TW, Zadrozny DB, Harrington T (1989) The benefits of early enteral jejunal hyperalimentation in the head-injured patient. Neurosurgery 25:729–735
13. Minard G, Kudsk KA (1994) Is early feeding beneficial? How early is early? New Horizons 2:156–163
14. Heyland DK, Cook DJ, Winder B, et al (1993) Enteral nutrition in the critically ill patient: A prospective survey. Crit Care Med 23:1055–1060
15. Shelley MP, Church JJ (1987) Bowel sounds during intermittent positive pressure ventilation. Anaesthesia 42:207–209
16. Reissman P, Teoh T-A, Cohen SM, et al (1995) Is early oral feeding safe after elective colorectal surgery? A prospective randomized trial. Ann Surg 222:73–77
17. Carr CS, Ling E, Boulos P, Singer M (1996) Randomised trial of safety and efficacy of immediate postoperative enteral feeding in patients undergoing gastrointestinal resection. Br Med J 312:869–871
18. McClave SA, Greene LM, Snider HL, et al (1997) Comparison of the safety of early enteral vs parenteral nutrition in mild acute pancreatitis. J Parent Enteral Nutr 21:14–20
19. Barnett JL, Owyang C (1988) Serum glucose concentration as a modulator of interdigestive gastric motility. Gastroenterology 94:739–499
20. Ott L, Young B, Phillips R, et al (1991) Altered gastric emptying in the head-injured patient: Relationship to feeding intolerance. J Neurosurg 74:738–742
21. Wysowski DK, Bacsanyi J (1996) Cisapride and fatal arrhythmia. N Engl J Med 335:290–291
22. Adam S, Batson S (1997) A study of problems associated with the delivery of enteral feed in critically ill patients in five ICUs in the UK. Intensive Care Med 23:261–266
23. Zaloga GP, Roberts P (1994) Permissive underfeeding. New Horizons 2:257–263
24. Weltz CR, Morris JB, Mullen JL (1992) Surgical jejunostomy in aspiration risk patients. Ann Surg 215:140
25. Payne-James JJ, Rana SK, Bray MJ, et al (1992) Retrograde (ascending) bacterial contamination of enteral diet administration systems. J Parent Enteral Nutr 16:369–373
26. Griffiths RD, Jones C, Palmer TEA (1997) Six month outcome of critically ill patients given glutamine supplemented parenteral nutrition. Nutrition 13:295–302
27. Beale R, Bryg D (1997) Clinical effects of immunonutrition on intensive care patients – a meta-analysis. Intensive Care Med 23 (suppl 1):S128 (Abst)
28. Alverdy JC, Aoys BS, Moss GS (1990) Effect of commercially available chemically defined liquid diets on the intestinal microflora and bacterial translocation from the gut. J Parent Enteral Nutr 14:442–447
29. Mowatt-Larssen CA, Brown RO, Wojtysiak SL, et al (1992) Comparison of tolerance and nutritional outcome between a peptide and a standard enteral formula in critically, hypoalbuminaemic patients. J Parent Enteral Nutr 16:20–24
30. Al-Saady NM (1994) Does dietary manipulation influence weaning from artificial ventilation? Intensive Care Med 20:463–465
31. Bower RH, Cerra, FB, Bershadsky B, et al (1995) Early enteral administration of a formula (Impact) supplemented with arginine, nucleotides, and fish oil in intensive care unit patients: results of a multicentre prospective randomized clinical trial. Crit Care Med 23:436–449
32. Atkinson S, Sieffert E, Bihari D (1998) A prospective randomised double-blind controlled clinical trial of enteral immunonutrition in the critically ill. Crit Care Med (in press)

33. Chandra RK, Whang S, Au B (1992) Enriched feeding formula and immune responses and outcome after Listeria monocytogenes challenge in mice. Nutrition 8:426–429
34. Moore FA, Moore EE, Kudsk KA, et al (1994) Clinical benefit of an immune enhancing diet for early postinjury enteral feeding. J Trauma 37:607–615
35. Kudsk KA, Minard G, Croce MA, et al (1996) A randomised trial of isonitrogenous enteral diets after severe trauma – an immune enhancing diet reduces septic complications. Ann Surg 224:531–543
36. Freund H, Ryan JR, Fischer JE (1978) Amino acid derangement in patients with sepsis: Treatment with branched-chain amino acid rich infusions. Ann Surg 188:423–430
37. Freund J, Hoover HC, Atamian S, et al (1979) Infusion of the branched-chain amino acids in postoperative patients. Ann Surg 190:18–23
38. Roth E, Funovics J, Muhlbacher F, et al (1982) Metabolic disorders in severe abdominal sepsis: glutamine deficiency in skeletal muscle. Clin Nutr 1:25–41
39. Ziegler TR, Young LS, Benfell K, et al (1992) Clinical and metabolic efficacy of glutamine-supplemented parenteral nutrition after bone marrow transplantation. Ann Int Med 116:821–828
40. Stehle P, Zander J, Mertes N, et al (1989) Effect of parenteral glutamine peptide supplements on muscle glutamine loss and nitrogen balance after major surgery. Lancet 1:231–233
41. Nirgiotis JG, Hennessey PJ, Andrassy RJ (1991) The effects of an arginine-free enteral diet on wound healing and immune function in the postsurgical rat. J Pediatr Surg 26:936–941
42. Gottschlich MM, Jenkins M, Warden GD, et al (1990) Differential effects of three enteral dietary regimens on selected outcome variables in burn patients. J Parent Enteral Nutr 14:225–236
43. Kulkarni AD, Fanslow WC, Rudolph FB, et al (1986) Effect of dietary nucleotides on response to bacterial infections. J Parent Enteral Nutr 17:148–152
44. Ziegler TR, Young LS, Ferrari-Balivera E, et al (1990) Use of human growth hormone combined with nutritional support in a critical care unit. J Parent Enteral Nutr 14:574–581

Immunonutrition in Cancer Surgical Patients

M. Braga, L. Gianotti, and A. Vignali

Introduction

Both major surgery and other types of injury are associated with severe alterations of the host's defense mechanisms and with an exuberant inflammatory response, making the patients highly susceptible to morbidity and mortality [1]. Nutritional support after injury may modulate immune, inflammatory and metabolic responses, gut function and clinical outcome of critically ill subjects. Early enteral versus parenteral feeding in traumatized and surgical patients is gaining wide consensus after promising results showing good tolerance and significant reduction of septic morbidity [2–6].

Research in this field has advanced with the addition to standard enteral and parenteral formulations, of specific nutritional substrates capable of affecting host defense, inflammatory response, intestinal barrier function, tissue oxygenation, nitrogen metabolism, ischemia/reperfusion injury, etc., which could theoretically lead to better outcome [7–17]. This new category of dietary compounds, namely "immunonutrients", has been shown to have peculiar properties. Among the most interesting and carefully investigated are:

1) Arginine which improves macrophage and natural tumor cytotoxicity, bactericidal activity, and vasodilatation through production of nitric oxide; stimulates T-cell proliferation and activation; and modulates nitrogen balance/protein synthesis and cytokine production [18]
2) Omega-3 polyunsaturated fatty acids, derived from fish oil, which are potent anti-inflammatory agents through the modulation of eicosanoid synthesis; regulate the fluidity of cell membranes; intervene in the pathway of coagulation; and up-regulate the immune response [14]
3) Glutamine which is known to facilitate the transport of nitrogen between organs; to reduce the skeletal and intestinal protein waste during stress; to enhance macrophage and neutrophil phagocytosis, and lymphocyte function; and to preserve intestinal permeability, by being the major fuel for different cell types [19]

All these substrates, tested separately or in different combinations improved morbidity and mortality in septic animal models [8–10, 20–22].

Postoperative Immunonutrition

Several clinical trials have evaluated the effect of dietary supplementation with arginine, n-3 fatty acids and nucleotides on the host immune response after injury or surgery. The administration of supplemented diets improved the host defense mechanisms and helped patients to overcome post-surgical immune depression more rapidly than standard diets. However, this enhancement was a delayed event. In fact, in the first days after surgery a similar impairment of phagocytosis ability, alteration of cytokine profiles, reduction of immunoglobulin levels, number of activated T and B cells and lymphocyte mitogenesis was found by comparing patients fed with supplemented or standard diets [5, 6, 23–26].

We investigated the potential effects of an enriched diet on host defense mechanisms and re-prioritization of protein synthesis in cancer patients who were candidates for elective curative surgery, to better understand the pathophysiologic mechanisms of immunonutrition. During surgery, after the tumor was resected, patients were randomized into three groups to receive: i) A standard enteral formula; ii) the same enteral diet enriched with arginine, omega-3 fatty acids, and RNA (Impact®, Novartis Nutrition, Bern, Switzerland); iii) total parenteral nutrition. The three regimens were processed to deliver the same amount of calories and nitrogen over the 7 days of postoperative treatment. Regardless of the type of artificial nutrition, all patients had an early, significant postoperative drop in polymorphonuclear neutrophil (PMN) phagocytosis and cell-mediated immune response, as measured by skin tests, confirming the immunosuppressive effect of surgical trauma. A significant amelioration of these immune parameters and of the levels of circulating interleukin (IL)-2 receptor was obtained in patients receiving the supplemented diet but only after a week of feeding [27]. The delayed recovery in the immune response might explain why supplemented diets given solely in the postoperative course led to variable improvements in outcome [6, 23, 27–29]. Our data also suggest that surgical trauma affects protein synthesis with an evident switch from constitutive proteins such as pre-albumin to acute-phase proteins such as IL-6. After a week of feeding with the enriched formula the trend was opposite with an increase in pre-albumin and a reduction of IL-6. To which specific nutritional component these beneficial effects should be attributed is difficult, but recent *in vitro* experiments suggest that eicosapentanoic acid (a major component of fish oil) added to the cell culture of hepatocytes increases spontaneous synthesis of pre-albumin and reverses the inhibitory effect of interleukin-6 (IL-6) on pre-albumin production [30]. Arginine, as well, may be involved in stabilizing reprioritization of hepatic protein synthesis [31].

Eight prospective randomized studies have investigated the potential advantages of immunonutrition on outcome [21, 23, 27–29, 32–34]. Five of them reported a significant reduction in infection in the patients fed with immuno-enhancing diets [21, 23, 29, 32, 34]. A recent multicenter study from Germany [28] showed that 22% of patients in the immunonutrition group versus 31% in the control group experienced postoperative infections (p = NS). When the authors stratified complications occurring after postoperative day 5 the difference between the two groups reached statistical significance.

In our experience [27, 35] the early postoperative administration of the supplemented diet significantly reduced both the severity of infections and postoperative stay, but the infection rate was not significantly lower than in the group fed with the standard diet (Fig. 1). A suitable explanation of these findings is that however early postoperative feeding is started, the amount of substrate given over the first days and the time required to reach adequate plasma and tissue substrate concentrations

Fig. 1. Clinical outcome in patients fed in the postoperative period by different routes and composition of the nutritional support. LOS: Length of stay; †: p = 0.06 vs Total parenteral nutrition; *: p < 0.05 vs Standard enteral and total parenteral nutrition

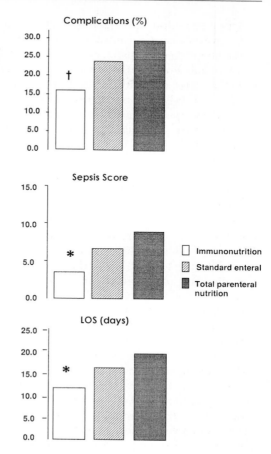

might be insufficient to allow a prompt burst of the immune system and an effective bacterial clearance shortly after surgery. The logical consequence of the above hypothesis is to commence administration of this immuno-enhancing diet before operation to obtain efficacious concentration of immunonutrients at the time of surgical injury.

Perioperative Immunonutrition

Experimental studies have strongly suggested the value of immunonutrition given both before and after injury [8–10]. In burned animals a significant reduction of overall mortality was found only when the administration of immunonutrients began 5 days before injury and continued afterwards [11, 12]. These data stimulated us to evaluate possible benefits of perioperative administration of supplemented diets in patients with gastrointestinal cancer who were candidates for major surgery [36].

Before operation patients were randomized to drink one litre per day, for seven consecutive days, of a control or a supplemented liquid diet (Impact®). In addition to the liquid diet, the patients of both groups were allowed to consume standard hospital food. Postoperative enteral feeding with either a supplemented or a control diet was started 6 hours after surgery with a jejunal infusion rate of 10 ml/h which was progressively increased to reach the full nutritional regimen (25 kcal/kg/day). In the first three postoperative days intravenous saline and electrolytes were administered according to clinical requirement as volume integration to the enteral diet.

Immune Response

Perioperative supplementation with immunonutrients prevented the early postoperative depression of both PMN and lymphocyte function which play a key role in the control of postoperative infections [36]. The two groups had similar baseline PMN phagocytosis abilities which did not significantly change throughout the week of pre-surgical feeding. A significant drop in phagocytosis was observed on postoperative days 1 and 4 in the control group. Conversely, in patients receiving the supplemented diet phagocytosis ability did not decrease after surgery, remaining similar to the preoperative values.

Concerning the variations in lymphocytes, a significant postoperative drop of natural killer (NK) cells was observed in both groups, which recovered on postoperative day 4 and 8 only in the supplemented group. The percentage of the CD8 subset increased on postoperative day 1 in the control group, while it decreased in the supplemented group. Also, throughout the first week after operation the patients fed with the supplemented diet had a higher CD4/CD8 ratio than the control group. The prompt and effective immune response observed in the supplemented group might be due to adequate plasma and tissue concentrations of specific nutrients such as arginine, n-3 fatty acids and RNA already available at the time of surgical stress. Part of the arginine effects may be mediated by the arginine-nitric oxide (NO) pathway. In fact, in experimental models the administration of arginine before and after trauma improved host survival by enhancing bacterial clearance and this protective effect was reversed when NO inhibitors were administered [8, 37].

Inflammatory Response

In patients receiving the supplemented formula the postoperative increase of IL-6 was significantly lower than in the control group. This was paralleled by the postoperative variations of C-reactive protein (CRP), whereas the synthesis of pre-albumin and RBP after operation was significantly improved in the supplemented group [36]. This might mean a switch from acute phase protein to visceral protein synthesis.

Inflammation has long been known to be an essential part of the healing and immune processes and to aid successful recovery after injury. Recently, an exuberant systemic and uncontrolled inflammatory response has been recognized to lead to organ dysfunction and adverse outcome through the massive release of pro-inflammatory cytokines such as tumor necrosis factor (TNF)-α, IL-1, and IL-6 [13]. This may be associated with a rapid decrease in the nitrogen balance, loss of lean body mass and catabolism. N-3 fatty acids exert anti-inflammatory, vasodilatatory and immunomodulatory properties through their ability to modulate the synthesis of different eicosanoids [14, 15]. Both pre and postoperative administration of diets enriched in n-3 fatty acids showed reduced plasma and tissue levels of specific leukotrienes, thromboxanes and prostaglandins (or their metabolites) with pro-inflammatory, immunosuppressive and vasoconstrictive effects [16, 17, 29]. Other clinical studies documented lower plasma levels of IL-6 and TNF-α when surgical patients were fed with similar supplemented diets [5, 6, 25, 26].

Gut Function

Operative gut microperfusion, measured by the laser Doppler flowmetry technique, was significantly different in the two groups. The patients receiving the supplemented diet had a higher small bowel and colon perfusion at the beginning of operation than the control patients. Furthermore, in the control group there was a significant reduction of microperfusion at the end of surgery. The patients fed with the supplemented formula finished surgery with values still higher than the baseline values of the control patients [36].

Postoperative jejunal tonometry is reported in Fig. 2. The higher values of jejunal intramucosal pH (pHi) in the supplemented group suggested that an adequate splanchnic blood flow promoted a good tissue oxygen tension, delivery and utilization. In other words, a higher intestinal microperfusion paralleled a better gut mucosa oxidative metabolism. Deficient blood flow and gut oxygenation could be a detrimental event particularly during abdominal surgery where intestinal anastomoses are frequently performed. Moreover, the detrimental sequelae observed following

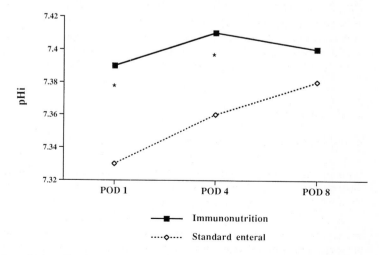

Fig. 2. Intramucosal intestinal pH (pHi) in patients fed perioperatively with different enteral diets. POD: Postoperative day; * $p < 0.05$

splanchnic hypoperfusion in the critically ill may be mediated by translocated endo-toxin and bacteria, which has been shown in several experimental models to activate pro-inflammatory and catabolic responses, organ failure and septic morbidity and mortality [38–40]. It is reasonable to hypothesize that the increased splanchnic microperfusion observed at laparotomy in the supplemented group is due to the constitutive component of NO because too short a time elapsed to allow for inducible NO synthesis.

Conclusion

The administration of immunonutrients both before, and after, surgery counteracts the early postoperative depression of the immune response, reduces the production of inflammatory cytokines and proteins and improves postoperative gut function. The maintenance of adequate gut microperfusion and mucosal oxygen metabolism, and the modulation of immune and inflammatory responses by perioperative immunonutrition would leave the host far better equipped to handle the surgical insult.

References

1. Meakins JL (1988) Host defense mechanisms in surgical patients: effect of surgery and trauma. Acta Chir Scand (suppl 550):43–53
2. Moore FA, Feliciano DV, Andrassy RJ, et al (1992) Early enteral feeding, compared with parenteral, reduces postoperative septic complications. Ann Surg 216:172–183
3. Kudsk KA, Croce MA, Fabian TC, et al (1992) Enteral versus parenteral feeding. Effects on septic morbidity after blunt and penetrating trauma. Ann Surg 215:503–513
4. Hasse JM, Blue LS, Liepa G, et al (1995) Early enteral nutrition support in patients undergoing liver transplant. J Parent Enteral Nutr 19:437–443
5. Braga M, Vignali A, Gianotti L, Cestari A, Profili M, Di Carlo V (1996) Immne and nutritional effects of early enteral nutrition after major abdominal operations. Eur J Surg 162:105–112
6. Braga M, Vignali A, Gianotti L, Cestari A, Profili M, Di Carlo V (1995) Benefits of early postoperative enteral feeding in cancer patients. Infusionther Transfusionmed 22:280–284
7. Barbour AG, Allred CO, Solberg SO, et al (1980) Chemiluminescence by polymorphonuclear leukocytes from patients with active bacterial infection. J Infect Dis 141:14–26
8. Gianotti L, Alexander JW, Pyles T, Fukushima R (1993) Arginine-supplemented diets improve survival in gut-derived sepsis and peritonitis by modulating bacterial clearance: the role of nitric oxide. Ann Surg 217:644–654
9. Gianotti L, Alexander JW, Gennari R, Pyles T (1995) Effect of oral glutamine on gut barrier function following thermal injury and immunosuppression. J Parent Enteral Nutr 19:69–74
10. Gennari R, Alexander JW, Eaves-Pyles T (1995) Effect of different combinations of dietary additives on bacterial translocation and survival in gut-derived sepis. J Parent Enteral Nutr 19:319–325
11. Braga M, Gianotti L, Costantini E, et al (1994) Impact of enteral nutrition on intestinal bacterial translocation and mortality in burned mice. Clin Nutr 13:256–261
12. Gianotti L, Braga M, Vaiani R, Profili M, Socci C, Di Carlo V (1996) Effect of composition of enteral solutions and timing of administration on outcome and bacterial translocation. Riv Ital Nutr Parent Enteral 14:191–195
13. Bone RC (1994) Sepsis and its complications: the clinical problem. Crit Care Med 22:S8–S11
14. Kinsella JE, Lokesh B, Broughton S, Whelan J (1990) Dietary polyunsaturated fatty acids and eicosanoids: potential effect on the modulation of inflammatory and immune cells: an overview. Nutrition 6:24–44

15. Mascioli EA, Iwasa Y, Trimbo S, Leader L, Bristian BR, Blackburn GL (1989) Endotoxin challange after menhaden oil diet: effect on survival of guinea pigs. Am J Clin Nutr 49:277–282
16. Wachtler P, Axel R, König W, Bauer H, Kemen M, Köller M (1995) Influence of a preoperative enteral supplementation on functional activities of peripheral leukocytes from patients with major surgery. Clin Nutr 14:275–282
17. Kenler AS, Swails WS, Driscoll DF, et al (1996) Early feeding in postsurgical cancer patients. Fish oil structured lipid-based polymetric formula versus a standard polymetric formula. Ann Surg 223:316–333
18. Raynold JV, Daly JM, Zhang S, et al (1988) Immunomodulatory mechanisms of arginine. Surgery 104:141–151
19. Hall JC, Heel K, McCauley R (1996) Glutamine. Br J Surg 83:305–312
20. Gianotti L, Alexander JW, Pyles T, et al (1996) Dietary fatty acids modulate host bactericidal response, microbial translocation and outcome following blood transfusion and thermal injury. Clin Nutr 15:291–296
21. Gottschlich MM, Jenkins M, Warden GD, et al (1990) Differential effects of three dietary regimens on selected outcome variables in burn patients. J Parent Enteral Nutr 14:225–236
22. Cerra FB, Lehmann S, Kostantinides N, et al (1991) Improvement in immune function in ICU patients by enteral nutrition supplemented with arginine, RNA and menhaden oil is independent of nitrogen balance. Nutrition 7:193–199
23. Daly JM, Lieberman MD, Goldfine J, et al (1992) Enteral nutrition with supplemental arginine, RNA, and omega 3 fatty acids in patients after operation. Immunologic metabolic and clinical outcome. Surgery 112:56–67
24. Vignali A, Braga M, Gianotti L, Cestari A, Profili M, Di Carlo V (1995) Impact of an enriched enteral formula on immune function and nutritional status in caner patients following surgery. Riv Ital Nutr Parent Enteral 13:25–31
25. Kemen M, Senkal M, Homann HH, et al (1995) Early postoperative enteral nutrition with arginine-omega 3 fatty acids and ribonucleic acid-supplemented diet versus placebo in cancer patients: an immunologic evaluation of Impact®. Crit Care Med 23:652–659
26. Senkal M, Kemen M, Homann HH, et al (1995) Modulation of postoperative immune response by enteral nutrition with a diet enriched with arginine, RNA, and omega-3 fatty acids in patients with upper gastrointestinal cancer. Eur J Surg 161:115– 122
27. Gianotti L, Braga M, Vignali A, et al (1997) Effect of route of delivery and formulation of postoperative nutritional support in patients undergoing major operations for malignant neoplasms. Arch Surg 132:1222–1229
28. Senkal M, Mumme A, Eickhoff U, et al (1997) Early postoperative enteral nutrition: clinical outcome and cost-comparison analysis in surgical patients. Crit Care Med 25:1489–1496
29. Daly JM, Weintraub FN, Shou J, Rosato EF, Lucia M (1995) Enteral nutrition during multimodality therapy in upper gastrointestinal cancer patients. Ann Surg 221:327–338
30. Wigmore SJ, Fearon KCH, Ross JA (1997) Modulation of human hepatocyte acute phase protein production by n-3 and n-6 polyunsaturated fatty acids. Ann Surg 225:103–111
31. Daly JM, Reynolds J, Thom A (1988) Immune and metabolical effect of arginine in surgical patients. Ann Surg 208:512–523
32. Moore FA, Moore EE, Kudsk KA, et al (1994) Clinical benefits of an immune-enhancing diet for early postinjury enteral feeding. J Trauma 37:607–615
33. Bower RH, Cerra FB, Bershadsky B, et al (1995) Early enteral administration of a formula (Impact®) supplemented with arginine, nucleotides and fish oil in intensive care unit patients: Results of a multicenter, prospective, randomized clinical trial. Crit Care Med 23:436–449
34. Kudsk KA, Minard G, Croce MA, et al (1996) A randomized trial of isonitrogenous enteral diets after severe trauma. An immuno-enhancing diet reduces septic complications. Ann Surg 224:531–543
35. Braga M, Gianotti L, Vignali A, et al (1998) Artificial nutrition after abdominal surgery: Impact of route of administration and composition of the diet. Crit Care Med (in press)
36. Braga M, Gianotti L, Cestari A, et al (1996) Gut function, immune and inflammatory responses in patients perioperatively fed with supplemented formulas. Arch Surg 131:1257–1265
37. Saito H, Trocki O, Wang SL, et al (1987) Metabolic and immune effects of dietary arginine supplementation after burn. Arch Surg 122:784–789

38. Fukushima R, Gianotti L, Alexander JW, Pyles T (1992) The degree of bacterial translocation is a determinant factor for mortality after burn injury and is improved by prostaglandin analogs. Ann Surg 216:438–445
39. Fukushima R, Alexander JW, Gianotti L, Pyles T, Ogle CK (1995) Bacterial translocation-related mortality may be associated with neutrophil-mediated organ damage. Shock 3:323–328
40. Gianotti L, Nelson JW, Alexander JW, et al (1994) Postinjury hypermetabolic response and magnitude of bacterial translocation. Prevention by early enteral nutrition. Nutrition 10:225–231

The Gut

Ischemia/Reperfusion of the Gut

M. Siegemund, W. Studer, and C. Ince

Introduction

The blood supply of the gut is compromised during different forms of shock to sustain the blood supply to the essential organs; the heart, brain and lung [1, 2]. Even in hyperdynamic septic shock with normal to supranormal superior mesenteric artery blood flow, ischemic regions due to an inhomogenous perfusion of the microcirculation have been found [3]. Ischemia of the gut also occurs during various surgical procedures, where a temporary cessation of the intestinal blood supply is necessary, or where low flow states are used, as in cardiac and vascular surgery [4]. Ischemia of the gut has been implicated as potentially hazardous due to bacterial translocation and/or inflammatory reactions which can initiate or perpetuate sepsis leading to multiorgan failure [5–7]. The dimension and duration of this oxygen depletion determines the severity of the resulting cellular dysfunction or necrosis. A reduction of intestinal blood supply of greater than 50% has been found to induce relevant tissue damage [8, 9].

Following the restoration of nutritive blood flow a second insult takes place which leads to further tissue injury. That reperfusion *per se* causes tissue injury in excess of that induced by ischemia alone, was first shown by Parks and Granger [10] with the observation that the histologic changes of injury after 3 hours of feline intestinal ischemia followed by one hour of reperfusion, were far worse than the changes after 4 h of ischemia alone. It is now known that reactive oxygen metabolites and inflammatory leukocytes play a major role in the pathogenesis of this reperfusion injury [6, 11, 12]. The impact of impaired microvascular oxygenation on the pathophysiology of ischemia/reperfusion is still a subject of intense research.

Despite reperfusion injury being a well documented disorder, the true extent of this problem in clinical settings is as yet not fully known. Several animal and human studies have shown that pharmacologic modulation of the reperfusion has a beneficial effect on the integrity and function of intestinal tissue and on the clinical course of critically ill patients. In vascular surgery, and especially in critically ill patients with repeated episodes of intestinal low flow, eliminating the harmful effects of nutritive blood supply during the reperfusion phase may be of potential advantage. This setting has the great advantage that the duration of ischemia and the beginning of reperfusion are known, and the clinician is able to apply some form of prophylactic therapy. In this paper a brief review of the pathophysiology of ischemia/reperfusion of the gut is given and therapeutic maneuvers directed at attenuating ischemia/reperfusion injury are discussed.

Mechanisms of Ischemia and Reperfusion Injury

The architecture of the microcirculation in the intestinal villi makes it especially vulnerable to hypoxia [8]. Each villus is supplied by a single central artery which is surrounded by a coat of subepithelial venules and capillaries draining blood from the top of the villus. The small distance between these vessels, and the countercurrent flow results in shunting of the oxygen supply to the gut microcirculation, especially in low flow conditions like hemorrhagic, cardiogenic or septic shock [2, 8, 13, 14]. Perfusion of the gastrointestinal tract can be further compromised by activation of the renin-angiotensin system causing splanchnic vasoconstriction [5, 15, 16].

The metabolic consequence of ischemia is a progressive decrease of adenosine triphosphate (ATP) production, despite the ongoing use of this energy-rich phosphate. Consequently, energy-rich phosphates are degraded from ATP to adenosine monophosphate (AMP) and further to adenosine. Anaerobic glycolysis will be activated to maintain the intracellular ATP level and leads to intracellular acidosis. The energy-rich phosphates are degraded to adenosine, which is further metabolized to inosine and hypoxanthine after rapid diffusion to the interstitial space where it is the major source of reactive oxygen metabolites [11]. In an animal model of non-occlusive intestinal ischemia, a 2 hour period of ischemia reduced ATP concentrations by 40% with a consecutive increase of AMP and hypoxanthine concentrations in intestinal tissue [17]. This potentially harmful condition can, as expected be reversed by resuscitation procedures.

The two beneficial consequences of reperfusion, restoring the energy supply and clearing toxic metabolites, are coupled with deleterious mechanisms. First, there is the generation of toxic oxygen free radicals from an interaction between arriving molecular oxygen and the hypoxanthine and xanthine from the degradation of purines [11, 18]. These reactive oxygen metabolites and cellular components such as membrane lipids, nucleic acids, enzymes, and receptors, lead to degradation of the microstructure of intestinal tissues and to loss of function, known collectively as reperfusion injury [18–20]. Furthermore polymorphonuclear neutrophils (PMN) generate reactive oxygen metabolites by themselves and directly interact with vascular endothelial cells, leading to microcirculatory disturbances associated with inflammation. This ischemia/reperfusion cascade leads to a collapse of the normal digestive and nutritional functions of the gut and ultimately to loss of barrier function to intraluminal toxic bacterial products [5, 19].

Reactive Oxygen Metabolites

A reactive oxygen metabolite is defined as a free radical derived from molecular oxygen and contains one or more unpaired electrons. They are energetically unstable, highly active and short lived molecules, which destroy cell membranes and their components by oxidation, to achieve more stability and a lower energy state by pairing of the free electron [21].

Under normal conditions xanthine dehydrogenase (XDH) is the enzyme responsible for the degradation of hypoxanthine to uric acid, the last step in the metabolism of purines. In non-ischemic cells the XDH uses nicotinamide adenine dinucleotide (NAD$^+$) instead of molecular oxygen as an electron acceptor in a reaction converting NAD$^+$ to NADH. During tissue ischemia, however, XDH is converted to the reactive oxygen metabolite producing xanthine oxidase (XO) [12, 22]. The two different paths of conversion, either reversible oxidation or irreversible proteolysis, to XO occur at different rates in individual tissues, although the amount of conversion is proportional to the duration of ischemia [22].

During ischemia, accumulation of hypoxanthine, from the degradation of purines, and its metabolizing enzyme XO, takes place. On reperfusion of the intestine the other substrate of the enzyme (molecular oxygen) is introduced, and XO degrades hypoxanthine to uric acid [17]. After the restoration of nutritive blood flow electrons are no longer transferred to NAD$^+$ but to molecular oxygen, resulting in the production of superoxide radical (O_2^-) or hydrogen peroxide (H_2O_2). These two reactive oxygen metabolites are also present under physiologic conditions, but are kept under control by intracellular antioxidant mechanisms such as superoxide dismutase (SOD) and catalase (Table 1). After ischemia the greater amount of O_2^- and H_2O_2 present makes these protective mechanisms ineffective. In addition the two radicals act as precursors for the hydroxyl radical (HO•), the most potent known oxidizing agent, probably responsible for most of the cellular damage that occurs from reperfusion injury [12, 18, 20]. The generation of hydroxyl radicals in the Haber-Weiss reaction also takes place under physiologic conditions at very low rates. During reperfusion this reaction is accelerated due to the presence of transition iron and copper ions released during ischemia, containing unpaired electrons acting as a template for the formation of the hydroxyl radical [18, 23]. In this scheme the superoxide radical reduces H_2O_2 to hydroxyl radical. The observation that the powerful iron-chelating agent desferrioxamine interrupts the generation of hydroxyl radical shows the influence of iron in reperfusion injury.

A further highly destructive reactive oxygen metabolite is generated by reaction of nitric oxide (NO) and O_2^-, producing peroxynitrite (ONOO$^-$). The endothelium derived NO shows vasodilating, anti-adhesive, and antithrombotic properties, is inactivated by superoxide and has been shown to be protective against intestinal reperfusion injury [12, 24]. Relatively small increases in superoxide and nitric oxide,

Table 1. Oxygen reactive metabolite generating reactions involved in intestinal ischemia-reperfusion

Name	Reaction	Radical	Structure
Hypoxanthine degradation	Hypoxanthine $+ 2O_2 + H_2O \rightarrow$ Xanthine $+ O_2^- + H_2O_2$	Oxygen superoxide	O_2^-
Xanthine degradation	Xanthine $+ 2O_2 + H_2O \rightarrow$ Uric acid $+ O_2^- + H_2O_2$	Hydrogen peroxide	H_2O_2
Fenton reaction	$Fe^{++} + H_2O_2 \rightarrow Fe^{+++} + OH^- + OH•$	Hydroxyl radical	OH•
Haber-Weiss-reaction	$O_2^- + H_2O_2 \rightarrow O_2 + OH^- + OH•$		
NO degradation	$NO + O_2^- \rightarrow ONOO^-$	Peroxynitrite	ONOO$^-$
Myeloperoxidase	$H_2O_2 + Cl^- + H^+ \rightarrow HOCl + H_2O$	Hypochlorus	HOCl

which appears to have beneficial vasodilatory effects on the microvasculature, may greatly increase the rate of peroxynitrite formation, to potentially cytotoxic levels [18, 25]. In a feline animal model of ischemia/reperfusion Payne and Kubes [26] showed that exogenous sources of NO like nitroprusside and L-arginine can reduce reperfusion induced mucosal barrier dysfunction independent of alterations in intestinal blood flow.

The XO inhibitors allopurinol, oxypurinol, and pterin aldehyde all dramatically attenuate both the epithelial cell necrosis and the increased microvascular permeability ofthe ishemic bowel [12, 27, 28]. In addition, the inactivation of XO with a specific molybdenum-deficient, tungsten-supplemented diet results in an attenuation of the reperfusion induced increase in microvascular permeability [29, 30]. Together with the observation in experimental animals that the intra-arterial infusion of hypoxanthine and xanthine oxidase results in increased intestinal permeability [31], these results suggest a central role for XO in the generation of reperfusion-induced reactive oxygen metabolites.

PMNs contain the enzymes, nicotinamide adenine dinucleotide phosphate (NADPH) oxidase and myeloperoxidase, needed for production of the reactive oxygen metabolites used for functional activity of destruction of pathogenic microorganisms. NADPH oxidase reduces O_2 to O_2^- and myeloperoxidase catalyzes the formation of hypochlorus acid from chloride ions and hydrogen peroxide. The hypochlorus acid by itself is about 100 times more reactive than H_2O_2 and reacts with primary amines of N-chloro derivatives, which are also potent oxidizing agents [6, 32]. These reactive oxygen metabolites, especially hydroxyl radicals, react aggressively with biologic substances, such as membrane phospholipids, protein, polysaccharides, nucleic acids, and polyunsaturated fatty acids. Enzymes and membrane proteins are inactivated by oxidation of sulfhydryl groups, and may be fragmented, cross-linked or aggregated, leading to inactivated ion channels and receptors, and to failure of mitochondrial respiration. Strand breaks and destruction of bases and deoxyribose sugars are the result of damage to DNA [19, 21]. The most damaging effect of reactive oxygen metabolites is probably the lipid peroxidation of polyunsaturated fatty acids in cell membranes. Following initiation by a single radical, in the presence of oxygen, long chains of lipid peroxides or lipid hyperoxides may be generated by a rapid chain reaction causing serious disruption of the cell membrane function and ultimately disintegration of the cell [21]. The increased permeability and plasma extravasation out of capillaries and venules may be a result of this free radical mediated lipid peroxidation [11, 33].

Leukocytes

Post-ischemic intestinal tissue generates large quantities of chemoattractants like leukotriene B_4 (LTB$_4$), platelet-activating factor (PAF) and activated complement factor 5 (C5a), associated with infiltration of neutrophils. Enhanced neutrophil adhesion to endothelium is seen in postcapillary venules during ischemia and to a much greater extent following reperfusion [34–36]. Accumulation of activated leukocytes in the microvasculature is associated with local and systemic tissue damage and results in depletion of circulating neutrophils. Therapy with monoclonal antibodies to prevent neutrophil adhesion to endothelial cells has been reported to prevent increased permeability and edema formation [37, 38].

The release of reactive oxygen metabolites results in a rise of intracellular calcium which can lead to activation of plasma phospholipase A_2 (PLA_2) and a subsequent generation of arachidonic acid products. PLA_2 is the primary enzyme in the generation of arachidonic acid and further cytokines that catalyze the hydrolytic splitting of free fatty acids from membrane phospholipids [6, 39]. Special forms of these fatty acids are chemically modulated to PAF. The high concentration of PLA_2 in the intestinal mucosa, the activation and potentiation of PLA_2 by reactive oxygen metabolites, the generation of PLA_2 and subsequent PAF formation are likely consequences of splanchnic ischemia/reperfusion [40–42]. The products, derived from cell membrane phospholipids through PLA_2 activation, PAF and leukotriene B_4, are recognized as essential neutrophil primers, and elevated levels of PAF have been found within the intestinal mucosa and the circulation after intestinal reperfusion [43–47]. Reperfusion but not ischemia led to an increase in mucosal LTB_4 levels [47, 48]. Pre-treatment with LTB_4 receptor antagonist or with a lipoxygenase inhibitor attenuates the adhesion of neutrophils to the endothelium [47]. Exogenously administered LTB_4, on the other hand, copies the microvascular alterations induced by ischemia/reperfusion.

The neutrophil membrane glycoprotein CD11a–c/CD18 has been shown to play an important role in mediating adhesion between leukocytes and endothelial cells (Fig. 1). Inflammatory mediators such as LTB_4 and PAF induce a rapid (1–2 min) expression of CD11b/CD18 on neutrophils, thereby allowing for rapid adhesion to endothelial cells [28, 49]. L-selectin, another adhesion molecule located on circulating

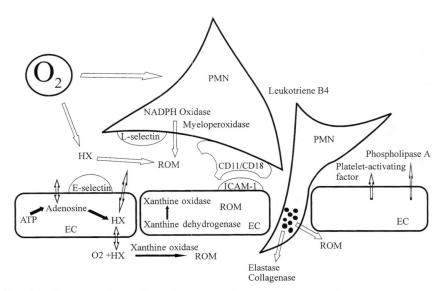

Fig. 1. Reactions between polymorphonuclear neutrophils (PMN) and endothelial cells (EC) involved in the ischemia/reperfusion injury. ROM: reactive oxygen metabolite; ICAM-1: intracellular adhesion molecule 1; CD11/CD18: leukocyte adhesion glycoprotein; HX: hypoxanthine

leukocytes, is responsible for the weak adhesive interactions manifest during leuko-cyte rolling [49]. This rolling is increased in low flow states, where the decreased shear stress makes it easier for leukocytes to create tight bonds with the endothelial cells [50]. Another effect of low blood flow and shear rate is the accumulation of in-flammatory mediators, and granulocyte derived proteins, like elastase and collage-nase, being generated by the leukocytes. Activated endothelial cells also produce two types of selectin molecules (selectin P and E), mediating the adhesion process. Var-ious stimuli like histamine and H_2O_2 lead to a rapid expression of selectin P on en-dothelial cells, whereas the cytokine induced expression of selectin E is slow [51]. The intracellular adhesion molecule-1 (ICAM-1) serves as a ligand for the above mentioned CD11/CD18 adhesion glycoproteins on leukocytes. The expression of ICAM-1 is also stimulated by cytokines over a period of several hours [52]. Different studies of monoclonal antibodies against the adhesion molecules have elucidated the contribution of single molecules to endothelial leukocyte adhesion, showing that antibodies against CD18 could nearly abolish the leukocyte adherence and emigra-tion, whereas the CD11 subunit and ICAM-1 antibodies reduce adherence only par-tially [34, 53, 54]. These animal experiments are consistent with CD11/CD18 interac-tions with ICAM-1 on the endothelial cell surface playing a major role in mediating close adherence and emigration of leukocytes [28].

Neutrophils are rapidly recruited to sites of inflammation where they are activat-ed, express their adhesion molecules, adhere to and migrate across the endothelium, and cause local destruction of cell membranes by release of their intracellular con-tents. Once neutrophils have entered the tissue they do not return to the blood stream, and either die by activation and release of intracellular contents or they are removed by macrophages [55]. The secretion of proteolytic enzymes and neutrophil-generated reactive oxygen metabolites results in the lysis of essential structural ma-trix proteins in the intestinal tissue, leading to increased microvascular permeability.

Measurements with intravital videomicroscopy and the monitoring of different granulocyte-specific enzymes have shown that the intensity of leukocyte accumula-tion elicited by ischemia/reperfusion is directly related to the magnitude and dura-tion of the ischemia [28, 35, 56]. Large numbers of neutrophils in capillaries can al-so lead to capillary plugging. Apart from the increase in adhesive potential, activa-tion of neutrophils also causes a rapid increased rigidity, trapping them either at the pre-capillary sphincter or the post-capillary venule. This effect in combination with tissue edema and cellular swelling may contribute to the so-called "no-reflow phe-nomena" of post-ischemic tissue [57, 58]. Indeed, in animals rendered either neutro-penic or which receive antibodies against adhesion molecules, this no-reflow phe-nomenon is significantly attenuated [58–60].

Massive intestinal ischemia/reperfusion injury can also cause tissue damage at distant organ sites. Studies on the influence of modulating reactive oxygen metab-olites, XO and activated PMNs in distal organ injury, like non-cardiogenic pulmo-nary edema, following splanchnic ischemia and reperfusion have shown this effect [61–66]. The lung may serve as a filter of activated neutrophils because of its low per-fusion pressure and the special microvascular architecture, where the white blood cells must pass through a series of capillary segments able to trap the cells by me-chanical or adhesive mechanisms possibly contributing to the development of acute respiratory distress syndrome (ARDS) [55].

Ischemia/Reperfusion Therapies and the Gut

The avoidance of prolonged periods of ischemia, remains the best way to avoid the accumulation of large quantities of hypoxanthine and XO. Clinical strategies have been developed aimed at the different components of evolving reperfusion injury. These include free radical scavenging, inhibition of reactive oxygen metabolite production, and neutrophil inhibition.

Anti-oxidant Therapy

A major problem of anti-oxidant therapy in clinical settings is to determine the appropriate time of administration, due to the short life-time of reactive oxygen metabolites following reperfusion with oxygenated blood. The deleterious mechanisms following reperfusion start immediately. Under conditions where the time of reperfusion can be anticipated, such as in aortic surgery, anti-oxidant therapy can be well timed. However in conditions of cardiogenic and hypovolemic shock where splanchnic ischemia starts immediately, and immediate resuscitation is required, the timing of anti-oxidant therapy is difficult. The end of intestinal hypoperfusion is also difficult to determine because the reduced blood flow may persist despite circulating blood volume and normalized systemic hemodynamics.

Allopurinol is oxidized to its active metabolite oxypurinol, a structural analog of hypoxanthine which in turn inhibits XO. It has been shown that allopurinol diminish the severity of histologically apparent mucosal lesions and the extent of microvascular damage induced by mesenteric ischemia/reperfusion [17, 27, 67, 68]. In studies in experimental animals with hemorrhagic shock-induced mucosal injury, allopurinol decreased the incidence of bacterial translocation [29, 30]. In addition allopurinol pre-treatment of animals has been shown to significantly attenuate the increase in leukocyte adherence and emigration observed after reperfusion [35].

Folic acid and pterin aldehyde also competitively inhibit XO, thereby preventing O_2^- production [69, 70]. The conversion of XDH to XO can be prevented by soybean trypsin inhibitor and this has been found to prevent microvascular and mucosal damage after intestinal reperfusion [71].

Chelation of iron may also be of great value due to its role in the generation of hydroxyl radicals during the Fenton and Haber-Weiss reactions [21]. Desferroxamine is a powerful iron-chelating agent, effectively sequestering Fe^{3+} from participation in the hydroxyl radical forming reactions, and was shown to be useful during ischemia/reperfusion. Desferroxamine is well tolerated in relatively high doses and is commonly used in iron-overload diseases like thalassemia [21]. Mannitol and albumin, two clinically used plasma substitutes, are also able to scavenge either hydroxyl radicals or lipid hydroperoxides [72, 73]. The advantage of desferroxamine over these two agents is that it prevents radical generation. Because the hydroxyl radical is very reactive, reacting with the first available molecule, hydroxyl scavengers would have to be present in very high concentrations in the tissues where radicals are actually being produced.

Tirilazad, a 21-aminosteroid, has been shown to scavenge O_2^-, inhibit lipid peroxidation, as well as preventing the release of arachidonic acid [71]. In animal experiments of intestinal ischemia/reperfusion, tirilazad has prevented lipid peroxidation but was not able to prevent injury of the gut mucosa [74]. In a more recent study with a 21-aminosteroid however, the application of the drug to animals with total occlusion of the superior mesenteric artery showed endothelial protective actions, lipid peroxidation inhibition, and a better rate of survival [75].

Modulation of Leukocyte Function

Neutrophil accumulation in the microvasculature following reperfusion augments tissue injury by the generation of further oxygen radicals and other inflammatory mediators. Inhibition of free radical production by neutrophils, or prevention of chemoattraction or neutrophil adherence, may modify reperfusion injury.

Monoclonal antibodies against the CD11/CD18 glycoprotein complex, which mediates the neutrophil endothelial interaction, have been shown to inhibit neutrophil chemotaxis and adherence, thereby ameliorating reperfusion injury [34, 37, 38, 53, 54]. In an animal model of intestinal occlusion/reperfusion, monoclonal antibodies against CD18 and CD11b nearly abolished the reperfusion-induced recruitment of adherent and emigrated leukocytes [76]. This therapy may be important in trauma patients, in whom a recent study has shown that the degree of metabolic acidosis after severe injury is directly correlated with the CD11b expression on circulating neutrophils, and maybe with the neutrophil activation and tissue injury [76]. However clinical studies in traumatized patients with monoclonal antibodies against neutrophil antigens may be difficult because of immunologic problems and the possible disruption of the natural neutrophil reaction to injury.

Several pro-inflammatory agents are involved in the ischemia/reperfusion injury of the gut. The rate of leukocyte adherence and emigration during the reperfusion period were greatly attenuated by PAF- and LTB_4-receptor antagonists [47]. Inhibitors of gut phospholipase A_2, like quinacrine, abrogate reperfusion-induced neutrophil infiltration in the intestinal mucosa and subsequent lung leak [65, 77].

The remote consequence of ischemia/reperfusion can be non-cardiogenic pulmonary edema, an early manifestation of ARDS. This is secondary to neutrophil mediated abnormal permeability of the lung microvasculature. It is assumed that the larger the mass of ischemic tissue, and the longer the ischemic time, the more likely it is that remote lung injury will occur. Experimental models suggest that this injury can also be caused by the sequestration of activated neutrophils within the pulmonary microvasculature, because both neutrophil depletion and the use of inhibitors of neutrophil activation effectively prevent the resulting pulmonary edema [39]. The increased pulmonary vascular permeability due to reperfusion of ischemic intestine can also be abolished by antibodies against PAF, P-selectin and CD18 [64, 78, 79].

Conclusion

In this review the underlying mechanisms involved in ischemia/reperfusion, their effects on the gastrointestinal tract and the modulation of these effects by therapy have been discussed. In summary, it can be said that ischemia/reperfusion injury is a relevant and important clinical topic which needs to be resolved. However, no consensus on a preferred therapy has been reached. The importance of the time of administration of anti-oxidant medications like allopurinol or desferroxamine makes their use difficult. Although the use of leukocyte modulating agents, like monoclonal antibodies, do not share this time dependency their use may be limited by non-specific immunologic effects. A final and more fundamental question in ischemia/reperfusion is the expected effect of blocking one step in the cascade of injury by therapeutic strategies, but leaving other pathways unaffected. It is clear that much fundamental and clinical research will need to be carried out to resolve these problems associated with ischemia/reperfusion injury of the gut.

References

1. Rowell LB, Detry JMR, Blackmon JR, Wyss C (1972) Importance of the splanchnic vascular bed in human blood pressure regulation. J Appl Physiol 32:213–220
2. Takala J (1996) Determinants of splanchnic blood flow. Br J Anaesth 77:50–58
3. Noeldge-Schomburg GFE, Priebe HJ, Armbruster K, Pannen B, Haberstroh J, Geiger K (1996) Different effects of early endotoxaemia on hepatic and small intestinal oxygenation in pigs. Intensive Care Med 22:795–804
4. Gelman S (1995) The pathophysiology of aortic cross-clamping and unclamping. Anesthesiology 82:1026–1060
5. Arranow JS, Fink MP (1996) Determinants of intestinal barrier failure in critical illness. Br J Anaesth 77:71–81
6. Biffl WL, Moore EE (1996) Splanchnic ischaemia/reperfusion and multiple organ failure. Br J Anaesth 77:59–70
7. Dantzker DR (1993) The gastrointestinal tract: the canary of the body? JAMA 270:1247–1248
8. Haglund U (1994) Gut ischaemia. Gut 35 (suppl 1):S73–S76
9. Bulkley GB, Kvietys PR, Parks DA, Perry MA, Granger DN (1985) Relationship of blood flow and oxygen consumption to ischemic injury in the canine small intestine. Gastroenterology 89:852–857
10. Parks DA, Granger DN (1986) Contributions of ischemia and reperfusion to mucosal lesion formation. Am J Physiol 250:G749–G753
11. Schoenberg MH, Berger HG (1993) Reperfusion injury after intestinal ischemia. Crit Care Med 21:1376–1386
12. Zimmerman BJ, Granger DN (1994) Oxygen free radicals and the gastrointestinal tract: role in ischemia-reperfusion injury. Hepato Gastroenterol 41:337–342
13. Ince C, Thio S, Van Iterson M, Sinaasappel M (1996) Microvascular PO_2 measured by Pd-porphine quenching of phophorescence in a porcine model of slowly developing sepsis. In: Bennett D (ed) 9th European Congress on Intensive Care Medicine, Glasgow (UK) Monduzzi, pp 133–139
14. Shepherd AP, Kiel JW (1992) A model of countercurrent shunting of oxygen in the intestinal villus. Am J Physiol 262:H1136–H1142
15. McNeill JR, Stark RD, Greenway CV (1970) Intestinal vasoconstriction after hemorrhage: roles of vasopressin and angiotensin. Am J Physiol 219:1342–1347
16. Reilly PM, MacGowan S, Miyachi M, Schiller HJ, Vickers S, Bulkley GB (1992) Mesenteric vasoconstriction in cardiogenic shock in pigs. Gastroenterology 102:1968–1979
17. Schoenberg MH, Fredholm BB, Haglund IJ, et al (1985) Studies on the oxygen radical mechanism involved in small intestinal reperfusion damage. Acta Physiol Scand 124:581–589
18. Grace PA (1994) Ischaemia-reperfusion injury. Br J Surg 81:637–647
19. Fink MP (1991) Gastrointestinal mucosal injury in experimental models of shock, trauma, and sepsis. Crit Care Med 19:627–641
20. Weiss SJ (1986) Oxygen, ischemia, and inflammation. Acta Physiol Scand 548 (suppl):9–38
21. Maxwell SRJ (1995) Prospects for the use of antioxidant therapies. Drugs 49:345–361

22. Parks DA, Williams TK, Beckman JS (1988) Conversion of xanthine dehydrogenase to oxidase in ischemic rat intestine: a reevaluation. Am J Physiol 254:G768–G774
23. Halliwell B, Guttridge JMC (1986) Oxygen free radicals and iron in relation to biology and medicine: some problems and concepts. Arch Biochem Biophys 246:501–514
24. Rubanyi G, Vanhoutte PM (1986) Superoxide anions and hyperoxia inactivate endothelium-derived relaxing factor. Am J Physiol 252:H822–H827
25. Beckman JS, Beckman TW, Chen J, Marshall PA, Fremann BA (1990) Apparent hydroxyl radical production by peroxynitrite: implications for endothelial injury from nitric oxide and superoxide. Proc Natl Acad Sci USA 87:1620–1624
26. Payne D, Kubes P (1993) Nitric oxide donors reduce the rise in reperfusion-induced intestinal mucosal permeability. Am J Physiol 265:G189–G195
27 Parks DA, Granger DN (1983) Ischemia-induced vascular changes: role of xanthine oxidase and hydroxyl radicals. Am J Physiol 245:G285–G289
28. Granger DN, Kothuis RJ (1995) Physiologic mechanisms of postischemic tissue injury. Annu Rev Physiol 57:311–332
29. Deitch EA, Bridges W, Ma JW, et al (1990) Hemorrhagic shock-induced bacterial translocation: the role of neutrophils and hydroxyl radicals. J Trauma 30:942–948
30. Deitch EA, Bridges W, Baker J, et al (1988) Hemorrhagic shock-induced bacterial translocation is reduced by xanthine oxidase inhibition or inactivation. Surgery 104:191–198
31. Parks DA, Shah AK, Granger DN (1984) Oxygen radicals: effects on intestinal vascular permeability. Am J Physiol 247:G167–G170
32. Zimmerman BJ, Granger DN (1992) Reperfusion injury. Surg Clin North Am 72:65–83
33. DelMaestro RF, Bjoerk J, Arfors KE (1982) Increase in microvascular permeability induced by enzymatically generated free radicals. Microvasc Res 22:255–270
34. Suzuki M, Inauen W, Kvietys PR, et al (1989) Superoxide mediates reperfusion-induced leukocyte-endothelial cell interactions. Am J Physiol 257:H1740–H1745
35. Granger DN, Benoit JN, Suzuki M, Grisham MB (1989) Leukocyte adherence to venular endothelium during ischemia-reperfusion. Am J Physiol 257:G683–G688
36. Grisham MB, Hernandez LA, Granger DA (1986) Xanthine oxidase and neutrophil infiltration in intestinal ischemia. Am J Physiol 251:G567–G574
37. Schoenberg MH, Poch B, Younes M, Schwarz A, Baczako K (1991) Involvement of neutrophils in postischemic damage to the small intestine. Gut 32:905–912
38. Hernandez LA, Grisham MB, Twohig B, Arfors KE, Harlan JM, Granger DN (1987) Role of neutrophils in ischemia-reperfusion-induced microvascular injury. Am J Physiol 253:H699–H703
39. Welbourn CR, Goldman G, Paterson IS, Valeri CR, Shepro D, Hechtman HB (1991) Pathophysiology of ischaemia reperfusion injury: central role of the neutrophil. Br J Surg 78:651–655
40. Chakraborti S, Gurtner GH, Michael JR (1989) Oxidant-mediated activation of phopholipase A_2 in pulmonary endothelium. Am J Physiol 257:L430–L437
41. Anderson BO, Moore EE, Banerjee A (1994) Phospholipase A_2 regulates critical inflammatory mediators of multiple organ failure. J Surg Res 56:199–205
42. Ambrosio G, Oriente A, Napoli C, et al (1994) Oxygen radicals inhibit human plasma acetylhydrolase, the enzyme that catabolizes platelet activating factor. J Clin Invest 93:2408–2416
43. Lewis MS, Whatley RE, Cain P, McIntyre TM, Prescott SM, Zimmerman GA (1988) Hydrogen peroxide stimulates the synthesis of platelet-activating factor by endothelium and induces endothelial cell-dependent neutrophil adhesion. J Clin Invest 82:2045–2055
44. Kubes P, Ibbotson G, Russell J, Wallace JL, Granger DN (1990) Role of platelet-activating factor in reperfusion-induced leukocyte adherence. Am J Physiol 259:G300–G305
45. Kubes P, Suzuki M, Granger DN (1990) Platelet-activating factor-induced microvascular dysfunction: role of adherent leukocytes. Am J Physiol 258:G158–G163
46. Filep J, Herman F, Braquet P, Mozes T (1989) Increased levels of platelet-activating factor in blood following intestinal ischemia in the dog. Biochem Biophys Res Commun 158:353–359
47. Zimmerman BJ, Guillory DJ, Grisham MB, Gaginella TS, Granger DN (1990) Role of leukotriene B_4 in granulocyte infiltration into the postischemic feline intestine. Gastroenterology 99:1358–1363
48. Mangino MJ, Anderson CB, Murphy MK, Brunt E, Turk J (1989) Mucosal arachidonate metabolism and intestinal ischemia-reperfusion injury. Am J Physiol 257:G299–G307
49. Kishimoto TK, Jutila MA, Berg EL, Butcher EC (1991) Neutrophil Mac-1 and MEL-14 adhesion proteins are inversely regulated by chemotactic factors. Science 245:1238–1241

50. Perry MA, Granger DN (1991) Role of CD11/CD18 in shear rate-dependent leukocyte-endothelial cell interactions in cat mesenteric venules. J Clin Invest 87:1798–1804
51. McEver RP (1991) Selectins: novel receptors that mediate leukocyte adhesion during inflammation. Thromb Haemost 65:223–228
52. Springer T (1990) Adhesion receptors of the immune system. Nature 346:425–434
53. Kurose I, Anderson DC, Miyaska M, et al (1994) Molecular determinants of reperfusion-induced leukocyte adhesion and vascular protein leakage. Circ Res 74:336–343
54. Perry MA, Granger DN (1992) Leukocyte adhesion in local versus hemorrhage-induced ischemia. Am J Physiol 263:H810–H815
55. Adams DH, Nash GB (1996) Disturbance of leukocyte circulation and adhesion to the endothelium as factors in circulatory pathology. Br J Anaesth 77:17–31
56. Zimmerman BJ, Holt JW, Paulson JC, et al (1994) Molecular determinants of lipid mediator-induced leukocyte adherence and emigration in rat mesenteric venules. Am J Physiol 266:H847–H853
57. Engler RL, Dahlgren MD, Morris DD, Peterson MA, Schmid-Schoenbein GW (1986) Role of leukocytes in response to acute myocardial ischemia and reflow in dogs. Am J Physiol 251:H314–H323
58. Barroso-Arranda J, Schmid-Schoenbein GW, Zweifach BW, Engler RL (1988) Granulocytes and the no-reflow phenomenon in irreversible hemorrhagic shock. Circ Res 63:437–447
59. Jerome SN, Dore M, Paulson JC, Smith CW, Korthuis RJ (1994) P-selectin and ICAM-1 dependent adherence reactions: role in the genesis of postischemic capillary no-reflow. Am J Physiol 266:H1316–H1321
60. Carden DL, Smith JK, Korthhuis RJ (1990) Neutrophil-mediated microvascular dysfunction in postischemic canine skeletal muscle: role of granulocyte adherence. Circ Res 66:1436–1444
61. Nielsen VG, McCammon AT, Tan S, Kirk KA, Samuelson PN, Parks DA (1995) Xanthine oxidase inactivation attenuates postocclusion shock after descending thoracic aorta occlusion and reperfusion in rabbits. J Thorac Cardiovasc Surg 110:715–722
62. Nielsen VG, Tan S, Weinbroum A, et al (1996) Lung injury after hepatoenteric ischemia-reperfusion: role of xanthine oxidase. Am J Respir Crit Care Med 154:1364–1369
63. Nielsen VG, Tan S, Baird MS, Samuelson PN, McCammon AT, Parks DA (1997) Xanthine oxidase mediates myocardial injury after hepatoenteric ischemia-reperfusion. Crit Care Med 25:1044–1050
64. Carden DL, Young JA, Granger DN (1993) Pulmonary microvascular injury following intestinal ischemia-reperfusion: role of P-selectin. J Appl Physiol 75:2529–2534
65. Koike K, Moore EE, Moore FA, Kim FJW, Carl VS, Banerjee A (1995) Gut phospholipase A$_2$ mediates neutrophil priming and lung injury after mesenteric ischemia-reperfusion. Am J Physiol 268:G397–G403
66. Koike K, Moore FA, Moore EE, Read RA, Carl VS, Banerjee A (1993) Gut ischemia mediates lung injury by a xanthine oxidase-dependent neutrophil mechanism. J Surg Res 54:469–473
67 Parks DA, Bulkley DN, Granger SR, Hamilton SR, McCord JM (1982) Ischemic injury in the cat small intestine: role of superoxide radicals. Gastroenterology 82:9–15
68. Granger DN, McCord JM, Parks DA, Hollwarth ME (1986) Xanthine oxidase inhibitors attenuate ischemia-induced vascular permeability changes in the cat intestine. Gastroenterology 90:80–84
69. Parks DA, Granger DN (1986) Role of oxygen radicals in gastrointestinal ischemia. In: Rotilio G (ed) Superoxide and superoxide dismutase in chemistry, biology, and medicine. Elsevier, Amsterdam, pp 614–617
70. Hernandez LA, Grisham MB, Granger DN (1987) A role of iron in oxidant-mediated ischemic injury to intestinal microvasculature. Am J Physiol 1987:G49–G53
71. Schiller HJ, Reilly PM, Bulkley GB (1993) Antioxidant therapy. Crit Care Med 21 (suppl):S92–S102
72. Pirsino R, DiSimplicio P, Ignesti G, et al (1988) Sulfhydryl groups and peroxidase-like activity in albumin as scavenger of organic peroxides. Pharmacol Res Com 20:545–552
73. Freeman BA, Crapo JS (1982) Biology of disease, free radicals and tissue injury. Lab Invest 47:412–426
74 Park P-O, Gerden B, Haglund U (1994) Effects of a novel 2-aminosteroid on methylprednisolone in experimental total intestinal ischemia. Arch Surg 129:857–860
75. Squadrito F, Altavilla D, Ammendolia L, et al (1995) Improved survival and reversal of endothelial dysfunction by the 21-aminosteriod, U-74389 G in splanchnic ischaemia-reperfusion injury in the rat. Br J Pharmacol 115:395–400

76. Botha AJ, Moore FA, Moore EE, Peterson VM, Goode AW (1997) Base deficit after major trauma directly relates to neutrophil CD11b expression: a proposed mechanism of shock induced organ injury. Intensive Care Med 23:504–509
77. Otamiri T, Lindahl M, Tagesson C (1988) Phospholipase A_2 inhibition prevents mucosal damage associated with small intestinal ischemia in rats. Gut 29:489–494
78. Carter MB, Wilson MA, Wead WB, Garrison N (1996) Platelet-activating factor mediates pulmonary macromolecular leak following intestinal ischemia-reperfusion. J Surg Res 60:403–408
79. Hill J, Lindsay T, Valeri CR, Shepro D, Hechtman HB (1993) A CD18 antibody prevents lung injury but not hypotension after intestinal ischemia reperfusion. J Appl Physiol 74:659–664

Stress Ulceration in the Critically Ill Population

J. Eddleston

Introduction

Acute deterioration in the gastrointestinal (GI) mucosa was first recognized in critically ill patients approximately 25 years ago. At that time gastric endoscopy demonstrated that between 80–100% of patients would have acute mucosal damage within 24 hrs of admission [1, 2]. The term "stress-related" was borne. Bleeding at that time was not common, but if it occurred, mortality rates as high as 80% were reported [1]. Even at that time certain subsets of patients were thought to be more at risk. These included patients with severe burns, head injuries, circulatory shock, respiratory failure, sepsis and multiple organ failure [1, 3]. Some pathologic states had specific names given to the associated acute upper GI mucosal changes such as Cushing's ulcers in patients with intracranial pathology [4].

Following these revelations, substantial effort over the last several decades has been directed to reducing the incidence of these acute mucosal changes without necessarily unraveling the pathologic mechanism underlying the injury. Generally there is a belief that intragastric acidity is a key factor in the pathogenesis. Consequently an accepted aim of prophylaxis has been to elevate intragastric pH to >4. Initial studies reported significant reductions in upper GI bleeding rates with the use of prophylactic agents [5–7], thereby paving the way for universal pharmacologic prophylaxis.

The utility of this approach has been recently questioned, because the incidence and severity of "stress-related" hemorrhage has decreased, most likely due to improvements in intensive care unit (ICU) care [8, 9] and one has become aware of the increased risk of nosocomial pneumonia associated with elevation of intragastric pH [10]. Cook et al. [11] recently have quantified the current risk of "stress-related" hemorrhage for patients admitted for ICU care as only 0.1% further fueling the debate about cost effectiveness.

Accurate assessment of the incidence of acute mucosal change can only be obtained by endoscopy. While the incidence of hemorrhage has continued to decline, endoscopy has consistently demonstrated that these acute upper GI mucosal changes are not rare [10, 12, 13], and continue to increase with time. Our knowledge of the changes which occur in perfusion of the gut and in particular its mucosal layer, coupled to the emerging pathophysiologic mechanisms underlying ischemia/reperfusion injury in animal models provide food for thought in understanding the basis for so-called "stress" ulceration.

Structural Basis for Gut Susceptibility

Unfortunately, the vascular structure of intestinal villi enhances the deleterious effects of a reduction in gut blood flow [14]. Blood is provided to each villus through a centrally located arteriole which does not branch until it reaches the villus tip. Venules return blood in a sub-epithelial network. These afferent and efferent blood vessels are located so close together that an effective counter-current exchange network is possible [15]. If one then considers the changes in hematocrit which occur along the length of the villus from base to tip, secondary to the phenomenon of plasma skimming [16], it is understandable why the villi are so extraordinarily sensitive to a reduction in gut blood flow, even in the face of unaltered oxygen consumption.

Furthermore, inflammatory states such as sepsis are known to be associated with a significant increase in gut and hepatic oxygen consumption [17]. In addition to increasing oxygen consumption, inflammatory states will adversely influence the regulation of microcirculatory blood flow in the gut. Nitric oxide (NO) has been implicated in this loss of vasoregulation and studies employing various inhibitors of inducible NO synthase (iNOS) have reported conflicting results [18, 19]. Induction of iNOS occurs following acute injury in models of acute inflammation [20]. *In vitro* it

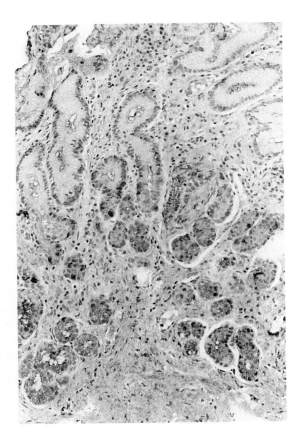

Fig. 1. "Diffuse" cytoplasmic positivity for inducible nitric oxide synthase in basal and mid-cryptal region of gastric antrum. Upper cryptal cells are negative (× 100)

produces nano-molar amounts of NO which are cytotoxic to a wide variety of cells [21], though it is as yet unclear whether the net effect of NO release is cytotoxic *in vivo*. The pattern and distribution of iNOS expression, namely diffuse and focal and located in the mid-cryptal region of the villus, is similar in critically ill patients [22] to that documented in a rodent model following induction of endotoxic shock [23] (Figs. 1, 2).

Another structural factor, the presence of pre-capillary or capillary sphincters, particularly in the gut mucosal layer, may also play a role in its susceptibility to any reduction in oxygen delivery [24]. Because few, or no sphincters are found in the muscularis layer, regulatory signals that cause these sphincters to constrict will preferentially cause mucosal ischemia. Their location distal to the resistance vessels means that sphincter constriction will not necessarily be reflected in measurements of total vascular resistance in the gut.

The sequence of events following any reduction in oxygen delivery to the gut is undoubtedly complex and appears to differ depending on the model studied but any reduction in blood flow that is followed by a restoration of flow raises the specter of reperfusion injury.

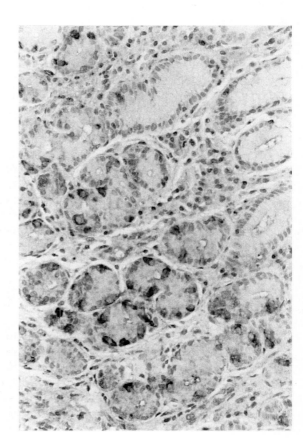

Fig. 2. "Focal" strong cytoplasmic positivity for inducible nitric oxide synthase in mid-cryptal cells of gastric antrum. Cells adjacent to the strongly positive cells show weak "diffuse" cytoplasmic positivity (× 200)

Monitoring of Gastrointestinal Mucosal Blood Flow and Relationship to Outcome

There are a number of research-based tools that are available to monitor and detect gut mucosal ischemia but few are of practical use to the clinician. The only current-ly available clinical monitor is the GI tonometer. Great debate continues about the relevance of calculating intramucosal gastric pH (pHi) from the tonometer PCO_2 and the use of arterial/tonometer CO_2 gap but these are outside the scope of this chapter and will not be discussed; suffice to say that evidence exists to correlate a poor outcome in ICU patients with a low pHi [25–28].

In patients undergoing urgent/emergency major abdominal surgery, even after hemodynamic optimization, reduction in pHi is common practice with commence-ment of surgery [22], reaching its lowest point at the end of surgery. Those patients who ultimately die experience the greatest fall in pHi at the time of surgery. Fiddian-Green et al. [29] used pHi to investigate "stress" ulceration and found that the pres-ence of a low pHi was the most powerful independent predictor of bleeding from the upper GI tract, whereas the intraluminal pH had no predictive power.

Intestinal Ischemia/Reperfusion Injury

The intestinal mucosa is rich in xanthine oxidase. During ischemia, adenosine tri-phosphate (ATP) is catabolized to hypoxanthine which is then oxidized in the pres-ence of molecular oxygen to form reactive O_2 species during reperfusion. Conver-sion of hypoxanthine dehydrogenase to the oxidase form takes place very swiftly, and even partial ischemia of the gut for periods as little as one hour, is sufficient to produce considerable conversion of the dehydrogenase form.

There is a growing body of evidence suggesting an important role for polymor-phonuclear (PMN) leukocytes or neutrophils in mediating the tissue injury and dys-function associated with ischemia/reperfusion of the GI tract. The evidence to sup-port this contention includes the fact that neutrophils infiltrate into post-ischemic intestinal tissues, and preventing neutrophil infiltration in part affords protection from tissue injury. The first evidence to demonstrate that neutrophils infiltrate into post-ischemic intestine was based on tissue myeloperoxidase (MPO) measurements [30, 31]. This enzyme is restricted primarily to neutrophils, and therefore gives a rea-sonable estimate of neutrophil levels within the affected tissue. Neutrophil influx differs in the different layers of the wall of the intestine. MPO activity in the mucosa has been quantified as doubling during ischemia and increasing four-fold with re-perfusion [32], though it must be remembered that baseline mucosal MPO levels are far greater in the mucosa than in other layers of the intestine. Considerable effort has been directed to unraveling ischemia/reperfusion injury in animal models. Work performed by our group [22] in patients undergoing major urgent/emergency ab-dominal surgery demonstrated significant increases in MPO activity in the gastric mucosa 72 hrs post-surgery. Whether this tissue injury is reflective of an ischemia/reperfusion injury or merely a reponse to tissue hypoxia is not clear.

Neutrophil influx into tissues is a complex series of events that includes initial contact with the endothelium, rolling, firm adhesion, and ultimately migration into surrounding tissues [33]. It has been suggested that recruitment of neutrophils by mast cells is the initiating event. Stabilization of mucosal mast cells in a rat model with doxantrazole, a stabilizer of both mucosal and connective tissue mast cells prevented the rise in rat mast cell protease II (RMCP II) and reduced the myeloperoxidase activity in the post-ischemic intestine [34]. RMCP II is a protease specific to mucosal mast cells in the rat. The degranulation of mucosal mast cells in animal models would appear to occur very quickly once reperfusion of an ischemic intestine begins [33]. Our group [22] was unable to locate any mast cells within the mucosa which had not already degranulated even minutes after induction of anesthesia. These patients had all received hemodynamic optimization prior to induction of anesthesia.

The identity of the mediator that activates mast cells to degranulate and recruit neutrophils in the post-ischemic intestine is still not clear. Evidence, however, would suggest that it is the increased flux of oxidants such as superoxide and hydrogen peroxide [36] that may be responsible for the mast cell activation. Although the source of the oxidants remains unknown, Boros et al. [36] demonstrated that allopurinol blocked histamine release from the post-ischemic gut by 87%, thereby suggesting an important role for the oxidant-generating enzyme xanthine oxidase in ischemia/reperfusion induced mast cell activation.

Role for Dopexamine?

Dopexamine is a new synthetic catecholamine with dopaminergic receptor agonist properties both at the dopamine 1 and dopamine 2 receptors and has potent β_2-adrenergic receptor agonist activity. It has no α or direct β_1 effects [37, 38]. Boyd et al. [39], when administering dopexamine in a randomized, prospective trial of high-risk surgical patients, suggested that the reduced mortality they observed could be due to an agent specific anti-inflammatory effect. More precise evidence of an anti-inflammatory effect attributable to dopexamine was described by Schmidt et al. [40]. This group evaluated the influence, in Wistar rats, of dopexamine on leukocyte adherence and vascular permeability in post-capillary venules during endotoxemia. Dopexamine, 120 mins after induction of endotoxemia, significantly reduced leukocyte adherence and plasma extravasation.

In addition, our group [22] has demonstrated a protective anti-inflammatory effect of dopexamine in patients undergoing major urgent/emergency intrabdominal surgery. We demonstrated that the preoperative, perioperative and postoperative administration of dopexamine up to 24 hrs post-surgery significantly reduced gastric mucosal MPO activity. This effect was independent of mast cell or iNOS activity, suggesting a direct effect of dopexamine on PMN infiltration.

Beneficial anti-inflammatory properties of dopexamine have also been reported by Tighe et al. [41] in their porcine model of sepsis. They tested the hypothesis that increasing cardiac output and oxygen consumption in porcine peritonitis (using dobutamine, dopexamine or colloid) could afford protection to the hepatic ultrastructure. Dopexamine offered agent specific anti-inflammatory protection to the hepatic ultrastructure, independent of hemodynamic or oxygen transport variables.

Conclusion

Acute deterioration in the upper GI tract still occurs, despite the incidence of overt bleeding continuing to fall. We must not be lured into a false sense of security and should now direct our efforts to understanding the pathophysiologic mechanism behind the injury. We know that critically ill patients undergo significant changes to their mucosal blood flow as part of their critical illness, and that the injury in man is characterized by an increased presence of MPO, signaling an increased presence of PMN within the gastric mucosa. The extent to which ischemia/reperfusion injury is responsible for mucosal injury as opposed to tissue hypoxia in the villus cannot be stated with assurance at this time. Either, or both, will result in structural damage to the mucosa.

References

1. Lucas CE, Sugawa C, Riddle J, et al (1971) Natural history and surgical dilemma of stress gastric bleeding. Arch Surg 102:266–273
2. Pleura DA (1978) Stress-related mucosal damage, an overview. Am J Med 83 (suppl 6A):3–6
3. Skillman JJ, Bushnell LS, Goldman H, et al (1969) Respiratory failure, hypotension, sepsis, and jaundice: A clinical syndrome associated with lethal hemorrhage from acute stress ulceration of the stomach. Am J Surg 117:523–530
4. Cushing H (1932) Peptic ulcer and the interbrain. Surg Gynecol Obs 55:1–34
5. McAlhany JC Jr, Czaja AJ, Pruitt BA Jr (1976) Antacid control of complications from acute gastroduodenal disease after burns. J Trauma 16:645–649
6. MaxDougall BRD, Bailey RJ, Williams R (1977) H2-receptor antagonists and antacids in the prevention of acute gastrointestinal hemorrhage in fulminant hepatic failure: Two controlled trials. Lancet 1:617–619
7. Hastings PR, Skillman JJ, Bushnell LS, et al (1978) Antacid titration in the prevention of acute gastrointestinal bleeding. N Engl J Med 298:1041–1045
8. Lacroix J, Infante-Rivard C, Jenicek M, et al (1989) Prophylaxis of upper gastrointestinal bleeding in intensive care units: A meta-analysis. Crit Care Med 17:862–869
9. Groll A, Simon JB, Wigle RD, et al (1986) Cimetidine prophylaxis for gastrointestinal bleeding in an intensive care unit. Gut 27:135–140
10. Eddleston JM, Vohra A, Scott P, et al (1991) A comparison of the frequency of stress ulceration and secondary pneumonia in sucralfate- or ranitidine-treated intensive care unit patients. Crit Care Med 19:1491–1496
11. Cook DF, Fuller HD, Guyatt GH, et al (1994) Risk factors for gastrointestinal bleeding in critically ill patients. N Engl J Med 330:377–381
12. Reusser P, Gyr K, Scheidegger D, et al (1990) Prospective endoscopic study of stress erosions and ulcers in critically ill neurosurgical patients: Current incidence and effect of acid-reducing prophylaxis. Crit Care Med 18:270–274
13. Eddleston JM, Pearson RC, Holland J, Tooth JA, Vohra A, Doran BH (1994) Prospective endoscopic study of stress erosions and ulcers in critically ill adult patients treated with either sucralfate or placebo. Crit Care Med 22:1949–1954
14. Goldfarb RD (1997) Inotropic treatment and intestinal tissue oxygenation in a model of porcine endotoxaemia. Crit Care Med 25:1108–1109
15. Casely-Smith R, Gannon BJ (1984) Intestinal microcirculation: Spatial organisation and fine structure. In: Shepherd AP, Granger DN (eds) Physiology of the intestinal circulation. Raven Press, New York, pp 9–31
16. Fink MP (1991) Gastrointestinal mucosal injury in experimental models of shock, trauma and sepsis. Crit Care Med 19:627–641
17. Dahn MS, Lange P, Hans B, Jacobs LA, Mitchell RA (1987) Splanchnic and total body oxygen consumption differences in septic and injured patients. Surgery 101:69–80

18. Schumaker PT, Kazaglis J, Connolly HV, et al (1995) Systemic and gut oxygen extraction during endotoxaemia. Role of NO synthesis. Am J Respir Crit Care Med 141:107–115
19. Kilbourn RG, Szabó C, Traber DL (1997) Beneficial versus detrimental effects of NOS inhibitors in circulatory shock: Lesson learned from experimental and clinical studies. Shock 7:235–246
20. Ialenti A, Ianaro A, Moncada S, Di Rosa M (1992) Modulation of acute inflammation by endogenous nitric oxide. Eur J Pharm 211:177–182
21. Nathan C (1992) Nitric oxide as a secretory product of mammalian cells. FASEB J 6:3051–3064
22. Byers RJ, Eddleston JM, Pearson RC, Bigley G, McMahon RFT (1998) Dopexamine reduces the incidence of acute inflammation in the gut mucosa following abdominal surgery in high risk patients. Crit Care Med (in press)
23. Cook HT, Bune AJ, Jansen AS, Taylor GM, Loi RK, Cattell V (1994) Cellular localisation of inducible nitric oxide synthase in experimental endotoxic shock in the rat. Clin Sci 87:179–186
24. Bohlen HG (1980) Intestinal tissue PO_2 and microvascular responses during glucose exposure. Am J Physiol 238:H164–H171
25. Gutierrez G, Palizas F, Doglio G, et al (1992) Gastric intramucosal pH as a therapeutic index of tissue oxygenation in critically ill patients. Lancet 339:195–199
26. Marik P (1993) Gastric intramucosal pH: a better predictor of multiple organ dysfunction syndrome and death than oxygen-derived variables in patients with sepsis. Chest 104:225–229
27. Maynard N, Taylor P, Bihari D, Mason R (1992) Gastric intramucosal pH in predicting outcome after surgery for ruptured abdominal aortic aneurysm. Br J Surg 80:517–532
28. Friedman G, Berlot G, Kahn RJ, Vincent JL (1995) Combined measurements of blood lactate concentrations and gastric intramucosal pH in patients with severe sepsis. Crit Care Med 23:1184–1193
29. Fiddian-Green RG, McGough E, Pittenger G, Rothman ED (1983) Predictive value of intramural pH and other risk factors for massive bleeding from stress ulceration. Gastroenterology 85:613–620
30. Hernandez LA, Grisham MB, Twohig B, Arfos KE, Harlan JM, Granger DN (1987) Role of neutrophils in ischaemia-reperfusion-induced microvascular injury. Am J Physiol 253:H699–H703
31. Grisham MB, Hernandez LA, Granger DN (1986) Xanthine oxidase and neutrophil infiltration in intestinal ischaemia. Am J Physiol 251:G567–G574
32. Kurtel H, Tso P, Granger DN (1992) Granulocyte accumulation in different layers of small intestine during ischaemia-reperfusion (I/R): Role of leukocyte adhesion glycoprotein CD11/CD18. Am J Physiol 262:C878–882
33. Kubes P (1996) Intestinal ischemia/reperfusion: A role for mast cells and neutrophils. In: Vincent JL (ed) Yearbook of intensive care and emergency medicine. Springer-Verlag, Berlin, Heidelberg, New York, pp 197–207
34. Kanwar S, Kubes P (1994) Mast cells contribute to ischemia/reperfusion-induced granulocyte infiltration and intestinal dysfunction. Am J Physiol 267:G316–G321
35. Blum H, Summers JJ, Schnall MD, et al (1986) Acute intestinal ischaemia studies by phosphorous nuclear magnetic resonance spectroscopy. Ann Surg 204:83–88
36. Boros M, Kaszaki J, Nagy S (1989) Oxygen free radical-induced histamine release during intestinal ischemia and reperfusion. Eur Surg Res 21:297–304
37. Brown RA, Dixon J, Farmer JB, et al (1985) Dopexamine: A novel agonist at peripheral dopamine receptors and beta 2-adrenoceptors. Br J Pharmacol 85:599–608
38. Brown RA, Farmer JB, Hall JC, et al (1985) The effects of dopexamine on the cardiovascular system of the dog. Br J Pharmacol 85:609–619
39. Boyd O, Grounds RM, Bennett ED (1993) A randomized clinical trial of the effect of deliberate perioperative increase of oxygen delivery on mortality in high risk surgical patients. JAMA 270:2699–2707
40. Schmidt W, Schmidt H, Hacker A, Gebhard M, Martin E (1998) Influence of dopexamine on leukocyte adherence and vascular permeability in postcapillary venules during endotoxemia. Intensive Care Med (in press)
41. Tighe D, Moss R, Heywood G, Al-Saady N, Webb A, Bennett D (1995) Goal-directed therapy with dopexamine, dobutamine, and volume expansion: Effects of systemic oxygen transport on hepatic ultrastructure in porcine sepsis. Crit Care Med 23:1997–2007

Hemodynamic Management of Gastric Intramucosal Acidosis in Septic Patients

E. Silva, D. De Backer, and J.-L. Vincent

Introduction

Although sepsis is typically characterized by normal or increased systemic blood flow and decreased oxygen extraction [1], regional hypoperfusion and tissue hypoxia may be present [2]. Systemic parameters currently monitored during resuscitation may not reflect regional blood flow abnormalities and ongoing hypoperfusion in specific organ system beds may lead to subsequent organ failure even when global blood flow is restored or increased [3–5]. A logical approach is to focus on assessment of regional oxygenation. Gastric tonometry is a possible tool to assess gastric perfusion. However, we need to understand better the meaning of a high gastric mucosal carbon dioxide tension (PCO_2) or a low gastric intramucosal pH (pHi) to adequately interpret studies assessing hemodynamic management guided by these measurements.

Physiology of Gastric Intramucosal Hypercapnia

Tonometry is a relatively non-invasive technique allowing measurement of gastric or intestinal mucosal PCO_2 from the equilibration between the PCO_2 in a balloon and that in the mucosal interstitial fluid [6]. From this measurement, the pHi can be calculated. The gastric intramucosal PCO_2 (PCO_2i) is directly influenced by the systemic arterial PCO_2 ($PaCO_2$). In normal volunteers, $PaCO_2$ is normal, so that this does not have to be considered to interpret an abnormal PCO_2i. In contrast, in critically ill patients PCO_2i must be corrected for abnormalities in $PaCO_2$ by calculating the gastric-arterial PCO_2 difference (PCO_2i-$PaCO_2$).

Mucosal acidosis may result from hemodynamic alterations associated with an imbalance between oxygen supply and demand to the gastric mucosa with or without an absolute reduction in gastric blood flow. Schlichtig and Bowles [7] showed that intestinal pHi remained relatively constant as regional oxygen delivery (DO_2) decreased to a point where oxygen consumption (VO_2) became supply dependent. Below this critical level, the pHi fell precipitously. In endotoxemic dogs, Vallet et al. [8] showed that despite restoration of splanchnic blood flow in the gut, VO_2 and pHi remained low and lactate output high, suggesting considerable blood flow redistribution within the gut wall.

In addition, mucosal acidosis may be related to direct metabolic alterations incluced by endotoxin that are not mediated by hemodynamic alterations [9]. If a low pHi may also reflect cellular metabolic alterations associated with altered cellular

Table 1. Causes of increased gastric intramucosal PCO_2 in septic patients

Physiologic influence
• Systemic arterial PCO_2
• Low gastric mucosal blood flow (stagnant flow)
• Increased CO_2 production by aerobic metabolism*
• Increased CO_2 production by anaerobic metabolism*
• Inhibition of pyruvate dehydrogenase*

* without proportional increase in gastric mucosal blood flow

oxygen metabolism, increasing hepato-splanchnic blood flow with vasoactive agents may fail to restore PCO_2i or pHi to normal values.

Table 1 summarizes the principal factors influencing gastric intramucosal PCO_2.

Adrenergic Agents

In septic patients, a variety of pharmacologic agents have been shown to decrease PCO_2i through systemic or local properties, including an increase in cardiac index and/or in gastric mucosal blood flow.

Dopamine

Dopamine affects all adrenergic receptor types. In low doses (< 3 µg/kg/min), the dopaminergic effects added to the β-adrenergic effects may selectively increase blood flow in the splanchnic and renal regions, but as the dose is increased, these effects are rapidly masked by α_1-receptor stimulation resulting in vasoconstriction.

Several studies have indicated that dopamine administration can increase splanchnic blood flow in septic patients. Ruokonen et al. [5] studied the effects of dopamine and norepinephrine in 10 patients with hyperdynamic septic shock and 11 patients after cardiac surgery (control group). The patients were randomly assigned to receive either agent, with the aim of restoring the mean arterial pressure to above 70 mmHg. All patients treated with norepinephrine also received low-dose dopamine to maintain renal perfusion. Dopamine consistently increased splanchnic blood flow, determined by the indocyanine green (ICG) clearance. The increase in splanchnic DO_2 was associated with an increase in regional VO_2. Meier-Hellman et al. [10] studied the effects of low-dose dopamine (2.8–3.0 µg/kg/min) combined with norepinephrine in patients with hyperdynamic septic shock. Dopamine selectively increased hepato-splanchnic flow (also determined by the ICG clearance method) in those patients who initially had a fractional hepato-splanchnic flow within the normal range. In this study, also, there was a significant increase in VO_2 in the hepato-splanchnic region. Whether this was the result of improved tissue oxygenation or the calorigenic effect of dopamine remains uncertain. Increasing the dosage of dopamine increased hepato-splanchnic VO_2 more than DO_2, which might be interpreted as a deleterious effect of dopamine on splanchnic oxygenation [11, 12].

Studies involving pHi measurement in septic patients have not shown beneficial effects with dopamine administration. Maynard et al. [13] studied 25 patients with the so-called systemic inflammatory response syndrome (SIRS), and observed that low doses of dopamine (2.5 µg/kg/min) had no effect on pHi. In this study, dopamine had no effect on splanchnic blood flow, as studied by ICG clearance and monoethylglycinexylidide (MEGX) concentration. Marik and Mohedin [14] reported that dopamine infusion during hyperdynamic septic shock increased DO_2 and VO_2, but decreased pHi, suggesting an imbalance between oxygen demand and supply in the splanchnic region. It is noteworthy that in this study, the doses of dopamine infused were very large (mean 26 µg/kg/min). In another study in severe sepsis patients, Nevière et al. [15] reported that dopamine decreased gastric mucosal blood flow as assessed by laser Doppler flowmetry, but had no effect on pHi or gastric intramucosal pCO_2. Olson et al. [16] also reported that low-dose dopamine administration did not increase pHi in septic patients. Recently, Meier-Hellmann et al. [10] demonstrated that low-doses of dopamine increased splanchnic DO_2 principally in patients with an initial fractional splanchnic blood flow less than 0.30. However, pHi and regional lactate did not change during the study.

In summary, although dopamine can increase splanchnic blood flow and decrease intestinal vascular resistance it does not improve gastric mucosal perfusion, perhaps because it redistributes flow away from the gastric mucosa. In septic patients, dopamine may increase splanchnic blood flow, but does not increase pHi.

Dopexamine

Dopexamine hydrochloride is a synthetic catecholamine with structural and pharmacologic similarities to dopamine. It has predominant dopaminergic (DA_1) and β_2-adrenergic receptor agonist activity. It may have an advantage over dopamine in that it does not stimulate α-adrenergic receptors, so that it has no vasoconstricting properties.

Several experimental studies have shown that dopexamine can improve gut oxygenation. In rabbits with septic shock, Lund et al. [17] reported that dopexamine improved oxygenation of gut, liver, and muscle, as reflected by an increase in tissue PO_2 and normalization of PO_2 distribution types. In a model of porcine peritonitis, Tighe et al. [18] observed that dopexamine may preserve hepatic ultrastructure by mechanisms other than an increase in oxygen supply. Cain and Curtis [19] studied the effects of dopexamine on gut metabolism in endotoxic dogs. Whereas the gut initially took up lactate, after endotoxin injection it became a significant lactate producer. In the dopexamine-treated group, gut lactate uptake decreased but it never converted to lactate production. As a result, the gut lactate flux was significantly lower in dopexamine-treated animals than in control animals at nearly all times during the experiment.

A few studies have reported the effects of dopexamine on pHi in critically ill patients [13, 20–22]. In a prospective, cross-over placebo-controlled study, Trinder et al. [20] randomized a heterogenous group of acutely ill patients with a low pHi to receive either dopexamine with colloid, or 5% dextrose for three hours prior to cross-over. Dopexamine administration failed to correct gastric intramucosal acidosis. Similar results were obtained by Kuhly et al. [21] with dopexamine failing to increase pHi and sigmoid mucosal pH. Investigators at Guy's hospital reported different re-sults. In one study involving patients with SIRS who also had a low pHi, Maynard et al. [13] observed that the addition of dopexamine at a dose of 1 µg/kg/min did not increase systemic oxygen delivery, but increased pHi, ICG clearance, and MEGX for-mation from lidocaine, suggesting a selective effect of dopexamine on hepato-splanchnic blood supply. In another study [22] involving a more specific group of septic patients, dopexamine increased pHi from 7.21 to 7.29. Hepatic blood flow, es-timated by ICG clearance, increased slightly but not significantly. Unlike the increase in pHi, the improvement in hepatic blood flow was not maintained following dopex-amine withdrawal.

In summary, experimental studies have shown that dopexamine can improve splanchnic oxygenation, and clinical studies also support an effect of dopexamine on splanchnic blood flow. However, the effects of dopexamine on pHi are not conclu-sive. Studies involving septic patients are scarce and inconsistent.

Dobutamine

With its predominant β_1- and β_2-adrenergic properties, dobutamine has become the more frequently used inotropic agent. Dobutamine has also been used to in-crease DO_2 even when cardiac output is not reduced [23]. Dobutamine does not have dopaminergic effects and is not supposed to significantly alter the distribution of blood flow.

In endotoxic pigs, Fink et al. [24] demonstrated that infusion of hetastarch plus dobutamine improved lipopolysaccharide-induced mucosal acidosis (ileal pHi) more than hetastarch alone. De Backer et al. [25] observed in endotoxic dogs that the administration of 10 µg/kg/min of dobutamine could increase mesenteric blood flow and DO_2 and prevented the increase in the pH-gap observed in the control group. In a fluid-resuscitated porcine model of endotoxic shock, Nevière et al. [26] demonstrated that dobutamine plus saline increased pHi, and mucosal perfusion as-sessed by laser Doppler flowmetry.

Some studies have reported the effects of dobutamine on splanchnic perfusion in septic patients. In septic shock patients, Duranteau et al. [27] studied the effects of epinephrine, norepinephrine, and norepinephrine plus dobutamine on gastric mu-cosal blood flow measured by laser-Doppler probe. Epinephrine and norepineph-rine with dobutamine increased gastric mucosal blood flow more than norepineph-rine alone, suggesting a proper vasodilating effect of dobutamine on gastric muco-sal vasculature. Meier-Hellmann et al. [28] also showed that septic patients treated with a combination of dobutamine and norepinephrine had greater splanchnic per-fusion (and cardiac output) than those treated with norepinephrine alone. In septic patients concomitantly treated with norepinephrine, Reinelt et al. [29] observed that dobutamine increased hepato-splanchnic DO_2 but not VO_2 or glucose uptake. In stable septic patients, De Backer et al. [30] observed that dobutamine increased he-pato-splanchnic blood flow, determined by the ICG clearance method, and this ef-fect was associated with significant increases in hepato-splanchnic DO_2 and VO_2. However, Ruokonen et al. [31] observed that dobutamine administration failed to in-crease hepato-splanchnic blood flow in 10 patients with severe pancreatitis.

Gutierrez et al. [32] studied the effects of dobutamine on pHi in 21 patients with sepsis syndrome with an initial pHi ≤ 7.32. The pHi increased, but systemic VO_2 did not change significantly, suggesting a selective effect of the drug on the splanchnic circulation. These results were consistent with a retrospective study by Silverman and Tuma [33] comparing the effects of dobutamine and packed red blood cell transfusions on pHi and indicating that only dobutamine increased pHi in the sub-group of patients with an initial low pHi. In patients with dopamine-resistant septic shock, Levy et al. [34] showed that a low-dose dobutamine infusion in association with norepinephrine increased pHi much faster than epinephrine alone. Creteur et al. [35] and Esen et al. [36] also reported an increase in pHi during dobutamine administration in patients with severe sepsis. Recently, in patients with severe sepsis Nevière et al. [15] observed that dobutamine increased pHi and gastric mucosal blood flow as assessed by Doppler techniques.

In summary, experimental and clinical studies concur to indicate that dobutamine can significantly increase splanchnic blood flow. Overall, dobutamine administration consistently increased pHi in septic patients.

Norepinephrine and Epinephrine

Norepinephrine is commonly used in the treatment of septic shock to restore arterial pressure. With its strong α-adrenergic mediated vasopressor effects, norepinephrine may threaten hepatosplanchnic perfusion. Some experimental studies have indicated that adrenergic agents may not significantly alter blood flow distribution in septic shock [38–40]. However, Zhang et al. [41] showed that during endotoxic shock in dogs, norepinephrine improved whole body and liver oxygen extraction capabilities. The authors postulated that the α-adrenergic effects, restoring the vascular tonus, contributed to this result.

In patients with septic shock, Ruokonen et al. [5] reported that norepinephrine increased splanchnic blood flow assessed by ICG clearance and splanchnic VO_2. However, the effects of norepinephrine on splanchnic blood flow were not uniform. In a pilot study comparing the effects of norepinephrine to those of dopamine on systemic and splanchnic oxygen utilization in patients with hyperdynamic sepsis, Marik and Mohedin [14] showed that norepinephrine increased pHi, whereas dopamine decreased it. As mentioned earlier, Levy et al. [34] reported that norepinephrine plus dobutamine increased pHi in patients with septic shock resistant to dopamine. Conversely, Meier-Hellmann et al. [28] in patients with septic shock showed that norepinephrine decreased the hepatic venous oxygen saturation, indicating a possible deterioration in splanchnic oxygenation. Recently, these same authors [42] showed that splanchnic blood flow was greater in patients with septic shock than in those with severe sepsis, although all patients with septic shock were treated with norepinephrine to maintain mean arterial pressure above 70 mmHg. However, pHi values were low in both groups and there was no correlation between splanchnic VO_2 and pHi or between splanchnic DO_2 and pHi. These results could indicate that although norepinephrine can increase splanchnic blood flow in septic shock, inadequate splanchnic oxygenation may remain even in the absence of splanchnic hypoperfusion.

At low doses, epinephrine acts predominantly on the peripheral β_1- and β_2-adrenergic receptors, whereas at moderate to high doses, α_1-receptor-mediated vasoconstrictor effects predominate. Epinephrine has variable effects on splanchnic blood flow [43–45]. Some studies have observed reduced intestinal blood flow in response to epinephrine, whereas others have observed increased blood flow. Most of the variability is probably related to differences in experimental models. In a newborn piglet model, Cheung et al. [46] reported that epinephrine decreased portal venous blood flow, total hepatic blood flow, and hepatic oxygen delivery with an increase in calculated mesenteric vascular resistance. Systemic and mesenteric oxygen extraction were not affected by epinephrine. In patients with septic shock, Meier-Hellmann et al. [47] demonstrated that changing the adrenergic support from a combination of dobutamine and norepinephrine to epinephrine alone increased the gradient between mixed venous and hepatic venous oxygen saturations (SvO_2-$ShvO_2$ gap), indicating a selective decrease in splanchnic perfusion. The same authors [48] recently reported that epinephrine decreased pHi and fractional splanchnic blood flow, and increased hepatic venous lactate when compared with dobutamine plus norepinephrine. Similar results were found by Levy et al. [34], who reported in 30 patients with septic shock that treatment with epinephrine transiently decreased pHi compared to treatment with norepinephrine plus dobutamine. Furthermore, epinephrine infusion was associated with an increase in systemic lactate levels, while norepinephrine plus dobutamine decreased them.

In summary, the findings concerning the effects of norepinephrine on splanchnic perfusion are inconsistent. In non-septic conditions and in the absence of severe hypotension, norepinephrine can decrease splanchnic perfusion. In septic patients norepinephrine showed variable effects on splanchnic oxygenation and pHi. Although the data available on the effects of epinephrine on pHi are still limited, they suggest a deleterious effect on gastric mucosal DO_2.

Non-Adrenergic Agents

Prostacyclin

Prostacyclin (PGI_2) combines vasodilating, antiplatelet aggregating and cytoprotective properties. PGI_2 has been shown to selectively increase splanchnic blood flow in animal models of hemorrhagic [49] and endotoxic [50] shock, and also to have protective effects on intestinal microcirculation .

The effects of PGI_2 on hepato-splanchnic blood flow have been studied by Radermacher and colleagues [51–53]. In septic shock patients who had been resuscitated with volume replacement, blood transfusion, and dobutamine infusion, these investigators found that PGI_2 increased pHi, suggesting that PGI_2 may improve splanchnic oxygenation even after conventional resuscitation goals have been achieved [51]. They further reported that PGI_2 administered in an aerosolized form [52] to septic shock patients could increase splanchnic blood flow (determined by ICG clearance) and pHi, while avoiding any detrimental effects on systemic hemodynamics. In patients undergoing major abdominal surgery, the protective effects of prostaglandins on intestinal function were also supported by the observation of increased bacterial translocation to mesenteric lymph nodes following ibuprofen administration [53]. Although these encouraging observations need to be confirmed, PGI_2 may find a place in the future as an adjuvant drug to improve splanchnic oxygenation.

Nitric Oxide and Nitric Oxide Synthase Inhibitors

Nitric oxide (NO) plays an important role in the regulation of blood pressure and organ blood flow distribution in normal conditions. It helps to maintain basal vasodilation in the mesenteric vasculature and the hepatic artery but not in the portal vein [54]. In rats, exogeneous supplementation of NO preserved blood flow and attenuated endotoxin-induced macroscopic jejunal damage [55]. The administration of the NO donor SIN-1 has been shown to increase superior mesenteric blood flow in endotoxic shock [56]. Increased NO availability may improve tissue perfusion not only by a vasodilating effect but also by inhibitory effects on platelet adhesion and aggregation, activation of leukocytes, mast cells, and other cellular elements involved in the inflammatory response [57, 58].

On the other hand, NO synthase (NOS) inhibitors have been shown to decrease blood flow to the splanchnic bed following endotoxemia [59, 60]. Hutcheson et al. [61] and Wright et al. [62] observed that N^G-monomethyl-L-arginine (L-NMMA) pre-treatment enhanced intestinal damage and increases in vascular permeability, and decreased hepatic blood flow. However, this may not be true for methylene blue (MB) which at low-to-moderate doses, selectively increased superior mesenteric blood flow following endotoxemia in fluid resuscitated dogs [63].

Some experimental studies have demonstrated that NO may be deleterious to splanchnic oxygenation. In a porcine model of endotoxic shock, Offner et al. [64] reported that the NOS inhibitor N-nitro-L-arginine methyl ester (L-NAME) decreased mesenteric blood flow less than carotid or renal blood flow. Furthermore L-NAME reversed the lipopolysaccharide-induced reduction in pHi. Salzman et al. [9] elegantly demonstrated that endotoxin may induce mucosal acidosis, perhaps because NO can alter the adenosine triphosphate (ATP) content of intestinal epithelial cells.

In septic shock patients, Eichelbrönner et al. [52] showed that, in contrast to aerosolized PGI_2, NO inhalation did not influence the pHi or ICG clearance.

The degree of release of NO, type of resuscitation, time of infusion, dose of NOS inhibitor or MB, variation in cardiac output, and method used to evaluate splanchnic oxygenation or perfusion can all influence the results and account for the lack of consistent findings.

N-acetylcysteine

N-acetylcysteine (NAC), an oxygen free radical scavenger which also enhances NO activity, exerts potent vasodilating and platelet inhibiting effects. NAC has been shown to improve oxygen extraction capabilities in endotoxic shock but did not influence fractional blood flow to the splanchnic region [65]. In a prospective, randomized, double-blind study, Spies et al. [66] observed that patients with septic shock who increased VO_2 during NAC infusion also showed an increase in pHi and an increase in DO_2. In septic patients, the same group showed that NAC prevented deterioration of oxygenation in gastric mucosal tissue during hyperoxia [67]. In a prospective, randomized, double-blind study which included 60 septic shock patients, Michel et al. [68] recently reported that liver blood flow increased with NAC administration, but this effect was proportional to the increase in cardiac index. Thus, NAC may increase pHi in septic patients, but these data need to be confirmed.

Conclusion

Many questions remain unanswered regarding the interpretation of a low pHi or a high gastric PCO_2. Clearly there can be a discrepancy between measurements of hepato-splanchnic or intestinal blood flow and pHi, and interventions that increase hepato-splanchnic blood flow may not consistently increase pHi [69, 70]. In patients with sepsis, additional factors complicate the issue. In these patients, high splanchnic blood flow may not guarantee adequate cellular oxygen availability for two reasons. First, there may be an imbalance between oxygen demand and supply such that demand exceeds supply, and second, there may be a redistribution of blood flow in the splanchnic area away from the mucosa, thus limiting oxygen supply to this region despite overall high blood flow.

Interpretation of the pHi is not straightforward. A low pHi may reflect poor mucosal perfusion but probably also metabolic abnormalities [71]. Hence, an increase in pHi following vasoactive drug administration in septic patients may be the result of increased gastric mucosal blood flow, improved oxygen extraction, anti-inflammatory properties of these drugs, or a combination of all these aspects. However, any vasoactive agents that increase gastric mucosal blood flow will decrease gastric mucosal PCO_2 because flow is the main determinant of its concentration.

Furthermore, the net desired effect of vasoactive agents is to decrease relative or absolute splanchnic ischemia, increasing the splanchnic and gastric mucosal blood flow. Although dopaminergic effects can increase splanchnic blood flow dopamine usually decreases pHi, suggesting a blood flow redistribution away from the gastric mucosa. Dobutamine increases splanchnic blood flow and tends to increase pHi in septic patients. Dopexamine has been shown to increase splanchnic oxygenation in sepsis, but these effects have not been systematically reported. Data on norepinephrine are more limited but suggest that norepinephrine could increase pHi in patients with septic shock. Prostacyclin and NAC may find a place as adjuvant drugs to improve splanchnic oxygenation. The role of NO is especially complex. At present, dobutamine seems to increase pHi most consistently in critically ill patients.

Progress in this area will depend on techniques that address not only total splanchnic blood flow, but also inter-organ flow distribution, intra-organ flow distribution, and other microcirculatory or metabolic malfunctions.

References

1. Schumacker PT, Cain SM (1987) The concept of a critical oxygen delivery. Intensive Care Med 13:223–229
2. Gutierrez G, Bismar H, Dantzker DR, Silva N (1992) Comparison of gastric mucosal pH with measures of oxygen transport and consumption in critically ill patients. Crit Care Med 20:451–457
3. Astiz ME, DeGent GE, Lin RY, Rackow EC (1995) Microvascular function and rheologic changes in hyperdynamic sepsis. Crit Care Med 23:265–271
4. Dahn MS, Lange MP, Wilson RF, Jacobs LA, Mitchell RA (1990) Hepatic blood flow and splanchnic oxygen consumption measurements in clinical sepsis. Surgery 107:295–301
5. Ruokonen E, Takala J, Kari A, Saxen H, Mertsola J, Hansen EJ (1993) Regional blood flow and oxygen transport in septic shock. Crit Care Med 21:1296–1303
6. Clark CH, Gutierrez G (1992) Gastric intramucosal pH: a noninvasive method for the indirect measurement of tissue oxygenation. Am J Crit Care 1:53–60
7. Schlichtig R, Bowles AS (1994) Distinguishing between aerobic and anaerobic appearance of dissolved CO_2 in intestine during low flow. J Appl Physiol 76:572–577
8. Vallet B, Lund N, Curtis SE, et al (1994) Gut and muscle tissue PO_2 in endotoxemic dogs during shock and resuscitation. J Appl Physiol 76:793–800
9. Salzman AL, Menconi MJ, Unno N, et al (1995) Nitric oxide dilates tight junctions and depletes ATP in cultured Caco-2BB intestinal epithelial monolayers. Am J Physiol 268:G361–G373
10. Meier-Hellmann A, Bredle DL, Specht M, et al (1997) The effects of low-dose dopamine on splanchnic blood flow and oxygen uptake in patients with septic shock. Intensive Care Med 23:31–37
11. Pawlik W, Sheperd AD, Jacobson ED (1975) Effects of vasoactive agents on intestinal oxygen consumption and blood flow in dogs. J Clin Invest 56:484–490
12. Royblat L, Gelman S, Bradley EL, et al (1990) Dopamine and hepatic oxygen supply-demand relationship. Can J Physiol Pharmacol 68:1165–1169
13. Maynard ND, Bihari DJ, Dalton RN, et al (1995) Increasing splanchnic blood flow in the critically ill. Chest 108:1648–1654
14. Marik PE, Mohedin J (1994) The contrasting effects of dopamine and norepinephrine on systemic and splanchnic oxygen utilization in hyperdynamic sepsis. JAMA 272:1354–1357
15. Nevière R, Mathieu D, Chagnon JL, et al (1996) The contrasting effects of dobutamine and dopamine on gastric mucosal perfusion in septic patients. Am J Respir Crit Care Med 154:1684–1688
16. Olson D, Pohlman A, Hall JB (1996) Administration of low-dose dopamine to nonoliguric patients with sepsis syndrome does not raise gastric intramucosal pH nor improve creatinine clearance. Am J Respir Crit Care Med 154:1664–1670
17. Lund N, de Asla RJ, Cladis F, et al (1995) Dopexamine hydrochloride in septic shock: effects on oxygen delivery and oxygenation of gut, liver, and muscle. J Trauma 38:767–775
18. Tighe D, Moss R, Heywood G, et al (1995) Goal-directed therapy with dopamine, dobutamine, and volume expansion: effects of systemic oxygen transport on hepatic ultrastructure in porcine sepsis. Crit Care Med 23:1997–2007
19. Cain SM, Curtis SE (1991) Systemic and regional oxygen uptake and delivery and lactate flux in endotoxic dogs infused with dopexamine. Crit Care Med 19:1552–1560
20. Trinder TJ, Lavery GG, Fee PH, et al (1995) Correction of splanchnic oxygen deficit in the intensive care unit: dopexamine and colloid versus placebo. Anaesth Intens Care 23:178–182
21. Kuhly P, Oschmann G, Hilpert J, et al (1996) Dopexamine does not change gastric and sigmoid mucosal pH in critically ill patients. Clin Intensive Care 7:58 (Abst)
22. Smithies M, Yee TH, Jacson L, et al (1994) Protecting the gut and the liver in the critically ill: effects of dopexamine. Crit Care Med 22:789–795
23. Leier CV, Underferth DV (1983) Dobutamine. Ann Intern Med 99:490–496
24. Fink MP, Kaups KL, Wang H, et al (1991) Maintenance of superior mesenteric arterial perfusion prevents increased intestinal mucosal permeability in endotoxic pigs. Surgery 110:154–161
25. De Backer D, Zhang H, Manikis P, et al (1994) Dobutamine can increase mesenteric blood flow during endotoxic shock in dogs. Am Rev Respir Dis 149:A19 (Abst)
26. Nevière R, Chagnon JL, Vallet B, et al (1997) Dobutamine improves gastrointestinal mucosal blood flow in a porcine model of endotoxic shock. Crit Care Med 25:1371–1377

27. Duranteau J, Sitbon P, Teboul JL, et al (1996) Compared effects of epinephrine (E), norepinephrine (NE) and norepinephrine-dobutamine combination (NE + Dobu) on the gastric mucosal blood flow in patients with septic shock. Am J Respir Crit Care Med 156:A832 (Abst)
28. Meier-Hellmann A, Reinhart K (1994) Influence of catecholamines on regional perfusion and tissue oxygenation in septic shock patients. In: Reinhart K, Eyrich K, Sprung C (eds) Sepsis. Current perspectives in pathophysiology and therapy. Springer-Verlag, Berlin, Heidelberg, New York, pp 274–291
29. Reinelt H, Radermacher P, Fischer G, et al (1997) Effects of a dobutamine-induced increase in splanchnic blood flow on hepatic metabolic activity in patients with septic shock. Anesthesiology 86:818–824
30. De Backer D, Creteur J, Smail N, et al (1996) Dobutamine increases hepatosplanchnic blood flow in septic patients. Am J Respir Crit Care Med 153:A125 (Abst)
31. Ruokonen E, Uusaro A, Alhava E, Takala J (1997) Effect of dobutamine infusion on splanchnic blood flow and oxygen transport in patients with acute pancreatitis. Intensive Care Med 23: 732–737
32. Gutierrez G, Clark C, Brown SD, et al (1994) Effect of dobutamine on oxygen consumption and gastric mucosal pH in septic patients. Am J Respir Crit Care Med 150:324–329
33. Silverman H, Tuma P (1992) Gastric tonometry in patients with sepsis: Effects of dobutamine infusions and packed red blood cell transfusions. Chest 102:184–188
34. Levy B, Bollaert PE, Charpentier C, et al (1997) Comparison of norepinephrine and dobutamine to epinephrine for hemodynamics, lactate metabolism, and gastric tonometric variables in septic shock. Intensive Care Med 23:282–287
35. Creteur J, De Backer D, Noordally O, et al (1996) Prognostic value of gastric mucosal PCO_2 in septic patients. Intensive Care Med 22 (suppl 2):S310 (Abst)
36. Esen F, Telci L, Çakar N, et al (1996) Evaluation of gastric intramucosal pH measurements with tissue oxygenation indices in patients with severe sepsis. Clin Intensive Care 7:180–189
37. Reinelt H, Fischer G, Wiedeck H, et al (1996) Effects of increased regional blood flow on splanchnic metabolism. Intensive Care Med 22 (suppl 1):S75 (Abst)
38. Bersten AD, Hersch M, Cheung H, et al (1992) The effect of various sympathomimetics on the regional circulations in hyperdynamic sepsis. Surgery 112:549–561
39. Breslow MJ, Miller CF, Parker SD, et al (1987) Effect of vasopressors on organ blood flow during endotoxin shock in pigs. Am J Physiol 252:H291–H300
40. Revelly JP, Liaudet L, Frascarolo P, et al (1997) The effect of norepinephrine on global and mesenteric blood flow during porcine endotoxic shock. Br J Anaesth 78 (suppl 2):A370 (Abst)
41. Zhang H, Smail N, Cabral A, Rogiers P, Vincent JL (1997) Effects of norepinephrine on regional blood flow and oxygen extraction capabilities during endotoxic shock. Am J Respir Crit Care Med 155:1965–1971
42. Meier-Hellmann A, Specht M, Hannemann L, et al (1996) Splanchnic blood flow is greater in septic shock treated with norepinephrine than in severe sepsis. Intensive Care Med 22: 1354–1359
43. Giraud GD, MacCannell KL (1984) Decreased nutrient blood flow during dopamine and epinephrine induced intestinal vasodilation. J Pharmacol Exp Ther 230:214–220
44. Kvietys PR, Granger DN (1982) Vasoactive agents and splanchnic oxygen uptake. Am J Physiol 243:G1–G9
45. Granger DN, Richardson PDI, Kvietys PR, et al (1980) Intestinal blood flow. Gastroenterology 78:837–863
46. Cheung JY, Barrington KJ, Pearson J, et al (1997) Systemic, pulmonary and mesenteric perfusion and oxygenation effects of dopamine and epinephrine. Am J Respir Crit Care Med 155:32–37
47. Meier-Hellmann A, Hannemann L, Specht M, et al (1994) The relationship between mixed venous and hepatic venous O_2 saturation in patients with septic shock. In: Vaupel P (ed) Oxygen transport to the tissues XV. Plenum Press, New York, pp 701–707
48. Meier-Hellmann A, Reinhart K, Bredle DL, et al (1997) Epinephrine impairs splanchnic perfusion in septic shock. Crit Care Med 25:399–404
49. Seelig RF, Kerr JC, Hobson RW, et al (1981) Prostacyclin (epopeostenol) – Its effect on canine splanchnic blood flow during hemorrhagic shock. Arch Surg 116:428–430
50. Rasmussen I, Arvidsson D, Zak A, et al (1992) Splanchnic and total body oxygen consumption in experimental fecal peritonitis in pigs: Effects of dextran and iloprost. Circ Shock 36:299–306

51. Radermacher P, Buhl R, Klein M, et al (1995) The effects of prostacyclin on gastric intramucosal pH in patients with septic shock. Intensive Care Med 21:414–421
52. Eichelbrönner O, Reinelt H, Wiedeck H, et al (1996) Aerosolized prostacyclin and inhaled nitric oxide in septic shock – different effects on splanchnic oxygenation? Intensive Care Med 22: 880–887
53. Brinkmann A, Wolf CF, Berger D, et al (1996) Perioperative endotoxemia and bacterial translocation during major abdominal surgery: Evidence for the protective effect of endogenous prostacyclin? Crit Care Med 24:1293–1301
54. Ayuse T, Brienza N, Revelly JP, et al (1995) Role of nitric oxide in porcine liver circulation under normal and endotoxemic conditions. J Appl Physiol 78:1319–1329
55. Boughton-Smith NK, Hucheson IR, Deaking AM (1994) Protective effect of S-nitroso-N-acetyl-penicillamine in endotoxin-induced acute intestinal damage in the rat. Eur J Pharmacol 191: 485–488
56. Zhang H, Rogiers P, Friedman G, et al (1996) Effects of nitric oxide donor SIN-1 on oxygen availability and regional blood flow during endotoxic shock. Arch Surg 131:767–774
57. Gauthier TW, Davenpeck KL, Lefer AM (1994) Nitric oxide attenuates leukocyte-endothelial interaction via P-selectin in splanchnic ischemia-reperfusion. Am J Physiol 267:G562–G568
58. Nishida J, McCuskey RS, McDonnell D, et al (1994) Protective role of NO in hepatic microcirculatory dysfunction during endotoxemia. Am J Physiol 267:G1135–G1141
59. Meyer J, Hinder F, Stothert J, et al (1994) Increased organ blood flow in chronic endotoxemia is reversed by nitric oxide synthesis inhibition. J Appl Physiol 76:2785–2793
60. Mulder MF, Lambalgen AA, Huisman E, et al (1994) Protective role of NO in the regional hemodynamic changes during acute endotoxemia in rats. Am J Physiol 266:H1558–H1564
61. Hutcheson IR, Whittle BJR, Boughton-Smith NK (1990) Role of nitric oxide in maintaining vascular integrity in endotoxin-induced acute intestinal damage in the rat. Br J Pharmacol 101: 815–820
62. Wright CH, Rees DD, Moncada S (1992) Protective and pathological roles of nitric oxide in endotoxin shock. Cardiovasc Res 26:48–57
63. Zhang H, Rogiers P, Preiser JC, et al (1995) Effects of methylene blue on oxygen availability and regional blood flow during endotoxic shock. Crit Care Med 23:1711–1721
64. Offner PJ, Robertson FM, Pruitt BA (1995) Effects of nitric oxide synthase inhibition on regional blood flow in a porcine model of endotoxic shock. J Trauma 39:338–343
65. Zhang H, Spapen H, Nguyen DN, et al (1995) Effects of N-acetyl-L-cysteine on regional blood flow during endotoxic shock. Eur Surg Res 27:292–300
66. Spies CD, Reinhart K, Witt I, et al (1994) Influence of N-acetylcysteine on indirect indicators of tissue oxygenation in septic shock patients: results from a prospective, randomized, double-blind study. Crit Care Med 22:1738–1746
67. Reinhart K, Spies CD, Meier-Hellmann A, Hannemann L, et al (1995) N-acetylcysteine preserves oxygen consumption and gastric mucosal pH during hyperoxic ventilation. Am J Respir Crit Care Med 151:773–779
68. Michel C, Sanft C, Schaffartzik W, et al (1997) N-acetylcysteine (NAC) increases liver blood flow in septic patients. Crit Care Med 25 (suppl):A117 (Abst)
69. Uusaro A, Ruokonen E, Takala J (1995) Gastric intramucosal pH does not reflect changes in splanchnic blood flow after cardiac surgery. Br J Anaesth 74:149–154
70. Parviainen I, Ruokonen E, Takala J (1995) Dobutamine induced dissociation between changes in splanchnic blood flow and gastric intramucosal pH after cardiac surgery. Br J Anaesth 74: 277–282
71. Fink MP (1996) Does tissue acidosis in sepsis indicate tissue hypoperfusion? Intensive Care Med 22:1144–1146

Intra-Abdominal Hypertension and Intensive Care

M. Sugrue and K. M. Hillman

Introduction

Intra-abdominal pressure (IAP) is an important indicator of a patient's underlying physiologic status. It is simple to measure, giving a reliable indicator of potentially serious intra-abdominal problems as well as other complications. IAP measurement is not a new concept to medicine, but it is only in recent years that the significance of the abdomen as a unique compartment is being realized. IAP has become one of the most important prognostic indicators in postoperative patients and is increasingly being used as part of routine patient monitoring in many intensive care units (ICU).

Historical Perspectives

IAP has become an increasingly important physiologic concept in intensive care. It was probably Wendt [1] as early as 1876, who first described the association between raised abdominal pressure and renal impairment. However, until the early part of this century, there was a poor understanding of the concept of IAP. Most investigators felt that the IAP was negative or sub-atmospheric. Emerson [2] first recognized that the pressure was usually positive and found that significant rises in IAP caused cardiac failure. Subsequently it has been found that increases in IAP are associated with significant physiologic alteration in cardiovascular and renal function.

One of the more outstanding pieces of research was conducted on human volunteers in 1947 by Bradley and Bradley [3] at Massachusetts Memorial Hospital. They were aware of the previous studies in the 1920s and 1930s which showed that increasing IAP above 15 mmHg reduced urine output and at levels above 30 mmHg, renal failure supervened [4]. Their experiment in 17 young healthy males found that increased IAP resulted in a reduction in the renal blood flow and glomerular filtration as a result of increases in venous pressures. They [3] concluded that such a uniform elevation of pressure throughout the abdominal cavity supported the concept that the abdomen and its contents should be considered as relatively non-compressible and fluid in character, and therefore behaved in accordance with Pascal's law. Recent studies in patients undergoing colonoscopy have confirmed that the transmission of pressure within the abdomen is in accordance with the laws of fluid mechanics [5]. In 1982, Harman et al. [6] confirmed that renal vascular resistance was probably the single most important contributor to renal dysfunction.

Technique of Measurement

A wide variety of innovative techniques have been used to measure IAP. IAP measurements have been performed in nearly every part of the abdominal cavity, including the stomach, urinary bladder, rectum, uterus, liver, inferior vena cava, and intraperitoneal cavity. Rectal pressure measurement was experimentally popular in the early part of this century, using a Miller Abbott tube [3]. Intra-gastric measurement was also used in the early part of this century with a Hamilton manometer [3]. More recently, nasogastric tubes with an attached gastric tonometer have been utilized [7]. The intra-gastric route has two specific advantages. It can be used when there has been trauma to the bladder or where the patient does not have a urinary catheter in place. Gastric pressures are also very useful when there is a tense pelvic hematoma following trauma, as vesicle pressures in this instance may not reflect the abdominal compartment pressures. Simultaneous urinary and gastric readings have found the mean difference between the two techniques to be marginal (0.35 mmHg; 95% confidence interval 3.8 to − 3.1 mmHg) [7].

Direct cannulation of the peritoneal cavity has been used experimentally but it has no advantage over more accessible and simple techniques [8]. Because of the fluid dynamics in the abdominal cavity, IAP can also be measured through a central line if its tip is in the inferior vena cava.

The gold standard for IAP measurement is undoubtedly the intravesical technique [9]. We have modified the technique slightly and our current technique is according to the following protocol. The patient is positioned flat in the bed. A standard Foley catheter is used with a T piece bladder pressure device attached between the urinary catheter and the drainage tubing. This piece is then connected to a pressure transducer, on-line to the monitoring system. The pressure transducer is placed in the mid-axillary line and the urinary tubing is clamped. Approximately 50 mls of isotonic saline is inserted into the bladder via a three-way stopcock. After zeroing, the pressure on the monitor is recorded. Guidelines for IAP measurement are summarized in Table 1. The incidence of raised IAP in the seriously ill is high, with approximately 30% of postoperative general surgery patients having IAPs greater than 20 mmHg [10]. After emergency surgery the incidence is even higher [10].

Pathophysiology

The abdominal cavity is defined superiorly by the diaphragms, anteriorly and posteriorly by the abdominal wall and inferiorly by the pelvic floor. Physiologic pressures can vary tremendously, depending on physical activity. At rest in the supine position, the normal IAP is 0–10 mmHg. During coughing and strenuous activity, values in excess of 150 mmHg can be recorded. The pressure is primarily determined by the volume of the viscera and the intra-compartment fluid load. The abdominal cavity pressure-volume curve has been studied in animals. Postmortem evaluation of human pressure-volume curves may not be reliable due to the postmortem loss of abdominal wall compliance. In general, the abdominal cavity exhibits a great tolerance to fluctuating volumes with little rise in IAP [11]. The compliance of the abdominal cavity can be seen at laparoscopy where it is possible to instill up to 5

Table 1. Some guidelines for IAP measurement

- A strict protocol and staff education on the technique and interpretation of IAP is essential
- Very high pressures (especially unexpected ones) are usually caused by a blocked urinary catheter
- The size of the urinary catheter does not matter
- The volume of saline instilled into the bladder is not critical
- A central venous pressure (CVP) manometer system can be used but it is more cumbersome than on-line monitoring
- If the patient is not laying flat, IAP can be measured from the pubic symphysis

liters of gas into the peritoneal cavity without exerting any significant influence on the IAP [7]. In a previous evaluation of IAP during laparoscopy we found that the mean volume of gas required to generate a pressure of 20 mmHg was 8.8 ± 4.3 l [7]. Adaptation can occur over time and this is seen clinically in patients with ascites, large ovarian tumors and, of course, pregnancy. The concept of a chronic abdominal compartment syndrome (ACS) has been proposed in morbidly obese patients, who have been found to have significantly increased IAP, predisposing perhaps to chronic venous stasis, urinary incontinence, incisional hernia and intracranial hypertension [12, 13].

The causes of acutely increased IAP are usually multifactorial. The first clinical postoperative reported cases of increased IAP were often after aortic surgery with postoperative hemorrhage from the graft suture line [14, 15]. In patients with peritonitis and intra-abdominal sepsis, tissue edema and ileus are the predominant causes of increased IAP. Raised IAP in trauma patients is often due to a combination of both blood loss and tissue edema. The common causes of increased IAP are shown in Table 2.

The concept of the ACS was first reported by Fiestman et al. [15], in four patients bleeding following aortic surgery. A precise definition of ACS is difficult. It has previously been defined as present when the peak inspiratory pressures are > 85 cmH$_2$O with hypercarbia and in the presence of abdominal distension [16]. This definition is probably unworkable as an increasing number of ICUs now adopt a more permissive approach to hypercapnia and such airway pressures are now considered dangerous. ACS has also been categorized in degrees from grade I to IV based on actual IAP measurements [17]. ACS is probably best described as occurring when adverse physiologic effects have resulted from increased IAP. However, it is not clear at exactly what levels of IAP negative physiologic IAP effects begin to occur.

Table 2. Causes of increased IAP

- Tissue edema secondary to insults such as ischemia and sepsis
- Ileus
- Intraperitoneal or retroperitoneal hematoma
- Ascites
- Pneumoperitoneum

Effect of Raised IAP on Individual Organ Function

Renal

Renal dysfunction in association with increased IAP has been recognized for over 100 years but it is only recently that its effects on large series of patients have been reported. In 1945, Bradley and Bradley [3] in a study of 17 volunteers demonstrated that there was a reduction in renal plasma flow and glomerular filtration rate (GFR) in association with increased IAP. In 1982, Harman et al. [6] showed that as IAP increased from 0 to 20 mmHg in dogs, the GFR decreased by 25%. At 40 mmHg, the dogs were resuscitated and their cardiac output returned to normal. However their GFR and renal blood flow did not improve, indicating a local effect on renal blood flow. The situation in seriously ill patients may, however, be different and the exact cause of renal dysfunction in the ICU is not clear, due to the complexity of critically ill patients. In a recent study [18], we found that out of 20 patients with increased IAP and renal impairment, 13 already had impairment before the IAP increased.

The most likely direct effect of increased IAP is an increase in the renal vascular resistance, coupled with a moderate reduction in cardiac output. Pressure on the ureter has been ruled out as a cause, as investigators have placed ureteric stents with no improvement in function [4]. Other factors which may contribute to renal dysfunction include humoral factors and intra-parenchymal renal pressures. In a canine study, increased antidiuretic hormone levels have been found in association with increases in IAP [19, 20]. The concept of renal decapsulation, on the basis of raised intrarenal pressure, was popular some decades ago, but now is rarely practiced.

The absolute value of IAP that is required to cause renal impairment has not been established. Some authors have suggested that 10–15 mmHg is a critical cut-off point [21, 22]. Others have found little renal impairment below 20 mmHg [10]. Maintaining adequate cardiovascular filling pressures in the presence of raised IAP also seems to be important [23, 24].

Cardiovascular

Increased IAP reduces cardiac output as well as increasing central venous pressure (CVP), systemic vascular resistance, pulmonary artery pressure and pulmonary artery wedge pressure [6, 24]. It should be remembered, however, that due to the associated rise in intra-pleural pressure, some of the rises seen in CVP may not reflect the intravascular volume and may be misleading when assessing the patient's volume status. Cardiac output is affected mainly by a reduction in stroke volume, secondary to a reduction in preload and an increase in afterload. This is further aggravated by hypovolemia. Paradoxically, in the presence of hypovolemia an increase in IAP can be temporarily associated with an increase in cardiac output [8]. The normal left atrial/right atrial pressure gradient may be reversed during raised IAP [25]. It has been observed that venous stasis occurs in the legs of patients with abdominal pressures above 12 mmHg [26]. In addition, recent studies in patients undergoing laparoscopic cholecystectomy show up to a four-fold increase in renin and aldosterone levels [27].

Respiratory

Both animal and human experiments have shown that IAP exerts a significant effect on pulmonary function. In association with increased IAP, there is diaphragmatic stenting, exerting a restrictive effect on the lungs with reduction in ventilation, decreased lung compliance, increase in airway pressures, and reduction in tidal volumes. These changes can occasionally be seen during laparoscopy, where lung compliance has been shown to be reduced once the IAP exceeds 16 mmHg. Respiratory changes related to increased IAP are aggravated by increased obesity and other physiologic conditions such as severe hemorrhage. There is also some adverse effect on the efficiency of gas exchange [28]. Often patients with raised IAP are acidotic and while initially this may be metabolic in origin, the effect of raised IAP adds a respiratory component. In critically ill ventilated patients the effect on the respiratory system can be significant, resulting in reduced lung volumes, impaired gas exchange and high ventilatory pressures. Hypercarbia can occur and the resulting acidosis can be exacerbated by simultaneous cardiovascular depression as a result of raised IAP. The effects of raised IAP on the respiratory system in ICU patients can sometimes be life-threatening, requiring urgent abdominal decompression.

Visceral Perfusion

Interest in visceral perfusion has increased with the popularization of gastric tonometry and there is an association between IAP and visceral perfusion as measured by gastric pH [7]. This has been confirmed recently in 18 patients undergoing laparoscopy, where reduction of between 11% and 54% in blood flow was seen in the duodenum and stomach respectively at an IAP of 15 mmHg [29]. Animal studies suggest that reduction in visceral perfusion is selective, affecting intestinal blood flow before, for example, adrenal blood flow [30]. We [10] have demonstrated in a study of 73 post-laparotomy patients that IAP and pHi are strongly associated, suggesting that early decreases in visceral perfusion are related to levels of IAP as low as 15 mmHg. Increasing IAPs may result in visceral hypoperfusion and secondary bacterial translocation as well as affecting wound healing. Both abnormal pHi and IAP predict the same adverse outcome with increased risk of hypotension, intra-abdominal sepsis, renal impairment, need for re-laparotomy and death [18].

Intracranial Contents

Raised IAP can have a marked effect on intracranial pathophysiology and cause severe rises in intracranial pressure (ICP) [24, 31]. It appears to cause raised ICP and decreased cerebral perfusion pressure by increasing intrathoracic pressure which, in turn, impedes cerebral venous drainage [24]. There may also be an added effect secondary to reduced systemic blood pressure as a result of decreased preload and impaired cardiovascular function [31]. The effect of raised IAP on ICP is especially relevant in multi-trauma when head injury with possible increased ICP and raised IAP can co-exist. Laparoscopy in trauma patients should be undertaken at as low a pressure as possible [32]. When this occurs there must be a decreased level of suspicion for early intervention to surgically decompress the abdomen in order to reduce the IAP and ICP.

Treatment

General Support

The precise management of IAP remains somewhat clouded by many published anecdotal reports and uncontrolled series. Aggressive non-operative intensive care support is critical to prevent the complications of ACS. This involves careful monitoring of the cardiorespiratory system and aggressive intravascular fluid replacement especially if this is associated with hemorrhage [33], maintenance of gas exchange with minimum ventilatory pressures and careful monitoring of renal function. Simple measures such as nasogastric decompression are, of course, mandatory.

Reversible Factors

The second aspect of management is to correct any reversible cause of raised IAP, such as intra-abdominal bleeding. Massive retroperitoneal hemorrhage is often associated with a fractured pelvis and consideration should be given to measures which would control hemorrhage such as pelvic fixation or vessel emobilization. In some cases, severe gaseous distension or acute colonic pseudo-obstruction can occur in ICU patients (unpublished observations). This may respond to drugs such as neostigmine (unpublished observations) but if it is severe, surgical decompression may be necessary. A common cause of raised IAP in ICUs is related to ileus. There is little that can be actively done in these circumstances apart from optimizing the patient's cardiorespiratory status and serum electrolytes. Occasionally, drugs such as metoclopramide have also been used. Tension pneumoperitoneum [35] can also cause an acute rise in IAP and may have to be surgically decompressed as a matter of urgency [36].

Increased IAP is often a symptom of an underlying problem. In a prospective review of 88 post-laparotomy patients, those with an IAP of greater or equal to 20 mmHg had an odds ratio for intra-abdominal sepsis of 3.9 (95% CI 0.7–22.7) [10]. Abdominal evaluation for sepsis is a priority and this obviously should include a rectal examination as well as investigations such as ultrasound and computed tomography (CT) scan. Surgery is usually the only treatment in patients whose rise in IAP is due to postoperative bleeding. In general, these patients, with the exception of the end-stage coagulopathic group, should do well.

Surgery for Raised IAP

As yet, there are few guidelines for exactly when surgical decompression is required in the presence of raised IAP. At one end of the spectrum, some studies have stated that abdominal decompression is the only treatment and that it should be performed early in order to prevent ACS [17]. The indications for abdominal decompression are related to correcting pathophysiologic abnormalities as much as achieving a precise and optimum IAP. For example, if gas exchange is being increasingly compromised with collapse of the lung bases and/or ventilatory pressures are increasing, abdominal decompression should be strongly considered. Similarly, if cardiovascular or renal function is being compromised and raised IAP is suspected, then decompression should be considered early. Unfortunately, visceral hypoperfusion is very difficult to predict, apart from gastric tonometry, and guidelines for surgical intervention would have to rely on levels of IAP which have been shown to correlate with visceral ischemia.

The approaches to abdominal decompression also vary. Temporary abdominal closure (TAC) has been popularized as a mechanism to reverse many of the sequelae of increased IAP. The theoretical benefits of abdominal decompression and TAC are therefore attractive and some authors have advocated the prophylactic use of TAC to decrease postoperative complications and facilitate planned re-exploration. However, it may be hard to justify this approach until a subgroup of high risk patients are more accurately identified. Burch et al. [17] has stated that abdominal decompression can reverse the sequelae of the ACS. Intra-abdominal pressure levels have been advocated as a guide to closure of the abdominal wall, especially in children. However, the existing literature currently has few prospective studies. Wittman et al. in two separate studies [36, 37] in 1990 and 1994, prospectively evaluated outcomes in 117 and 95 patients, respectively. A multi-institutional study [37] of 95 patients concluded that a staged approach to abdominal repair with TAC was superior to conventional techniques for dealing with intra-abdominal sepsis. Torrie and colleagues [38] have recently retrospectively reported their experience with 64 patients (median APACHE II score 21) undergoing TAC and found the mortality to be 49%. Some indications for TAC are listed in Table 3.

A large number of different techniques have been used to facilitate TAC, including intravenous (IV) bags, velcro, silicone, zips. Whatever technique, it is important that effective decompression be achieved with adequate incisions. Consideration should also be given to the use of silos, as approximately 25% of patients with TAC have post-TAC pressures greater than 20 mmHg (unpublished data). Silos provide potential room for increased intra-abdominal volume to expand and are fashioned out of various synthetic materials. Existing literature suggests that polytetrafluoroethylene (PTFE) and polypropylene (PP) are both useful materials for TAC [39, 40]. The cheapest method is using a sterile 3 l IV bag, cutting along three sides and sewing to the edges of the wound. This has the advantage that at subsequent operations, the plastic can be incised and re-sutured for an indefinite number of times. The PFTE

Table 3. Some indications for performing TAC

- Abdominal decompression
- To facilitate re-exploration in abdominal sepsis
- Inability to close the abdomen
- Potentially prevents abdominal compartment syndrome

Table 4. Some guidelines for surgical decompression for raised IAP

- Early investigation and correction of the cause of raised intra-abdominal pressure
- Ongoing abdominal bleeding with raised IAP requires urgent operative intervention
- Reduction in urinary output is a late sign of renal impairment in patients with increased IAP. Gastric tonometry may provide earlier information on visceral perfusion
- Abdominal decompression requires a full length abdominal incision
- The surgical dressing should be closed using a sandwich technique using 2 suction drains placed laterally to facilitate fluid removal from the wound
- Do not take the dressing down. If it leaks, reapply under full sterile condition
- If the abdomen is very tight, pre-closure with a silo should be considered

tissue patch with micro meshed holes, allows fluid to permeate through, facilitating ongoing decompression of the abdomen. It has been suggested that PTFE may be associated with fewer side-effects than PP, although in the presence of obvious contamination, PTFE should not be used. Moreover PP patches are associated with erosion into viscera and this can occur months and even years after insertion.

Unfortunately, clinical infection is common in the open abdomen and the infection is usually polymicrobial. Particular care needs to be taken in patients post-aortic surgery as the aortic graft may become colonized. The mesh in this situation should be removed and the abdomen left open. It is desirable to close the abdominal defect as soon as possible. This is often not possible due to persistent tissue edema. Some guidelines for surgical decompression are listed in Table 4.

Conclusion

The concept of IAP measurement and its significance is increasingly important in the ICU and is rapidly becoming part of routine care. Patients with raised IAP require close and careful monitoring, aggressive resuscitation and a low index of suspicion for surgical abdominal decompression.

References

1. Wendt E (1867) Über den Einfluss des Intraabdominalen Druckes auf die Absonderungsgeschwindigkeit des Harnes. Arch Physiologische Heilkunde 525–527
2. Emerson H (1911) Intra-abdominal pressures. Arch Intern Med 7:754–784
3. Bradley SE, Bradley GP (1947) The effect of increased intra-abdominal pressure on renal function in man. J Clin Invest 26:1010–1022
4. Thorington JM, Schmidt CF (1923) A study of urinary output and blood-pressure changes resulting in experimental ascites. Am J Med Science 165:880
5. Tzelepis GE, Nasiff L, McCool FD, Hammond J (1996) Transmission of pressure within the abdomen. J Appl Physiol 81:1111–1114
6. Harman KP, Kron IL, McLachlan DH, et al (1982) Elevated intra-abdominal pressure and renal function. Ann Surg 196:594–597
7. Sugrue M, Buist MD, Lee A, et al (1994) Intra-abdominal pressure measurement using a modified nasogastric tube: description and validation of a new technique. Intensive Care Med 20:588–603

8. Motew M, Ivankovich AD, Bieniarz J, et al (1972) Cardiovascular effects and acid base and blood gas changes during laparoscopy. Am J Obstet Gynecol 115:1002–1012

9. Kron IL, Harman PK, Nolan SP (1984) The measurement of intraabdominal pressure as a criterion for abdominal re-exploration. Ann Surg 196:594–597

10. Sugrue M, Buist MD, Hourihan F, Deane S, Bauman A, Hillman K (1995) Prospective study of intra-abdominal hypertension and renal function after laparotomy. Br J Surg 82:235–240

11. Salkin D (1934) Intraabdominal pressure and its regulation Am Rev Tuberculosis 30:436–457

12. Bump RC, Sugarman HJ, Fantl JA, et al (1992) Obesity and lower urinary tract function in women: Effect of surgically induced weight loss. Am J Obstet Gynecol 167:392–399

13. Amaral JF, Tsiaris W, Morgan T, et al (1987) Reversal of benign intracranial hypertension by surgically induced weight loss. Arch Surg 122:946–949

14. Platell CF, Hall J, Clarke G, et al (1990) Intra-abdominal pressure and renal function after surgery to the abdominal aorta. Aust NZ J Surg 60:213–216

15. Fietsam R, Villalba M, Glover JL, et al (1989) Intra-abdominal compartment syndrome as a complication of ruptured abdominal aortic aneurysm repair. Am J Surg 55:396–402

16. Morris JA, Eddy VA, Blinman TA, Rutherford EJ, Sharp KW (1993) The staged celiotomy for trauma. Issue in unpacking and reconstruction. Ann Surg 217:576–586

17. Burch J, Moore E, Moore F, Franciose R (1996) The abdominal compartment syndrome. Surg Clin North Am 76:833–842

18. Sugrue M, Jones F, Lee A, et al (1996) Intraabdominal pressure and gastric intramucosal pH: Is there an association? World J Surg 20:988–991

19. Le Roith D, Bark H, Nyska M, et al (1982) The effect of abdominal pressure on plasma antidiuretic hormone in the dog. J Surg Res 32:65–69

20. Bloomfield GL, Blocher CR, Fakhry IF, Sica DA, Sugerman HJ (1997) Elevated intra-abdominal pressure increases plasma renin activity and aldosterone levels. J Trauma 42:997–1005

21. Pusajo J, Bumaschny E, Agurrola A, et al (1994) Postoperative intra-abdominal pressure: its relation to splanchnic perfusion, sepsis, multiple organ failure and surgical intervention. Intensive Crit Care Digest 13:2–7

22. Lacey JB, Brooks SP, Griswald J, et al (1987) The relative merits of various methods of indirect measurement of intraabdominal pressure as a guide to closure of abdominal wall defects. J Pediatr Surg 22:1207–1211

23. Kashtan J, Green JF, Parsons EQ, Holcroft JW (1981) Haemodynamic effects of increased abdominal pressure. J Surg Res 30:249–255

24. Bloomfield GL, Ridings PC, Blocher CR, Marmarou A, Sugerman HJ (1996) Effects of increased intra-abdominal pressure upon intracranial and cerebral perfusion pressure before and after volume expansion. J Trauma 40:936–943

25. Iwase K, Kamikke W, Uchikoshi F, Takenka H (1996) Effect of pneumoperitoneum on interatrial pressure gradient during laparoscopic cholecystectomy. World J Surg 20:234–237

26. Jorgensen JO, Lalak NJ, North L, Hanel K, et al (1994) Venous stasis during laparoscopic cholecystectomy. Surg Lap Endo 4:128–133

27. O'Leary E, Hubbard K, Tormey W, Cunningham AJ (1996) Laparoscopic cholecystectomy: haemodynamic and neuroendocrine responses after pneumoperitoneum and changes in position. Br J Anaesth 75:640–644

28. Kelman GR, Swapp GH, Smith, et al (1972) Cardiac output and arterial blood gas tension during laparoscopy. Br J Anaesth 44:1155–1161

29. Schilling MK, Redaelli C, Krahenbuhl L, Signer C, Buchler MW (1997) Splanchnic microcirculatory changes during CO_2 laparoscopy. J Am Coll Surg 184:378–382

30. Caldwell CB, Ricotta JJ (1987) Changes in visceral blood flow with elevated intra-abdominal pressure. J Surg Res 43:14–20

31. Bloomfield GL, Ridings PC, Blocher CR, Marmarou A, Sugerman HJ (1997) A proposed relationship between increased intra-abdominal, intrathoracic, and intracranial pressure. Crit Care Med 25:496–503

32. Este-McDonald JR, Josephs LG, Birkett DH, Hirsch EF (1995) Changes in intracranial pressure associated with apneumic retractors. Arch Surg 130:362–365

33. Simon RJ, Friedlander MH, Ivtury RR, DiRaimo R, Machiedo GW (1997) Haemorrhage lowers the threshold for intra-abdominal hypertension-induced pulmonary dysfunction. J Trauma 42:398–403

34. Hillman KM (1982) Pneumoperitoneum – a review. Crit Care Med 10:476–481
35. Higgins JRA, Halpin MG, Midgley AK (1988) Tension pneumoperitoneum: a surgical emergency. Brit J Hosp Med 160–161
36. Wittmann D, Aprahamian C, Bergstein J (1990) Etappenlavage: Advanced diffuse peritonitis managed by planned multiple laparotomies utilising zippers, slide fastener and velcro analogue for temporary abdominal closure. World J Surg 14:218–226
37. Wittmann D, Bansal N, Bergstein J, et al (1994) Staged abdominal repair compares favourably with conventional operative therapy for intra-abdominal infections when adjusting for prognostic factors with a logistic model. Theor Surg 9:201–207
38. Torrie J, Hill AA, Streat S (1996) Staged abdominal repair in critical illness. Anaesth Intensive Care 24:368–374
39. Bleichrodt R, Simmermacher R, van der Lai B, Schakenraad JM (1993) Expanded polytetrafluoroethylene patch versus polypropylene mesh for the repair of contaminated defects of the abdominal wall. Surg Gynecol Obstet 176:18–24
40. Brown GL, Richardson D, Malangoni MA, Tobin GR, Ackerman D, Polk HC (1985) Comparison of prosthetic materials for abdominal wall reconstruction in the presence of contamination and infection. Ann Surg 201:705–711

Head Trauma

Pharmacological Augmentation of Endogenous Neuroprotective Responses after Traumatic Brain Injury

P. M. Kochanek and R. S. B. Clark

Introduction

Much of the investigative work in both the experimental and clinical approaches to the optimal management of patients with severe traumatic brain injury has focused on optimization of supportive care. In addition, a variety of contemporary pharmacologic approaches have been evaluated in both laboratory models [1] and in clinical studies [2]. As a result, a variety of promising agents have been identified. No pharmacologic approach has, however, been successfully applied in a clinical trial in patients with severe traumatic brain injury [2]. These pharmacologic approaches have, for the most part, focused on either the attenuation of acute post-traumatic excitotoxicity [1, 2] or the inhibition of oxidant damage [3] in the injured brain using specific inhibitors.

We have focused our efforts on the development of novel therapeutic approaches in the treatment of traumatic brain injury. To this end, we have applied two basic strategies: Evaluating novel mechanisms of secondary damage and related inhibitors of these mechanisms; and defining and augmenting endogenous neuroprotective responses. This second approach, augmenting endogenous neuroprotective responses, is a relatively unique one [3, 4], and is the focus of this chapter. In this review, two relatively unexplored mechanisms of potential pharmacologic neuroprotection after traumatic brain injury are addressed. Both laboratory and clinical studies by our group, along with the work of other investigators, are presented to provide, as much as possible, a bench-to-bedside state of the art review. These two novel areas currently under investigation by our group include:
1) Ameliorating energy failure by augmenting the local adenosine response; and
2) augmenting posttraumatic anti-apoptotic defense mechanisms.

Ameliorating Energy Failure by Augmenting the Local Adenosine Response

Numerous studies, in both experimental models and in patients, have suggested that excitotoxicity contributes to the development of secondary damage after severe traumatic brain injury [1, 2, 5]. Immediately after injury, a massive increase in interstitial levels of the excitatory amino acids glutamate and aspartate are observed in experimental models of traumatic brain injury [6]. Similar increases in glutamate and aspartate have been reported during secondary insults, such as delayed spikes of intracranial hypertension or jugular venous desaturation episodes in humans [6].

Much of this excitotoxicity may be mediated via post-synaptic receptors such as the n-methyl-D-aspartate (NMDA) and α-amino-3-hydroxy-5-methyl-4-isoxazole (AMPA) receptors [1, 5]. Post-traumatic events such as neuronal depolarization, spreading depression, and ischemia produce these increases in interstital levels of excitatory amino acids. Much of the focus of neuroprotective pharmacologic strategies for the prevention of secondary damage after traumatic brain injury has focused on antagonists of the NMDA or AMPA receptor. For example, activation of the NMDA receptor by glutamate or aspartate results in agonist-mediated calcium accumulation, activation of a variety of toxic cascades including proteases and neuronal nitric oxide synthase (NOS), results in neuronal necrosis or apoptosis [5, 7]. Another mechanism that may contribute to secondary damage after traumatic brain injury is acute inflammation. We, and others, have demonstrated a robust acute inflammatory response to traumatic brain injury in both experimental animal models and in humans. This response includes cytokine production [8], adhesion molecule expression [9, 10], and leukocyte accumulation [11]. Toumond et al. [12] recently demonstrated a reduction in lesion volume using an anti-inflammatory strategy, namely administration of an antagonist to interleukin-1 (IL-1), in a rat model of traumatic brain injury. One endogenous defense system which appears to have important attenuating effects on both excitotoxicity and inflammation, and is thus a potential therapeutic target, is the production of adenosine during the dephosphorylation of adenosine triphosphate (ATP) to lower energy compounds.

Adenosine may be an important endogenous neuroprotectant in the traumatically injured brain. This potential is best seen by examining the effects of adenosine binding to its A_1 and A_2 receptors. Adenosine binding the A_1 receptor, localized in neurons, decreases K^+ and Cl^- conductances, producing hyperpolarization of the neuronal membrane and reduces pre-synaptic excitatory amino acid release, resulting in a reduction in both neuronal activation and accompanying metabolic activity [13, 14]. Remarkably, the distribution of the A_1 receptor is spatially similar to that of the NMDA receptor [15], thus the neuroprotective potential of this pathway is obvious. Adenosine binding to the A_2 receptor on cerebral blood vessels and the cerebrovascular endothelium has the potential to produce a variety of neuroprotective effects including local vasodilation and the inhibition of leukocyte activation [16]. This could improve blood flow to injured and compromised brain regions, those with blood flow inadequate to meet metabolic demands [17], and attenuate the acute inflammatory response [11]. The affinity of adenosine for the A_1 receptor is much greater than for the A_2 receptor, since nanomolar concentrations of adenosine reduce neuronal activity *in vitro* [18, 19], while micromolar concentrations are required to induce vasodilation at the A_2 receptor [16]. The actions of adenosine at the A_3 receptor in the central nervous system are less well defined. A theoretical scheme of the scenarios resulting in adenosine production and the potential neuroprotective effects of augmenting the adenosine response for the traumatically injured brain are shown in Fig. 1.

The neuroprotective potential of augmenting the effects of adenosine have been demonstrated in a variety of experimental paradigms pertinent to brain injury, including cell culture, hippocampal slice preparations, and ischemia models [20, 21]. Studies of the role of adenosine in either laboratory models of traumatic brain injury or in patients with severe head injury, however, have been rather limited.

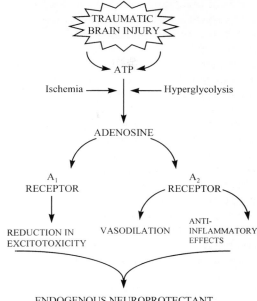

Fig. 1. Theoretical schematic illustrating the potential pathways resulting in endogenous neuroprotectant effects of adenosine in the injured brain

Specific to traumatic brain injury, Nilsson et al. [22] reported 20–30-fold increases in brain interstital adenosine accompanying large increases in glutamate, aspartate and lactate after weight-drop-induced brain injury in rats. These increases were demonstrated using cerebral microdialysis techniques. Headrick et al. [23] reported 60-fold increases in adenosine in brain interstital fluid after experimental traumatic brain injury produced by fluid-percussion in rats. This increase in adenosine was, however, more transient in nature than the duration of energy failure as assessed by phosphorous magnetic resonance spectroscopy. Intracerebroventricular administration of the adenosine agonist 2-chloroadenosine attenuated these metabolic disturbances. We [24] recently reported similar large, but transient, increases in brain interstital levels of adenosine and related purine metabolites in a contemporary model of cerebral contusion produced by controlled cortical impact in rats.

The participation of adenosine in human brain injury has received very limited attention. Recently, we reported significant increases in adenosine in cerebrospinal fluid of both adults [25] and children [26] after severe head injury, compared to controls. A variety of other parameters were measured in these patients including cerebral blood flow, cerebral metabolic rate for oxygen, cerebrospinal fluid lactate, and outcome. Univariate and multivariate analyses of the adult data revealed that the increase in adenosine was significantly associated with both uncoupling of cerebral blood flow and oxidative metabolism, and with mortality. One possible explanation for this finding is that adenosine is attempting to defend the traumatically injured brain by supporting the hyperglycolysis recently reported by Bergsneider and co-workers [27]. Oxidative metabolism is markedly inhibited after severe traumatic brain injury in patients and it is proposed that glycolytically-controlled maintenance of ionic homeostasis by astrocytes is a key mechanism driving this process [28]. Consistent with this hypothesis, in our series of patients exhibiting an association between increased cerebrospinal fluid adenosine and mortality, cerebrospinal fluid lactate levels were increased during the period of reduced oxidative metabolism and uncoupling, providing further support for a possible role for adenosine as an endogenous neuroprotectant molecule after human head injury. We recently published a preliminary report showing significant increases in adenosine and xanthine in brain interstital human from humans during episodes of jugular venous desaturation [29]. This finding suggests a possible role of adenosine in defending the brain during episodes of secondary hypoxia/ischemia episodes such as delayed spikes of intracranial hypertension, local expansion of mass lesions, or secondary hypotension or hypoxemia. Thus a putative role for adenosine both in the early post-injury phase and during delayed episodes of secondary injury in the intensive care unit is supported.

A variety of potential strategies are available to augment the endogenous adenosine response after head injury including administration of adenosine analogs [23], inhibitors of enzymes involved in the metabolism of adenosine, such as adenosine deaminase and adenosine kinase, or agents that enhance adenosine binding to the A_1 receptor [20, 21, 30, 31]. The administration of the adenosine kinase inhibitor deoxy-iodotubercidin was recently shown to reduce infarct size in a model of focal cerebral ischemia/reperfusion in rats [31] and in a model of experimental epilepsy [32]. Therapeutic evaluation of these agents in experimental models of traumatic brain injury, and additional descriptive studies of adenosine in human head injury are needed in this promising area of investigation.

Augmenting Post-traumatic Anti-Apoptotic Defense Mechanisms

After traumatic brain injury neuronal cell death occurs in both an immediate and a delayed fashion. Delayed neuronal death may be an irreversible consequence of secondary brain injury after trauma; however, increasing evidence suggests that at least a portion of this delayed neuronal death may be regulated by specific genes that are induced or become activated after injury [33, 34]. Thus, manipulating programmed cell death, or apoptosis [35, 36], offers a possible therapeutic target for attenuating secondary brain injury after trauma.

Apoptosis is a form of programmed cell death that is characterized by delayed energy failure, the requirement for new protein synthesis, DNA fragmentation by endonucleases, condensation of nuclear material, and cytoplasmic and nuclear shrinkage. In contrast, necrosis is characterized by primary energy failure, inhibition of protein synthesis, direct DNA damage, cytoplasmic swelling, and rupture of cellular, nuclear, and organelle membranes [35, 36]. There have been several recent reports showing apoptosis as well as necrosis after traumatic brain injury in multiple experimental models [33, 37–40] and in humans [41]. Rink et al. [37], were the first to report apoptotic cell death after experimental traumatic brain injury using a fluid-percussion model in rats. These investigators identified DNA fragmentation *in situ* after injury using terminal deoxynucleotidyl-transferase mediated dUTP nick-end labeling (TUNEL). Neurons with characteristics of both apoptosis and necrosis were seen in regions that are selectively vulnerable to delayed cell death in this model. We have reported similar findings using a clinically relevant model of controlled cortical impact with secondary insult (moderate hypoxemia and mild hypotension) [39]. Apoptosis is also seen after controlled cortical impact without secondary insult [38], but it is less extensive compared with controlled cortical impact with secondary insult.

In embryogenesis and in the normal maintenance and development of adult tissues which have a high degree of cell turnover, apoptotic cell death plays an integral role and is tightly regulated by specific genes and their translated proteins [35, 36, 42]. These include genes that suppress apoptosis such as the *bcl-2* gene family members *bcl-2* and *bcl-x$_L$*; genes that accelerate apoptosis such as the *bcl-2* gene family members *bax* and *bcl-x$_S$* [43]; and proteins that execute the apoptotic program such as the cysteine proteases interleukin-1β converting enzyme (ICE; caspase 1) and cpp32 (caspase 3) [33]. These apoptosis-regulatory genes and proteins are also likely involved in the ultimate degree of cell survival after ischemic [44], excitotoxic [45], and traumatic brain injury. We have recently shown that the anti-apoptotic gene *bcl-2* is induced in surviving neurons after traumatic brain injury in rats [34]. Importantly, inhibiting the apoptotic process using cysteine protease inhibitors reduces neurologic dysfunction after traumatic brain injury in rats [33]. In addition, attenuating apoptotic cell death by administering neurotrophins after traumatic brain injury is associated with a reduction in cholinergic neuronal cell loss and cognitive dysfunction [40]. Potential therapeutic targets aimed at reducing apoptotic cell death after traumatic brain injury are shown in Fig. 2.

Although pharmacologic agents designed to specifically manipulate apoptotic cell death after injury are limited, novel therapies have been developed and tested in

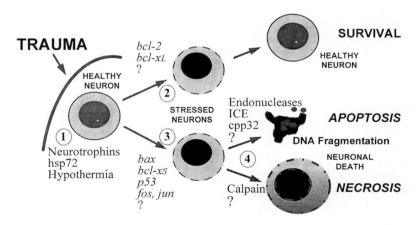

Fig. 2. Potential therapeutic targets aimed at reducing apoptotic neuronal death after traumatic brain injury. 1) Non-specific therapies that reduce primary cellular injury and attenuate signals triggering the apoptotic cascade. 2) Therapies augmenting anti-apoptotic endogenous neuroprotective genes. 3) Therapies inhibiting pro-apoptotic genes. 4) Therapies targeting effectors of cell death such as proteases and endonucleases. Overall neuronal cell survival/death may depend in part upon the balance of anti- and pro-apoptotic forces

experimental models. Relevant to brain injury, these include agents that have many effects which include reducing apoptotic cell death, such as the neurotrophins [40] and anti-inflammatory agents [46], as well as more selective inhibitors of apoptosis such as the cysteine protease inhibitors. Newer therapies are also being developed which have highly specific effects, and can be used to investigate mechanisms of apoptotic cell death as well as for future clinically relevant treatments. Antisense oligonucleotides, which can specifically block translation of single proteins, are promising agents [47]. There are limitations to the use of antisense oligonucleotides [48], however, their further development may provide powerful tools for blocking apoptosis at certain points along the programmed cell death cascade. While it is tempting to hypothesize that manipulating the expression of a single apoptotic-regulatory protein will significantly alter downstream effects and improve outcome after traumatic brain injury, it is likely that multiple proteins will need to be targeted. Indeed, therapies with multiple beneficial effects that include the attenuation of apoptotic cell death, such as hypothermia or neurotrophin replacement, may be necessary to improve outcome.

The role of apoptosis and the apoptotic process after human head injury is even less well defined. Thomas and colleagues [41] have reported TUNEL-positive cells in the brain after traumatic brain injury. In a preliminary report, we have shown that the apoptosis-regulatory proteins bcl-2, bcl-x_L, bax, and ICE can be detected in brain tissue specimens removed during emergent surgical decompression for the treatment of life-threatening intracranial hypertension [49]. These proteins have also been detected in brains from patients with a variety of other pathologic states, including Parkinson's disease [50] and Alzheimer's disease [51]. Finally, a provocative study by Stocker et al. [52], has reported an association between the apoptosis-related soluble Fas ligand in cerebrospinal fluid and intracranial pressure and cerebral perfusion pressure after severe head injury. Further investigation is required to determine whether specifically augmenting the anti-apoptotic response improves histopathologic and functional outcome after traumatic brain injury. In addition, the contribution of apoptotic cell death to ultimate outcome after traumatic brain injury in experimental models and in humans remains to be defined.

Conclusion

Current therapies for the treatment of human head injury are limited to largely supportive care, and additional treatments are needed [2]. Augmenting endogenous neuroprotectant mechanisms represents a potentially promising approach to the treatment of head injury. Evidence has been presented that two of these endogenous neuroprotective pathways, the production of adenosine, and the expression of anti-apoptotic genes are logical candidates for further investigation in this regard. A variety of other endogenous defense pathways such as the immediate early response gene expression, the neurotrophic response, selected beneficial aspects of the acute inflammatory response, and anti-oxidant systems may represent additional pathways to be similarly augmented. Further study of this intriguing new approach is needed.

References

1. McIntosh TK (1993) Novel pharmacologic therapies in the treatment of experimental traumatic brain injury: A review. J Neurotrauma 10:215–261
2. Bullock R, Doppenberg EMR (1997) Clinical neuro-protection trials in severe traumatic brain injury: Lessons from previous studies. J Neurotrauma 14:71–76
3. Muizelaar JP, Marmarou A, Young HF, et al (1993) Improving the outcome of severe head injury with the oxygen radical scavenger polyethylene glycol-conjugated superoxide dismutase: A phase II trial. J Neurosurg 78:375–382
4. Mattson MP, Scheff SW (1994) Endogenous neuroprotection factors and traumatic brain injury: Mechanisms of action and implications for therapy. J Neurotrauma 11:3–33
5. Lipton SA, Rosenber PA (1994) Excitatory amino acids as a final common pathway for neurological disorders. N Engl J Med 330:613–620
6. Zauner A, Bullock R (1996) The role of excitatory amino acids in severe brain trauma: Opportunities for therapy: A Review. In: Bandak FA, Eppinger RH, Ommayas AK (eds) Traumatic brain injury, bioscience and mechanics. Mary Ann Liebert Publishers, New York, pp 97–104
7. Portera-Cailliau C, Price DL, Martin LJ (1997) Non-NMDA and NMDA receptor-mediated excitotoxic neuronal deaths in adult brain are morphologically distinct: Further evidence for an apoptosis-necrosis continuum. J Comp Neurol 378:88–104
8. Goss J, Styren S, Miller P, et al (1995) Hypothermia attenuates the normal increase in interleukin 1b RNA and nerve growth factor following traumatic brain injury in the rat. J Neurotrauma 12:159–167
9. Whalen M, Carlos T, Bell M, Carcillo J (1997) Soluble adhesion molecules in CSF are increased in children with severe head injury. Crit Care Med 25 (suppl 1):A20 (Abst)
10. Carlos TM, Clark RSB, Franicola-Higgins D, Schiding JK, Kochanek PM (1997) Expression of endothelial adhesion molecules and recruitment of neutrophils following traumatic brain injury in rats. J Leuk Biol 61:279–285
11. Clark RSB, Schiding JK, Kaczorowski SL, Marion DW, Kochanek PM (1994) Neutrophil accumulation after traumatic brain injury in rats: Comparison of weight-drop and controlled cortical impact models. J Neurotrauma 11:499–506
12. Toulmond S, Rothwell NJ (1995) Interleukin-1 receptor antagonist inhibits neuronal damage caused by fluid percussion injury in the rat. Brain Res 671:261–266
13. Segal M (1982) Intracellular analysis of a postsynaptic action of adenosine in the rat hippocampus. Eur J Pharmacol 79:193–199
14. Siggins GR, Schubert P (1981) Adenosine depression of hippocampal neurons in vitro: an intracellular study of dose dependent actions on synaptic and membrane potentials. Neurosci Lett 23:55–60
15. Bowery NG, Wong EHF, Hudson AL (1988) Quantitative autoradiography of (3H) MK-801 binding sites in mammalian brain. Br J Pharmacol 93:948–954
16. Cronstein BN (1994) Adenosine, an endogenous anti-inflammatory agent. J Appl Physiol 76:5–13
17. Hovda DA, Lee SM, Smith ML, et al (1995) The neurochemical and metabolic cascade following brain injury: Moving from animal models to man. J Neurotrauma 12:903–906
18. Londos C, Cooper DMF, Wolff J (1980) Subclasses of external adenosine receptors. Proc Natl Acad Sci USA 77:2551–2554
19. Van Calker D, Muller M, Hampriecht B (1979) Adenosine regulates via two different types of receptors. The accumulation of cyclic amp in cultured brain cells. J Neurochemistry 11:999–1005
20. Miller LP, Hsu C (1992) Therapeutic potential for adenosine receptor activation in ischemic brain injury. J Neurotrauma 9 (suppl 2):S563–S577
21. Gidday JF, Fitzgibbons JC, Shah AR, Kraujalis MJ, Park TS (1995) Reduction in cerebral ischemic injury in the newborn rat by potentiation of endogenous adenosine. Pediatr Res 38:306–311
22. Nilsson P, Hillered L, Ponten U, Ungerstedt U (1990) Changes in cortical extracellular levels of energy-related metabolites and amino acids following concussive brain injury in rats. J Cereb Blood Flow Metab 10:631–637
23. Headrick JP, Bendall MR, Faden AI, Vink R (1994) Dissociation of adenosine levels from bioenergetic state in experimental brain trauma: Potential role in secondary injury. J Cereb Blood Flow Metab 14:853–861

24. Bell M, Jackson E, Carcillo J, et al (1996) Interstitial adenosine is increased after controlled cortical impact (CCI) in rats. J Neurotrauma 13:596 (Abst)

25. Clark RSB, Carcillo JA, Kochanek PM, et al (1998) Cerebrospinal fluid adenosine concentration and uncoupling of cerebral blood flow and oxidative metabolism after severe head injury in humans. Neurosurgery (in press)

26. Bell M, Adelson PD, Jackson E, et al (1996) Adenosine concentrations in cerebrospinal fluid after severe traumatic brain injury in children. Crit Care Med 24 (suppl 1):A136 (Abst)

27. Bergsneider M, Hovda DA, Shalmon E, et al (1997) Cerebral hyperglycolysis following severe traumatic brain injury in humans: a positron emission tomography study. J Neurosurg 86:241–251

28. Pellerin L, Magistretti PJ (1994) Glutamate uptake into astrocytes stimulates aerobic glycolysis: A mechanism coupling neuronal activity to glucose utilization. Proc Natl Acad Sci USA 91:10625–10629

29. Bell MJ, Robertson CS, Kochanek PM, et al (1997) Interstitial accumulation of purine metabolites after traumatic brain injury (TBI) in humans: Evidence for energy failure during jugular venous desaturation. Soc Neurosci Abstr 23:1124

30. Halle JN, Kasper CE, Gidday JM, Koos BJ (1997) Enhancing adenosine A_1 receptor binding reduces hypoxic-ischemic brain injury in newborn rats. Brain Res 759:309–312

31. Miller LP, Jelovich LA, Yao L, DaRe J, Ugarkar B, Foster AC (1996) Pre- and peristroke treatment with the adenosine kinase inhibitor, 5′-deoxyiodotubercidin, significantly reduces infarct volume after temporary occlusion of the middle cerebral artery in rats. Neurosci Lett 220:73–76

32. Zhang G, Franklin PH, Murray TF (1993) Manipulation of endogenous adenosine in the rat prepiriform cortex modulates seizure susceptibility. J Pharmacol Exp Therap 264:1415–1424

33. Yakovlev AG, Knoblach SM, Fan L, Fox GB, Goodnight R, Faden AI (1997) Activation of CPP32-like caspases contributes to neuronal apoptosis and neurologic dysfunction after traumatic brain injury. J Neurosci 17:7415–7424

34. Clark RSB, Chen J, Watkins SC, et al (1998) Apoptosis suppressor gene bcl-2 expression after traumatic brain injury in rats. J Neurosci (in press)

35. Saunders JW (1966) Death in embryonic systems. Science 154:604–612

36. Kerr JFR, Wyllie AH, Currie AR (1972) Apoptosis: A basic biological phenomenon with wide-ranging implications in tissue kinetics. Br J Cancer 26:239–257

37. Rink A, Fung K-M, Trodanowksi JQ, Lee VMY, Neugebauer E, McIntosh TK (1995) Evidence of apoptotic cell death after experimental traumatic brain injury in the rat. Am J Pathol 147:1575–1583

38. Colicos MA, Dash PK (1996) Apoptotic morphology of dentate gyrus granule cells following experimental cortical impact injury in rats: possible role in spatial memory deficits. Brain Res 739:120–131

39. Clark RSB, Kochanek PM, Dixon CE, et al (1997) Early neuropathologic effects of mild or moderate hypoxemia after controlled cortical impact injury in rats. J Neurotrauma 14:179–189

40. Sinson G, Perri BR, Trojanowski JQ, Flamm ES, McIntosh TK (1997) Improvement of cognitive deficits and decreased cholinergic neuronal cell loss and apoptotic cell death following neurotrophin infusion after experimental traumatic brain injury. J Neurosurg 86:511–518

41. Thomas LB, Gates DJ, Richfield EK, O'Brien TF, Schweitzer JB, Steindler DA (1995) DNA end labeling (TUNEL) in Huntington's disease and other neuropathological conditions. Exp Neurol 133:265–272

42. Steller H (1995) Mechanisms and genes of cellular suicide. Science 267:1445–1449

43. Hockenbery DM (1995) bcl-2, a novel regulator of cell death. BioEssays 17:631–638

44. MacManus JP, Linnik MD (1997) Gene expression induced by cerebral ischemia: an apoptotic perspective. J Cereb Blood Flow Metab 17:815–832

45. Graham SH, Chen J, Stetler RA, Zhu RL, Jin KL, Simon RP (1996) Expression of proto-oncogene bcl-2 is increased in the rat brain following kainate-induced seizures. Restorative Neurol Neurosci 9:243–250

46. Chopp M, Li Y, Jiang N, Zhang RL, Prostak J (1996) Antibodies against adhesion molecules reduce apoptotis after transient middle cerebral artery occlusion in rat brain. J Cereb Blood Flow Metab 16:578–584

47. Crooke ST, Bennett CF (1996) Progress in antisense oligonucleotide therapeutics. Annu Rev Pharmacol Toxicol 36:107–129

48. Stein CA (1995) Does antisense exist? Nature Med 11:1119–1121
49. Clark RSB, Kochanek PM, Chen J, et al (1997) Expression of cell death regulatory proteins cpp32, bax, and bcl-xL after traumatic brain injury in rats. J Cereb Blood Flow Metab 17 (suppl):S22 (Abst)
50. Mogi M, Harada M, Kondo T, et al (1996) bcl-2 protein is increased in the brain from parkinsonian patients. Neurosci Lett 215:137–139
51. Su JH, Satou T, Anderson AJ, Cotman CW (1996) Up-regulation of bcl-2 is associated with neuronal DNA damage in Alzheimer's disease. Neuroreport 7:437–440
52. Stocker KM, Imhof HG, Trentz O, Ertel W (1997) Significance of apoptosis-induced fas antigen-fas ligand system for post-traumatic brain edema. Langenbecks Arch Chir 114:481–483

Experimental and Clinical Neuroprotection: An Update

C. Werner

Introduction

Cerebral ischemia, and or hypoxia, may occur as a consequence of shock, vascular stenosis or occlusion, vasospasm, neurotrauma, and cardiac arrest. The ischemic/hypoxic insult evokes a cascade of pathophysiologic processes which may consecutively result in neuronal necrosis. The first level of the ischemic cascade is the accumulation of lactic acid due to anaerobic glycolysis. This leads to increased membrane permeability and in turn accumulation of perivascular and intracellular fluids. Since the anaerobic metabolism is insufficient to maintain cellular energy states, the adenosine triphosphate (ATP)-stores deplete and failure of energy-dependent membrane ion pumps occurs. This produces membrane depolarization, increases in excitatory neurotransmitter concentration (i.e., glutamate, aspartate) and activation of NMDA- (N-methyl-D-aspartate), AMPA- (α-amino-3-hydroxy-5-methyl-4-isoxazolpropionate), and voltage dependent Ca^{++}- and Na^{+}-channels. The consecutive massive Ca^{++} and Na^{+} influx leads to activation of several catabolic intracellular processes. Ca^{++} activates lipid peroxidases, proteases, and phospholipases which in turn increase the intracellular concentration of free fatty acids (FFA) and free radicals. Consecutively, membrane degeneration of vascular and cellular structures leads to cellular death.

The strategies to protect the brain from ischemic/hypoxic insults are based on the understanding of these pathophysiologic processes. Maintenance of normal to high cerebral perfusion pressure, normoxia, and surgical decompression are by far the most important and effective neuroprotective interventions. Besides these treatment modalities, concepts of physical and pharmacologic brain protection include interventions to increase cerebral blood flow (CBF) in the ischemic territory, reduction of cerebral metabolism and intracranial pressure (ICP), inhibition of lactic acid accumulation and excitatory neurotransmitter activity, prevention of Ca^{++}-influx, inhibition of lipid peroxidation, and free radical scavenging.

Physical Neuroprotection

Hyperventilation

Therapeutic hyperventilation is one of the traditional methods of reducing ICP in mechanically ventilated patients. Hyperventilation is supposed to reduce secondary brain injury by the following mechanisms: 1) Increasing interstitial and intracellular pH; 2) increasing perfusion to ischemic territories by redistribution of blood (inverse steel effect); 3) reduction of cerebral blood volume and ICP.

During ischemia, neuronal acidosis occurs as a function of anaerobic glycolysis with accumulation of lactic acid. Hyperventilation produces respiratory compensation of ischemic acidosis. However, respiratory alkalosis is only effective for a period of less than 24 hours due to compensatory loss of bicarbonate ions [1]. Additionally, hyperventilation to $PaCO_2$ values < 25 mmHg increases the extent of ischemia. Together there is no experimental or clinical evidence which supports the use of hyperventilation to decrease infarct size or improve neurologic outcome.

Hyperventilation may theoretically improve perfusion in ischemic territories by hypokapnic vasoconstriction in non-ischemic tissues (inverse steel effect). This hypothesis is based on observational reports indicating recovery of the electroencephalogram (EEG) or cerebral perfusion with hyperventilation [2]. In contrast, controlled experimental and clinical studies suggest that hypocapnic vasoconstriction increases, rather than decreases, the degree of cerebral ischemia [1, 3]. This indicates that hypocapnic cerebrovascular constriction is ineffective in redistributing perfusion in favor of ischemic territories and may even aggravate neuronal injury.

In patients with transient but critical elevations of ICP (e.g., plateau waves), acute hyperventilation ($PaCO_2$: 30–34 mmHg) still represents a life-saving treatment until more specifc interventions are initiated to reduce the intracranial hypertension. With recovery of ICP, hyperventilation must be carefully reversed to maintain normocapnia ($PaCO_2$: 36–40 mmHg). However chronic hyperventilation may have adverse effects on outcome in patients with head injury as hypocapnic vasoconstriction produces further reductions in CBF and worsens outcome despite decreases in ICP. This aspect of hyperventilation is particularly important in patients with pre-existing cerebral ischemia following head injury, while hyperventilation may be beneficial in patients with relative or absolute hyperemia [4, 5]. As a consequence chronic hyperventilation to $PaCO_2$ values < 30 mmHg is never indicated even in the presence of permanent intracranial hypertension as this concept does not reduce ICP over time but may worsen neurologic outcome in patients with head injury [5].

Hypothermia

Deep hypothermia ($< 28\,°C$) protects against both focal and global ischemia. In recent years, increasing interest has developed concerning the cerebral effects of mild ($29\,°C$–$32\,°C$) and moderate ($33\,°C$–$36\,°C$) hypothermia. This is due to observations in laboratory animals and humans showing brain protection with small reductions in brain temperature during increased ICP and cerebral ischemia. It has been suggested that hypothermic protection is related to suppression of major biochemical processes such as decreases in cerebral metabolism, reduction of excitatory neurotransmitter release, and inhibition of accumulation of lipid peroxidation products and free radical generation. Other studies indicate that small changes in temperature economize CBF and prevent post-ischemic hyper- and hypoperfusion and formation of brain edema.

Hypothermia During Cerebral Ischemia: In rats, hypothermia (33 °C–30 °C) induced during focal or global cerebral ischemia with reperfusion produced decreases in infarct size and improved neurologic outcome in a temperature-dependent fashion. In contrast, hypothermia was not protective during permanent focal ischemia [6]. In a cardiac resuscitation model histopathologic damage was reduced with mild (34 °C) or moderate hypothermia (32 °C–30 °C); however, deep hypothermia (28 °C–15 °C) did not improve neurologic outcome due to generation of toxic metabolites and myocardial depression [7]. This suggests a temperature threshold below which there will be no beneficial effect of hypothermia in the setting of cerebral ischemia.

Hypothermia Following Cerebral Ischemia: In rats subjected to focal cerebral ischemia, post-ischemic mild hypothermia (34 °C) reduced infarct size and improved neurologic outcome [8]. Similarily, mild hypothermia (34 °C) induced immediately following cardiopulmonary resuscitation and maintained for 1 h effectively reduced histopathologic and functional damage. In rats and dogs subjected to a fluid percussion injury or epidural compression, post-traumatic moderate hypothermia (31 °C–30 °C) reduced mortality and improved neurofunctional behaviour in surviving animals [9]. However, neuroprotection was inducible only if hypothermia was initiated within a time window of 15–90 minutes after the insult.

Hypothermia and Clinical Neuroprotection: Between 1958 and 1962, mild to moderate hypothermia (28 °C–34 °C) was initiated in 116 patients with severe head injury within the first 12–24 h following trauma, for a period of 2 to 10 days. In these studies mortality was 43% to 72% and the majority of deaths occurred during re-warming. Despite the subjective impression of neuronal protection by hypothermia, no conclusion could be drawn from these investigations due to the lack of control patients. Recently, three prospective, controlled, and randomized phase-II-studies have shown that neurologic deficit and mortality related to head injury were significantly reduced when mild to moderate hypothermia was induced within 6 to 24 h following the injury and maintained for 24 to 48 h [10–12]. Currently a prospective, controlled, and randomized phase-III-trial is being conducted to confirm these results as the following aspects on therapeutic hypothermia still have to be defined: Timing of the initiation of hypothermia; optimal temperature; duration of hypothermia; and the optimal regimen of re-warming. However, hyperthermia must be treated aggressively in patients with cerebral ischemia [13].

Pharmacologic Brain Protection (Table 1)

Thrombolysis

Studies in models of acute thrombembolic stroke have shown that thrombolytic treatment using recombinant tissue plasminogen activator (rt-PA), urokinase, single-chain urokinase plasminogen activator (scu-PA) or streptokinase is effective in reperfusing ischemic territories. Unfortunately, early clinical studies failed to confirm the beneficial effects of thrombolytic treatment in acute stroke due to poor control of physiologic variables, violations of the protocol, and inadequate radio-

Table 1. Partial list of brain protection drugs in or near clinical trials

Drug	Action
SNX-111	Ca^{++}-channel blocker
Aptiganel	NMDA-receptor blocker
Fosphenytoin/lamotrigine	Na^+-channel blocker
Clomethiazole	stimulates inhibitory GABA receptors
bFGF	growth factor
Insulin-like growth factor-1	growth factor
nNOS-blockade	reduces $NO^{\cdot} + O_2^{\cdot -}$ and $ONOO^-$
Cu-Zn SOD, Mn-SOD	scavenging of free radicals
N-t-butyl-α-phenylnitrone	scavenging of free radicals
ICE-like protease-inhibitors	suppression of apoptosis
ICAM-1 inhibitors	reduction of PMN-activity

nNOS: neuronal nitric oxide synthase; SOD: superoxide dismutase; ICE: interleukin converting enzyme; PMN: polymorphonuclear neutrophils

logic diagnostics. Following identification of adverse effects of thrombembolic treatment, five placebo-controlled, prospective multicenter trials were conducted to confirm the neuroprotective effect of thrombolysis. Three of these trials using streptokinase (MAST-E, MAST-I, ASK) were prematurely terminated due to increased intracranial hemorrhages and mortality. In contrast the European Cooperative Acute Stroke Study (ECASS-I) as well as the National Institute of Neurological Disorders and Stroke rt-PA Stroke Study Group found an increase in favorable outcome despite a higher incidence of intracranial hemorrhage in patients treated with rt-PA within 3–6 hours following the onset of neurologic symptoms [14, 15]. As a consequence of adverse side effects, the ECASS-II study investigates the effectiveness of lower concentrations of rt-PA in parallel with meticulous control of the protocol requirements.

Anesthetics

The proposed mechanisms of anesthetic protection include reduction of cerebral metabolism and intracranial pressure, suppression of seizures and sympathetic discharge, and a re-set of the thermoregulatory threshold. Additionally, anesthetics may reduce intracellular Ca^{++}- and free radical accumulation. However, the clinical and experimental data remain controversial.

Volatile Anesthetics

Isoflurane, sevoflurane and desflurane produce maximum cerebral metabolic suppression in parallel at concentrations >2 MAC end-tidal. This effect suggests that volatile anesthetics may correct for the imbalance between oxygen supply and demand during focal cerebral ischemia. Animal studies with focal or incomplete hemispheric ischemia have shown that isoflurane, sevoflurane, and desflurane may decrease infarct size and improve neurologic outcome when given prior to the ischemic challenge [16]. These experimental data are consistent with studies in isoflurane anesthetized patients undergoing carotid endarterectomy showing increased tolerance to lower levels of CBF with preserved neuronal function during carotid cross-clamping when compared to enflurane or halothane background anesthesia [17]. In contrast, volatile anesthetics have no neuroprotective properties in the setting of global cerebral ischemia and when given after the insult.

Hypnotics

Numerous studies in laboratory animals have shown that barbiturates as well as propofol reduce infarct size and improve neurologic outcome following focal or incomplete global cerebral ischemia as long as physiologic variables were controlled during the experiments [18]. While experimental data support the preventive neuroprotective effects of hypnotic agents, the clinical evidence is less convincing. In patients undergoing cardiac surgery with normothermic cardiopulmonary bypass the infusion of thiopental [total dose during extracorporeal circulation (ECC) 39.5 ± 8.4 mg/kg iv] was able to reduce postoperative neuropsychologic deficits [19]. In contrast, barbiturates infused to comatose patients within the first hour following cardiopulmonary resuscitation were ineffective in reducing mortality as well as neurological deficits in survivors compared to standard intensive care unit (ICU) treatment [20]. These data are consistent with the view that the infusion of hypnotics prior to focal, but not global, ischemic insults may increase the ischemic tolerance of neurons. Barbiturates may also be beneficial in patients with severe head injury and refractory intracranial hypertension. This conclusion is related to a series of clinical studies where infusion of barbiturates was effective in reducing ICP and likely the mortality rate following brain trauma, as long as systemic hemodynamic stability was maintained [21].

Benzodiazepines

Midazolam and diazepam reduce neurologic deficit and increase survival rate following incomplete global ischemia and hypoxia. Likewise, intraoperative administration of diazepam reduced the incidence and extent of postoperative neuropsychologic deficits in patients undergoing cardiopulmonary bypass [22]. Despite the modest neuroprotective potential of benzodiazepines, midazolam and diazepam are not first choice agents in patients with cerebral ischemia due to their extended duration of recovery along with a delayed neurologic examination.

Plasma Glucose Concentration

Studies in laboratory animals and humans have shown that hyperglycemia is associated with worsened outcome following stroke or neurotrauma. The mechanisms by which normoglycemia may protect neuronal tissue include decreases in intracellular lactic acidosis along with decreases in membrane permeability and reduced edema of endothelial cells, neuroglia, and neurons [23]. As a consequence, plasma glucose concentrations should be assayed every 2 hours and maintained within the range of 100–150 mg/dl.

Calcium-Channel Blocker

Ca^{++} may enter the intracellular space by action of agonist controlled Ca^{++}-channels (e.g., glutamate, NMDA) or by activation of pre-synaptic voltage-dependent L-, T-, N-, P-, and Q-type Ca^{++}-channels with consecutive release of excitatory neurotransmitters, nitric oxide, and activation of catabolic processes (proteases, nucleases, lipases). The proposed mechanisms of neuronal protection by Ca^{++}-channel blockers include cerebral vasodilation, prevention of vasospasm, reduced Ca^{++}-influx and modulation of free fatty acid metabolism. Unfortunately, the results in animal models are rather contradictory. While several studies found decreases in neuronal injury and improved outcome following focal ischemia, others have failed to produce protection with Ca^{++}-channel blockers. Only the N-type Ca^{++}-antagonist SNX-111, an omega-conopeptide, was extremely neuroprotective in animal models of focal and global cerebral ischemia even when infused within 24 hours following the insult [24]. Several clinical trials have tested the neuroprotective effects of the L-Typ Ca^{++}-channel blocker, nimodipine, in patients with acute ischemic stroke and aneurysmal or traumatic subarachnoid hemorrhage. According to a meta-analysis [25] of 9 placebo-controlled trials with a total of 3700 patients with acute stroke, oral administration of nimodipine appears to be associated with a favorable outcome as long as the treatment commences within the first 12 hours following the onset of the symptoms. This is consistent with the results from a meta-analysis [26] of 8 placebo-controlled studies in 1202 patients with aneurysmal subarachnoid hemorrhage demonstrating an improved chance of developing a favorable outcome, and reduced incidence of cerebral vasospasm with the prophylactic administration of nimodipine. Patients with traumatic subarachnoid hemorrhage may also benefit from the infusion of nimodipine [27]. However, Ca^{++}-channel blockers may induce arterial hypotension below the individual ischemic threshold of the patients and any relevant decrease in arterial blood pressure will reverse any potentially neuroprotective effects of the intended treatment.

NMDA and AMPA Receptor Antagonists

Glutamate and aspartate are known as excitatory neurotransmitters which stimulate NMDA receptors (Ca^{++}- and Na^{+}-influx) and AMPA receptors (Na^{+}-influx). Since the activation of these receptors initiates catabolic intracellular processes, blockade of NMDA and AMPA receptors may protect cerebral tissue.

NMDA Receptor Antagonists: Ketamine, MK-801 (dizocilpine), aptiganel, dextromethorphan, dextrorphan, and Mg^{++} represent non-competitive NMDA-receptor antagonists. In animal models of focal (but not global) cerebral ischemia and head injury ketamine as well as MK-801 reduced neuronal injury and improved outcome [28].

Likewise, infusion of the competetive NMDA receptor antagonist CGS 19 755 (selfotel) reduced infarct size following focal and global ischemia. Clinical trials using MK-801 were terminated due to toxic side effects and the induction of mitochondrial vacuolization. The clinical development of the anti-tussive agents dextromethorphan and dextrorphan, was also terminated because of side effects such as hallucination, agitation, and sedation. Clinical phase-III-trials in patients with acute stroke and head injury using aptiganel (Cerestat, CNS-1102) are currently in process but the safety committee has indicated major concerns because of the induction of severe hallucinations with this NMDA receptor blocker. Four clinical trials in patients with acute stroke or head injury were also prematurely terminated because of adverse effects of the competetive NMDA receptor antagonist CGS 19 755 (selfotel) [29].

AMPA Receptor Antagonists: Studies in laboratory animals have shown that the competetive and non competetive AMPA receptor antagonists NBQX und GYKI 52 466 reduce histopathologic damage even when infused within 12 hours after induction of ischemia. Unfortunately, the current class of these compounds is still too toxic and thus not available for clinical use.

Lazaroids

The term lazaroids is frequently used to describe compounds such as lipid peroxidase inhibitors, anti-oxidants, and free radical scavengers. The proposed mechanisms by which these drugs reduce neuronal injury include increased order of lipid bilayers, free radical scavenging and prevention of FFA-accumulation by inhibition of lipid peroxidation.

Glucocorticoids

Studies in patients with acute stroke or following resuscitation could not demonstrate a significant reduction in infarct size or improvement in neurologic outcome with the infusion of glucocorticoids (e.g., dexamethasone or methylprednisolone) despite some positive effects in experimental preparations. Likewise, controlled clinical trials could not exclude moderate beneficial nor moderate harmful effects in patients with head injury receiving either dexamethasone or methylprednisolone [30]. However, rather than banning these agents, it is more likely that there are sub-groups of patients with acute ischemic or traumatic brain lesions who may improve from lipid peroxidase inhibition. In contrast to stroke or head injury high doses of methylprednisolone (30 mg/kg bolus; 5,4 mg/kg/23 h) given within the first 8 hours following spinal cord injury may reduce motor deficit and improve function of sensory tracts [31].

21-Aminosteroids

Tirilazad mesylate (U-74006F) is a potent inhibitor of oxygen free radical-induced lipid peroxidation. Most of the laboratory investigations have shown that tirilazad reduces infarct size and improves neurologic outcome in models of transient or permanent focal or global cerebral ischemia even when infused after the insult [32]. In contrast, phase III clinical trials in patients with acute stroke, subarachnoid hemorrhage, and head injury failed to confirm the experimental neuroprotective evidence [33]. Currently, the phase III multicenter study from Europe, Australia and New-Zealand in patients with subarachnoid hemorrhage is the only investigation demonstrating a reduction in mortality with administration in male patients, while female patients did not benefit from tirilazad [34].

Radical Scavengers

During ischemia and reperfusion molecular oxygen is reduced to the following oxidants: Superoxide radicals, hydrogen peroxide, and hydroxyl radicals. Oxygen free radicals represent a highly reactive species which rapidly interact with cellular membranes, nuclear acids, receptors and enzymes, and induce lysis in these structures. Superoxide dismutase (SOD) is a physiological free radical scavenger which exists in two isoforms: Cytosolic copper-zink-SOD and mitochondrial manganese-SOD. Studies in cell cultures and transgenic mice have shown that SOD produces a maximum reduction in cellular oxidative stress. Unfortunately, SOD has an extremely low penetration through the blood brain barrier and cellular membranes. Consequently, SOD was conjugated with polyethyleneglycol (PEG) to enhance its bioavailability. In patients with severe head injury (phase II trial) PEG-SOD reduced mortality when given in high concentrations. However, a consecutive phase III trial in 463 head-injured patients failed to confirm the neuroprotective effects of PEG-SOD [35]. In patients with aneurysmal subarachnoid hemorrhage (phase III trial) the hydroxyl-scavenger AVS (nicaraven) reduced neurologic deficits [36].

Conclusion

Normal to high cerebral perfusion pressure, normoxia, and surgical decompression are by far the most important and effective neuroprotective treatments. Interventions to increase CBF in the ischemic territory, reduction of cerebral metabolism, lactic acidosis and excitatory neurotransmitter activity, prevention of Ca^{++} influx, inhibition of lipid peroxidation, and free radical scavenging, have been proposed to be protective in cerebral ischemia. However, only a few of these treatments have been proven to be efficacious in the setting of experimental or clinical ischemia. With current knowledge, the following physical and pharmacologic interventions seem to be protective in a variety of different pathophysiologic states:

1) Chronic normoventilation ($paCO_2$: 36–40 mmHg) in head injured patients with normal or moderately elevated ICP. Transient hyperventilation ($paCO_2$: 30–34 mmHg) in patients with acute intracranial hypertension may be appropriate until other interventions will reduce ICP

2) Mild to moderate hypothermia prevents experimental neuronal necrosis and improves neurologic outcome when induced before, during, or after cerebral ischemia. In patients, mild to moderate hypothermia seems to improve neurologic

outcome following head injury. However, the precise degree of hypothermia, the duration and the re-warming technique still have to be defined

3) Infusion of recombinant tissue plasminogen activator (rt-PA) increases the chance of a favorable neurologic outcome in patients with acute stroke

4) Anesthetics given prior to ischemic challenges appear to extend the ischemic tolerance of neurons. Barbiturates may decrease elevated ICP and improve neurologic outcome

5) Hyperglycemia is associated with worsened outcome following stroke or neurotrauma and plasma glucose concentrations should be assayed every 2 hours and maintained within the range of 100–150 mg/dl

6) According to two meta-analyses on patients with acute stroke or subarachnoid hemorrhage from ruptured aneurysms, nimodipine improves neurologic outcome, reduces the incidence of cerebral vasospasm, and appears to decrease the occurrence of delayed neurological deficits. Patients with traumatic subarachnoid hemorrhage may also benefit from the infusion of nimodipine

7) In general, glucocorticoids have no significant positive or negative effect in patients with head injury or acute stroke. High-dose methylprednisolone slightly improves sensory and motor function following spinal cord injury

References

1. Ruta TS, Drummond JC, Cole DJ (1993) The effect of acute hypocapnia on local cerebral blood flow during middle cerebral artery occlusion in isoflurane anesthetized rats. Anesthesiology 78:134–140
2. Artru AA, Merriman HG (1989) Hypocapnia added to hypertension to reverse EEG changes during carotid endarterectomy. Anesthesiology 70:1016–1018
3. Cold GE (1989) Does acute hyperventilation provoke cerebral oligaemia in comatose patients after acute head injury. Acta Neurochir 96:100–106
4. Obrist WD, Langfitt TW, Jaggi JL, Cruz J, Gennarelli TA (1984) Cerebral blood flow and metabolism in comatose patients with acute head injury. J Neurosurg 61:241–253
5. Muizelaar JP, Marmarou A, Ward JD, et al (1991) Adverse effects of prolonged hyperventilation in patients with severe head injury: a randomized clinical trial. J Neurosurg 75:731–739
6. Morikawa E, Ginsberg MD, Dietrich WD, et al (1992) The significance of brain temperature in focal cerebral ischemia: histopathological consequences of middle cerebral artery occlusion in the rat. J Cereb Blood Flow Metab 12:380–389
7. Weinrauch V, Safar P, Tisherman S, Kuboyama K, Radovsky A (1992) Beneficial effect of mild hypothermia and detrimental effect of deep hypothermia after cardiac arrest in dogs. Stroke 23:1454–1462
8. Hoffman WE, Werner C, Baughman VL, Thomas C, Miletich DJ, Albrecht RF (1991) Postischemic treatment with hypothermia improves outcome from incomplete cerebral ischemia in rats. J Neurosurg Anesth 3:34–38
9. Clifton GL, Jiang JY, Lyeth BG, Jenkins LW, Hamm RJ, Hayes RL (1991) Marked protection by moderate hypothermia after experimental traumatic brain injury. J Cereb Blood Flow Metab 11:114–121
10. Clifton GL, Allen S, Barrodale P, et al (1993) A phase II study of moderate hypothermia in severe brain injury. J Neurotrauma 10:263–271
11. Marion DW, Penrod LE, Kelsey SF, et al (1997) Treatment of traumatic brain injury with moderate hypothermia. N Engl J Med 336:540–546
12. Shiozaki T, Sugimoto H, Taneda M, et al (1993) Effect of mild hypothermia on uncontrollable intracranial hypertension after severe head injury. J Neurosurg 79:363–368
13. Reith J, Jørgensen HS, Pedersen PM, et al (1996) Body temperature in acute stroke: relation to stroke severity, infarct size, mortality, and outcome. Lancet 347:422–425

14. Hacke W, Kaste M, Fieschi C, et al (1995) Intravenous thrombolysis with recombinant tissue plasminogen activator for acute hemispheric stroke. The European Cooperative Acute Stroke Study (ECASS). JAMA 274:1017–1025

15. The National Institute of Neurological Disorders and Stroke rt-PA Stroke Study Group (1995) Tissue plasminogen activator for acute ischemic stroke. N Engl J Med 333:1581–1587

16. Werner C, Möllenberg O, Kochs E, Schulte am Esch J (1995) Sevoflurane improves neurological outcome following incomplete cerebral ischaemia in rats. Br J Anaesth 75:756–760

17. Messick JM, Casement B, Sharbrough FW, Milde LN, Michenfelder JD, Sundt TM (1987) Correlation of regional cerebral blood flow (rCBF) with EEG changes during isoflurane anesthesia for carotid endarterectomy: critical rCBF. Anesthesiology 66:344–349

18. Warner DS, Takaoda S, Wu B, et al (1996) Electroencephalographic burst suppression is not required to elicit maximal neuroprotection from pentobarbital in a rat model of focal cerebral ischemia. Anesthesiology 84:1475–1484

19. Nussmeier NA, Arlund C, Slogoff S (1986) Neuropsychiatric complications after cardiopulmonary bypass: cerebral protection by a barbiturate. Anesthesiology 64:165–170

20. Brain resuscitation clinical trial I study group (1986) Randomized clinical study of thiopental loading in comatose survivors of cardiac arrest. N Engl J Med 314:397–403

21. Bullock R, Chesnut RM, Clifton G, et al (1996) The use of barbiturates in the control of intracranial hypertension. J Neurotrauma 13:711–714

22. Marana E, Cavaliere F, Beccia F, et al (1982) Cerebral protection during extracorporeal circulation. Resuscitation 10:89–100

23. Woo J, Lam C, Kay R, Wong A, Teoh R, Nicholls M (1990) The influence of hyperglycemia and diabetes mellitus on immediate and 3-month morbidity and mortality after acute stroke. Arch Neurol 47:1174–1177

24. Buchan AM, Gertler SZ, Li H, et al (1994) A selective N-type Ca^{++}-channel blocker prevents CA1 injury 24 h following severe forebrain ischemia and reduces infarction following focal ischemia. J Cereb Blood Flow Metab 14:903–910

25. Mohr JP, Orgogozo JM, Harrison MJG, et al (1994) Meta-analysis of oral nimodipine trial in acute ischemic stroke. Cerebrovasc Dis 4:197–203

26. Barker FG, Ogilvy CS (1996) Efficacy of prophylactic nimodipine for delayed ischemic deficit after subarachnoid hemorrhage: a metaanalysis. J Neurosurg 84:405–414

27. Harders A, Kakarieka A, Braakman R, et al (1996) Traumatic subarachnoid hemorrhage and its treatment with nimodipine. J Neurosurg 85:82–89

28. Hoffman WE, Pelligrino D, Werner C, Kochs E, Albrecht RF, Schulte am Esch J (1992) Ketamine decreases plasma catecholamines and improves neurologic outcome from incomplete cerebral ischemia in rats. Anesthesiology 76:755–762

29. Grotta J, Clark W, Coull B, et al (1995) Safety and tolerability of the glutamate antagonist CGS 19755 (selfotel) in patients with acute ischemic stroke. Stroke 26:602–605

30. Alderson P, Roberts I (1997) Corticosteroids in acute traumatic brain injury: systematic review of randomised controlled trials. Br Med J 314:1855–1859

31. Bracken MB, Shepard MJ, Collins WF, et al (1990) A randomized, controlled trial of methylprednisolone or naloxone in the treatment of acute spinal-cord injury. N Engl J Med 322:1405–1411

32. Smith SL, Scherch HM, Hall ED (1996) Protective effects of tirilazad mesylate and metabolite U-89678 against blood brain barrier damage after subarachnoid hemorrhage and lipid peroxidative neuronal injury. J Neurosurg 84:229–233

33. Haley EC, Kassell NF, Apperson-Hansen C, et al (1997) A randomized double-blind, vehicle controlled trial of tirilazad mesylate in patients with aneurysmal subarachnoid hemorrhage: a cooperative study in North America. J Neurosurg 86:467–474

34. Kassell NF, Haley EC, Apperson-Hansen C, et al (1996) A randomized double-blind, vehicle controlled trial of tirilazad mesylate in patients with aneurysmal subarachnoid hemorrhage: a cooperative study in Europe, Australia, and New Zealand. J Neurosurg 84:221–228

35. Young B, Runge JW, Waxman KS, et al (1996) Effects of pegorgotein on neurologic outcome of patients with severe head injury. JAMA 276:538–543

36. Asano T, Takakura K, Sano K, et al (1996) Effects of a hydroxyl radical scavenger on delayed ischemic neurological deficits following aneurysmal subarachnoid hemorrhage: results of a multicenter, placebo-controlled double-blind trial. J Neurosurg 84:792–803

Cerebral Extraction Monitoring in Brain Injury

N. Stocchetti, S. Rossi, and S. Rotelli

Introduction

Jugular saturation monitoring has gained increasing acceptance in neurointensive care. Several therapeutic decisions are currently based on the internal jugular vein (IJ) content of oxygen or metabolites [1–6]. This is based on the assumption that a reliable sample of mixed venous blood can be drawn from the IJ. In fact many investigators have sampled from the IJs, and a number of reports have been published, based on the assumption that information obtained from one side of the neck is identical, or at least very close, to the data which can be measured in the opposite side [3, 6–8].

The similarity of the venous content in the two jugular veins has been questioned [9–11]. As far as we know this issue was first discussed in 1945 [12], in a review of 25 cases. It was examined later in 1948 [13], showing that "two thirds of the blood supplied to one hemisphere through an internal carotid artery is actually drained through the ipsilateral IJ" and in 1959 [14], suggesting that in many cases the differences are quite small, while in others they are more pronounced. Discrepancies between the two IJs have been documented in head injured patients [11] and confirmed by other groups [9, 10]. Additional limitations, such as the occurrence of the Bohr effect [15] or the possibility of inadequate recognition of focal lesions [16, 17] have been reported. Despite that, an increasing number of investigators are currently engaged in research and clinical applications focused on the saturation detected on only one side.

In the present chapter we will address some potentially helpful points to assist in the choice of which side should be cannulated. We will briefly review the anatomic basis of the venous drainage from the brain, and discuss the degree of discrepancy between the two IJs that may be expected based on available studies. We will suggest a practical approach to the choice of side for IJ cannulation, and, finally, we will discuss the interpretation of IJ saturation data considering the risk of discrepancies.

Venous Drainage from the Brain

On the convex and medial surface of the brain there are 8–12 pairs of veins passing to the superior sagittal sinus. These so-called cortical veins dip deep into the brain, well below the cortical layer, and establish free communication with the internal, or deep, cerebral veins. The inferior half of the brain has many large veins, the principal one being the middle cerebral vein, which runs in the sylvian fissure and ends in the cavernous sinus. This large vessel also communicates with the superior sagittal sinus through the great anastomotic vein of Trolard and with the transverse sinus through the large vein of Labbè. The veins on the inferior surface of the frontal lobe pass partly to the inferior sagittal sinus and partly to the cavernous sinus. The inferior temporal veins supply partly the transverse and partly the superior petrosal sinus, the latter joining the lateral sinus to form the jugular bulb. The inferior occipital surface has a large vein (posterior cerebral vein) passing over the cerebral peduncle to join the great cerebral vein (of Galen) just before the latter enters the straight sinus.

The deep, or central, veins are drained principally through the great cerebral vein into the straight sinus. However, the free communications with the so-called cortical veins are not to be ignored. The paired internal cerebral veins, one from each hemisphere, form the great cerebral vein; this receives the posterior cerebral vein and veins from the upper surface of the cerebellum and then flows into the straight sinus. These paired internal cerebral veins are formed by the confluence of the choroid vein and the vena terminalis. The posterior cerebral vein also receives the basal vein, the thalamic vein and veins from the choroid plexus of the third ventricle, corpus callosum, pineal region and area at the posterior horn of the lateral ventricle. The terminal vein drains the region of the corpus striatum, thalamus, fornix, septum pellucidum and anterior horn of the lateral ventricle. The choroid vein drains the choroid plexus of the lateral ventricle, the hippocampus, the inferior horn of the lateral ventricle, the fornix and, in part, the corpus callosum. The basal vein drains the insula, opercular gyri, corpus striatum, anterior cerebral vein and interpeduncular structures.

The cerebellar veins are divided into a superior and an inferior group. The latter, larger than the former, pass partly to the petrosal and transverse sinuses and partly to the occipital sinus. The superior cerebellar veins pass partly to the straight sinus and partly to the transverse and superior petrosal sinuses. The veins of the medulla and pons terminate in the inferior petrosal and transverse sinuses.

The principal dural sinuses, collecting blood from the aforementioned sources, join to form the torcular Herophili. Thus, the superior sagittal sinus and the straight sinus, the latter representing the junction of the inferior sagittal sinus and the great cerebral vein, adjoin. The two lateral sinuses take origin from the region of the torcular, ultimately to reach the jugular bulbs. The cavernous and circular sinuses, at the base of the brain, have equally free communication from side to side through the petrosal sinuses to the jugular bulbs, and via the basilar plexus to the longitudinal veins in the spinal canal.

The venous drainage of the brain has numerous, but small, communications with extracerebral pathways. These are the so-called emissary veins, the most prominent being the mastoid emissary vein, the less constant parietal emissary vein, the veins passing through the foramens of the base of the skull and the orbits and the veins which communicate with the pterygoid plexus. Problems can arise from this extracerebral contamination of the venous drainage, but in quantitative terms this contribution to the overall flow is negligible (approximately 2%). The main concern is related to the degree of mixing. In comatose severely head injured patients, it has been shown using the intravenous xenon (Xe) 133 method [18], that 65% of cases have significant hemispherical and/or regional cerebral blood flow (CBF) differences. Using the stable Xe/computerized tomography technique Marion and co-workers [19] have recently shown that in almost half of their studies regional CBF was different from the global value by at least 25%. If some anatomic basis exists for a separate drainage of regions of the brain we would expect some difference in the hemoglobin saturation when the relationships between oxygen supply and consumption are not constant in different regions of the brain.

There are different views about the anatomo-physiologic pattern of cerebral venous outflow. For Lazorthes and Gibbs [12, 20] the right IJ drains the cortical areas, while the left collects blood flowing from the sub-cortical regions, at least in some subjects. Shenkin et al. [13], suggests that two thirds of the blood in each IJ flows from the ipsilateral hemisphere and just one third is mixed, the many tributary veins passing directly to the lateral and petrous sinuses. An incomplete mixing is, therefore, expected by all these investigators.

Discrepancy Between the Two Internal Jugular Veins

One practical way of evaluating the degree of mixing is to look directly at the content of the cerebral blood flowing in the two jugular veins. In the case of incomplete mixing, significant differences should be detected, and from a clinical perspective this is the most relevant point, since an estimate of the reliability of our data can be directly obtained.

We have investigated 32 head injured patients who were admitted to our intensive care unit (ICU) in coma. Patients with known or suspected artero-venous fistulas were excluded. The patients underwent a standard treatment protocol. Both IJs were cannulated and catheter position was verified by antero-posterior and lateral X-rays. The lateral film was obtained in a position slightly less than perpendicular to the neck to allow visualization of both catheters. The correct placement of the catheters was indicated by the projection of the catheter tips into the superior jugular bulb. Blood samples were taken simultaneously from the two IJs and immediately processed using a Co-Oximeter (Instrumentation Laboratory 482 Co-Oximeter). Based on the hypothesis that it is the depth of lesions, rather than the side where the lesion is located, that could explain differences in oxygen saturation, we developed a grading for the analysis of computerized tomography (CT) of the head. Each lesion, regardless of density, was identified in 3 slices of the CT scan: Upper (the slice above the last where the frontal horns of lateral ventricles were identifiable); medium (where the body and the frontal horns of the lateral ventricles were fully visible); and lower (at the level of the perimesencephalic cistern). In each slice the lesions were assigned to two areas: Cortical (up to 1 cm from the surface) or deep (more than 1 cm from the surface).

Statistical analysis was performed in two steps. Firstly, we analyzed the degree of agreement between the hemoglobin saturation measured in the two veins. The analysis of agreement was done according to the measurement of bias proposed by Bland and LaManthia [21, 22]. Secondly, we analyzed the maximum differences between the two IJs in order to extrapolate from the sample examined the range of variability in the real population. This was done using a "summary measures method" [23] with confidence limits calculation. The hemoglobin saturation measured in this investigation was the fractional saturation, i.e., the ratio of oxygenated hemoglobin to total hemoglobin. The percent saturation of the hemoglobin in both IJs was measured and one side compared with the other.

The total number of samples processed was 342, with an average of 5.34 paired samples from each patient. The mean duration of bilateral catheterization was 64.12 hours (SD 28.69) for standard catheters and 62.4 hours (SD 15.64) for fiberoptic catheters. The first paired sample was done after radiologic confirmation of the correct position of the catheters, usually within a couple of hours after insertion.

Fifteen patients showed differences in hemoglobin saturation greater than 15% (i.e., 60% on one side and 76% on the other); 3 more patients showed differences in hemoglobin saturation greater than 10% at some point during the investigation. Only 8 patients had differences less than 5%. The mean value of the difference between the right and left side was 5.32 with a standard deviation of 5.15. Thirteen patients had higher hemoglobin saturations in the right IJ, and 16 had higher values in the left. Three patients had no differences between the two sides. These data are summarized in Fig. 1.

Each patient was classified into one of two groups according to their CT scan: Patients with unilateral lesions (21 cases); and patients with bilateral lesions (11 cases). Among those patients with unilateral lesions, eleven had lesions of the right hemisphere, and 6 of these had differences between the two IJs greater than 5%. The left side had a higher hemoglobin saturation in two cases. Seven patients had left hemisphere lesions and 6 of them developed a difference between the two IJs greater than 5%. Three of these patients had a higher hemoglobin saturation in the right IJ. Among the eleven patients with bilateral lesions, we detected a difference between the two IJs greater than 10% in five cases, and between 6 and 10% in three additional patients.

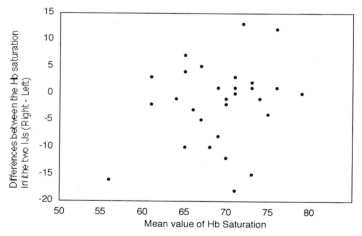

Fig. 1. Differences in hemoglobin (Hb) saturation between the 2 jugular veins are plotted in this chart. According to Bland and Altman [21] differences are plotted against the best reference value available, which is the average of the two contralateral measurements

The question we have raised in our previous paper was: How would our understanding of the patient's situation differ, using data obtained from one side as opposed to the other? In other words, would our diagnosis and treatment be different if the catheter was placed on one side instead of the other? For this reason statistical analysis was carried out looking at the maximum difference as the "summary measure" for each patient and calculating the bias. We arbitrarily chose the thresholds of 5, 10 and 15% of hemoglobin saturation because in our opinion a difference of 5% is acceptable, a difference of 10% is highly suspicious and a difference of 15% or more can completely mislead judgement, and is therefore unacceptable. A patient with an IJ hemoglobin saturation of 60% is still within normal limits, but most intensivists will intervene strongly when the value falls under 45%. Similarly, the ventilation management should be changed if the hemoglobin saturation is above 85%. Our data suggest a 95% probability that between 30 and 64% of patients could have, at some point during monitoring, a difference greater than 15% between the two IJs and this is of major concern. The bias of the data is not marked, ranging from -4.77 to 15.41%, although the implication of that data changes if we want to use the actual reading for a fast, effective treatment.

The comparison made using continuous recording through fiberoptic catheters showed an additional problem. In two cases the side with the greater saturation changed over time and gave readings lower than the other side. Due to the limited number of cases recorded we cannot measure the incidence of this finding, that could be anecdotal. Additional concern comes from data obtained through intermittent samples; they seldom show the same inversion of saturation. However these dynamic changes represent the exception, not the rule, since they occur in less than 3% of samples.

Practical Approach to the Choice of the Side for IJ Cannulation

Based on our data, we were not able to identify a consistent relationship between the CT scan findings of bilateral, predominantly monolateral, cortical or deep lesions and understandable patterns in the IJ saturation data. However, notwithstanding these theoretical considerations, the attending physician has the responsability of choosing the appropriate side for IJ cannulation and a practical approach should be drawn. This approach is not based on conclusive data, and it should be treated with appropriate caution.

It has been suggested that the IJ catheter should be placed in the side of most severe injury or in the right side in case of diffuse lesions [5]. We believe that the main goal expected from cerebral O_2 monitoring has to be identified in advance, as it may guide the choice between left or right, or even bilateral, cannulation.

Generally speaking, a clear distinction between diffuse damage or predominantly focal lesions is necessary. In cases of diffuse damage it is not possible to predict a side of deeper cerebral disturbance and there is no point in targeting a side for IJ. If there are no reasons for cannulating one specific side, then the easier side makes sense. The easier side is where the larger IJ is, since a larger vein increases the probability of successful cannulation. Dearden [4] has suggested selecting the appropriate side from a functional viewpoint, assessing the relative effect on intracranial pressure (ICP) produced by compressing each IJ. Alternatively, a comparison of the two jugular foramina can be made on the CT scan. The biggest IJ corresponds to the biggest foramen, and the most appropriate side for monitoring can be identified at no cost, on a routine CT scan, without any increase in ICP. Some help in identifying the dominant IJ can be provided by ultrasound evaluation of the neck, using Doppler devices which are available on the market.

In focal lesions, on the other hand, the goal of cerebral O_2 monitoring may change. In these cases, as in ischemic hypodense areas, the main goal of monitoring and treatment becomes the restoration of adequate perfusion in such areas. Information gathered from portions of the cerebral tissue as close as possible to those areas is more likely to be useful than data coming from structures located in far regions. It is therefore our suggestion that the IJ vein should be cannulated on the side corresponding to the main focal lesion of interest.

Based on these assumptions, we believe that bilateral monitoring is normally not necessary, and may be reserved for patients in whom bilateral focal lesions are detected. Alternatively, bilateral cannulation may be suitable when, after an initial IJ has been cannulated, a focal contralateral lesion is identified in subsequent CT scans.

Conclusion

We do not recommend inserting a catheter in both IJs on a routine basis, as this would double costs and complications. We believe instead that any judgment based on IJ data must be carefully weighed, aware of the high probability of inaccurate data. The data provided by the hemoglobin saturation should be considered together with all other available information, as is customary in intensive care. An important point, however, should be addressed. Assuming that low values of IJ saturation are associated with situations of inadequate oxygen delivery any occurrence of IJ desaturation has to be considered (and treated) seriously. Even in the event that the sample we have processed is not representative of the global ratio between cerebral blood flow and metabolism, a low saturation level means that "somewhere in the brain" there is ischemia. While we can not be overconfident of apparently good data, as they do not rule out pathologic values on the other side, we should vigorously treat any case of documented desaturation.

References

1. Cruz J (1992) Jugular venous oxygen saturation monitoring. J Neurosurg 77:162–163
2. Cruz J, Gennarelli TA, Alves WM (1992) Continuous monitoring of cerebral hemodynamic reserve in acute brain injury: relationship to change in brain swelling. J Trauma 32:629–635
3. Cruz J, Miner ME, Allen SJ, Alves WM, Gennarelli TA (1991) Continuous monitoring of cerebral oxygenation in acute brain injury: assessment of cerebral hemodynamic reserve. Neurosurgery 29:743–749
4. Dearden NM (1991) Jugular bulb venous oxygen saturation in the management of severe head injury. Curr opin Anaesthesiology 4:279–286
5. Robertson CS, Narayan RK, Gokaslan ZL, et al (1989) Cerebral arteriovenous oxygen difference as an estimate of cerebral blood flow in comatose patients. J Neurosurg 70:222–230

6. Sheinberg M, Kanter MJ, Robertson CS, Contant CF, Narayan RK, Grossman RG (1992) Continuous monitoring of jugular venous oxygen saturation in head-injured patients. J Neurosurg 76: 212–217
7. Bullock R, Stewart L, Rafferty C, Teasdale GM (1993) Continuous monitoring of jugular bulb oxygen saturation and the effect of drugs acting on cerebral metabolism. Acta Neurohir Suppl Wien: 113–118
8. Gibbs EL, Lennox WG, Nims LF, Gibbs FA (1942) Artenal and cerebral venous blood. Arterial-venous differences in man. J Biol Chem 144: 325–332
9. Chieregato A, Targa L, Mantovani G, Droghetti L, Zatelli R (1994) Cerebral arteriovenous oxygen difference and lactate-oxygen index: a case of bilateral monitoring. J Neurosurg Anesthesiol 6: 43–47
10. Inagawa H, Okada Y, Suzuki S, Ono K, Maekawa K (1994) Bilateral jugular bulb oximetry. In: Tsubokawa T, Marmarou A, Robertson C, Teasdale G (eds) Neurochemical monitoring in the intensive care unit. Springer-Verlag, Tokyo, pp 113–119
11. Stocchetti N, Paparella A, Bridelli F, Bacchi M, Piazza P, Zuccoli P (1994) Cerebral venous oxygen saturation studied with bilateral samples in the internal jugular veins. Neurosurgery 34: 38–44
12. Gibbs EL, Lennox WG, Gibbs FA (1945) Bilateral internal jugular blood. Comparison of A-V differences, oxygen-dextrose ratios and respiratory quotients. Am J Psychiatry 102: 184–190
13. Shenkin HA, Harmel MH, Kety SS (1948) Dynamic anatomy of the cerebral circulation. Arch Neurol Psychiatry 60: 240–252
14. Lassen NA (1959) Cerebral blood flow and oxygen consumption in man. Physiol Rev 39: 183–238
15. Cruz J, Gennarelli TA, Hoffstad OJ (1992) Lack of relevance of the Bohr effect in optimally ventilated patients with acute brain trauma. J Trauma 33: 304–311
16. Chieregato A, Targa L, Zatelli R (1996) Limitations of jugular bulb oxyhemoglobin saturation without intracranial pressure monitoring in subarachnoid hemorrhage. J Neurosurg Anesthesiol 8: 21–25
17. Andrews PA, Murugavel S, Deehan S (1996) Conventional multimodality monitoring failure to detect ischemic cerebral blood flow. J Neurosurg Anesthesiol 8: 220–226
18. Obrist WD, Langfitt TW, Jaggi JL, Cruz J, Gennarelli TA (1984) Cerebral blood flow and metabolism in comatose patients with acute head injury. J Neurosurg 61: 241–253
19. Marion DW, Darby J, Yonas H (1991) Acute regional cerebral blood flow changes caused by severe head injuries. J Neurosurg 74: 407–414
20. Lazorthes G, Gouazè A, Salamon G (1978) La regulation de la circulation veineuse. In: Lazorthes G, Gouazè A, Salamon G (eds) Vascolarisation et circolation de l'encèphale. Masson, Paris, pp 59–62
21. Bland JM, Altman DG (1986) Statistical methods for assessing agreement between two methods of clinical measurement. Lancet 8: 307–310
22. LaManthia KR, O'Connor T, Barash PG (1990) Comparing methods of measurement: an alternative approach. Anesthesiology 72: 781–783
23. Matthews JNS, Altman DG, Campbell MJ, Royston P (1990) Analysis of serial measurements in medical research. Br Med J 300: 230–235

Surgery and Obstetrics

Pediatric Problems in Heart Surgery

A. J. van Vught, N. Sreeram, and C. H. Schröder

Introduction

Advances in pediatric cardiology, heart surgery and cardio-anesthesiology have made either complete repair or long-term palliation of even very complex congenital heart diseases possible [1–5]. The majority of congenital heart defects are now treated on a routine basis and most patients pass their postoperative phase without difficulty. Nevertheless, complex heart surgery is sometimes associated with significant problems in organ systems other than the cardiovascular system and challenges pediatric intensive care to employ its most recent acquisitions in medical knowledge and technology when dealing with these often young children.

Following heart surgery, problems in other organ systems may arise from adverse preoperative conditions, from postoperative circulatory failure and from the adverse effects of long term disease and intensive supportive treatment. These problems are excellently discussed in recent textbooks [6]. In this chapter we will summarize the essentials of preoperative evaluation and postoperative hemodynamic assessment in neonates with congenital heart disease and will briefly discuss the most common complications in the early postoperative course outside the cardiovascular system; respiratory failure, electrolyte disturbances and renal failure. Other postoperative problems such as neurologic, gastroenterologic and infectious complications will just be mentioned. For a more in depth discussion the reader is referred to the recent literature.

Preoperative Condition

A heart defect may be associated with other congenital defects or may be part of a more complex combination of congenital anomalies [7]. These associated anomalies may complicate the postoperative course or, in view of the future outlook for that individual, may change the decision to intervene immediately or to be more conservative. In addition, the genetic background of congenital heart disease is now gradually being revealed, making counseling of the parents more and more possible [8–13]. Therefore, each newborn with a congenital heart defect must have a thorough investigation for additional, or genetically determined, defects before surgery. Sometimes the results of such investigations are not available prior to instituting surgical therapy. Nevertheless, blood samples must be obtained even before any blood transfusions have been given, because this may disturb chromosomal examination and im-

Table 1. Screening for additional congenital anomalies in neonates with congenital heart defects

1. Physical examination:
   - Apart from general physical examination pay particular attention to overt or submucosal palatal clefts, to anomalies of the spinal column and to anal patency.
   - Check choanal patency on both sides and check gastro-esophageal continuity. Keep a high level of suspicion for tracheo-esophageal fistulas.
2. Consult the clinical geneticist.
3. Echographic examinations:
   - Brain.
   - Abdomen (kidneys, urinary tract, liver, spleen).
4. Radiological examination:
   - Spinal column on thoracic X-ray.
   - Complete spinal column examination if there are abnormalities on inspection or if there are renal anomalies.
5. Chromosomal analysis:
   - Standard karyogram.
   - If suspected DiGeorge syndrome or velo-cardio-facial syndrome (see text): FISH for 22q11-.
6. If suspected DiGeorge syndrome:
   - Immunological analysis: number and function of T cells and thymus dependent markers on lymphocytes.
7. If the child dies before a complete diagnosis has been made, take a skin biopsy for fibroblast culture.

FISH: fluorescent *in situ* hybridization

munological tests. Table 1 presents a checklist for such a preoperative investigation.

Chromosomal abnormalities occur in approximately 5% of all patients with congenital heart defects; trisomy 21 (Down's syndrome) being by far the most frequent [7]. In Down's syndrome, apart from heart defects, the majority being atrioventricular or ventricular septal defects, other associated major congenital anomalies are infrequent. However, tracheo-esophageal fistula, duodenal stenosis and renal dysgenesis may sometimes occur and may be difficult to diagnose. Structural lung abnormalities in infants with Down's syndrome are now increasingly recognized [14–16] and may complicate postoperative respiratory management. Their pulmonary vascular bed appears to be more reactive than in other infants [17], and in order to prevent post-extubation laryngeal edema and stenosis, they need more careful handling of the upper airways during intubation [18].

The CHARGE association comprises a number of associated anomalies: Coloboma oculi, heart disease, atresia choanae, retarded growth and development, genital anomalies, ear anomalies and/or deafness. The VACTER association includes vertebral anomalies, anal atresia, cardiac defects, tracheal, ear and renal anomalies. Both syndromes may be incomplete. The DiGeorge syndrome and velo-cardio-facial syndrome will be discussed separately.

Failure to thrive and malnutrition, hypoxia, circulatory and metabolic derangements may put subsequent surgery at direct risk and lay the basis for postoperative organ failure, apart from associated congenital defects. If possible these disturbances should be corrected before surgery. However, the severity of these disturbances and the time needed to correct them must be balanced against the possible deleterious effects of any delay in surgery. This particularly applies to obstructive lesions in the systemic circulation and cyanotic defects in the neonate when the clinical condition deteriorates in spite of maximal prostaglandin administration.

DiGeorge Syndrome

A syndrome with important implications for pre- and postoperative care is the DiGeorge syndrome. The DiGeorge syndrome is a combination of a cardiac anomaly with absence or hypoplasia of the parathyroids and the thymus and sometimes with facial dysmorphology (Table 2) [19, 20]. However, the clinical expression may vary considerably and may be incomplete. The heart defect is usually, but not exclusively, a conotruncal defect, most frequently an interrupted aortic arch or a truncus arteriosus. But it can also include transposition of the great arteries, tetralogy of Fallot, or hypoplastic left heart syndrome. In some published cohorts up to 68% of the patients with interrupted aortic arch and 33% of the patients with truncus arteriosus had important features of the DiGeorge syndrome [21]. The DiGeorge syndrome is associated with abnormalities in the chromosomal 22q11 region especially with deletions in that region [22, 23]. These deletions can be detected with the so called FISH technique, fluorescent *in situ* hybridization. With this technique a very specific part of the chromosomal DNA can be detected with a so-called probe. The probe consists of a complement piece of DNA which is labeled with a fluorescent marker. There is a clinical and cytogenetic overlap with the velo-cardio-facial syndrome (Shprintzen syndrome) and with other syndromes, in particular the CHARGE association [23, 24]. On the other hand, in one series 29% of patients with a conotruncal defect had a 22q11 deletion without any other syndromal feature [25]. It appears that the extent of the lesion in the 22q11 region determines the severity and extent of the congenital disorder, which varies from virtually no clinical signs to severe and lethal syndromes [23].

Apart from the other associated abnormalities the main importance of the DiGeorge syndrome is its association with immunological abnormalities. Transfused donor lymphocytes may immunologically attack the patient. In the setting of severe

Table 2. DiGeorge Syndrome

1. Congenital heart defect
   Interrupted aortic arch
   Truncus arteriosus
   Transposition of great arteries, tetralogy of Fallot
2. Agenesis/hypoplasia of parathyroids
   Hypocalcemia (< 2.00 mmol/l), sometimes associated with tetany or convulsions.
3. Agenesis/hypoplasia of thymus
   Low number of T lymphocytes, poorly functioning lymphocytes, defective expression of thymus dependent markers on lymphocytes.
4. Facial dysmorphology
Overlap with velo-cardio-facial syndrome (Shprintzen)
   CHARGE association

T cell dysfunction, the patient's own T cells are not able to beat off this attack. This may lead to a potentially fatal graft-versus-host disease after blood transfusion. Therefore, in patients suspected of having DiGeorge syndrome only irradiated blood, this also for pump-priming, must be used, until it has been determined that the number of T cells are sufficient and the T cells are functioning normally [19]. T cell function must be checked routinely in all patients with an interrupted aortic arch and a truncus arteriosus and in other patients with additional features of the DiGeorge syndrome, the velo-cardio-facial syndrome or the CHARGE association.

Postoperative Problems

Cardiopulmonary bypass itself, with or without circulatory arrest and hypothermia, may have a significant impact on myocardial and other organ function. This may be mediated by hypoxia, ischemia and subsequent reperfusion damage, complement activation and other inflammatory and immunological mechanisms [26–32]. The impact of cardiopulmonary bypass is directly related to time on bypass and is usually reversible in 3 to 7 days.

After recovery from the surgical procedure, organ failure is almost exclusively the result of circulatory failure. This applies to respiratory failure, fluid and electrolyte disorders, and renal failure as well as to other organ dysfunction. Therefore, close attention should be paid to postoperative hemodynamics, to ensure adequate heart function and early diagnosis of residual heart defects. Only then will supportive treatment be successful.

Circulatory Assessment

As organ failure after recovery from surgery is almost exclusively the result of circulatory failure, low cardiac output must primarily be ruled out or corrected. Low cardiac output in infants is indicated by a low peripheral temperature (central to peripheral temperature difference, or ΔT, $> 5\,^{\circ}C$), a drop in blood pressure of $> 10\%$ of the predicted value, absent pedal pulses, urinary output of < 0.5 ml/kg/h, lactacidosis (arterial lactate > 5 mmol/l) or serum potassium > 5 mmol/l.

Cardiac output is determined by heart rate and stroke volume. Of these, heart rate is the most important variable in infants. Heart rate can be increased nearly fourfold, stroke volume can at best be doubled. Therefore, it must be decided if there is sinus rhythm (defined as a positive P wave in electrocardiogram (EKG) lead II) and if there is an appropriate tachycardia. If not, the heart must be paced. Stroke volume is determined by preload, afterload and myocardial function. Basically preload is the muscle fibre length at end diastole. Notwithstanding the physiologic objections, preload is, in clinical practice, best reflected by the central venous pressure (CVP). Generally a CVP of 10–15 mmHg is considered to provide optimal preload. Above 18 mmHg cardiac output may decline because of myocardial fiber overstretch. However, in some situations a CVP as high as 23 mmHg may be required to maintain adequate cardiac output. It is unknown how much positive end-expiratory pressure (PEEP) or mean airway pressure in ventilated patients contributes to the rise in the

Table 3. Diagnostic steps in postoperative low cardiac output

1. Assess heart rhythm and heart rate.
   If not in sinus rhythm or if heart rate is not appropriate, pace the heart.
2. Assess preload.
   If too low, give fluid.
3. Assess afterload.
   If too high, give vasodilator.
4. Assess myocardial function.
   For myocardial dysfunction, give inotropes.
5. Exclude cardiac tamponade.
   Be aware of tamponade without fluid.
6. Exclude technical failures.
   Decide whether reoperation is required for residual shunts, obstructions or leaks.

CVP and therefore, these values are generally neglected. Afterload is the force the ventricle must deploy during systole. It is best reflected by intraventricular systolic pressure and therefore, in the absence of outflow obstruction, by systolic blood pressure. Afterload can be diminished by vasodilators such as nitroglycerin, nitroprusside and ketanserin. These are indicated if after adequate filling the ΔT remains $>5\,°C$ or if arterial blood pressure is $>30\%$ above the predicted value. Myocardial function can be determined by echocardiography. Myocardial function can be supported by inotropes such as dopamine, dobutamine, dopexamine, (nor)epinephrine and phosphodiesterase inhibitors such as milrinone. A discussion of the different effects and side effects of these drugs is beyond the scope of this overview.

In low cardiac output states echocardiography is also indicated to exclude technically unsatisfactory surgical repair with residual shunts, residual obstruction or residual leaks and to diagnose cardiac tamponade. In cardiac tamponade the patient characteristically has come from the operating room in good condition, but after a clinically stable period deteriorates suddenly. Usually CVP rises rapidly and arterial blood pressure falls suddenly. Sometimes drains which have been producing substantial volumes suddenly run dry. Apart from this classical clinical picture, in which the diagnosis of pericardial fluid can be made easily by echocardiography, tamponade without any fluid may occur if the heart itself has swollen and is compressed within the pericardium or within the closed chest after difficult and long operations. Increasingly, the sternum is electively left open to prevent this complication, and to allow easier decompression of the heart. Table 3 summarizes the diagnostic steps in postoperative low cardiac output in infants.

Respiratory Failure

The most common reason for prolonged stay in the intensive care unit (ICU) is persistent respiratory insufficiency. A number of postoperative complications may cause respiratory failure (Table 4). Acute respiratory distress syndrome (ARDS) defined as a pulmonary capillary leakage syndrome, occasionally occurs after cardiopulmonary bypass procedures and affects lung compliance and causes ventilation-

Table 4. Causes of respiratory failure after heart surgery

1. Cardiac failure
2. Acute respiratory distress syndrome (ARDS)
3. Pleural effusion
   – Ascites
   – Thoracic soft tissue edema
   – Pneumothorax, pulmonary interstitial emphysema
4. Airway hypersecretion
   – Respiratory infection
   – Bronchospasm
5. Paralysis of the diaphragm
6. Lobar emphysema
7. Malnutrition

perfusion mismatch [26]. Pleural effusion, ascites, thoracic soft tissue edema and pulmonary air leakage impede adequate ventilatory pump function. Small airway obstruction mainly restricts lung emptying, giving rise to airtrapping and increased work of breathing [33]. Paralysis of the diaphragm interferes with respiratory movements and mechanics [34]. Lobar emphysema caused by airway compression of dilated heart chambers or great vessels may become manifest after surgery in connection with the onset of artificial ventilation and may inhibit weaning of the ventilator [35]. Malnourished patients with wasted respiratory muscles may have insufficient strength to breath spontaneously. All these factors can, to a variable degree, contribute to postoperative respiratory failure. Their relative contribution is often difficult to determine. However, among all these possible factors heart failure may be the major, albeit hidden, factor causing ventilator dependency.

The mechanisms by which heart failure leads to respiratory failure are only partially understood. Fig. 1 summarizes the mechanisms by which spontaneous respiration may compromise heart function, and by which the compromised heart function may compromise spontaneous breathing, eventually leading to a vicious circle ending in overt respiratory failure [36]. During spontaneous inspiration the intrathoracic pressure becomes more negative. This negative intrathoracic pressure sucks blood to the right side of the heart which then pumps it into the lungs. The negative intrathoracic pressure also increases the pressure across the ventricular wall. This transmural pressure is physiologically the pressure against which the ventricle must employ its systolic force. Therefore, the increased negative intrathoracic pressure exerts an increased afterload on the left ventricle [37]. If the left ventricle is not able to deal with this increased afterload, blood accumulates in the lungs, increasing lung water and decreasing lung compliance. To overcome this decreased lung compliance, the respiratory muscles must generate more negative intrathoracic pressure to maintain adequate tidal volume. More negative intrathoracic pressure is followed by increased venous return to the right heart and imposes more afterload on the left ventricle. Herewith the vicious circle is closed and the system collapses. The lower part of Fig. 1 expresses these events graphically in a so called Campbell diagram [38]. In a Campbell diagram lung volume on the Y-axis is plotted against the expanding pressure on the X-axis. The dotted P_c line is the thoracic wall compliance curve.

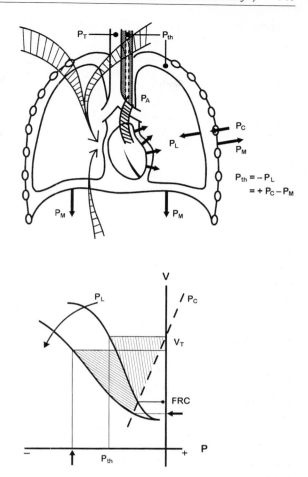

Fig. 1. Mechanisms by which spontaneous breathing compromises heart function. Upper part: schematic picture of the physiologic events. Lower part: Campbell diagram. See text for explanation. P_T tracheal pressure, P_A alveolar pressure, P_{th} intrathoracic pressure, P_L retractive force of the lung, P_c thoracic recoil force, P_M muscle force, V_T tidal volume, FRC functional residual capacity

The solid P_L line is the lung compliance curve. The surface area between both lines P_c and P_L, from functional residual capacity (FRC) to tidal volume, represents the elastic work of breathing. When lung water increases, because of the increased venous return the left heart cannot cope and lung compliance falls. As a consequence FRC diminishes, pulmonary right-to-left shunting increases, work of breathing increases and more negative intrathoracic pressure is needed to generate and maintain tidal volume. Finally the system collapses.

It is evident that mechanical ventilation may reverse these events by decreasing venous return and decreasing left ventricle afterload [39], and in addition diminishing the oxygen need of the overburdened respiratory muscles. Conversely, discontinuation of mechanical ventilation in heart surgery patients can result in overt or subclinical heart failure with subsequent respiratory distress and problems with the weaning process. Treatment should primarily be directed to heart function and not to respiratory function. Ventilatory support in these cases is symptomatic and may at most be a bridge to circulatory recovery.

Chylothorax

The postoperative course after heart surgery is sometimes complicated by chylothorax [40, 41]. The diagnosis is made by pleural effusion of a milky fluid, characterized by the presence of lymphocytes, fat globules, a protein content of at least half the serum protein level and a high amount of triglycerides (>5 g/l or 6 mmol/l). If no feeding is given, the effusions may remain clear with low levels of triglycerides. Then, chylothorax may become manifest after introduction of fat-containing enteral feeding. Chylothorax is usually caused by surgical damage to the large intrathoracic lymph channels, particularly on the left side. But it is often seen in lesions or repairs associated with a high right atrium and systemic venous pressures (e.g., the Fontan circulation) and can also appear as a result of heart failure [42]. The mechanism of the latter is not precisely known.

Chylothorax may result in the loss of large quantities of lymphatic fluid with subsequent loss of circulating volume, electrolytes, calories, immunoglobulins, complement, clotting factors and lymphocytes. Relieving the lymphatic flow by medium chain triglyceride-based feeding can be effective in slight leaks. In more severe cases abstaining from all oral intake will usually diminish or even stop the chyle production within a week. The loss of fluids and electrolytes must be carefully balanced and replaced. High calory total parenteral nutrition must compensate for caloric loss. Finally, immunoglobulins and lymphocytes must be checked weekly. When hypogammaglobulinemia occurs, intravenous immunoglobulins must be supplied. If lymphocytes fall below 500/mm^3, sensitivity to (viral) infections increases and appropriate measures to protect the patients are recommended. Sometimes albumin must be replaced too and in rare cases clotting factors. If the patient is carefully monitored and adequately compensated for the above mentioned losses, spontaneous recovery may be expected in 70–80% of the pediatric cases [40, 41]. In adult cases a more aggressive approach (thoracoscopic ligation of the thoracic duct, pleurodesis) is advocated to avoid the immune and nutritional consequences of large leaks [13]. Patients with chyle losses of more than 1 ml/kg/h are more difficult to manage in the long term and are at special risk. They may be considered for surgical exploration and ligation or diathermy coagulation of the leaking lymphatic duct.

Hyponatremia

The treatment of hyponatremia in cardiac patients, both pre- and postoperatively, may be difficult. Hyponatremia is a renal mediated response to decreased perfusion pressure (Fig. 2) [43]. Perfusion pressure, as it is perceived by the kidney, may be diminished either by a decrease in cardiac output or by an increased venous pressure. In an attempt to increase the perfusion pressure, at first salt together with water is retained, but subsequently more water is retained than salt. The serum sodium will then start to fall. Inappropriate water and salt prescriptions and use of diuretics may aggravate hyponatremia. Increased venous pressure causes edema and ascites. In this way, large amounts of water and salt are sequestrated without substantially increasing perfusion pressure. Diuretics are only of limited value; most diuretics act by

Fig. 2. Schematic picture of renal response to right heart failure. Increased venous pressure and decreased cardiac output diminish renal perfusion pressure. Increased venous pressure induces edema and ascites. Decreased renal perfusion pressure activates water and salt retention. When water retention surpasses salt retention hyponatremia occurs. R.A.A.S: renine-angiotensin-aldosterone system; ADH: antidiuretic hormone; ANF: atrial natriuretic factor; ?: other unknown factors

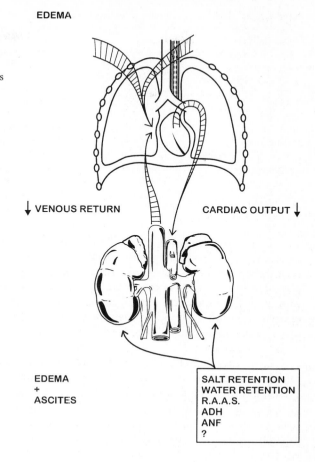

EDEMA

↓ VENOUS RETURN   CARDIAC OUTPUT ↓

EDEMA
+
ASCITES

SALT RETENTION
WATER RETENTION
R.A.A.S.
ADH
ANF
?

diminishing or blocking renal sodium reabsorption, thus causing natriuresis followed by water excretion. The treatment of heart failure with hyponatremia, and especially when renal failure is imminent, is vigorous support of heart function with inotropic agents and no increase in the dose of diuretics.

Renal Failure

Renal failure following heart surgery has been reported in 3–8% of patients [44–48], a figure that has remained virtually unchanged during the last 20 years. Except for the eventual concomitant occurrence of kidney disease, renal failure in postoperative patients is primarily caused by periods of renal hypoperfusion [44, 46, 48, 49]. Renal function follows heart function. On the other hand, renal failure may be worsened by nephrotoxic drugs such as aminoglycosides and high doses of furosemide. Renal failure may considerably disturb fluid and electrolyte management. When it complicates the postoperative course, mortality has been reported between

Table 5. Renal replacement therapy after heart surgery

Hemodialysis	Peritoneal dialysis	Continuous arterio-venous hemodiafiltration (CAVHD)	Continuous veno-venous hemodiafiltration (CVVHD)
> 10 kg	No age limitation	No age limitation	No age limitation
Very effective in fluid withdrawal and clearance	Less effective in fluid withdrawal and clearance	Effective in fluid withdrawal, less effective in clearance	Very effective in fluid withdrawal, more (?) effective in clearance than CAVH
Significant hemo-dynamic disorder	Hemodynamically well tolerated	Hemodynamically well tolerated	Hemodynamically well tolerated
Heparinization	No heparinization	Heparinization	Heparinization

30–65% [44–49]. However, renal failure is an indicator for high mortality rather than its main cause. Nevertheless, it must be treated vigorously [46, 47, 49–51]. Renal support therapy may be a lifesaving bridge to total or partial recovery of renal function, provided heart failure is overcome. Indications for renal replacement therapy are imminent fluid overload and hyperkalemia. There is no evidence for a beneficial effect of routine renal replacement therapy on the prevention or outcome of multiorgan failure, when this is not urged by otherwise untreatable fluid overload or electrolyte disturbances [52].

Table 5 summarizes the advantages and disadvantages of different types of renal replacement therapy. Hemodialysis is very effective in fluid withdrawal and clearing potassium, urea and creatinine. By an experienced team it can be performed in children down to 10 kg. In infants less than 10 kg, hemodialysis generally results in significant hemodynamic disorder even when they initially have an uncompromised circulation. Heparinization is necessary and specialized personnel are required. In the other 3 methods, peritoneal dialysis, continuous arterio-venous hemofiltration (CAVH) [53, 54] and continuous veno-venous hemofiltration (CVVH), there are no age or weight limitations. A poor perfusion pressure often impedes CAVH. With pump assisted CVVH a number of inconveniences and problems of CAVH can be avoided. Both methods are effective in fluid withdrawal, but are less effective in clearance, even if combined with a dialysate counterflow through the filter (hemodiafiltration). In both techniques heparinization is mandatory.

Until now, peritoneal dialysis has been the technique of first choice [51]. The peritoneal catheter is often already placed during surgery. It is generally well tolerated and easy to perform [55]. However, in hemodynamically unstable patients receiving high doses of inotropes it is less effective than in stable renal patients. In such patients, CVVH is the method of choice.

Other Complications

Central nervous system complications may arise from pre-, intra-, or postoperative hypoxia, ischemia or acid-base disorders [56]. They may affect subsequent neurologic development [57]. Convulsions or other motor disturbances are the primary manifestations [58, 59]. Electroencephalogram (EEG) manifestation of seizures has been reported in 20% of neonates undergoing correction of transposition of the great arteries, with only 6% having clinical convulsions [58]. The pathogenesis is only partially understood and probably comprises developmental characteristics of the neonatal brain in relation to cerebral hemodynamic regulation, metabolism and development of neuroreceptors. Convulsions in the postoperative period are treated with the usual anticonvulsant drugs.

Infants with heart defects may have significantly higher needs than healthy infants [60, 61]. Failure to meet these high energy needs will result in failure to thrive. Postoperative feeding difficulties may require early onset of parenteral nutrition. Not infrequently there are opposing needs for high calory intake and fluid restriction. Ultimately one has to recourse to peritoneal dialysis, CAVH or CVVH. The last two techniques, particularly, allow for the administration of relatively large amounts of fluids for parenteral nutrition [54].

Infection, either early or late onset, finally threatens every intensive care patient. Although all kinds of infection can be expected in postoperative cardiac patients, special attention should be paid to sepsis from contaminated intravascular lines [62, 63] and to endocarditis [64]. Careful bacteriologic surveys and rational antibiotic strategies form the basis of a well-conducted ICU. Fever alone is not sufficient to diagnose and treat a possible infection. Apart from preventive measures, a rational protocol for infection control in the postoperative phase should first comprise the appraisal of a suspicious serious or real infection, next the assessment of the site of infection and finally the identification of the infective agent and its sensitivity. Only then can a proper antibiotic therapy be selected. Sometimes, the results of diagnostic tests cannot be awaited and empiric therapy must be started on the basis of educated guesses. However, such a therapy must be reconsidered once the results of the bacteriologic tests have become available.

Conclusion

All neonates with congenital heart defects must be scrutinized carefully for additional congenital disorders before surgery. Pediatric problems after heart surgery are most probably the result of hemodynamic disturbances, or the consequence of a basic more complex disorder. They can only be treated in a successful way within a multidisciplinary team in which pediatric intensivists, heart surgeons, cardio-anesthesiologists and pediatric cardiologists can rely on a high standard of other pediatric disciplines.

Acknowledgment: The authors thank Professor J. F. Hitchcock for his critical remarks and Mr. G. Meijerman for designing Figures 1 and 2.

References

1. Emmanouilides GC, Riemenschneider TA, Allen HD, Gutgesell HP (eds) (1995) Heart disease in infants, children and adolescents (5th edn). Williams & Wilkins, Baltimore

2. Kirklin JW, Baratt-Boyes BG (eds) (1993) Cardiac surgery; morphology, diagnostic criteria, natural history, techniques, results, and indications (2nd edn). Churchill Livingstone, New York

3. Jonas RA (1995) Advances in surgical care of infants and children with congenital heart disease. Curr Opin Pediatr 7:572–579

4. Armstrong BE (1995) Congenital cardiovascular disease and cardiac surgery in childhood: Part 1. Cyanotic congenital heart defects. Curr Opin Cardiol 10:58–67

5. Armstrong BE (1995) Congenital cardiovascular disease and cardiac surgery in childhood: Part 2. Acyanotic congenital heart defects and interventional techniques. Curr Opin Cardiol 10: 68–77

6. Nichols DG, Cameron DE, Greeley WJ, Lappe DG, Ungeleider RM, Wetzel RC (eds) (1995) Critical heart disease in infants and children. Mosby, St. Louis

7. Kramer H-H, Majewski F, Trampisch HJ, Rammos S, Bourgeous M (1987) Malformation patterns in children with congenital heart disease. Am J Dis Child 141:789–795

8. Benson DW, Basson CT, MacRae CA (1996) New understandings in the genetics of congenital heart disease. Curr Opin Pediatr 8:505–511

9. Bristow J (1995) The search for genetic mechanisms of congenital heart disease. Cell Mol Biol Res 41:307–319

10. Olson EN, Srivastava D (1996) Molecular pathways controlling heart development. Science 272: 671–676

11. Buskens E, Grobbee DE, Frohn Mulder IM, Wladimiroff JW, Hess J (1995) Aspects of the aetiology of congenital heart disease. Eur Heart J 16:584–587

12. Johnson MC, Payne RM, Grant JW, Strauss AW (1995) The genetic basis of paediatric heart disease. Ann Med 27:289–300

13. Payne RM, Johnson MC, Grant JW, Strauss AW (1995) Toward a molecular understanding of congenital heart disease. Circulation 91:494–504

14. Yamaki S, Horiuchi T, Takahashi T (1985) Pulmonary changes in congenital heart disease with Down's syndrome: their significance as a cause of postoperative respiratory failure. Thorax 40: 380–386

15. Gyves-Ray K, Kirchner S, Stein S, Heller R, Hernanz-Schulman M (1994) Cystic lung disease in Down's syndrome. Pediatr Radiol 24:137–138

16. Gonzalez OR, Gomez IG, Recalde AL, Landing BH (1991) Postnatal development of the cystic lung lesions of Down syndrome: suggestion that the cause is reduced formation of peripheral air spaces. Pediatr Pathol 11:623–633

17. Hals J, Hagemo PS, Thaulow E, Sorland SJ (1993) Pulmonary vascular resistance in complete atrioventricular septal defect; a comparison between children with and without Down's syndrome. Acta Paediatr 82:595–598

18. de Jong AL, Sulek M, Nihill M, Duncan NO, Friedman EM (1997) Tenuous airway in children with trisomy 21. Laryngoscope 107:345–350

19. Greenberg F (1989) What defines DiGeorge anomaly. J Pediatr 115:412–413

20. Greenberg F (1993) DiGeorge syndrome: an historical review of clinical and cytogenetic features. J Med Genet 30:803–806

21. van Mierop LHS, Kutsche LM (1986) Cardiovascular anomalies in DiGeorge syndrome and importance of neural crest as a possible pathogenetic factor. Am J Cardiol 58:133–137

22. Driscoll D, Budarf ML, Emanuel BS (1992) A genetic etiology for DiGeorge syndrome: consistent deletions and microdeletions of 22q11. Am J Hum Genet 50:924–933

23. Scrambler PJ (1993) Deletions of human chromosome 22 and associated birth defects. Curr Opin Genet Dev 3:432–437

24. Driscoll D, Salvin J, Sellinger B, et al (1993) Prevalence of 22q11 microdeletions in DiGeorge and velocardiofacial syndromes: implications for genetic counselling and prenatal diagnosis. J Med Genet 30:813–817

25. Goldmunz E, Driscoll D, Budarf ML, et al (1993) Microdeletions of chromosomal region 22q11 in patients with congenital conotruncal cardiac defects. J Med Genet 30:807–812

26. Kern FH, Greeley WJ, Ungeleider RM (1995) Cardiopulmonary bypass. In: Nichols DG, Cameron DE, Greeley WJ, Lappe DG, Ungeleider RM, Wetzel RC (eds) Critical heart disease in infants and children. Mosby, St. Louis, pp 497–529

27. Kirklin JK, Blackstone EH, Kirklin JW (1987) Cardiopulmonary bypass: studies on its damaging effects. Blood Purif 5:168–178

28. Westaby S (1987) Organ dysfunction after cardiopulmonary bypass. A systemic inflammatory reaction initiated by the extracorporeal circuit. Intensive Care Med 13:89–95
29. Nilsson L, Brunnkvist S, Nilsson U, et al (1988) Activation of inflammatory systems during cardiopulmonary bypass. Scand J Thorac Cardiovasc Surg 22:51–53
30. Knudsen F, Andersen LW (1990) Immunological aspects of cardiopulmonary bypass. J Cardiothorac Anesth 4:245–258
31. Butler J, Rocker GM, Westaby S (1993) Inflammatory response to cardiopulmonary bypass. Ann Thorac Surg 55:552–559
32. Casey LC (1993) Role of cytokines in the pathogenesis of cardiopulmonary-induced multisystem organ failure. Ann Thorac Surg 56:S92–S96
33. van den Berg B, Aerts JGJV, Bogaard JM (1995) Effect of continuous positive airway pressure (CPAP) in patients with obstructive pulmonary disease (COPD) depending on intrinsic PEEP levels. Acta Anaesth Scand 39:1097–1102
34. Tonz M, von Segesser LK, Mihaljevic T, Arbenz U, Stauffer UG, Turina MI (1996) Clinical implications of phrenic nerve injury after pediatric cardiac surgery. J Pediatr Surg 31:1265–1267
35. Gordon I, Dempsey JE (1990) Infantile lobar emphysema in association with congenital heart disease. Clin Radiol 41:48–52
36. Miro AM, Pinsky MR (1994) Heart-lung interactions. In: Tobin MJ (ed) Principles and practice of mechanical ventilation. McGraw-Hill, New York
37. Richard Ch, Teboul J-L, Archambaud F, Hebert J-L, Michaut P, Auzepy P (1994) Left ventricular function during weaning of patients with chronic obstructive pulmonary disease. Intensive Care Med 20:181–186
38. Grassino AE, Roussos C, Macklem PT (1991) Static properties of the chest wall. In: Crystal RG, West JB (eds) The lung; scientific foundations. Raven Press, New York, pp 856–857
39. Pinsky MR, Matuschak GM, Klain M (1985) Determinants of cardiac augmentation by elevation of intrathoracic pressure. J Appl Physiol 58:1189–1198
40. Nguyen DM, Shum Tim D, Dobell AR, Tchervenkov CI (1995) The management of chylothorax/chylopericardium following pediatric cardiac surgery: a 10-year experience. J Card Surg 10:302–308
41. Bond SJ, Guzetta PC, Snyder ML, Randolph JG (1993) Management of pediatric postoperative chylothorax. Ann Thorac Surg 56:469–473
42. Villena V, de Pablo A, Martin Escribano P (1995) Chylothorax and chylous ascites due to heart failure. Eur Respir J 8:1235–1236
43. Berry PhL (1990) Nephrology for the pediatric cardiologist. In: Garson A, Bricker JT, McNamara DG (eds) The science and practice of pediatric cardiology. Lea & Febiger, Philadelphia, pp 2425–2444
44. Frost L, Pedersen RS, Lund O, Hansen OK, Hansen HE (1991) Prognosis and risk factors in acute, dialysis requiring renal failure after open heart surgery. Scand J Thorac Cardiovasc Surg 25:161–166
45. Shaw NJ, Brocklebank JT, Dickinson DF, Wilson N, Walker DR (1991) Long-term outcome for children with acute renal failure following cardiac surgery. Int J Cardiol 31:161–165
46. Hanson J, Loftness S, Clarke D, Campbell D (1989) Peritoneal dialysis following open heart surgery in children. Pediatr Cardiol 10:125–128
47. Rigden SPA, Barrat TM, Dillon MJ, de Leval M, Stark J (1982) Acute renal failure complicating cardiopulmonary bypass surgery. Arch Dis Child 57:425–430
48. Chesney RW, Kaplan BS, Freedom RM, Haller JA, Drummond KN (1975) Acute renal failure: an important complication of cardiac surgery in infants. J Pediatr 87:381–388
49. Giuffre RM, Tam KH, Williams WW, Freedom RM (1992) Acute renal failure complicating pediatric cardiac surgery: a comparison of survivors and nonsurvivors following acute peritoneal dialysis. Pediatr Cardiol 13:208–213
50. Vricella LA, de Begona JA, Gundry SR, Vigesaa RE, Kawauchi M, Bailey LL (1992) Aggressive peritoneal dialysis for treatment of acute kidney failure after heart transplantation. J Heart Lung Transplant 11:320–329
51. Mee RBB (1992) Dialysis after cardiopulmonary bypass in neonates and infants. J Thorac Cardiovasc Surg 103:1021–1022
52. Schetz M, Ferdinande P, van den Berghe G (1995) Removal of proinflammatory cytokines with renal replacement therapy: sense or nonsense? Intensive Care Med 21:169–176

53. Paret G, Cohen AJ, Bohn DJ, et al (1992) Continuous arteriovenous hemofiltration after cardiac operations in infants and children. J Thorac Cardiovasc Surg 104:1225–1230
54. Zobel G, Stein JI, Kuttnig M, Beitzke A, Metzler H, Rigler B (1991) Continuous extracorporeal fluid removal in children with low cardiac output after cardiac operations. J Thorac Cardiovasc Surg 101:593–597
55. Ryan CA, Hung O, Soder CM (1992) Hemodynamic effects of peritoneal dialysis in three children following open heart surgery. Pediatr Cardiol 13:30–32
56. Tasker RC (1995) Cerebral function and heart disease. In: Nichols DG, Cameron DE, Greeley WJ, Lappe DG, Ungeleider RM, Wetzel RC (eds) Critical heart disease in infants and children. Mosby, St. Louis, pp 157–184
57. Bellinger DC, Jonas RA, Rappaport LA, et al (1995) Developmental and neurological status of children after heart surgery with hypothermic circulatory arrest or low-flow cardiopulmonary bypass. N Engl J Med 332:549–555
58. Helmers SL, Wypij D, Constantinou JE, et al (1997) Perioperative electroencephalographic seizures in infants undergoing repair of complex cardiac defects. Electroencephalogr Clin Neurophysiol 102:27–36
59. Wong PC, Barlow CF, Hickey PR, et al (1992) Factors associated with choreoathetosis after cardiopulmonary bypass in children with congenital heart disease. Circulation 86 (suppl 5):118–126
60. Zuckerberg AL, Deutschman CS, Caballero B (1995) Nutrition and metabolism in the criticaly ill child with heart disease. In: Nichols DG, Cameron DE, Greeley WJ, Lappe DG, Ungeleider RM, Wetzel RC (eds) Critical heart disease in infants and children. Mosby, St. Louis, pp 415–436
61. Barton JS, Hindmarsh PC, Scimgeour CM, Rennie MJ, Preece MA (1994) Energy expenditure in congenital heart disease. Arch Dis Child 70:5–9
62. Jansen B (1993) Vascular catheter-related infection: aetiology and prevention. Curr Opin Infect Dis 6:526–531
63. Goldmann DA, Pier GB (1993) Pathogenesis of infections related to intravascular catheterization. Clin Microbiol Rev 6:176–192
64. Baltimore RS (1997) Cardiac and vascular infections. In: Long SS, Pickering LK, Prober ChG (eds) Principles and practice of pediatric infectious diseases. Churchill Livingstone, New York, pp 289–298

Crises in Pre-Eclampsia

D. Watson and J. Coakley

Introduction

Pre-eclampsia is a condition unique to pregnancy and complicates approximately 15% of primigravid pregnancies. Eclampsia complicates severe pre-eclampsia and occurs in approximately 0.04% of deliveries. Pre-eclampsia and eclampsia are the commonest causes of maternal death in the developed countries [1, 2]. Patients may also suffer significant morbidity from this multiple system disorder [3] and require intensive medical and nursing supervision of a multidisciplinary nature [4].

Eclampsia

Should a patient have a seizure the airway must be protected, oxygenation maintained and the seizure terminated with the administration of an intravenous benzodiazepine such as diazepam emulsion. Eclampsia complicates severe disease but is not necessarily associated with severe hypertension. In many instances tracheal intubation and mechanical ventilation are necessary in view of an altered level of consciousness. In addition to the immediate control of convulsions it is important to control raised blood pressure and then expedite delivery of the baby if the seizure has occurred antenatally.

A significant cause of morbidity and mortality in eclampsia is associated with accompanying cerebral oedema or intracerebral hemorrhage. If there are localizing neurological signs patients require urgent investigation with computerized tomography (CT) scanning or magnetic-resonance imaging (MRI). If associated with eclampsia, cerebral ischemia is thought to be attributable to cerebral vasoconstriction [5]. As with other neurologic emergencies thought to be secondary to vasospasm there have been reported improvements following nimodipine administration [6]. Cerebral vasodilation may also be a beneficial effect of magnesium sulfate administration either directly, or by increased endothelial production of prostacyclin. Guidelines for magnesium sulfate administration are given in Table 1. Serum magnesium concentrations may be measured directly or inferred from repeated clinical examinations. If reflexes are absent, respiratory performance depressed, or serum magnesium concentration is shown to be high then any magnesium infusion should be stopped. In the event of cardiorespiratory arrest complicating magnesium administration, calcium gluconate should be injected whilst continuing with advanced life support measures. It is important that anesthesiologists and pediatricians are

Table 1. Guidelines for magnesium sulfate dosage in the management of pre-eclampsia and eclampsia

1. Give a loading dose of 4 g magnesium sulfate as a 20% solution intravenously at a rate of 1 g/min during eclamptic seizures or over 10–15 minutes for seizure prophylaxis.
2. Start a continuous intravenous infusion of magnesium sulfate at the rate of 1–3 g/h and continue the infusion for at least 24 h after delivery.
3. If convulsions persist after 15 mins give 2–4 g magnesium sulfate intravenously at a rate no faster than 1 g/min. Measure serum magnesium concentration.
   - Normal range   0.75–1.25 (mmol/l)
   - Effective anticonvulsant   2–3.5 (mmol/l)
   - Reflexes disappear   5.00 (mmol/l)
   - Respiratory depression   7.50 (mmol/l)
   - Cardiac arrest   15.00 (mmol/l)

Examine carefully every four hours for the presence of limb reflexes, respiratory rate of at least 16/min and urinary output of at least 30 ml/h.

told that magnesium is being administered since it enhances the action of non-depolarizing muscle relaxants and may cause the newborn to be flaccid.

In the event of CT scanning demonstrating cerebral oedema then measures normally adopted in dealing with such a neurologic emergency should be implemented. The patient should be nursed approximately 30% head-up with a safe or secured airway. Hypoxia and hypercarbia should be avoided at all costs by supplemental oxygen administration and if necessary elective mechanical ventilation. Blood pressure control should avoid reductions in cerebral blood flow by tolerating a higher mean arterial pressure (MAP) of 80–100 mmHg. It is nevertheless advisable to treat diastolic blood pressures higher than 110 mmHg to minimize the risk of intracranial hemorrhage. Infusions of antihypertensive agents require invasive intra-arterial monitoring, central venous pressure assessment and consideration of pulmonary arterial catheterization in refractory cases. Crystalloid solutions should be restricted and colloid solutions should be considered if there is oliguria associated with low cardiac filling pressures. The largest study of untreated cases found that the cardiac output was low to normal [7] associated with increased systemic vascular resistance.

Acute Respiratory Distress Syndrome

Acute respiratory distress syndrome (ARDS) is considered comparable to intracerebral hemorrhage as an immediate cause of death in patients with hypertensive disorders of pregnancy [8]. Pulmonary aspiration of gastric contents may complicate tracheal intubation, over sedation or seizures and give rise to direct lung injury. Secondary lung injury may follow the systemic inflammatory response syndrome (SIRS) or injudicious fluid administration. It may also be a sequel to large volume hemorrhage complicating liver rupture or life-threatening coagulopathy. The incidence of ARDS complicating pregnancy appears to be increasing. This may be partly due to patients surviving longer and allowing time for the condition to become established. It may also be due to its more frequent demonstration at autopsy. Standard management protocols for this condition apply to the obstetric patient as for the non-pregnant woman.

Pulmonary Aspiration

In Mendelson's original series [9] women died from asphyxia not from the chemical pneumonitis that now carries his name. Aspiration of large volumes of acidic gastric contents is associated with hypoxia and hypovolemia. This may exacerbate generalized tissue hypoxia and precipitate splanchnic vasoconstriction. This in turn, may initiate the release of inflammatory mediators and give rise to SIRS and multiple organ dysfunction (MODS).

The management of pulmonary aspiration in obstetric patients should be the same as for the non-pregnant population. The airway must be secured and cleared of debris. Appropriate ventilatory support should be instituted early. Pulmonary artery catheterization should be undertaken to guide volume administration and hemodynamic support. For the severest and most florid cases with refractory hypoxemia and hypercarbia extracorporeal gas exchange or inhaled nitric oxide should be considered.

The severity of aspiration pneumonitis depends on the acidity of the gastric contents as well as the volume aspirated. A possibility therefore exists to prevent acid aspiration by neutralizing gastric contents prophylactically during childbirth. A regimen involving the regular prescription of oral ranitidine (150 mg 6-hourly) together with 30 mls of the non-particulate antacid, 0.3 M sodium citrate, has been shown to be an effective means of controlling the acidity and volume of the gastric contents [10]. National surveys in the United Kingdom reveal that routine prophylaxis now generally consists of such combinations of H_2-receptor blockade and antacid [11]. This practice remains important given that 75% of all eclamptic seizures still occur unexpectedly in hospital and some may arise only following delivery.

Hemorrhage

Liver rupture, intra-adrenal hemorrhage, obstetric hemorrhage complicating life-threatening coagulopathy or abruptio placentae are all possible sequelae of severe pre-eclampsia. Uncontrolled hypertension may also predispose to rupture of congenital intracerebral aneurysms. Typically a narrowing of the pulse pressure and sustained tachycardia with falling intravascular filling pressures and hematocrit complete the clinical picture.

In the case of surgical hemorrhage opportunities exist to minimize the delay to full tissue resuscitation. Recent consensus conference statements on the prevention and management of tissue dysoxia indicate that aggressive attempts to augment oxygen delivery to supranormal values are unwarranted. Nevertheless effective fluid resuscitation and rapid restoration of normal hemodynamics are essential [12]. This remains a contentious area [13] for the general surgical or trauma patient. It would seem logical nevertheless to extend these principles of critical care to obstetric patients with life-threatening hemorrhage but intensivists may not be convinced of the benefit of boosting oxygen delivery in even some critically ill patients. The impact of right heart catheterization has also not been settled in the general management of the critically ill [14, 15]. There is an overall lack of published physiologic data involving obstetric patients with life-threatening illnesses such as pre-eclampsia or hemorrhage. Nevertheless the development of protocols encompassing best nursing and medical practice for the management of this multisystem disorder is to be recommended [16–18].

HELLP Syndrome

A considerable proportion (4–20%) of the severest cases of pre-eclampsia are complicated by the spectrum of the HELLP syndrome (haemolysis, elevated liver enzymes, low platelet [19, 20]). This syndrome can be associated with significant fetomaternal morbidity and mortality. The clinical features of the condition are not necessarily those of pre-eclampsia. Hypertension and proteinuria may be mild. Women may complain of epigastric or right upper quadrant pain, nausea or vomiting. Laboratory investigations may reveal low grade hemolysis, low or falling platelet counts (less than $100000 \times 10^6/l$) and evidence of disseminated intra-vascular coagulation. Abnormalities in liver function tests include raised transaminase and lactate dehydrogenase concentrations and raised levels of unconjugated bilirubin. The principle differential diagnosis are hemolytic uremic syndrome and thrombocytopenic purpura. Alternatively HELLP syndrome can present as a life-threatening emergency with placental abruption, liver rupture or acute renal failure. The syndrome may also present or worsen in the postpartum period associated with hypertension, myocardial dysfunction and pulmonary edema of multifactoral etiology.

The management of the HELLP syndrome is to control vital signs and blood pressure in particular [21]. The coagulopathy should be corrected with fresh frozen plasma and platelet transfusions. This will facilitate the establishment of intra-vascular monitoring techniques and operative intervention. Women may require judicious colloid fluid administration given the associated features of pulmonary edema, renal insufficiency and whole-body capillary leak syndrome. Following delivery of the placenta the mainstay of treatment is supportive and symptomatic to temporise as far as possible until spontaneous resolution of the syndrome. Liver enzyme abnormalities appear to recover before low platelet concentrations. In the recovery phase investigations to exclude other diagnoses should be undertaken. It is noteworthy that HELLP syndrome, like pre-eclampsia, can recur in later pregnancies.

Acute Renal Failure

This is not commonly encountered in obstetric practice. It may complicate severe pre-eclampsia, the HELLP syndrome or obstetric hemorrhage. It should be managed using standard protocols. In the recovery phase investigations to exclude pre-existing renal disease should be undertaken by nephrologists.

Conclusion

Pre-eclampsia is a disorder of unknown etiology unique to pregnant or postpartum women. Early recognition and management of this condition may serve to avoid serious maternal complications. Maternal treatment revolves around delivery of the fetus and the placenta. Advanced stages of this disease result in classical multiple organ dysfunction which may be life-threatening to the mother and her baby. Complications of pre-eclampsia include severe hypertension, eclamptic seizures, cerebral edema, pulmonary edema, liver rupture, abruptio placentae, HELLP syndrome and acute renal failure. A multidisciplinary approach and the application of basic principles for the care of the critically ill are as warranted for the obstetric patient as for the non-pregnant population.

References

1. Department of Health (1966) Report on confidential enquiries into maternal deaths in the United Kingdom 1991–1993. HMSO, London
2. Kaunitz AM, Hughes JM, Grimes DA, Smith JC, Rochat RW (1990) Causes of maternal mortality in the United States, 1979–1986. Am J Obstet Gynecol 163:460–465
3. Williams DJ, de Swiet M (1997) The pathophysiology of pre-eclampsia. Intensive Care Med 23:620–629
4. Dildy GA, Cotton DB (1991) Management of severe pre-eclampsia and eclampsia. Crit Care Clin 7:829–850
5. Lewis LK, Hinshaw DB, Will AD, Hasso AN, Thompson JR (1988) CT and angiographic correlation of severe neurological disease in toxaemia of pregnancy. Neuroradiology 30:56–64
6. Horn EH, Filshie M, Kerslake RW, Jaspan T, Worthington BS, Rubin PC (1990) Widespread cerebral ischaemia treated with nimodipine in a patient with eclampsia. Br Med J 301:794
7. Wallenburg HCS (1988) Haemodynamics in hypertensive pregnancy. In: Rubin PC (ed) Hypertension Vol 10. Elsevier, Amsterdam, pp 66–101
8. Sibai BM, Mabie BC, Harvey CJ, Gonzalez AR (1987) Pulmonary edema in severe preeclampsia-eclampsia: analysis of thirty-seven consecutive cases. Am J Obstet Gynecol 156:1174–1179
9. Mendelson CL (1946) Aspiration of stomach contents into the lungs during obstetric anaesthesia. Am J Obstet Gynecol 52:191–205
10. Gillett GB, Watson JD, Langford RM (1984) Ranitidine and single-dose antacid therapy as prophylaxis against acid aspiration syndrome in obstetric practice. Anaesthesia 39:638–644
11. Tordoff SG, Sweeny BP (1990) Acid aspiration prophylaxis in 288 obstetric anaesthetic departments in the United Kingdom. Anaesthesia 45:776–780
12. Third European consensus conference in intensive care medicine (1996) Tissue hypoxia. How to detect, how to correct, how to prevent? Am J Respir Crit Care Med 154:1573–1578
13. Shoemaker WC, Belzberg H (1997) Maximizing oxygen delivery in high-risk surgical patients. Crit Care Med 25:714–715
14. Dalen JE, Bone RC (1996) Is it time to pull the pulmonary catheter? JAMA 276:916–918
15. Soni N (1996) Swan song for the Swan Ganz catheter? Br Med J 313:763–764
16. Redman CWG, Roberts JM (1993) Management of pre-eclampsia. Lancet 341:1451–1454
17. Robson SC, Redfern N, Walkinshaw SA (1992) A protocol for the intrapartum management of severe pre-eclampsia. Int J Obstet Anesth 1:222–229
18. The Eclampsia Trial Collaborative Group (1995) Which anti-convulsant for women with eclampsia? Evidence from the Collaborative Eclampsia Trial. Lancet 345:1455–1463
19. Weinstein L (1982) Syndrome of hemolysis, elevated liver enzymes and low platelet count: a severe consequence of hypertension. Am J Obstet Gynecol 142:159–167
20. Sibai BM, Ramadam MK, Usta I, Salama M, Mercer BM, Friedman SA (1993) Maternal morbidity and mortality in 442 pregnancies with hemolysis, elevated liver enzymes and low platelets (HELLP syndrome). Am J Obstet Gynecol 169:1000–1006
21. Watson D, Yau E, Hayes MA, Macklin SA (1996) Hemodynamic changes in the HELLP syndrome. In: van Zundert A, Ostheimer GW (eds) Pain relief and anesthesia in obstetrics. Churchill Livingstone, New York

ICU Performance – Evaluation

Performance of the ICU: Are We Able to Measure it?

R. Moreno

Introduction

In the last decades, there has been a worldwide expansion in the number and specification of intensive care units (ICUs). A better knowledge of the physiopathologic mechanisms in the critically ill patient together with an increase in the number and sophistication of the available therapeutic options have allowed the treatment of an increasing number of severely ill patients. Situations that just a few years ago were hopeless are nowadays routinely handled in the ICU.

This change has had a price, with the ICU presently being responsible for an increasing percentage of the hospital and health care budget. Thus, the evaluation of the effectiveness of the ICU has become an important and current issue, with intensivists being confronted with increasing pressure to critically analyze and justify the adequacy of employed practices. An important part of this problem is the evaluation of our performance, or, in other words, how well are we treating our patients.

The evaluation of the effectiveness of the ICU with strict scientific methods is a difficult task. According to standard methodologic criteria, such an evaluation should preferably be based on formal randomized double-blinded studies, for instance comparing the effectiveness of care in the ICU with standard care in general wards. However, such study proposals meet with opposition on the basis of ethical arguments in view of the general belief that ICU-treatment is appropriate and mandatory. As a matter of fact, even the appropriate evaluation of certain procedures of daily ICU practice has been hampered by such objections, as demonstrated recently by Connors et al. [1]. Other approaches have been used, such as studies using historic controls, but can be justly criticized on methodologic grounds. These facts imply that we have to live with the general assumption that the development of intensive care, with regard to its medical activities and indications, followed the path of multiple natural experiments. Consequently, we should compare the effectiveness of intensive care on the level of the individual ICU. In other words, the question to answer, is whether the outcome of the patients treated in one ICU is in accordance with the expected outcome? With this approach, the actual outcome in the population under analysis is compared to the outcome in a reference population while controlling for case mix factors, by using general outcome prediction models. We replace the question "how good are our results" with "are our results better (or worse) than others". The reference population can be chosen as a gold standard if the model used for prediction is based on data from outstanding ICUs, or just as a reference population if the model is based on non-selected or non-representative ICUs [2].

Several investigators have proposed the use of the ratio between observed and predicted deaths (standardized mortality ratio, SMR) as an indicator of the effectiveness of care in the ICU [3]. The assumption is that although ICUs may admit very heterogeneous groups of patients concerning relevant outcome markers, such as large differences in age, previous health status or acute health status, the existing outcome prediction models can account for most of these characteristics [3]. The use of this methodology requires, first, that the outcome of interest is relevant, clearly defined and susceptible to accurate measurement, and second, that the outcome prediction model is able to control for important patient baseline characteristics which, in turn, are related to the outcome of interest. Thus, a full understanding of prediction models including their methodologic limitations is essential for the clinicians and managers who use such models as a tool in the process of quality evaluation and quality control in the ICU.

The Use of General Outcome Prediction Models in the Evaluation of Performance

Developed more than 15 years ago, general outcome prediction models are today a methodologic cornerstone in the process of performance evaluation, since they allow the prediction of mortality in a given patient, based on the severity of his illness. The severity of illness is evaluated through the use of a severity of illness scoring system, that takes into account the most important factors related to prognosis, e.g., age, previous health status, diagnosis, presence and degree of physiologic derangement. For each of the analyzed parameters a numeric value is assigned depending on the degree of deviation from normality. The final result or score is the sum of the points attributed to each of the analyzed parameters. An equation then transforms the score into a probability of mortality, based on a reference population. The reference population is usually chosen from a large multinational database obtained in thousands of patients. The most frequently used models are the new simplified acute physiologic score (SAPS II) [4], the acute physiology and chronic health evaluation (APACHE II and III) [5, 6] and the new mortality probability models (MPM) [7].

To evaluate the performance of a given ICU we sum up the expected probabilities of death for all the patients in that ICU, in order to compute the expected mortality. The expected mortality is then compared with the observed mortality through the use of the SMR. If the observed mortality in the ICU is higher than the expected, we refer to its performance as poor; if the observed mortality is lower than the predicted, we refer to its performance as good. Assuming that the errors resulting from data collection are small and randomly distributed and that the model is well-calibrated, the supporters of this methodology attribute the differences between predicted and observed mortality to local variations in the quality of care [8].

It should be noted that the use of this methodology assumes that the relationship between severity of illness and performance is constant. In other words, that the performance of one ICU is the same in low- and high-risk patients. It has been advocated in the past on theoretic grounds that the performance of an ICU can vary according to the severity of the admitted patients [2, 9], but this approach had been used in only one study, containing a number of patients in the middle and high-risk groups too small to allow definitive analysis [9]. This approach has been recently used in the EURICUS-I study by Reis Miranda et al. [10] who demonstrated clearly that the performance can vary within each ICU according to the disease severity of the admitted patients.

The assumptions behind the use of the SMR have been challenged several times in the past years [11–14]. Diverse definitions of the variables used, inadequate intra- and inter-rater reliability of collected data and poor calibration of the models used, have all been shown to affect the performance of the equations used to predict mortality. In addition, our ability to control for case mix is increasingly questioned [15]. Even the choice of the outcome (usually hospital mortality) is subjected to debate since it may be prone to bias (some even speak of manipulation). It has been demonstrated that some hospitals tend to change the location of deaths (e.g., by discharging patients to die) whereas other hospitals discharge patients very early in the course of their disease [16]. Moreover, the use of the hospital outcome to evaluate the performance of the ICU implies that we are attributing to the ICU all the responsibilities for an event that depends also on the post-ICU care [17].

In this process, the evaluation of the applicability of the general outcome prediction model to the population under analysis is a crucial step. As stated by a recent consensus conference [18] "Mortality prediction models are almost always overspecific for the patient samples upon which they were developed, and thus performance usually deteriorates when models are applied to different population samples. ... For this reason, we recommend that mortality prediction models always be tested in patient samples distinct from those in which the models were developed".

The main question to be answered at this stage is the adequacy of outcome predictions when compared to actual outcomes. Three major issues must be evaluated [19]. The first is the model calibration or reliability, or how well the model predictions compare with the observed outcomes. The second is the model discrimination, refinement or spread, or how well the model distinguishes between observations with a positive or a negative outcome. A third source of model deviation can be the existence in the test set of subsets of observations in which the model does not perform well. Contrary to the first two factors, where a lot of research has been done and consensual techniques have emerged, there is little in the literature on how to identify these observations or what to do when the fit is unsatisfactory in some groups [19]. The evaluation of calibration and discrimination in the overall population has been named overall goodness-of-fit. The evaluation of the appropriateness of the predictions across sub-groups has been termed uniformity-of-fit. These issues will be reviewed in more detail below.

The evaluation of the overall goodness-of-fit comprises the evaluation of calibration and discrimination in the target population. Calibration evaluates the degree of correspondence between the estimated probabilities of mortality and the observed mortality in the sample under analysis. Four methods have been employed: Overall observed/expected (O/E) mortality ratios; Flora's Z score [20]; Hosmer-Lemeshow goodness-of-fit tests [21]; and calibration curves.

Overall O/E mortality ratios: These are computed by dividing the overall observed mortality rate (i.e., the actual number of deaths) by the predicted number of deaths (resulting from the sum of the individual probabilities of mortality assigned by the model); additional computations can be made to estimate the confidence interval for the ratio [22]. In a perfectly calibrated model this value should be one. Since this test evaluates the O/E mortality ratio in the overall sample it cannot detect deviations in only a certain subset of observations e.g., high-risk patients.

Flora's Z score: This is based on a statistical technique that compares the number of survivors observed in the given data set with the number that would be predicted from the baseline survival curve. The difference is then standardized and compared to a table of the normal distribution [20]. This approach suffers from the same drawbacks of the overall O/E ratios and has been infrequently used.

Hosmer-Lemeshow goodness-of-fit tests: These are two chi-square statistics proposed for the formal evaluation of the calibration of outcome prediction models [21]. In Hosmer-Lemeshow $\hat{H}$ test, patients are divided in 10 strata, according to their predicted probabilities: 0.0 to 0.1, 0.1 to 0.2 ... 0.9 to 1.0. Then, a chi-square statistic is used to compare the actual and the expected number of deaths and the actual and expected number of survivors in each of the strata. Large differences suggest that the model is not well calibrated. Hosmer-Lemeshow $\hat{C}$ test is similar, with the strata being formed based on deciles of the predicted mortality. The same authors demonstrated that the grouping method at the basis of the $\hat{C}$ statistic is preferable to the one based on fixed cut points, especially when many of the estimated probabilities are small [21]. These tests are currently regarded as an obligatory part of calibration evaluation [18], although they are also subject to criticism [23]. It should be noted that to have the statistical power needed for the detection of lack of fit the analyzed sample must have a certain dimension [24].

Calibration curves: These are also used for reporting information on the calibration of a model. This type of chart compares the observed mortality rate with the one expected by the model. They can be misleading since the number of patients in each group tends to go down from left to right (i.e., when moving from a low probability to a high probability of death) and as a consequence even small non-significant differences in the higher severity groups appear visually more important than significant differences in the low probability groups. These curves are not a formal statistical test of the adequacy of the model, being used only for information purposes. However, the publication of calibration curves has been recommended as part of the standard assessment of the validation of a model.

Discrimination evaluates how well the model can distinguish between observations with a positive or a negative outcome. This assessment can be done by a nonparametric test like Harrell's c-index, using the rank of the magnitude of the assessment error. This index measures the probability that for two randomly chosen patients, the one with the higher probability prediction has the outcome of interest. It has been shown that this index relates directly to the area under a receiver operating characteristic (ROC) curve and can be obtained as the parameter from the Mann-Whitney-Wilcoxon rank sum test statistic [25].

The concept of the area under the ROC curve derives from psychophysics and has been applied in signal processing. In a ROC curve, a series of two-by-two tables is constructed with cut points that vary from the lowest possible value to the highest possible value of the score. For each table, the true positive rate (or sensitivity) and the false positive rate (or 1 minus specificity) is computed. The final plot of all pairs of true positive rates versus false positive rates is the visual representation of the ROC curve. The interpretation of the area under the ROC curve is easy: A model with a perfect discrimination has an area of 1.0, and a model where discrimination is no better than chance has an area of 0.5. For the most frequently used outcome prediction models this area is usually over 0.80. Methods for comparing the areas under ROC curves have been described [26], but can lead to misleading conclusions if the shape of the curves is different [27]. It has been shown that this method is not as affected by the size of the sample as calibration measures [24].

Other measures have been used, based on classification tables, with authors reporting sensitivity, specificity, positive and negative predictive values and overall correct classification rates. They are, however, of limited utility in the validation of a model, because they have to use a fixed cut point (usually 10, 50 or 90%). Moreover, they depend on the mortality rate of the sample, with models usually having low values on sensitivity when the analyzed sample has a relatively high proportion of patients with low probability of mortality, since relatively few patients will have a probability of mortality greater than the chosen decision criteria.

The relative importance of calibration and discrimination varies with the use of the model, with some authors arguing that for research or quality assurance purposes (group comparisons) calibration is especially important and that for decisions about individual patients both descriptors are very relevant [28]. From a methodological point of view the poor calibration of a model can be corrected. However, there is almost nothing that can adjust a model when it presents poor discrimination [19].

The Application of General Outcome Prediction Models to Independent Populations

In recent years, a series of studies have tested the applicability of general outcome prediction models on independent populations. One of these was the Portuguese prospective multicenter study [29], testing the applicability of the SAPS II and the APACHE II models in a Portuguese cohort. During the study period, 19 Portuguese ICUs collected data on 1094 patients (after application of the exclusion criteria 982 patients entered the final analysis). Mean ($\pm$ standard deviation) severity scores were high (SAPS II score 41.4 ± 20.7; SAPS II probability 32.6 ± 29.9; APACHE II score 19.6 ± 9.9 and APACHE II probability 33.5 ± 27.4) with an overall mortality in the ICU of 24.5% and corresponding mortality in the hospital of 32.0%.

The results demonstrate that both models failed to accurately predict mortality. With respect to overall calibration, as measured by Hosmer-Lemeshow $\hat{H}$ and $\hat{C}$ tests, statistically significant differences were apparent between observed mortality and the mortality predicted by the models. This problem was more obvious for APACHE II than for SAPS II (SAPS II: $\hat{H}$ test 29.7, $\hat{C}$ test 28.3; APACHE II: $\hat{H}$ test 32.7, $\hat{C}$ test 49.7; $p < 0.01$ for all). The same was observed in the calibration curves, with both models overestimating mortality in the most severely ill patients. Discrimination was better for SAPS II than for APACHE II (0.817 versus 0.787, $p < 0.001$). It should be noted that the analyzed population was very different from the population represented in the European/North American database [4] or in Knaus et al.'s database [5], with a higher percentage of non-surgical patients, with a longer length of stay in the ICU, higher severity scores, and higher mortality. Nevertheless, the results challenge the validity of both models when applied to the Portuguese population.

Another recent example of the evaluation of the applicability of general outcome prediction models to independent populations is given by the EURICUS-I study, that explored the "effects of organization and management on the effectiveness and efficiency of ICUs in the countries of the European community" [10]. In this study, the necessity of a performance indicator at the ICU level led us to evaluate the applicability of the SAPS II and the admission MPM II_0 in a group of 16060 patients pooled from a total of 89 ICUs from 12 European Countries. The severity of illness, as described by the two scoring systems, showed large variation between ICUs, with a range of medians from 2.9% to 34.8% for the SAPS II probability (18 to 45 points in terms of score) and from 3.9% to 39.3% for the MPM II_0 probability. Mean ($\pm$ standard deviation) severity scores were 33.8 ± 17.8 for SAPS II score, 22.3 ± 25.0 for SAPS II probability and 23.6 ± 24.5 for MPM II_0 probability, with an overall mortality in the ICU of 24.5% and corresponding hospital mortality of 32.0%.

Concerning calibration, both SAPS II and MPM II_0 overestimated mortality. The Z statistic computed according to Flora's method was 10.42 for MPM II_0 and 6.82 for SAPS II. In both cases, the difference between predicted and observed number of survivors was statistically significant ($p < 0.001$). Figure 1 shows the calibration curves of SAPS II and MPM II_0. These curves demonstrate that as the predicted risk of hospital mortality (either by SAPS II or by MPM II_0) increased, the proportion of patients who died also increased. However, for SAPS II predicted risks $> 40\%$, the observed mortality within each risk group lay significantly below the diagonal line or, in other words, the model overestimates mortality in "sicker" patients. The same pattern was present in the MPM II_0 model with the shift becoming apparent at around the 30% predicted risk of death. The obvious discrepancy between the predicted and observed outcomes is also depicted by the Hosmer-Lemeshow goodness-of-fit $\hat{H}$- and $\hat{C}$-tests (SAPS II: $\hat{H}$ test 218.2, $\hat{C}$ test 208.4; MPM II_0: $\hat{H}$ test 437.1, $\hat{C}$ test 368.2; $p < 0.001$ for all).

For estimation of the discriminative power of the models the area under the ROC curve was used. The results were 0.822 (standard error 0.005) for SAPS II and 0.785 (standard error 0.006) for MPM II_0. The area for SAPS II was similar to the area of the original SAPS II model (0.8229); for MPM II_0 it was significantly lower (0.824), meaning that SAPS II presented better discriminative properties. Formal comparison of the two curves by the method of Hanley and McNeil [26] results in a very statistically significant difference ($p < 0.0001$). The results demonstrate that although the discriminative power was similar to the original database (lower for MPM II_0), both models calibrated badly in this population.

The Importance of the Uniformity-of-Fit

Until now, validation focused mainly on measures of overall discrimination and calibration. The evaluation of the impact of case mix not directly related to severity of illness on the performance of outcome prediction models has been subject to less in-

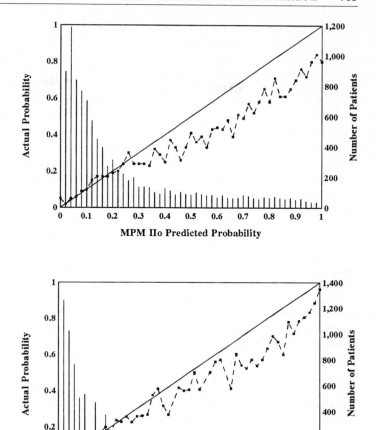

Fig. 1. Calibration curves in EURICUS-I database for the admission mortality probability model (MPM II$_0$) and the new simplified acute physiology score (SAPS II). The solid line represents perfect correspondence between actual and predicted risk of death and the dotted line the observed versus predicted risk of death. *Top:* data for MPM II$_0$. *Bottom:* data for SAPS II. In both panels, bars provide the distribution of patients in the analyzed groups

vestigation. Although some authors such as Rowan et al. [30] and Goldhill et al. [15] in the United Kingdom and Apolone et al. [13] in Italy have suggested that the performance of a model could depend to a large extent on the composition of the population being studied, no consensus exists regarding how to define or evaluate the behavior of a model in sub-populations.

We proposed the evaluation of these issues through a formal test of performance, comprising discrimination, calibration and O/E mortality ratios within clinically relevant subgroups, in order to identify whether the performance of the model is identical in all groups (uniformity-of-fit). To stratify patients, we used two different strategies: Patient-related criteria included in the models and which we would expect the models to take into account (age group and type of patient); and other criteria not included in the models (location in the hospital before ICU admission and diagnostic category). These last two were chosen since they represent important patient characteristics present at ICU admission and do not depend on therapeutic aspects. Together with severity of illness, this set of variables defined the baseline categories of patient characteristics.

Using these methods we explored the magnitude and extension of the impact of case mix on the performance of general outcome prediction models when using the SAPS II and the MPM II_0 models [31]. Our results demonstrate that very large differences in the predictive capability of SAPS II and MPM II_0 were apparent between subgroups, both in discrimination and in calibration. For example, when patients were stratified according to their location before admission to the ICU, both models presented a better discriminative power in patients admitted from the operating room/post-anesthesia room and emergency department than in patients admitted from the ward. Hosmer-Lemeshow $\hat{H}$ and $\hat{C}$ tests unveiled a poor calibration in all groups, although lower in patients admitted from the operating room/post-anesthesia room. The evaluation of the O/E mortality ratios showed that both models overestimated mortality in patients admitted from the operating room/post-anesthesia room and from the emergency department and underestimated mortality in patients admitted from the ward (Table 1).

Table 1. Uniformity of fit of the new simplified acute physiology score (SAPS II) and the admission mortality probability model (MPM II_0) in EURICUS-I database. Stratification by location of the patient before admission to the ICU

SAPS II

Location	N	ROC (SE)	$\hat{H}$ test	$\hat{C}$ test	O/E (95% CI)
Operating room/recovery room	3647	0.841 (0.010)	60.27[a]	54.87[a]	0.82 (0.76–0.88)
Emergency room	2912	0.838 (0.011)	154.14[a]	130.16[a]	0.76 (0.71–0.81)
Ward	1822	0.767 (0.012)	152.33[a]	142.35[a]	1.13 (1.08–1.19)
Others	1516	0.794 (0.013)	63.62[a]	62.91[a]	0.95 (0.88–1.02)

MPM II_0

Location	N	ROC (SE)	$\hat{H}$ test	$\hat{C}$ test	O/E (95% CI)
Operating room/recovery room	3647	0.797 (0.011)	123.42[a]	103.08[a]	0.79 (0.73–0.85)
Emergency room	2912	0.828 (0.010)	212.69[a]	190.03[a]	0.68 (0.63–0.73)
Ward	1822	0.707 (0.013)	209.01[a]	210.65[a]	1.13 (1.07–1.19)
Others	1516	0.759 (0.014)	102.22[a]	90.97[a]	0.87 (0.80–0.94)

[a] degrees of freedom $= 10$, $p < 0.001$

N: number of patients; ROC: area under the receiver operating characteristic curve; SE: standard error; $\hat{H}$ test: Hosmer-Lemeshow goodness-of-fit $\hat{H}$ test; $\hat{C}$ test: Hosmer-Lemeshow goodness-of-fit $\hat{C}$ test; O/E ratio: observed/expected mortality ratio; CI: confidence interval

The above findings seriously challenge the rationale underlying the use of the SMR for purposes of performance evaluation. How can we conclude that the performance of the ICUs in the EURICUS-I database was poor in patients admitted from the ward and very good when treating patients admitted from other locations? Similar results were obtained when the other grouping strategies were chosen, for example diagnostic category of admission. Problems in the design of the models, e.g., the omission from the regression equation of important variables, are more probable explanations for this phenomenon than variations in performance.

The dissimilar performance of the models in mutually exclusive subgroups can have serious consequences, since there is a trend to cluster similar types of patients in certain ICUs. For example, ICUs dealing mainly with medical patients will be more prone to receive patients from the ward than from the operating room, with non-operative diagnoses than with post-operative ones, and with an ICU length of stay (LOS) higher than ICUs dealing mainly with scheduled surgery patients. Even the longer LOS of certain types of patients can influence the predictive capabilities of the models, since it dramatically affects their discriminative capabilities.

The Influence of Length of ICU Stay on the Predictive Capability of General Outcome Prediction Models

In analyzing the factors that determine the LOS of critically ill patients, we were able to demonstrate a mixed influence of patient and hospital characteristics and not solely the severity of the illness. After correction for the severity of illness as evaluated by the SAPS II score, LOS was longer in medical patients, in patients admitted from other ICUs/other hospitals or from the ward, in patients with non-operative respiratory or trauma (non-operative or post-operative) diagnoses and in those admitted to university hospitals (unpublished data). The relationship between LOS and severity followed a non-linear pattern, resulting from a different relationship between LOS in survivors and non-survivors (Fig. 2). Of major concern is the drop in discriminative power of the SAPS II model with increasing LOS, with the model being hardly better than chance in patients with more than one week in the ICU (Fig. 3).

This work complements our previous analysis of the uniformity-of-fit. Again, a clustering of certain patient-types in certain ICUs was apparent, with different case mix of patients implying different performances and validity of the scores in different settings. However, can a perfect calibration of the models solve the problems?

Customizing a Model

We recently faced this situation when analyzing data from the EURICUS-I study. Since MPM II_0 was not able to adequately describe the population [14] we customized the model to better understand the reasons underlying this poor fit [32]. Two different strategies were chosen: The customization of the logit (first-level customization); and the customization of the variables (second-level customization). The impact of these two different strategies was evaluated using formal goodness-of-fit analysis, both in the overall sample and across relevant subgroups.

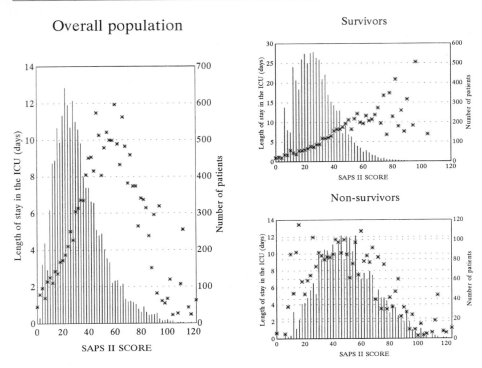

Fig. 2. Relationship between the length of stay in the ICU and the new simplified acute physiology score (SAPS II) in EURICUS-I database. *Left:* overall population; *Right-top:* survivors; *Right-bottom:* non-survivors. In each of the groups the bars indicate the number of patients in each group

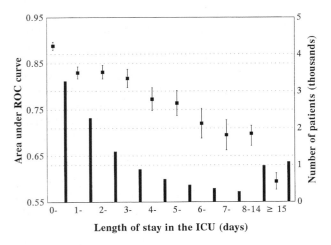

Fig. 3. Area under the receiver operating characteristics (ROC) curve for the new simplified acute physiology score (SAPS II) according to the length of stay in the ICU in EURICUS-I database. Point estimates are presented with respective standard errors; bars denote the number of patients in each group

In this study, data on 10 397 patients were available. Observed hospital mortality was 21.0%, and mean ($\pm$ standard deviation) predicted hospital mortality according to MPM II$_0$ was 24.2% $\pm$ 25.1%. Before the development of new logistic equations, the database was spliced randomly at the ICU level into two samples: Development (n = 6931); and validation (n = 3466). Basic demographic characteristics and baseline characteristics were not significantly different in development and validation samples.

For first-level customization, we developed a new logistic regression equation with hospital outcome as the dependent variable and the original logit of MPM II$_0$ as the independent variable. The equation was established as:

$$P_1 = \frac{e^{-0.4926 + 0.7502 \text{ (logit)}}}{1 + e^{-0.4926 + 0.7502 \text{ (logit)}}} \qquad (1)$$

where P_1 is the probability of hospital mortality computed after this first-level customization, logit is $\beta_0 + \beta_1 x_1 + \beta_2 x_2 \ldots \beta_{15} x_{15}$, and $\beta_0, \beta_1, \ldots \beta_{15}$ are the coefficients in the original MPM II$_0$ model.

For second-level customization, new maximum likelihood estimates for each of the 15 original variables were computed on the development sample and a new logit was calculated. The probability of hospital mortality, P_2, was established as:

$$P_2 = \frac{e^{\text{New Logit}}}{1 + e^{\text{New Logit}}} \qquad (2)$$

where the new logit is $\beta'_0 + \beta'_1 x_1 + \beta'_2 x_2 \ldots \beta'_{15} x_{15}$, and $\beta'_0, \beta'_1, \ldots \beta'_{15}$ are the new coefficients. Table 2 describes the new coefficients together with their respective odds ratios. Two variables (cardiac dysrhythmia and heart rate) were no longer significant at the multivariate level but were kept to maintain comparability with the original model. After the development of the new equations and the computation of the associated estimated probabilities of death, discrimination and calibration were evaluated both in the development and validation samples.

For estimation of the discriminative power of the models, the area under the ROC curve was used (Table 3). The discriminative capability of the models was only slightly affected by second-level customization, remaining lower than in the original description of the MPM II$_0$ (0.824). When comparing the customized model with the original model, a small improvement was seen with second-level customization but only in the development sample (development sample: Z = 1.67, p = 0.058; validation sample: Z = 0.74, p = 0.230).

The calibration curves for the three models are presented in Figure 4. These curves demonstrate that customization, either first or second level, was able to correct the deviations of the original model. Hosmer-Lemeshow goodness-of-fit $\hat{H}$ and $\hat{C}$ tests unveiled the same result (Table 3). The chi-square statistics after the second level-customization were lower than after the first-level customization (development sample, $\hat{H}$ test: 8.93 versus 10.88; $\hat{C}$ test: 5.92 versus 15.71; validation sample, $\hat{H}$ test: 22.24 versus 30.12; $\hat{C}$ test: 20.94 versus 21.68), suggesting a better overall fit.

The application of the original model yielded an overall O/E mortality ratio with 95% confidence intervals that did not encompass 1.0 (development sample 0.86, 95%

Table 2. New coefficients for each variable in the admission mortality probability model (MPM II$_0$) with their estimated coefficients, standard errors (SE), adjusted odds ratios and 95% confidence intervals (CI) for the adjusted odds ratios

Variable	Customized MPM II$_0$	
	β (SE)	Adjusted Odds Ratio (95 % CI)
Physiology		
Heart rate	0.0504 (0.1363)	1.1 (0.8–1.4)
Systolic blood pressure	0.7731 (0.0897)	2.2 (1.8–2.6)
Coma or deep stupor	0.7046 (0.0926)	2.0 (1.7–2.4)
Chronic diagnoses		
Chronic renal insufficiency	0.5019 (0.1384)	1.7 (1.3–2.2)
Cirrhosis	0.4779 (0.1944)	1.6 (1.1–2.4)
Metastatic neoplasm	0.7233 (0.1504)	2.1 (1.5–2.8)
Acute diagnoses		
Acute renal failure	1.2967 (0.1140)	3.7 (2.9–4.6)
Cardiac dysrhythmia	−0.1004 (0.0986)	0.9 (0.7–1.1)
Cerebrovascular incident	0.6198 (0.1380)	1.9 (1.4–2.4)
Gastrointestinal bleeding	0.6376 (0.1481)	1.9 (1.4–2.5)
Intracranial mass effect	0.5632 (0.1396)	1.8 (1.3–2.3)
Other		
CPR prior to ICU admission	0.8099 (0.1267)	2.2 (1.8–2.9)
Mechanical ventilation	0.7341 (0.0775)	2.1 (1.8–2.4)
Type of admission	1.1871 (0.1066)	3.3 (2.7–4.0)
Age (10-year odds ratio)	0.0316 (0.0023)	1.4 (1.3–1.4)
Constant	−5.3504	

CPR: cardiopulmonary resuscitation; ICU: intensive care unit

confidence interval 0.82 to 0.89; validation sample 0.89, 95% confidence interval 0.84 to 0.94); this fact implies that the model overestimates global mortality. After customization, this problem was corrected (Table 3).

Table 3. Discrimination and calibration of the admission mortality probability model (MPM II$_0$) before and after first- and second-level customization

Model	Sample	ROC (SE)	Ĥ test	Ĉ test	O/E ratio (95% CI)
Original	Development	0.803 (0.007)	220.50[a]	191.05[a]	0.86 (0.82–0.89)
Model	Validation	0.782 (0.009)	150.33[a]	133.76[a]	0.89 (0.84–0.94)
1st level	Development	0.803 (0.007)	10.88	15.71	1.00 (0.96–1.04)
customization	Validation	0.782 (0.009)	30.12[a]	21.68	1.04 (0.98–1.10)
2nd level	Development	0.810 (0.006)	8.93	5.92	1.00 (0.98–1.02)
customization	Validation	0.785 (0.009)	22.24	20.94	1.06 (1.00–1.11)

[a] p < 0.001

ROC: area under the receiver operating characteristic curve; Ĥ test: Hosmer-Lemeshow goodness-of-fit test Ĥ; Ĉ test: Hosmer-Lemeshow goodness-of-fit test Ĉ; O/E ratio: observed/expected mortality ratio; SE: standard error; CI: confidence intervals

Fig. 4. Calibration curves for the original and customized (first- and second-level) admission mortality probability model (MPM II$_0$). The solid line represents the perfect correspondence between actual and predicted risk of death; the dotted line the observed versus predicted risk of death on the development sample; and the dashed line the observed versus predicted risk of death on the validation sample. *Top:* data for original MPM II$_0$; *Middle:* data for the first-level customized MPM II$_0$. *Bottom:* data for second-level customized MPM II$_0$. In all panels, the left bars provide the distribution of patients in the analyzed groups in the development sample, and the right bars provide the distribution of patients in the analyzed groups in the validation sample

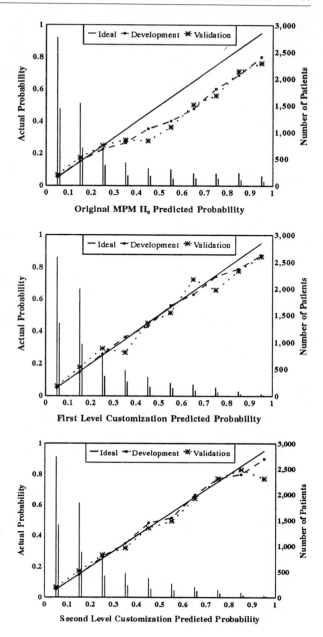

Concerning the uniformity-of-fit, customization corrected most, although not all deviations resulting from the application of the original MPM II$_0$. Problems remained in some groups, namely in patients admitted from the ward or with postoperative respiratory diagnoses.

Conclusion

Are the results of the above mentioned studies isolated results? If we review the literature, most of the published studies, no matter which outcome prediction model was used, unveiled similar results. Recent examples are the application of SAPS II in Italy [13] and Portugal [29], of the previous version of MPM in the United Kingdom [33], of APACHE II in the United Kingdom, [30], Japan [34] and Portugal [29], or APACHE III in Brazil [35].

This implies that even models developed in large multinational databases later failed when applied out of their development population. In some cases a potential explanation can be found, for example, asymmetry in the availability of technology [36]; in other cases, only differences in the definitions used, and measured and unmeasured case mix remain as explanation.

For the present time, the above mentioned results imply that the application of an outcome prediction model to an independent population should only be done after validation of the model in that population. If it does not correctly describe the population, then an appropriate investigation of the underlying causes is needed, complemented by customization of the model. This approach will restrain the evaluation of ICU performance to experimental or quasi-experimental settings. The alternative is to take the risk of attributing differences in case mix to differences in the performance and quality of care of the analyzed ICUs, but this is something that our colleagues and society expect us not to do.

References

1. Connors AF, Speroff T, Dawson NV, et al (1996) The effectiveness of right heart catheterization in the initial care of critically ill patients. JAMA 276:889–897
2. Teres D, Lemeshow S (1993) Using severity measures to describe high performance intensive care units. Crit Care Clin 9:543–554
3. Knaus WA, Draper EA, Wagner DP, Zimmerman JE (1986) An evaluation of outcome from intensive care in major medical centers. Ann Intern Med 104:410–418
4. Le Gall JR, Lemeshow S, Saulnier F (1993) A new simplified acute physiology score (SAPS II) based on a European/North American multicenter study. JAMA 270:2957–2963
5. Knaus WA, Draper EA, Wagner DP, Zimmerman JE (1985) APACHE II: a severity of disease classification system. Crit Care Med 13:818–829
6. Knaus WA, Wagner DP, Draper EA, et al (1991) The APACHE III prognostic system. Risk prediction of hospital mortality for critically ill hospitalized adults. Chest 100:1619–1636
7. Lemeshow S, Teres D, Klar J, Avrunin JS, Gehlbach SH, Rapoport J (1993) Mortality Probability Models (MPM II) based on an international cohort of intensive care unit patients. JAMA 270:2478–2486
8. Knaus WA, Wagner DP, Zimmerman JE, Draper EA (1993) Variations in mortality and length of stay in intensive care units. Ann Intern Med 118:753–761
9. Pollack MM, Alexander SR, Clarke N, et al (1990) Improved outcomes from tertiary center pediatric intensive care: a statewide comparison of tertiary and nontertiary care facilities. Crit Care Med 19:150–159
10. Reis Miranda D, Ryan DW, Schaufeli WB, Fidler V (1997) Organization and management of Intensive Care: a prospective study in 12 European countries. Springer-Verlag, Berlin, Heidelberg
11. Ferry-Lemonnier E, Landais P, Loirat P, Kleinknecht D, Brivet F (1995) Evaluation of severity scoring systems in ICUs: translation, conversion and definition ambiguities as a source of interobserver variability in Apache II, SAPS and OSF. Intensive Care Med 21:356–360

12. Rowan K (1996) The reliability of case mix measurements in intensive care. Curr Opin Crit Care 2:209–213
13. Apolone G, D'Amico R, Bertolini G, et al (1996) The performance of SAPS II in a cohort of patients admitted in 99 Italian ICUs: results from the GiViTI. Intensive Care Med 22:1368–1378
14. Moreno R, Reis Miranda D, Fidler V, Van Schilfgaarde R (1998) Evaluation of two outcome predictors on an independent database. Crit Care Med (in press)
15. Goldhill DR, Withington PS (1996) The effects of casemix adjustment on mortality as predicted by APACHE II. Intensive Care Med 22:415–419
16. Mckee M, Hunter D (1994) What can comparisons of hospital death rates tell us about the quality of care? In: Delamothe T (ed) Outcomes in clinical practice. British Medical Journal Press, London, pp 108–115
17. Reis Miranda D, Moreno R (1997) ICU models and their role in management and utilization programs. Curr Opin Crit Care 3:183–187
18. Hadorn DC, Keeler EB, Rogers WH, Brook RH (1993) Assessing the performance of mortality prediction models. CA, RAND/UCLA/Harvard Center for Health Care Financing Policy Research, Santa Monica
19. Miller ME, Hui SL (1991) Validation techniques for logistic regression models. Stat Med 10:1213–1226
20. Flora JD (1978) A method for comparing survival of burn patients to a standard survival curve. J Trauma 18:701–705
21. Hosmer DW, Lemeshow S (1989) Applied logistic regression. John Wiley & Sons, Inc., New York
22. Hosmer DW, Lemeshow S (1995) Confidence interval estimates of an index of quality performance based on logistic regression estimates. Stat Med 14:2161–2172
23. Champion HR, Copes WS, Sacco WJ, et al (1996) Improved predictions from a severity characterization of trauma (ASCOT) over trauma and injury severity score (TRISS): results of an independent evaluation. J Trauma 40:42–49
24. Zhu B-P, Lemeshow S, Hosmer DW, Klarm J, Avrunin J, Teres D (1996) Factors affecting the performance of the models in the mortality prediction model and strategies of customization: a simulation study. Crit Care Med 24:57–63
25. Hanley J, McNeil B (1982) The meaning and use of the area under a receiver operating characteristic (ROC) curve. Radiology 143:29–36
26. Hanley J, McNeil B (1983) A method of comparing the areas under receiver operating characteristic curves derived from the same cases. Radiology 148:839–843
27. Hilden J (1991) The area under the ROC curve and its competitors. Med Decis Making 11:95–101
28. Schuster DP (1992) Predicting outcome after ICU admission. The art and science of assessing risk. Chest 102:1861–1870
29. Moreno R, Morais P (1997) Outcome prediction in intensive care: results of a prospective, multicentre study. Intensive Care Med 23:177–186
30. Rowan KM, Kerr JH, Major E, McPherson K, Short A, Vessey MP (1993) Intensive Care Society's APACHE II study in Britain and Ireland – II: Outcome comparisons of intensive care units after adjustment for case mix by the American APACHE II method. Br Med J 307:977–981
31. Moreno R, Apolone G, Fidler V, Reis Miranda D (1996) Evaluation of the uniformity of fit of SAPS II and MPMo on an independent database. Intensive Care Med 22:S267 (Abst)
32. Moreno R, Apolone G (1997) The impact of different customization strategies in the performance of a general severity score. Crit Care Med 25:2001–2008
33. Rowan KM, Kerr JH, Major E, McPherson K, Short A, Vessey MP (1994) Intensive Care Society's acute physiology and chronic health evaluation (APACHE II) study in Britain and Ireland: A prospective, multicenter, cohort study comparing two methods for predicting outcome for adult intensive care patients. Crit Care Med 22:1392–1401
34. Sirio CA, Tajimi K, Tase C, et al (1992) An initial comparison of intensive care in Japan and United States. Crit Care Med 20:1207–1215
35. Bastos PG, Sun X, Wagner DP, Knaus WA, Zimmerman JE, The Brazil APACHE III Study Group (1996) Application of the APACHE III prognostic system in Brazilian intensive care units: a prospective multicenter study. Intensive Care Med 22:564–570
36. Bastos PG, Knaus WA, Zimmerman JE, Magalhães Jr A, Wagner DP, The Brazil APACHE III Study Group (1996) The importance of technology for achieving superior outcomes from intensive care. Intensive Care Med 22:664–669

Evidence-Based Medicine: The Wolf in Sheep's Clothing

H. A. Cassiere, M. Groth, and M. S. Niederman

Introduction

The concept of practising clinical medicine utilizing the current literature is a cornerstone of modern practice. Examples of this are plentiful in the medical literature with the use of thrombolytics in acute myocardial infarction and the use of inhaled corticosteroids in asthma being prime examples. This concept is not new and has its philosophical origins extending back to the mid-19th century, and its application appears to make sound logical, as well as, medical sense. The so called "new" field of evidence based medicine (EBM) is a discipline that uses the current "best evidence" in making decisions about the care of individual patients. Physicians systematically analyze the published literature and give guidance about which patient care interventions are likely to be beneficial. It is an attempt at applying clinical trials to specific patient encounters.

Evidence-Based Medicine: Strengths and Weaknesses

Although the fundamental principles of EBM are sound, in the realm of critical care medicine few clinical questions are easily answered by this method because of the complexity of the patient population. In addition, few well-performed, large, prospective, randomized trials are available to clarify complicated critical care patient issues. An example of the application of this new discipline was found in a recent review, where several authors used the principles of EBM to address the question of what practices are effective for the prevention of nosocomial pneumonia [1]. The intervention that was evaluated was the use of subglottic secretion drainage from specially designed endotracheal tubes. The analysis of benefit was derived from examining a previously published, prospective randomized clinical trial with the end point being to determine if this practice should be widely used as a ventilator-associated pneumonia prevention strategy. The discussion was insightful and served to remind us how the literature should be examined and pointed out the key features one should consider when designing a clinical trial or when reviewing whether the published literature is applicable to patient management decisions. The end result of this EBM exercise was the conclusion that more data are needed to recommend widespread use of this ventilator-associated pneumonia prevention tool.

This particular conclusion is cautious and clinically neutral. However, does it really help the clinician, or is it typical of what can be expected from EBM in the realm of critical care: Namely that very few therapies and interventions will be shown by this approach to be valid and worthy of widespread clinical use? The intensive care unit (ICU) is a complex environment filled with many variables and uncertainties (the "gray zone"). We wonder how much of what we do in the ICU is evidence based and would stand up to the rigors of EBM? An example that immediately comes to mind is the use of the pulmonary artery catheter. This device has been used in critical care for the last several decades without clear and convincing evidence that patients derive unequivocal benefits from its use. And its use has been identified as increasing mortality in a recent retrospective analysis [2]. Does this mean that its widespread use should be limited and not recommended? Should intensivists refrain from using this and other "unproven" therapies and interventions? Should insurance companies and health care organizations stop reimbursing critical care physicians for its use? Obviously, the answer to these questions is no.

The field of EBM is a double-edged sword, and one must realize its strengths and understand its weaknesses. Answering simple clinical questions may be the strength of this new discipline but its application to the critical care environment must be closely followed and scrutinized because of the complexity involved in caring for the critically ill patient. Those of us who take care of individuals in the ICU realize that no two patients are alike. Even within the same diagnostic group, such as cardiogenic shock, septic shock, or severe community-acquired pneumonia, no two patients are identical. An excellent example of this concept can be found in a recent study that evaluated the use of dobutamine in septic shock patients [3]. The authors found that some patients with septic shock on inotropic support have ongoing gut ischemia, a finding associated with detrimental effects. This may be no surprise to many but the point is that these patients could not ordinarily be distinguished, on usual clinical grounds, from the group that did not have gut ischemia. Even within the same patient populations, differences can be found that may be clinically, as well as therapeutically, significant. Large clinical trials, even those that are well designed and performed, cannot always account for this interpatient variability. The corollary to this is that systematically reviewing and categorizing these clinical trials does not, and cannot, account for this problem. This does not mean that data derived from clinical trials are inapplicable, it simply means that clinicians, both practising and those involved with the EBM genre, must realize the limitations of such data.

The review by Cook et al. [1] was useful, but we as practising critical care physicians still need to decide what place evidence-based medicine should have in our specialty and how the conclusions that it leads to should be incorporated into patient management decisions. The review by Cook et al. [1] shows us how to review the literature carefully and how to apply it to clinical questions. Included in the discussion are such key issues as: How do patients get randomized in a study? How should the randomization process be concealed? Why is an intent-to-treat analysis necessary? What is the difference between single, double and triple blinding of a study? How does one determine if the randomization process was successful in accounting for differences among patients? How can a treatment effect be estimated? What is the value of subgroup analysis when it yields different conclusions than those reached for the group as a whole? The discussion focused on how to analyze the published literature and was a useful primer for the interested reader.

Unfortunately the authors of this excellent review took the dangerous next step, one that appeared subtle at first but upon further analysis revealed itself as the wolf in sheep's clothing. Although the reader of this excellent review could be comforted by its logical and methodical analysis, the authors revealed their teeth by stating that conclusions from an EBM analysis can be used to define whether the results of a clinical trial should be applied to patient care. We believe that in doing this they have gone too far. In asking this question, the authors presume that a set of rules can be developed to tell us how to interpret the literature and how to apply it to the ideal management of specific patients. This is a dangerous and potentially damaging use of EBM, particularly to those of us involved with the care of critically ill patients. We as clinicians also review the medical literature and care for critically ill patients. Do our own unpublished conclusions count? Will parties interested in controlling critical care resources use these exercises in reviewing the medical literature as gospel? We think that there can be no substitute for a well-trained, experienced critical care physician. Reviewing the literature is a necessity, but being dictated by others' interpretations of it is dangerous. Medicine is an art as well as a science, albeit not an exact science.

While nobody would argue that clinical decisions should be guided by evidence from the literature, our concern is that EBM will tie our hands and prevent us from using "gray zone" interventions, i.e., those of marginal or questionable benefit, in critically ill patients. Even more concerning is that we will withhold potentially useful therapies because prospective, randomized controlled trials have not shown unequivocal evidence of benefit for a therapy, particularly a potentially life-saving but expensive therapy. In an imaginary discussion between Socrates and "Enthusiasticus" (aka. Meta-analyticus), Socrates warns that health care managers "see your beloved evidence based medicine as a means to shackle the doctors and bend them to their will. ... Beware Enthusiasticus, that you are not used as a dupe in a political game of health economics. Remember, hemlock may be down the line" [4].

The concept of "gray zone" issues is key to the critical care physician [5]. Many of the interventions that we perform in seriously ill patients have limited benefit and are costly. If EBM dominates our specialty, managed care organizations may try to prevent us from attempting to salvage certain patients. If a patient is admitted with severe community-acquired pneumonia, accompanied by hypotension and respiratory failure, mortality is predictably high, and the benefits of ICU care have been questioned [6]. Does this mean that we should not provide critical care to these patients until prospective randomized controlled trials show a benefit for this expensive and marginally beneficial therapy? As physicians, our obligation is to treat these patients with any reasonable modality, and we recognize that not all treated patients will benefit. Still, we would never use data from a prognostic scoring system (APACHE or MPM), that predicted a high chance of death, to prevent us from treating a patient with a potentially reversible process. Rather, we would use clinical judgment and experience to define how aggressively we will intervene in a patient with severe community-acquired pneumonia.

Is EBM going to be used to prevent critical care physicians from providing care that offers only a limited chance of benefit to critically ill patients? Will we be required to justify all our interventions with prospective randomized controlled trials of high quality, or can we develop effective patient care strategies from imperfect data, combined with clinical experience? An excellent example of this concept is the debate over whether ventilator-associated pneumonia (VAP) has a true "attributable mortality" [7]. Clearly some patients die with pneumonia, not from it, while others die as a direct result of pneumonia. Until we prove unequivocally that pneumonia has an attributable mortality, should we withhold antibiotic therapy since some patients will die regardless of how they are treated? Should we prove the existence of attributable mortality by randomizing patients with VAP to a therapy versus no therapy trial? Although this sounds ludicrous, it is based upon the basic principles of EBM and seems, at least to us, dangerous when applied to the critically ill. And again, this is only one of many examples where the data supporting a therapeutic intervention are based upon imperfect data. Even with our best therapies for VAP, not all patients recover, and mortality rates may exceed 50%. This suggests only a limited benefit to antibiotic therapy in VAP patients, yet clinicians still view such therapy as a necessity.

EBM asks that we do not make firm patient care recommendations without data from well performed clinical trials. Sometimes this is not possible and even impractical, and often those of us who care for the critically ill need to make decisions, even though the data available to us are imperfect. Again, the art of medicine shines through and shows us that caring for patients is more than following recommendations. For example, a multi-specialty group of physicians that included critical care, pulmonary and infectious disease physicians has written the American Thoracic Society's guidelines for the therapy of hospital-acquired pneumonia [8]. These guidelines were based on the best available data at the time and the experience of those involved. They give important direction and structure to clinicians that manage patients with this difficult clinical problem. Using EBM standards, maybe guidelines should not have been written at all since we still cannot agree on how to diagnose hospital-acquired pneumonia (clinically or bronchoscopically), and antibiotic recommendations are based on expected bacterial susceptibility patterns, and not on prospective randomized controlled trials [9]. In spite of these limitations, we believe that is it possible to write guidelines that give helpful and useful clinical direction. The idea that therapeutic recommendations cannot be made until we have amassed a mountain of prospective randomized controlled trial data to support them is an extreme view, and one of limited applicability to the ICU patient.

EBM presents other problems to the critical care physician. If unequivocal data in a prospective randomized controlled trial support a certain therapy, does this mean that you can apply the therapy successfully in your ICU? For example, if published data show wide variability in the success of a new therapy among different institutions and among different types of patients how will this therapy work in your institution? On the other hand, if your institution has locally collected data showing success with a new therapy that has not been as successful in broad clinical trials, should you abandon its use? By EBM standards, it might be argued that large-scale prospective randomized controlled trial data should take precedence over local experience and regional practice patterns. This failure to value local data or years of clinical experience, compared to published data, is one of the major concerns with EBM as a discipline.

Table 1. Problems with evidence-based medicine in critical care

- Many decisions involve "gray zone" issues
- Lack of unequivocal proof for a therapy may discourage reimbursement for its use
- Patients are heterogeneous and this may not be reflected in clinical trials
- Published clinical trials may be biased toward positive results
- The roles of clinical experience and local data are de-emphasized
- Published trials are often out of date: therapeutic issues may have changed i.e., antimicrobial resistance
- Clinical decisions and care must be provided even in the absence of concordance within published data

Conclusion

These concerns about the use of EBM to guide the practise of critical care should be discussed widely (Table 1). However, an even more pressing issue is how we will practise our specialty in the new era of managed care. Will the focus on only using evidence-based interventions that are "cost-effective" prevent us from caring for some potentially salvageable patients? A complicated critically ill patient absorbs more health care resources and is more expensive to an insurer than a patient who is admitted to the ICU and dies immediately. This is a harsh economic reality but one that is not calculated into the usual cost-effectiveness equation. If a therapy saves one life out of 100, is it cost-effective? Some would argue and say no, but can human life be quantified? Will we only be allowed to use therapies that are of proven benefit after multiple clinical trials? Going back to the example of subglottic secretion drainage, this is a simple, biologically plausible method for preventing early onset VAP, and if this method were widely available, we would use it. The intervention is not dangerous and has obvious potential benefit. While further studies of the topic are warranted, we would not, as suggested by Cook et al. [1] use an EBM analysis to reach the (not surprising and clinically not useful) conclusion that we need more confirmatory data to increase our confidence in this method. Critical care medicine is and will likely remain a field filled with clinical uncertainty. Data can help us deal with this uncertainty and guide clinical decision-making. However, decisions must be made by clinicians, not reviewers, who combine experience, judgment and a thoughtful review of the literature. Many of us do this now and do it well. We must resist any effort to restrain our use of "gray zone " interventions, particularly if the motivation for withholding such care is economic, under the guise that "we don't have enough evidence" to suggest an unequivocal benefit of therapy, the true wolf in sheep's clothing.

References

1. Cook DJ, Hebert PC, Heyland DK, et al (1997) How to use an article on therapy or prevention: Pneumonia prevention using subglottic secretion drainage. Crit Care Med 25:1502–1513
2. Connors AF, Speroff T, Dawson NV, et al (1996) The effectiveness of right heart catheterization in the initial care of critically ill patients. JAMA 276:889–897

3. Levy B, Bollaert PE, Lucchelli JP, et al (1997) Dobutamine improves the adequacy of gastric mucosal perfusion in epinephrine-treated septic shock. Crit Care Med 25:1649–1654
4. Grahame-Smith D (1995) Evidence based medicine: Socratic dissent. Br Med J 310:1126–1127
5. Naylor CD (1995) Grey zones of clinical practice: some limits to evidence-based medicine. Lancet 345:840–842
6. Hook EW, Horton CA, Schaberg DR (1983) Failure of intensive care unit support to influence mortality from pneumococcal bacteremia. JAMA 249:1055–1061
7. Fagon JY, Chastre J, Vaugnat A, Trouillet JL, Novara A, Gibert C (1996) Nosocomial pneumonia and mortality among patients in intensive care units. JAMA 275:866–869
8. Campbell GD, Niederman MS, Broughton WA, et al (1996) Hospital-acquired pneumonia in adults: Diagnosis, assessment of severity, initial antimicrobial therapy, and preventative strategies: A consensus statement. Am J Respir Crit Care Med 153:1711–1725
9. Niederman MS, Torres A, Summer W (1994) Invasive diagnostic testing is not needed routinely to manage suspected ventilator-associated pneumonia. Am J Respir Crit Care Med 150:565–569

Subject Index

Springer-Verlag
and the Environment

We at Springer-Verlag firmly believe that an international science publisher has a special obligation to the environment, and our corporate policies consistently reflect this conviction.

We also expect our business partners – paper mills, printers, packaging manufacturers, etc. – to commit themselves to using environmentally friendly materials and production processes.

The paper in this book is made from low- or no-chlorine pulp and is acid free, in conformance with international standards for paper permanency.